D0938181

AN ADVANCED REVIEW OF SPEECH–LANGUAGE PATHOLOGY

AN ADVANCED REVIEW OF SPEECH–LANGUAGE PATHOLOGY

Preparation for PRAXIS and Comprehensive Examination

Second Edition

Celeste Roseberry-McKibbin

M. N. Hegde

pro·ed
An International Publisher

8700 Shoal Creek Boulevard
Austin, Texas 78757-6897
800/897-3202   Fax 800/397-7633
www.proedinc.com

© 2006 by PRO-ED, Inc.
8700 Shoal Creek Boulevard
Austin, Texas 78757-6897
800/897-3202   Fax 800/397-7633
www.proedinc.com

All rights reserved. No part of the material protected by
this copyright notice may be reproduced or used in any
form or by any means, electronic or mechanical, including
photocopying, recording, or by any information storage
and retrieval system, without prior written permission of
the copyright owner.

Library of Congress Cataloging-in-Publication Data

Roseberry-McKibbin, Celeste.
   An advanced review of speech-language pathology : preparation for praxis
and comprehensive examination / by Celeste Roseberry-McKibbin & M. N.
Hegde.-- 2nd ed.
      p. cm.
   Includes bibliographical references and index.
   ISBN 1-4164-0127-X (softcover : alk. paper)
   1. Speech disorders--Outlines, syllabi, etc. 2. Language
disorders--Outlines, syllabi, etc. 3. Speech therapy--Outlines, syllabi,
etc. 4. Audiology--Outlines, syllabi, etc. I. Hegde, M. N. (Mahabalagiri
N.), 1941– II. Title.
RC423.R66 2006
616.85'50076--dc22
                        2005026160

Cover and book designed by Cinqué Hicks.

This book is designed in Minion, Meta, Lucida Sans, and Bawdy Italic.

Printed in the United States of America

1   2   3   4   5   6   7   8   9   10   09   08   07   06   05

We dedicate this book to our families: Mike McKibbin, Mark McKibbin, Prema Hegde, and Manu Hegde, with our love.

CONTENTS

15 APPENDIX

page 727

PREFACE

The idea for the first edition of this book was born back in 1996. I (Celeste Roseberry-McKibbin) was part of a team that was conducting workshops for speech–language pathologists who needed to pass the PRAXIS so that they could become licensed and certified in order to accommodate increasingly stringent professional state and federal requirements. These experienced clinicians, who had graduated from school 10–35 years ago, suddenly found themselves faced with the need to quickly learn (or retrieve from memory) a great deal of current information to pass a challenging examination. The task seemed formidable to many of them.

At the same time, M. N. Hegde and I were dealing with many graduate students who were experiencing great stress over the prospect of taking upcoming master's comprehensive examinations as well as the PRAXIS (usually taken within the same time period). All of these people needed current information covering the entire field of speech–language pathology. Many of them did not have time to go to libraries, check out books, read through each book, and extract the most relevant and up-to-date information that was likely to be asked on the PRAXIS and on comprehensive examinations in graduate programs. As we reflected upon this situation, an idea was born. Why not write a book that would meet those needs? Why not gather current, relevant material into one book that would help students and practitioners review for examinations that would open (or, sadly, close) career doors to them?

Several years later, the first edition of this book came together in one comprehensive package geared toward helping students and practitioners study for and pass the PRAXIS and comprehensive examinations in graduate programs. But there was, and still is, also a third purpose for the book. We intend it to be not only a study guide, but also a review for practitioners who want an update of the field for their professional growth. We have spoken with many practitioners in various professional settings, some of whom are aware that much of their knowledge has become dated but do not have the time or resources to obtain current knowledge in so many areas of an ever-expanding field. Thus, we have also written this book for experienced speech–language pathologists who would like to read current and comprehensive information for their own professional development.

It has been a joy to update a book that is unique in the field of speech–language pathology. No other book is written specifically to meet the needs of students taking comprehensive examinations and the PRAXIS, experienced practitioners taking the PRAXIS, and experienced practitioners who are seeking professional growth. When we have discussed the book with students and practitioners, the resounding response has been, "How soon will the book be out? I want to buy it! Please hurry and finish it!" (The last comment has also been heard from our spouses, but that is another story.) It is a great privilege for us to contribute the second edition of this book to our field, and we hope that it will open doors for those who are seeking further knowledge and opportunities.

The book includes unique pedagogical devices to facilitate the learning process. Each chapter has special features to help readers learn and retain the information presented. Each begins with a detailed "Preview Outline" to orient readers to its contents. Next, each chapter section consists of both a brief introduction and a summary to help readers (a) become aware of what they will read, (b) read it, and (c) review what they have just read. We believe that repetition is one of the keys to learning and retaining information. At the end of each chapter, "Chapter Highlights" reviews and summarizes the most pertinent information. Readers who are studying for examinations can, soon before the examination, refresh their memories by re-reading section introductions and summaries and chapter highlights.

At the end of each chapter, we also have put test questions in essay and multiple-choice formats. The multiple-choice questions are written in a manner similar to that of the questions on the PRAXIS to help prepare readers for those questions. One valid and constructive criticism of the multiple-choice questions in our first edition is that they were so easy that they did not truly reflect the questions on the PRAXIS. We agreed, and made the multiple-choice questions longer, more difficult, and far more representative of the questions on the actual PRAXIS exam. One difference between the multiple-choice questions in the first and second editions is that in the latter, we have included many more "case study"-type questions to reflect the current PRAXIS. Answers to multiple-choice test questions are at the very end of every chapter. For readers who want more information about certain topics within a chapter, we have included a comprehensive list of current references and recommended readings at the end of each chapter.

A unique and key feature of this book is the "Concepts to Consider" questions that are embedded in the body of each chapter. We believe that adults learn best when they can actively interact with information, not just passively read it. To that end, we have written short essay questions to help readers pause, think about, and integrate the information that they have just read. We believe that answering those questions in writing will greatly assist readers in integrating and retaining the information in each chapter.

In the second edition of this book, we have also made some content updates. We have incorporated more information about speech science, literacy, contemporary theories of phonological development, and other areas. We have split the old Chapter 13, "Special Topics in Speech–Language Pathology," into two separate chapters. Chapter 13 in the current edition covers the topics of counseling, medical speech–language pathology, and craniofacial anomalies and genetic syndromes. Information about a greater number of genetic syndromes has also been added. Chapter 14 in this edition deals with the background and nature of ASHA and the professions, issues in certification and licensure, and legislation which impacts communicative disorders professionals in various settings. To this chapter, we have added information pertaining to speech–language pathology assistants, HIPAA, and other contemporary issues affecting our profession.

A new and special product that was not available when we published the first edition of this book is a CD that contains three practice PRAXIS exams. We could not have completed this CD without the extensive knowledge and expertise of Dr. Glen Tellis, a former student of ours. The CD and the second edition of this book are designed to go hand in hand to help readers gain both content knowledge and experience answering PRAXIS-type questions. Glen, we are thrilled to have you on board!

We were flattered by and most pleased with the success and acclaim that greeted the first edition of this book. Students and professionals from across the United States have thanked us for writing this book, and we feel blessed to know that our work is providing help and support for so many people. We have worked very hard to make this second edition even more useful for readers.

A book such as this never happens without the help of many people. We would like to thank Peggy Kipping, Dolly Jackson, and Matt Synatschk at PRO-ED and Cinqué Hicks at Thinkmark for their expert help, advice, and encouragement along the way. We also thank our families, especially Mike McKibbin, Prema Hegde, and Floyd and Beverly Roseberry for their unconditional love and support for us as we have worked on the second edition of this book. Lastly, I would like to thank Dr. James McCartney and Ms. Lynda Oldenburg at California State University, Sacramento for their understanding of my need to finish this book in a timely fashion and for helping arrange my schedule so I could do it. You guys are the best!

Again, it is a privilege for us to contribute this work to our field. Thanks to the help and support of many individuals listed above, we are able to offer the second edition of this book to students and practitioners from all over the United States. It is our hope that it will open doors to those very deserving individuals who have dedicated their lives to serving people with communicative disorders.

CHAPTER 1

ANATOMY,

NEUROANATOMY, AND

PHYSIOLOGY OF THE

SPEECH MECHANISM

The process of speech is one most people take for granted. However, speech depends on an intricate and complex system of structures and functions working together to allow human beings to communicate with one another. Respiration, or breathing, supplies the energy for speech. Phonation involves voicing and the structures and processes that create voice. Resonation, the process by which the voice or laryngeal tone is modified by various cavities and structures, is closely tied to articulation, the process of making speech sounds.

RESPIRATION: STRUCTURES AND PROCESSES

INTRODUCTION

Respiration, the process of breathing, is foundational to speech. The respiratory framework includes the lungs, bronchi, trachea, spinal column, sternum, and ribs. Respiration involves the cycle of inhalation (or inspiration) and exhalation (or expiration).

Respiration Patterns During Speech Production

- When we inhale, we bring oxygen to the blood. When we exhale, we get rid of mixed air and gases which result from respiratory metabolism (Nicolosi, Harryman, & Kresheck, 2004). When an excessive amount of carbon dioxide creates a need for oxygen, the *medulla oblongata* in the brain stem fires impulses to the respiratory muscles.

- *Respiration* is the exchange of gas between an organism and its environment (Seikel, King, & Drumright, 2000). Inhalation (also called inspiration) and exhalation (also called expiration) create the rhythmic cycle of respiration. Inhalation draws air into the lungs, where an exchange of oxygen and carbon dioxide takes place. Through the actions of the diaphragm and other respiratory muscles, we expand the chest cavity and thus the lungs to inhale air.

- As the lungs expand, the pressure within the lungs is reduced compared to the pressure outside the lungs. The air moves through the open laryngeal valve into the lungs, equalizing the pressure inside and outside the lungs.

- At that point, muscles contract to reduce the volume of the chest cavity, creating a positive pressure within the lungs. As a result, we exhale. In this manner, the cycle of inhalation and exhalation automatically continues.

- Respiration provides the air supply needed to set the vocal folds into vibration for speech. Because speech is typically produced on exhalation, the duration of exhalations during speech tends to be longer than the duration of exhalations during silent periods. Longer, louder utterances may require deeper inhalation than usual. Singers often inhale deeply.

- Compared to quiet breathing, breathing for speech is more consciously monitored and adjusted to meet the demands of speech in various daily situations. These adjustments are continuous and rapid. To make these rapid adjustments, people need to have intact respiratory structures.

Framework of Respiration

- Respiration is the foundation for speech. As previously stated, respiration involves inhalation and exhalation. Humans generally inhale and then speak on exhaled air. The basic process of inhalation can be summarized as follows:

  - inhale ➜ chest and lungs expand ➜ diaphragm lowers ➜ air flows in through the nose and mouth ➜ air goes down pharynx and between open vocal folds ➜ air continues downward through trachea and bronchial tubes ➜ air reaches final destination of lungs

- The above process of inhalation, as well as the processes in exhalation and speaking, is complex and requires the support of many structures, including the lungs, bronchi, trachea, spinal column, sternum, and ribs.

Lungs

- The previously mentioned exchange of gas in respiration is accomplished in the *lungs*. Healthy lungs are soft, spongy, porous, elastic, and pink. They have a rich vascular supply and numerous air sacs.
- When the respiratory system is at rest, the lungs are partially inflated to approximately 40% of their total lung capacity (Davenport & Sapienza, 2004).
- The lungs are located in the thoracic cavity and take up most of the cavity's space. The right lung is shorter and broader and bigger than the left lung because of the liver underneath it, which forces it upward slightly. The lungs are illustrated in Figure 1.1.

Bronchi

- The *bronchi* are tubes that extend from the lungs upward to the trachea. The bronchi are composed of cartilaginous rings bound together by fibroelastic tissue (Zemlin, 1998).
- In the lungs, the bronchi subdivide into *bronchioles*. The bronchioles repeatedly divide until

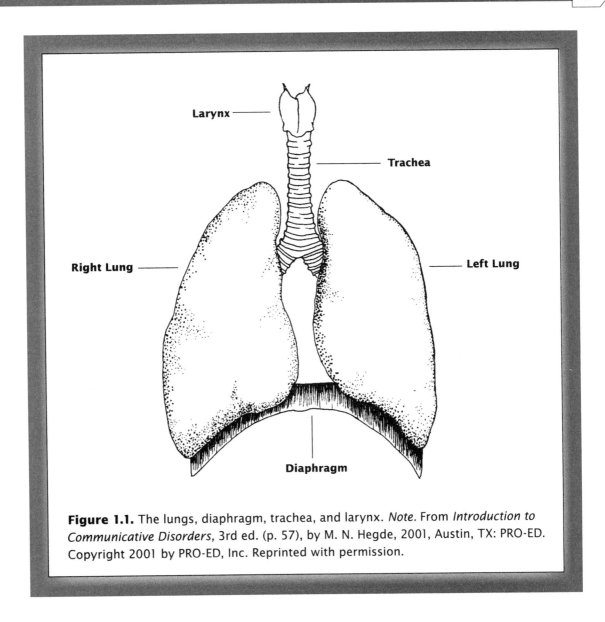

Figure 1.1. The lungs, diaphragm, trachea, and larynx. *Note.* From *Introduction to Communicative Disorders,* 3rd ed. (p. 57), by M. N. Hegde, 2001, Austin, TX: PRO-ED. Copyright 2001 by PRO-ED, Inc. Reprinted with permission.

they ultimately communicate with *alveolar ducts* that open into tiny air sacs in the lungs. As the bronchi and bronchioles divide, they become less cartilaginous and more muscular in composition.

Trachea

- As a person inhales, the air goes in through the larynx to the trachea to the lungs, which expand, as previously stated. When a person exhales, the air goes upward again through the *trachea,* a tube formed by approximately 20 rings of cartilage (illustrated in Figure 1.1).
- These rings of cartilage are incomplete in the back where the trachea comes into direct contact with the esophagus. The first tracheal cartilage is larger than the rest and connects to the inferior or bottom border of the cricoid cartilage.
- The trachea extends from the larynx, at the level of the sixth cervical vertebra, and the last tracheal ring splits in two or *bifurcates* into the left and right primary bronchi at the level of the fifth thoracic vertebra.

Spinal Column

- The *spinal column* consists of 32–33 individual vertebrae. These vertebrae are divided into five segments (see Figure 1.2):

    - 7 *cervical* vertebrae (C1–C7)
    - 12 *thoracic* vertebrae (T1–T12)
    - 5 *lumbar* vertebrae (L1–L5)
    - 5 *sacral* vertebrae (S1–S5)
    - 3–4 *coccygeal* vertebrae (fused together and called the coccyx)

- The thoracic vertebrae provide points of attachment for the ribs. The lumbar vertebrae are large, which makes them suitable for weight-bearing functions.

Sternum

- The *sternum,* also called the *breastbone,* is located on the superior, anterior thoracic wall. The sternum consists of three parts: the manubrium, body, and xiphoid process.
- The *manubrium* is the uppermost segment of the sternum. The manubrium provides the attachment for the clavicle and the first rib.
- The corpus or *body* of the sternum is long and narrow. The cartilages of ribs 2 through 7 attach to the body of the sternum.
- The *xiphoid process* is a small cartilaginous structure found at the bottom of the body of the sternum.

Rib Cage

- The *rib cage,* or *thoracic cage,* is usually called the chest. It consists of 12 pairs of ribs that form a cylindrical structure. The rib cage houses and protects such organs as the heart and lungs. Figure 1.3 shows a schematic of the rib cage.
- The rib cage is composed of several structures:

    - sternum in the anterior surface

CONCEPTS TO CONSIDER

Briefly describe three structures that are key to adequate respiration. What is the role of each structure?

_____

_____

_____

_____

_____

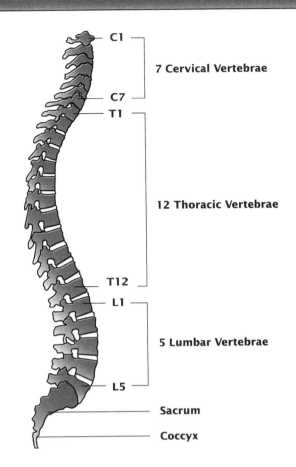

Figure 1.2. Components of the vertebral column: 7 cervical (C) vertebrae, 12 thoracic (T) vertebrae, 5 lumbar (L) vertebrae, 5 fused vertebrae of the sacrum (S), and the coccyx.

- 12 thoracic vertebrae in the posterior surface
- 12 pairs of ribs that connect laterally from the vertebrae to their individual *costal cartilages*

Muscles of Respiration

Thoracic Muscles of Inspiration

- The *diaphragm,* illustrated in Figure 1.1, is the floor of the chest cavity. It is a thick, dome-shaped muscle that separates the abdomen from the thorax. The *abdomen* houses structures such as the intestines, liver, and kidneys.
- Various abdominal muscles are critical in providing support for breathing. Because the lungs rest upon it, the diaphragm plays a major role in breathing.

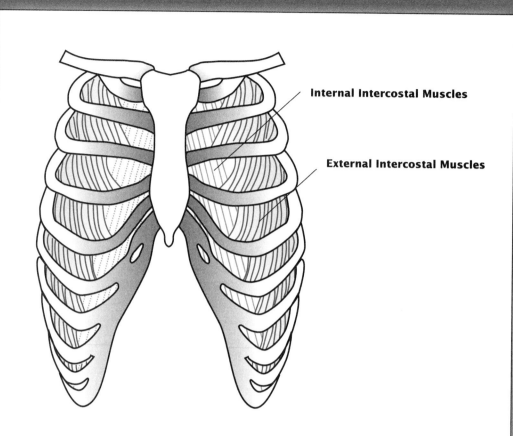

Internal Intercostal Muscles

External Intercostal Muscles

Figure 1.3. Rib cage with the internal and external intercostal muscles. External intercostals are absent near the sternum, allowing one to see the deeper internal intercostals within that region. On the left rib cage, the fascia covering the internal intercostals has been removed, whereas the fascia remains present and translucent on the right.

- The *intercostal muscles* (illustrated in Figure 1.3) between the ribs are also critical for respiration. The 11 paired *internal intercostals* pull the ribs downward to decrease the diameter of the thoracic cavity for exhalation, and the 11 paired *external intercostals* raise the ribs up and out to increase the diameter of the thoracic cavity for inhalation.
- Several other muscles also help elevate the rib cage. The *serratus posterior superior, levator costarum brevis, levator costarum longis,* and *external intercostal* muscles are all involved in rib cage elevation.
- These muscles and their innervations are summarized below (Seikel et al., 2000). (*Note:* The innervations basically arise from the vertebrae and their nerves and branches. For purposes of efficiency, only the vertebrae involved are listed—not the specific vertebral branches and nerves.)

Muscle and Innervation	Function
diaphragm (C3–C5)	distends abdomen, enlarges vertical dimension of thorax, depresses central tendon of diaphragm

Muscle and Innervation	Function
serratus posterior superior (C7, T1–T4)	elevates rib cage
levator costarum brevis (T2–T12)	elevates rib cage
levator costarum longis (T2–T12)	elevates rib cage
external intercostal (T2–T11)	elevates rib cage

- Accessory muscles of the neck are also involved in the process of respiration. Two of the key neck muscles are the sternocleidomastoid and the trapezius.
- The *sternocleidomastoid* elevates the sternum and thus, indirectly, the rib cage. The *trapezius* controls the head and elongates the neck, and thus also indirectly influences respiration.
- Muscles of the shoulder and upper arm also act to move the rib cage and increase or decrease its dimensions. These muscles include the *pectoralis major, pectoralis minor, serratus anterior,* and *levator scapulae.*
- These muscles and their innervations and functions are summarized below (Seikel et al., 2000). (*Note:* The innervations basically arise from the vertebrae and their nerves and branches. For purposes of efficiency, only the vertebrae involved are listed—not the specific vertebral branches and nerves.)

Muscle and Innervation	Function
pectoralis major (C4–T1)	increases transverse dimension of rib cage through elevation of sternum
pectoralis minor (C4–T1)	increases transverse dimension of rib cage
serratus anterior (C5–C7)	elevates ribs 1–9
levator scapulae (C3–C5)	elevates scapula, supports neck
rhomboideus major (C5)	stabilizes shoulder girdle
rhomboideus minor (C5)	stabilizes shoulder girdle
internal intercostal (T2–T11)	depresses ribs 1–11
innermost intercostal (T2–T11)	depresses ribs 1–11
transversus thoracicus (T2–T6)	depresses ribs 2–6

- Two posterior thoracic muscles are also involved in respiration. The *subcostal muscle* depresses the thorax. The *serratus posterior inferior muscles,* when contracted, pull the rib cage down and thus aid in exhalation.

Abdominal Muscles of Expiration

- Most muscles involved with breathing assist with inspiration. However, muscle action is also needed for exhalation of air. Muscles of expiration include the *latissimus dorsi, rectus abdominus, transversus abdominus, internal oblique abdominus,* and *quadratus lumborum.*
- These muscles, their innervations, and their functions are briefly summarized below (Seikel et al., 2000). (*Note:* The innervations basically arise from the vertebrae and their nerves and branches. For purposes of efficiency, only the vertebrae involved are listed—not the specific vertebral branches and nerves.)

Muscle and Innervation	Function
latissimus dorsi (C6–C8)	stabilizes the posterior abdominal wall for expiration
rectus abdominus (T7–T12)	flexes vertebral column

Muscle and Innervation	Function
transversus abdominus (T7–T12)	compresses abdomen
internal oblique abdominus (T7–T12)	compresses abdomen, flexes and rotates trunk
quadratus lumborum (T12, L1–L4)	supports abdominal compression through bilateral contraction, which fixes abdominal walls

SUMMARY

✓ Respiration, the process of breathing involving an exchange of gas between an organism and its environment, is necessary for life itself. It is also the foundation of speech.

✓ The framework of respiration supports the muscles necessary for respiration to take place. These muscles include two primary categories: the thoracic muscles of inspiration and the abdominal muscles of expiration.

✓ Respiration provides the foundation and energy for phonation.

PHONATION: STRUCTURES AND PROCESSES

INTRODUCTION

Commonly known as the voice box, the larynx lies at the top of the trachea and houses the vocal folds, which vibrate to produce voice. Optimal laryngeal function and voicing depend upon the integrity of key laryngeal cartilages as well as intrinsic and extrinsic laryngeal muscles. Certain neuroanatomical structures are also critical. These include cortical areas, the cerebellum, and cranial nerves VII and X.

Larynx

■ During speech, the lungs produce the necessary air for phonation. The air flows upward through the trachea and comes toward the larynx. The *larynx* (called the voice box by laypeople) lies at the top of the trachea in the anterior portion of the neck. It is a valving mechanism that opens and closes. The major structures of the larynx are shown in Figure 1.4.

■ The larynx houses the *vocal folds,* which vibrate to produce sound. The vocal folds *adduct* (move toward the midline) and *abduct* (move away from the midline) as they vibrate. When a person is breathing quietly, the vocal folds are abducted.

■ In addition to producing the sound needed for speech, the larynx has biological functions. These include (a) closure of the trachea so that food and other substances do not enter the lungs, (b) production of the cough reflex to expel foreign substances that accidentally enter the trachea, and (c) closure of the vocal folds to build subglottic pressure necessary for physical tasks such as excretion and lifting heavy items.

Laryngeal Structures and Cartilages

■ The larynx is suspended from the U-shaped *hyoid bone,* which floats under the mandible or lower jaw. The muscles of the tongue and various muscles of the mandible, skull, and larynx are attached to the hyoid bone.

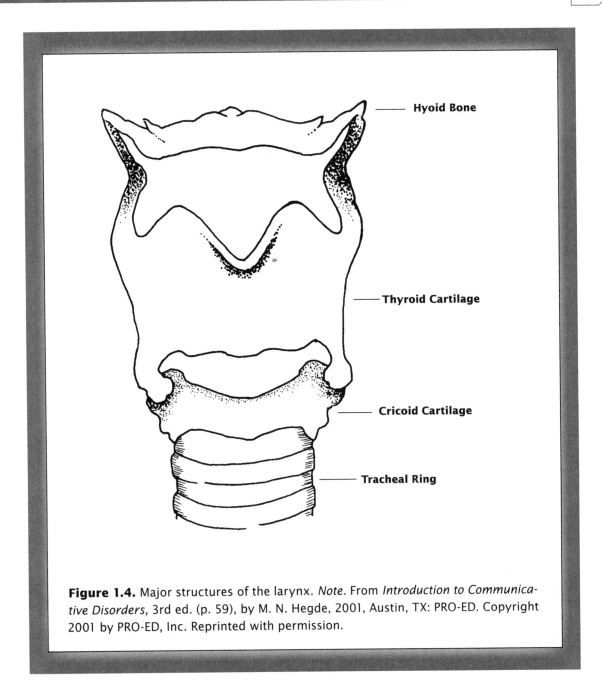

Figure 1.4. Major structures of the larynx. *Note.* From *Introduction to Communicative Disorders,* 3rd ed. (p. 59), by M. N. Hegde, 2001, Austin, TX: PRO-ED. Copyright 2001 by PRO-ED, Inc. Reprinted with permission.

■ The *epiglottis,* a protective structure, is a leaf-shaped piece of cartilage medial to the thyroid cartilage and hyoid bone. During swallowing, the epiglottis drops to cover the orifice of the larynx (Seikel et al., 2000). Figure 1.5 illustrates the epiglottis and other key laryngeal structures.

■ Key cartilages of the larynx include the thyroid, cricoid, and arytenoid cartilages. The *thyroid cartilage* forms the anterior and lateral walls of the larynx and protects the larynx.

■ The *cricoid cartilage,* which some view as the uppermost tracheal ring, is linked with the thyroid cartilage and the paired arytenoid cartilages. The cricoid cartilage completely surrounds the trachea.

Figure 1.5. A front and back view of key laryngeal structures. *Note.* From *Introduction to Communicative Disorders*, 3rd ed. (p. 233), by M. N. Hegde, 2001, Austin, TX: PRO-ED. Copyright 2001 by PRO-ED, Inc. Reprinted with permission.

■ The *arytenoid cartilages* are small, pyramid-shaped cartilages connected to the cricoid through the *cricoarytenoid joint,* which permits sliding and circular movements.

■ The small, cone-shaped *corniculate cartilages* sit on the apex of the arytenoids. They assist in reducing the laryngeal opening when a person is swallowing. The tiny cone-shaped *cuneiform cartilages* are located under the mucous membrane that covers the aryepiglottic folds (defined later). The cuneiform cartilages serve to stiffen or tense the aryepiglottic folds (Nicolosi et al., 2004).

Intrinsic Laryngeal Muscles

■ The *intrinsic laryngeal muscles* are primarily responsible for controlling sound production (Zemlin, 1998). The intrinsic muscles of the larynx are the thyroarytenoids, lateral cricoarytenoids, transverse arytenoids, oblique arytenoids, cricothyroids, and posterior cricoarytenoids.

■ The *thyroarytenoids* are attached to the thyroid and arytenoid cartilages. The thyroarytenoid muscles are divided into two muscle masses: the internal thyroarytenoids and the external thyroarytenoids.

■ The internal thyroarytenoids are the primary portions of the thyroarytenoid muscle that vibrate and produce sound. Some people also refer to them as the *vocalis muscle, vocal folds,* and *vocal cords.* The vocal folds are illustrated in Figure 1.6.

■ Adductor muscles include the *lateral cricoarytenoids, transverse arytenoids,* and *oblique arytenoids.* These muscles act to bring the vocal folds together. The lateral cricoarytenoids increase medial compression.

■ The *cricothyroid muscle* is attached to the cricoid and thyroid cartilages. It lengthens and tenses the vocal folds.

■ Figure 1.7 illustrates the *posterior cricoarytenoid* muscle and the *oblique* and *transverse arytenoid* muscles. Vocal fold adduction is supported when the oblique and transverse arytenoid muscles contract and pull the arytenoids closer together. Abduction of the vocal folds is accomplished when the posterior cricoarytenoid muscle contracts.

■ The following lists provide a simple summary of the intrinsic laryngeal muscles, the number of the cranial nerves that innervate them (e.g., "X"), the attachments of each muscle pair, and their functions. (*Note:* Most intrinsic laryngeal muscles are innervated by the recurrent laryngeal nerve branch of cranial nerve X, the vagus nerve. An exception is the cricothyroids,

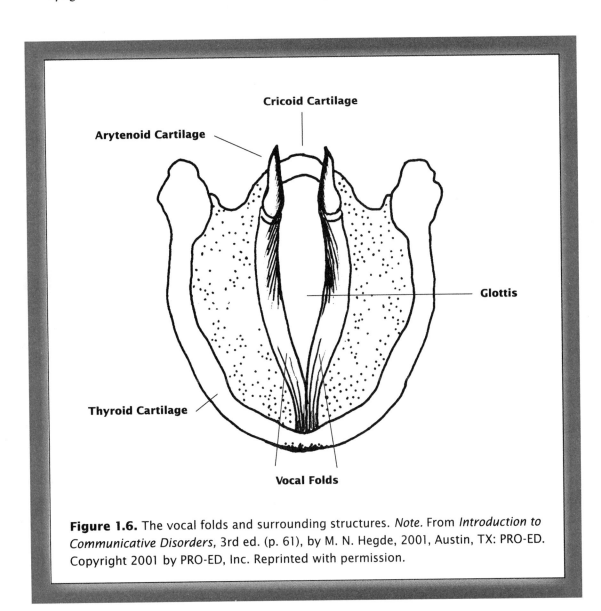

Figure 1.6. The vocal folds and surrounding structures. *Note.* From *Introduction to Communicative Disorders,* 3rd ed. (p. 61), by M. N. Hegde, 2001, Austin, TX: PRO-ED. Copyright 2001 by PRO-ED, Inc. Reprinted with permission.

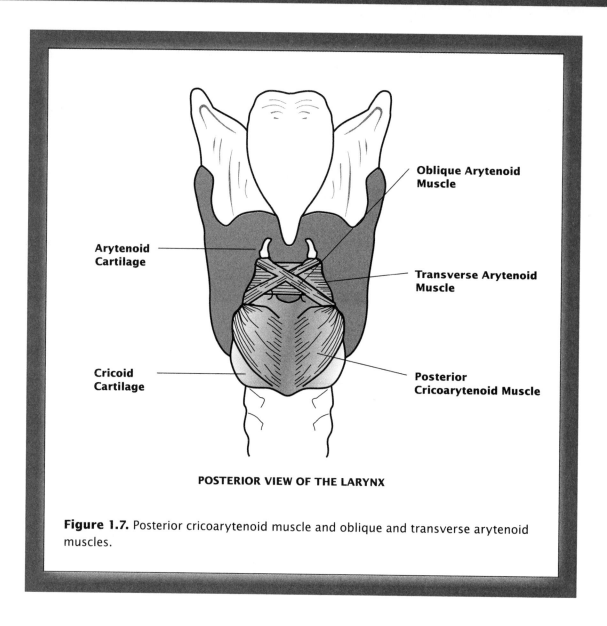

POSTERIOR VIEW OF THE LARYNX

Figure 1.7. Posterior cricoarytenoid muscle and oblique and transverse arytenoid muscles.

which are innervated by the external branch of the superior laryngeal nerve branch of the vagus.)

Muscles and Innervation	Function
thyroarytenoids (X)	internal thyroarytenoids are primary portion of vocal folds that vibrate and produce sound
lateral cricoarytenoids (X)	adduct vocal folds, increase medial compression
transverse arytenoids (X)	adduct vocal folds
oblique arytenoids (X)	pull apex of arytenoids in a medial direction
cricothyroids (X)	lengthen and tense vocal folds
posterior cricoarytenoids (X)	abduct vocal folds

- When the vocal folds are abducted, a small opening is created, which is called the *glottis*. The glottis is not an anatomical structure; it is merely the name of that space.

Extrinsic Laryngeal Muscles

- The primary function of the *extrinsic laryngeal muscles* is to support the larynx and fix its position (Zemlin, 1998). The extrinsic laryngeal muscles have one attachment to a structure within the larynx and one attachment to a structure outside the larynx. All extrinsic muscles are attached to the hyoid bone and lower or raise the position of the larynx within the neck.

- The *elevators,* or *suprahyoid muscles,* lie above the hyoid bone. Their primary function is elevation of the larynx. The suprahyoid muscles are the *digastrics, geniohyoids, mylohyoids,* and *stylohyoids, hyoglossus,* and *genioglossus.*

- The *depressors,* or *infrahyoid muscles,* lie below the hyoid bone. Their primary function is depression of the larynx. The infrahyoid muscles are the *thyrohyoids, omohyoids, sternothyroids,* and *sternohyoids.*

- The following list provides a brief summary of the elevators and depressors, their locations, and their functions. Innervation of these muscles is generally provided by branches of cranial nerve V (trigeminal), cranial nerve VII (facial), cranial nerve X (vagus), cranial nerve XII (hypoglossal), and portions of cervical spinal nerves C1–C3. (For more detailed information, see Seikel et al., 2000.)

Elevators and Innervation	Depressors and Innervation
digastrics (V, VII)	thyrohyoids (XII, C1)
geniohyoids (XII, C1)	omohyoids (C1–C3)
mylohyoids (V)	sternothyroids (C1–C3)
stylohyoids (VII)	sternohyoids (C1–C3)
hyoglossus (XII)	
genioglossus (XII)	

Vocal Folds

- The vocal folds have three layers: (a) the *epithelium,* or outer cover; (b) the *lamina propria,* or middle layer (which actually consists of three layers); and (c) the *vocalis muscle,* or body, which provides stability and mass to the vocal fold.

- There are two other pairs of folds (see Figure 1.8):

  - *Aryepiglottic folds.* The aryepiglottic folds are composed of a ring of connective tissue and muscle extending from the tips of the arytenoids to the larynx. They separate the laryngeal vestibule from the pharynx and help preserve the airway.
  - *Ventricular,* or *false,* vocal folds. The ventricular folds vibrate only at very low fundamental frequencies and usually not during phonation in a normal speaker. The ventricular folds compress during such activities as coughing and lifting heavy items.

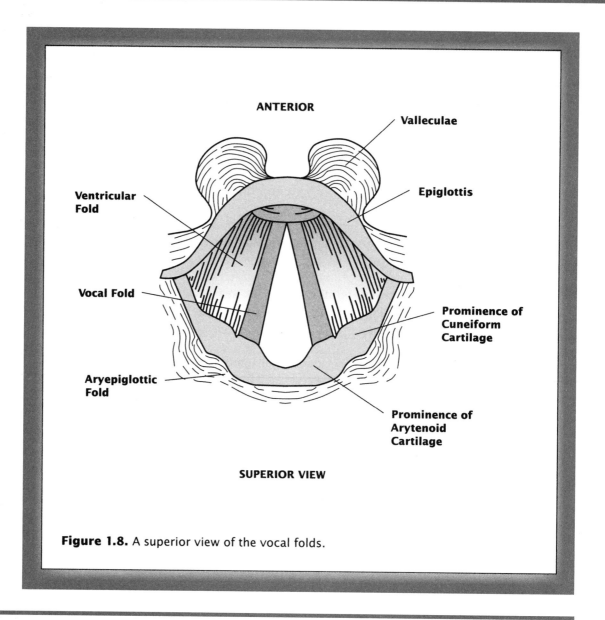

Figure 1.8. A superior view of the vocal folds.

Physiology of Phonation

Myoelastic–Aerodynamic Theory and Bernoulli Effect

- The *myoelastic–aerodynamic theory* states that the vocal folds vibrate because of the forces and pressure of air and the elasticity of the vocal folds.
- The air flowing out of the lungs is temporarily stopped by the closed (or nearly closed) vocal folds. This builds up subglottal air pressure, which eventually blows the vocal folds apart. During this process, the folds are set into vibration as well.
- The air then moves with increased velocity through the glottal opening. As the air moves swiftly through the open, but still somewhat constricted, vocal folds, the pressure between the edges of the vocal folds decreases, and consequently, the folds are sucked together.
- The *Bernoulli effect,* caused by the increased speed of air passing between the vocal folds, is the "sucking" motion of the vocal folds toward one another.
- Once again, the subglottal air pressure builds up and sets the folds in motion. Thus, there is a

cycle of opening and closing of the vocal folds; this cycle is repeated more than 100 times per second during vocalization.

CONCEPTS TO CONSIDER

Give a brief description of the myoelastic–aerodynamic theory and the Bernoulli effect.

_____

_____

_____

_____

_____

Mucosal Wave Action

- The mucosal wave is critical to vibration of the vocal folds. In *mucosal wave action,* the cover (epithelium and superficial lamina propria, Reinke's space) and the transition (intermediate and deep layers of the lamina propria) over the vocalis muscle slide and produce a wave.
- This wave travels across the superior surface of the vocal fold about two-thirds of the way to the lateral edge of the fold. Generally, the wave dissipates before reaching the inner surface of the thyroid cartilage. There is no vibration, and thus no phonation, without a mucosal wave.
- Vocal folds that have been stripped surgically, while being free of overt pathology such as nodules, may be stiff and have difficulty vibrating due to alteration of the normal mucosal wave.

Neuroanatomy of the Vocal Mechanism

Cortical Areas

- The primary cortical areas involved in speech motor control, including phonation, are:

  - area 4 (primary motor cortex)
  - area 44 (Broca's area)
  - areas 3, 1, 2 (somatosensory cortex)
  - area 6 (supplementary motor cortex)

Cerebellum

- The function of the cerebellum is to regulate motor movement. It is critical in the control of speech movement.

- The cerebellum is key to the coordination of the laryngeal muscles for adequate phonation. It is also key to the effective functioning of other speech systems such as respiration.

Cranial Nerves

- Cranial nerve VII (*the facial nerve*) innervates the posterior belly of the digastric muscle.
- Cranial nerve X (*the vagus nerve*) includes the following primary branches, which innervate the larynx:

    - *Superior laryngeal nerve (SLN)*. The superior laryngeal nerve has internal and external branches. The internal branch provides all sensory information to the larynx, and the external branch supplies motor innervation solely to the cricothyroid muscle.
    - *Recurrent laryngeal nerve (RLN)*. The recurrent laryngeal nerve supplies all motor innervation to the interarytenoid, posterior cricoarytenoid, thyroarytenoid, and lateral cricoarytenoid muscles. It supplies all sensory information below the vocal folds.

SUMMARY

✓ Air for speech comes from the lungs, through the trachea, to the larynx and sets the vocal folds in motion for voicing. Adequate voicing depends upon the integrity of many laryngeal structures.

✓ Key laryngeal structures and cartilages provide protection to the larynx and aid in the process of vocalization.

✓ There are two sets of laryngeal muscles. The intrinsic laryngeal muscles have both their attachments within the larynx. The extrinsic laryngeal muscles have one attachment inside the larynx and one attachment outside the larynx.

✓ The physiology of phonation can be explained by the myoelastic–aerodynamic theory and the phenomenon of the Bernoulli effect. Mucosal wave action is critical to vocal fold vibration.

✓ Key neuroanatomical structures involved in vocalization include cortical areas, the cerebellum, and cranial nerves VII (facial nerve) and X (vagus nerve).

RESONATION AND ARTICULATION: STRUCTURES AND PROCESSES

INTRODUCTION

Respiration provides the energy for voicing. As the laryngeal tone travels upward past the larynx, it must be resonated by various structures such as the pharynx, the oral cavity, and the nasal cavity. The resonated tone is shaped and modified further through articulation, or production of speech sounds. Key structures involved in articulation include the pharynx, the soft palate, the hard palate, the mandible, the teeth, the tongue, the lips, and the cheeks. Functioning of these structures depends in part upon innervation by various cranial nerves.

Fundamentals of Resonation

- The vocal folds vibrate to produce voice. *Resonation* is the process by which the voice, or laryngeal tone, is modified when some frequency components are dampened and others are enhanced. The resonators that serve to modify laryngeal tone are the pharynx, the nasal cavity, and the oral cavity.

■ The *pharynx*, or throat, is part of the upper airway. It is located superiorly and posteriorly to the larynx. The size and shape of the pharynx are modified by the position of the tongue in the mouth (forward or back) and the vertical positioning of the larynx in the neck (high or low) (Peña-Brooks & Hegde, 2000).

■ The *nasal cavity* has an important role in resonation. Only three sounds in English—/m/, /n/, and /ŋ/—are produced with *nasal resonance*. During the production of those sounds, the soft palate, or velum, is relaxed and lowered, as illustrated in Figure 1.9(A). Thus, there is *coupling* of the nasal and oral cavities; they are not separated from one another.

■ The velum is elevated and retracted for production of all other sounds in English. During production of those sounds, the velum is raised and retracted, or moved back, to make contact with the posterior pharyngeal wall, separating the oral cavity from the nasal cavity, as illustrated in Figure 1.9(B). The cavities are thus *uncoupled*. In this way, the sounds are produced primarily with *oral resonance*.

■ The *oral cavity* is the primary resonating structure for all English sounds, except /m/, /n/, and /ŋ/. The source-filter theory of vowel production provides a widely accepted description of how the oral cavity is capable of producing speech sounds.

■ According to the *source-filter theory*, the vocal tract is visualized as a series of linked tubes: the oral cavity, or mouth; the pharynx; and the nasal cavity (see Figure 1.10). These linked tubes

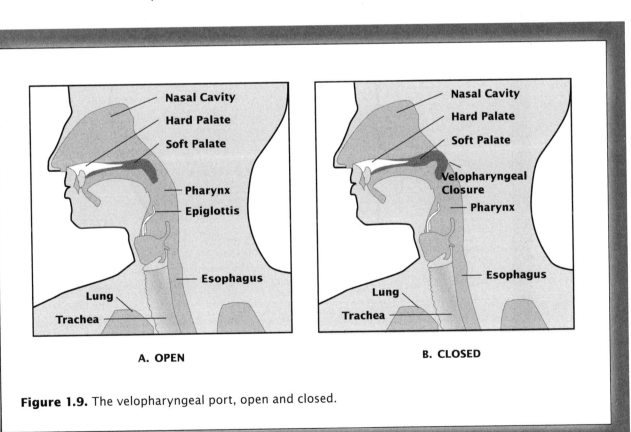

Figure 1.9. The velopharyngeal port, open and closed.

provide the variable resonating cavity that helps produce speech (Seikel et al., 2000).

■ The source-filter theory states that energy from the vibrating vocal folds (the *source*) is modified by the resonance characteristics of the vocal tract (the *filter*) (Kent, 1997).

■ The vocal folds generate a voicing source. This voicing source is routed through the vocal tract, where it is shaped into speech sounds. Those speech sounds may be vowels when the source is phonation, and consonants when the sources include the turbulence of frication or combinations of turbulence and voicing.

■ Changes in the configuration and shape of the articulators (described below) govern the resonance characteristics of the vocal tract. The resonances of the vocal tract determine the sound of each specific vowel. But whether consonants or vowels are produced, in each case the person produces a noise source and passes it through the filter of the oral cavity, which has been specifically configured for production of that sound (Seikel et al., 2000).

■ Structures within the oral cavity are shaped and moved to provide specific resonance for each sound. These structures are key in the process of articulation.

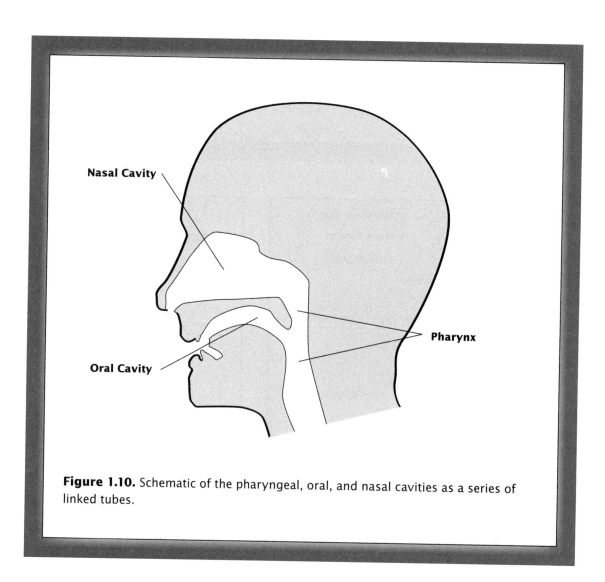

Figure 1.10. Schematic of the pharyngeal, oral, and nasal cavities as a series of linked tubes.

Fundamentals of Articulation

■ Articulation refers to the connection of movable parts or the joining of two elements. In speech, articulation refers to movements of speech structures to produce speech sounds. Articulation may also refer to the act of saying something clearly. In this section, the term *articulation* refers to the movement of joined anatomic parts as well as the production of speech sounds that result from such movements.

■ When a person is speaking, the larynx produces sound. The sound, as stated, travels through the pharynx and the oral cavity (and the nasal cavity for nasal sounds). In the oral cavity, important structures modify the sound into specific sounds for speech. These structures include the pharynx, the soft palate, the hard palate, the mandible, the teeth, the tongue, the lips, and the cheeks.

Pharynx

- The pharyngeal cavity is divided into three segments, which are illustrated in Figure 1.11:

    - the *laryngopharynx*, which begins immediately superior to the larynx and ends at the base of the tongue, is connected to the
    - *oropharynx*, which extends up to the soft palate and is connected to the
    - *nasopharynx*, which ends where the two nasal cavities begin.

- The laryngopharynx and the oropharynx add resonance to the sounds produced by the larynx. However, as previously stated, the nasopharynx adds noticeable resonance only to the nasals, /m/, /n/, and /ŋ/.
- The muscles of the pharynx are summarized in the following lists (Seikel et al., 2000). Most pharyngeal muscles are innervated by cranial nerve X (the vagus nerve) and cranial nerve XI (the spinal accessory nerve) via the pharyngeal plexus. The *pharyngeal plexus* is formed by the joining of cranial nerves X and XI; it supplies the upper pharyngeal musculature.

Muscle and Innervation	Function
salpingopharyngeus (X, XI)	elevates lateral pharyngeal wall
stylopharyngeus (IX)	elevates and opens pharynx
superior pharyngeal constrictor (X, XI)	constricts pharyngeal diameter, pulls pharyngeal wall forward
middle pharyngeal constrictor (X, XI)	narrows diameter of pharynx
inferior pharyngeal constrictor, cricopharyngeus (X, XI)	constricts superior orifice of esophagus
inferior pharyngeal constrictor, thyropharyngeus (X, XI)	reduces diameter of lower pharynx

Soft Palate

- The soft palate, also called the *velum*, is a flexible muscular structure at the juncture of the oropharynx and the nasopharynx. It is located in the posterior area of the oral cavity and hangs from the hard palate (roof of the mouth). The *uvula* is the small, cone-shaped structure

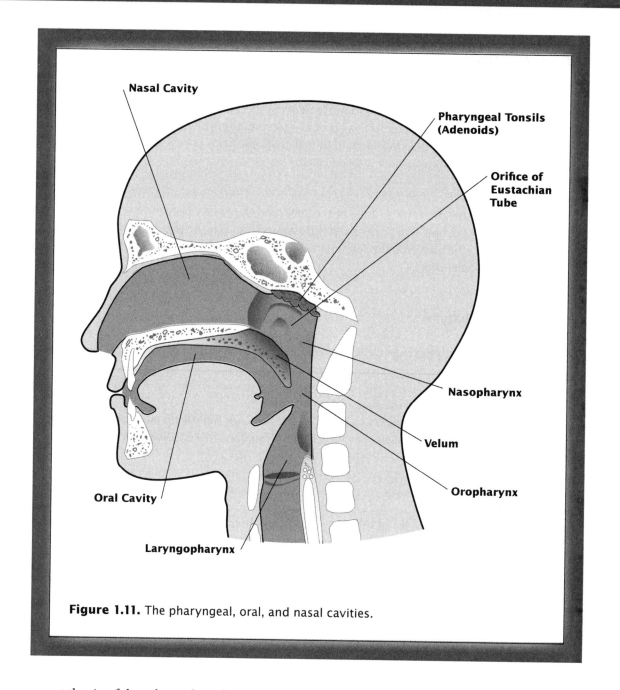

Figure 1.11. The pharyngeal, oral, and nasal cavities.

at the tip of the velum. The soft palate and other major structures of the oral cavity are shown in Figure 1.12.

- The soft palate is a dynamic structure of muscles that can be elevated or lowered. As previously stated, when the soft palate is lowered, there is coupling of the nasal and oral cavities for nasal sounds or quiet breathing through the nose.

- When the soft palate is raised and retracted, the muscles of the pharynx also move inward to meet the muscles of the soft palate. With this sphincter-like action, the nasal port is then closed. This action is called *velopharyngeal closure.*

- If the muscular bulk of the soft palate is inadequate, the nasal cavity may remain open to some extent. Speakers with this condition sound excessively nasal because sound energy passes through the nasal cavities when it should not.

- The soft palate is composed of a number of muscles (see Figure 1.13). These include the *levator veli palatini,* the *tensor veli palatini,* the *palatoglossus,* and the *palatopharyngeus* muscles.

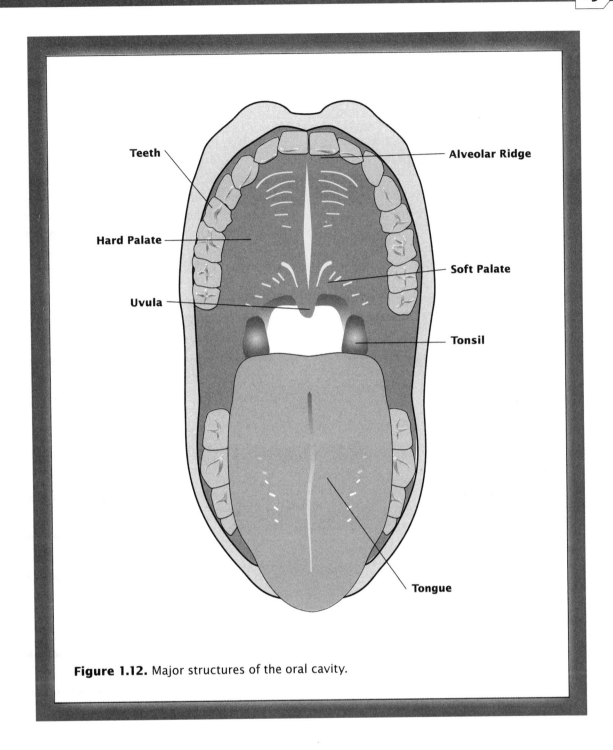

Figure 1.12. Major structures of the oral cavity.

These muscles and their functions and innervations are summarized in the lists below (Seikel et al., 2000). (*Note:* The innervation "X, XI" refers specifically to the pharyngeal plexus, a structure arising from cranial nerve X, the vagus nerve, and cranial nerve XI, the spinal accessory nerve.)

Muscle and Innervation	Function
levator veli palatini (X, XI)	primary elevator of velum
tensor veli palatini (V)	tenses velum, dilates Eustachian tube

Muscle and Innervation	Function
palatoglossus (X, XI)	elevates and depresses velum
palatopharyngeus (X, XI)	narrows pharyngeal cavity, lowers velum, may assist in elevating larynx

Hard Palate

- The bony hard palate is the roof of the mouth and the floor of the nose. It is part of the *maxillae,* or paired bones, which are the largest in the face and form the entire upper jaw (Zemlin, 1998). The maxillae are also referred to as the maxillary bone. The hard palate is illustrated in Figure 1.14.
- The front portion of the maxillary bone is called the *premaxilla.* The premaxilla houses the four upper front teeth known as the incisors.
- The portion of the maxillary bone that forms most of the hard palate is called the *palatine process.* The palatine process consists of two pieces of bone that grow and fuse at the midline

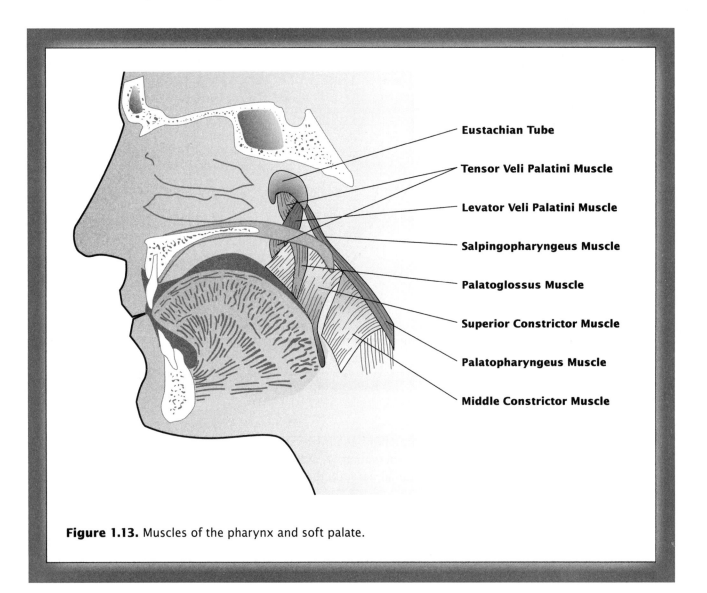

Figure 1.13. Muscles of the pharynx and soft palate.

during the fetal stage.

- The outer edges of the maxillary bone are called the *alveolar process,* which houses the molar, bicuspid, and cuspid teeth.
- For genetic and toxic environmental reasons, the premaxilla may fail to fuse with the maxillary bone. Also, the palatine process may fail to fuse at midline. These failures cause clefts of the palate in utero.
- Posteriorly, the maxillary bone joins with the *palatine bone* (different from the palatine process, which is part of the maxillary bone). The soft palate attaches to the palatine bone.

Mandible

- Also known as the lower jaw, the *mandible* is an important facial bone. It houses the lower teeth and forms the floor of the mouth. The mandible is formed by the fusion of two bones in the midpoint of the chin, but is considered to be one bone in adults.
- The *alveolar arch* is the part of the mandible that houses the teeth. The two arches of the mandible are hinged to the skull with a set of muscles and tendons. The mandible is attached to the temporal bone of the skull by a joint called the *temporomandibular joint.*
- The muscles of the mandible serve two major functions: (a) opening and closing the mouth, and (b) chewing food. Although its major task is to chew food, the mandible is important for speech because it houses the lower teeth, serves as a framework for the tongue and lower lip, and is an integral part of the oral cavity.

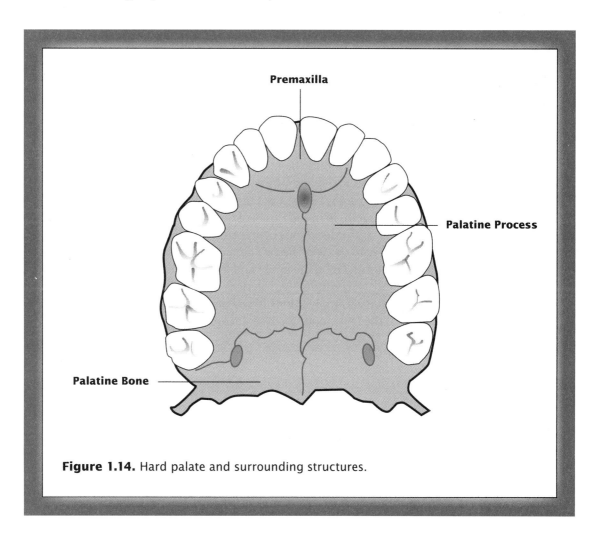

Figure 1.14. Hard palate and surrounding structures.

- The muscles of the mandible may be categorized as either elevators or depressors (Seikel et al., 2000). They arise from branches of cranial nerves V (trigeminal nerve), VII (facial nerve), and XII (hypoglossal nerve); the geniohyoid also rises from the C1 spinal nerve. These muscles are summarized below.

Elevators and Innervation	Function
masseter (V)	elevates mandible
temporalis (V)	elevates mandible, draws mandible back if protruded
medial (internal) pterygoid (V)	elevates mandible
lateral (external) pterygoid (V)	protrudes mandible

Depressors and Innervation	
anterior belly of digastric (V)	depresses mandible in conjunction with posterior belly of digastric; pulls hyoid forward
posterior belly of digastric (VII)	depresses mandible in conjuction with anterior belly of digastric; pulls hyoid back
geniohyoid (XII, C1)	depresses mandible
mylohyoid (V)	depresses mandible

Teeth

- The lower dental arch is part of the mandible, and the upper dental arch is part of the maxillary bone. The major function of the teeth is *mastication* (chewing), but the teeth also aid in production of some speech sounds. For example, the labiodental sounds /f/ and /v/ require the lower lip to come in contact with the upper teeth. Thus, the teeth are considered articulators.
- Teeth, illustrated in Figure 1.15, are called by different names (e.g., molars, bicuspids) depending upon their location in the mouth. *Deciduous teeth* are temporary teeth that appear in a baby, usually around 6–9 months of age. Babies normally have 20 deciduous teeth, 10 in each arch. Of the 10, 4 are incisors, 2 are canine, and 4 are molar.
- Adults have 32 teeth, 16 in each arch; of the 16 teeth, 4 are incisors, 2 are canine, 4 are premolar, and 6 are molar. The deciduous dental arch does not have premolars or the third molar.
- *Occlusion* refers to the way the two dental arches come together when a person "bites down." Occlusion is normal if (a) the upper and lower dental arches meet each other in a symmetrical manner, and (b) if the individual teeth in the two arches are properly aligned.
- *Malocclusions* include deviations in the positioning of individual teeth and the shape and relationship of the upper and lower dental arches. Types of malocclusions are further described in Chapter 5.

Tongue

- The tongue plays an important role in eating and in speech production. The taste buds of the tongue help people taste their food, and the muscles of the tongue help it to move food around in the oral cavity for efficient mastication and swallowing. Movements of the tongue are critical to articulation.
- For example, tongue movement is necessary to produce /k/, /ŋ/, and many other sounds. The tongue can also constrict the air passage and thus create the friction needed for sounds such as /ʃ/.

Figure 1.15. Types of teeth.

List three pharyngeal muscles, three soft palate muscles, and three mandibular muscles that are key in the process of articulation.

- Anatomically, the tongue is divided into four major parts: tip, blade, dorsum, and root (see Figure 1.16):

    - The *tip* is the thinnest and most flexible part of the tongue, and it plays an important role in articulation.
    - The *blade* is a small region adjacent to the tip; in a resting position, the blade is the portion of the tongue that lies just inferior to the alveolar ridge.
    - The *dorsum* is the larger area of the tongue that lies in contact with both the hard and soft palates.
    - The *root* is contained in the very back of the tongue.

- The *lingual frenulum* (or *frenum*) connects the mandible with the inferior portion of the tongue. This band of tissue may stabilize the tongue during movement (Seikel et al., 2000).
- There are two sets of important tongue muscles: intrinsic and extrinsic. Upon contraction, these muscles perform important functions in articulation. The tongue muscles are innervated by cranial nerve XII, the hypoglossal nerve.
- The *genioglossus muscle* forms the bulk of the tongue and allows it to move freely. Figure 1.17 illustrates the genioglossus and related muscles.

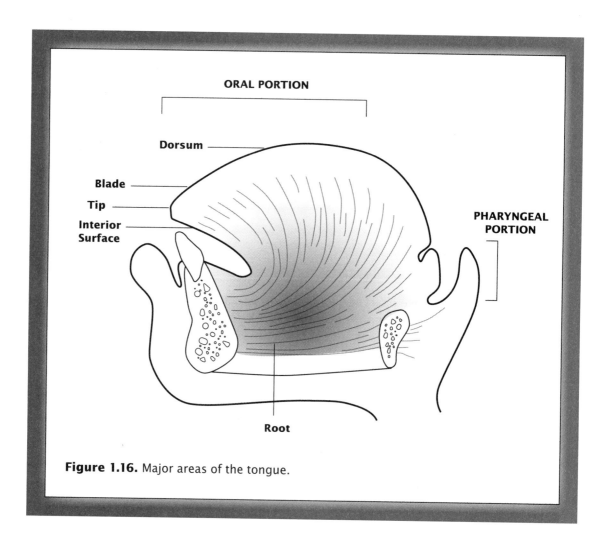

Figure 1.16. Major areas of the tongue.

Figure 1.17. The genioglossus and related muscles.

Intrinsic Tongue Muscles and Innervation	Function
superior longitudinal muscle (XII)	shortens tongue, turns tip upward, assists in turning lateral margins upward
inferior longitudinal muscle (XII)	shortens tongue, pulls tip downward, assists in retraction
transverse muscles (XII)	narrow and elongate tongue
vertical muscles (XII)	flatten the tongue
genioglossus (XII)	forms bulk of tongue; is able to retract tongue, draw tongue downward, draw entire tongue anteriorly to protrude tip or press tip against alveolar ridges and teeth
styloglossus (XII)	draws tongue up and back, may draw sides of tongue upward to help make dorsum concave
hyoglossus (XII)	retracts and depresses tongue
chondroglossus (XII)	depresses the tongue

Face: Lips and Cheeks

- Several major bones of the face have already been discussed. There are major facial muscles, involving the lips and cheeks, that are important for articulation (see Figure 1.18). These muscles assist in production of various sounds, especially the labial sounds /m/, /b/, and /p/.
- The primary muscle of the lips is the *orbicularis oris* muscle. The cheeks are primarily composed of the *buccinator* muscle, a large flat muscle whose inner surface is covered with mucous membrane.
- Most of the facial muscles are innervated by either the *buccal branches* or the *mandibular marginal branch* of cranial nerve VII, the facial nerve. These muscles are summarized in the following lists (Seikel et al., 2000).

Muscle and Innervation	Function
mentalis (VII)	pulls lower lip out, wrinkles and elevates chin
platysma (VII)	depresses mandible
risorius (VII)	retracts lips at corners
buccinator (VII)	constricts oropharynx; moves food onto grinding surfaces of molars
depressor labii inferioris (VII)	pulls lip down and out to dilate orifice
depressor anguli oris (triangularis) (VII)	helps to press lower and upper lips together; depresses corners of mouth
zygomatic minor (VII)	elevates upper lip
zygomatic major (VII)	retracts and elevates angle of mouth
orbicularis oris inferioris and superioris (VII)	pulls lips together, seals lips, serves as point of insertion for other muscles, interacts with other muscles to produce facial expressions
levator anguli oris (VII)	draws corner of mouth upward and toward medial
levator labii superioris (VII)	elevates upper lip
levator labii superioris alaeque nasi (VII)	elevates upper lip

SUMMARY

✓ Tones generated by the larynx travel upward and are resonated by the pharynx, oral cavity, and nasal cavity. This process of resonation is explained by the source-filter theory.

✓ Articulation refers to the movement of speech structures to produce sounds. It depends upon the integrity of the following structures: the pharynx, soft palate, hard palate, mandible, teeth, tongue, lips, and cheeks.

✓ The cranial nerves mostly involved with innervating the muscles involved in articulation include cranial nerve V (trigeminal), VII (facial), X (vagus), XI (spinal accessory), and XII (hypoglossal).

Figure 1.18. Muscles of the face.

NEUROANATOMY AND NEUROPHYSIOLOGY: THE NERVOUS SYSTEM

Neurology is the study of neurological disorders and diseases and their diagnosis and treatment. *Neuroanatomy* is a branch of neurology concerned with the study of *structures* of the nervous system. *Neurophysiology*, another branch of neurology, is concerned with the study of the *function* of the nervous system.

In this section, we discuss basic neuroanatomy and neurophysiology of speech, language, and hearing. It is assumed that the reader has taken coursework in these areas; thus, this section provides only a basic "refresher" of some foundational ideas.

This section covers neurons and neural transmission. It discusses basic facts about the workings of the peripheral and autonomic nervous systems, including information about the cranial nerves. The central nervous system is then described according to its general parameters: the brain stem, reticular activating system, diencephalon, basal ganglia, cerebellum, cerebrum, pyramidal system, extrapyramidal system, connecting fibers in the brain, cerebral ventricles, protective layers of the brain, and cerebral blood supply. (*Note:* The extrapyramidal system is not technically a part of the central nervous system; however, it is closely related to the central nervous system and is thus discussed in this section.)

NEURONS AND NEURAL TRANSMISSION

INTRODUCTION

The nervous system is composed of billions of specialized cells that function interconnectedly. Neurons are the most important of these cells. Sensory or afferent neurons carry sensory impulses toward the brain, whereas motor or efferent nerves transmit impulses away from the brain. Nerves may be organized into systems.

Anatomy and Physiology of Nerve Cells

- The central nervous system is made up of different types of cells. *Glial cells* or *neuroglia* include *Schwann cells* and *oliodendroglia,* which are related to myelin production, and *microglia,* which act as scavengers to remove dead cells and other waste (Freed, 2000).

- *Neurons* are the most important type of nerve cells. There are billions of neurons that receive information from other neurons, process that information, and then transmit the information to still other neurons.

- The neuron or nerve cell has two parts: (a) nerve fibers and (b) the soma, or cell body, which contains the nucleus. Figure 1.19 shows a typical nerve cell.

- The core of the cell body is called the *nucleus.* The cell body is covered with a membrane. The axons and dendrites are projections of the cell body and specialize in receiving and conducting stimuli.

- *Dendrites* are short fibers that extend from the cell body. They receive neural impulses generated from the axons of other cells, and they transmit those impulses to the cell body.

- Each cell has a single *axon,* which is wrapped in a myelin sheath (defined later). Axons are longer fibers than dendrites and have *terminal,* or *end, buttons* at the tip. The end button of one neuron either makes close contact with or actually touches the dendrite of another neuron. Axons send out impulses generated within the neuron; these impulses are sent away from the cell body to other neurons.

- Neurons communicate with each other through junctions called *synapses.* An axon branches out into several smaller fibers, which form terminals. These terminals connect to a synapse, although this neural junction includes a small gap or space. Thus, a synapse consists of the terminal button of one neuron, the receptive site of another neuron, and the synaptic cleft or space between the two (Peña-Brooks & Hegde, 2000).

- *Neural transmission* is a chemical process of information exchange at the level of the synapse. A *neurotransmitter,* a chemical contained within the terminal buttons, helps make contact between two cells by diffusing itself across the synaptic space.

- Such diffused neurotransmitters become bound to receptors in the postsynaptic membrane. The diffused neurotransmitter may cause the inhibition or excitation of the next neuron. *Dopamine* and *acetylcholine* are two important neurotransmitters in the motor system.

- Neurons have certain specialized functions. There are three basic types of neurons: *motor neurons, sensory neurons,* and *interneurons.*

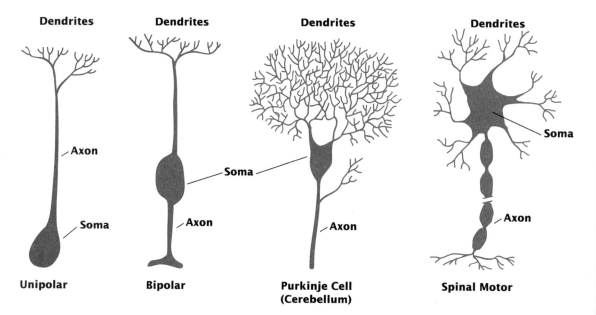

Figure 1.19. A typical neuron.

CONCEPTS TO CONSIDER

Describe neurons in terms of their key parts and their function in the human body.

_____

_____

_____

_____

_____

■ *Sensory neurons,* also called *afferent neurons,* carry sensory impulses from the peripheral sense organs *toward* the brain. *Motor neurons,* also called *efferent neurons,* transmit impulses *away* from the central nervous system. Motor neurons cause glandular secretions or muscle contractions (movement).

■ *Interneurons,* the most common type of neuron in the nervous system, link neurons with other neurons. Because they form connections with other neurons, interneurons play an important role in controlling movement (Freed, 2000).

■ Many axons, especially the larger axons of the central nervous system and those in the peripheral nervous system, have a white insulating sheath called *myelin* around them. Schwann cells and oliodendroglia provide the myelin sheath around the axon. The myelin has breaks at the junction between the cells to facilitate the impulse transfer.

■ Neurons are arranged in the form of fibers. A *nervous system,* on the other hand, is an organization of nerves according to specific spatial, structural, and functional principles. The peripheral, autonomic, and central nervous systems are often collectively referred to as the nervous system. In the next sections, each of these systems is explained.

SUMMARY

✓ Neurons, the central building blocks of the nervous system, are composed of a cell body, dendrites, and an axon.

✓ Some of these nerves have myelin sheaths around them. Various types of nerves transmit impulses to and from the central nervous system.

THE PERIPHERAL AND AUTONOMIC NERVOUS SYSTEMS

INTRODUCTION

The peripheral nervous system, a collection of nerves outside the spinal column and skull, carries sensory and motor impulses back and forth from the brain to various parts of the body. The 12 pairs of cranial nerves are part of the peripheral nervous system; some of them are critical to language, speech, and hearing. The 31 pairs of spinal nerves are indirectly involved with speech because they control automatic functions such as breathing. Part of the peripheral nervous system is the autonomic nervous system, with its sympathetic and parasympathetic branches, which may have an indirect effect upon speech in certain situations.

Peripheral Nervous System

Basic Principles

- The *peripheral nervous system* (PNS) is a collection of nerves that are outside the skull and spinal column. These nerves carry *sensory* impulses originating in the peripheral sense organs to the brain, and *motor* impulses originating in the brain to the glands and muscles of the body.
- The PNS contains three types of nerves: the spinal, the cranial, and the peripheral autonomic nerves. There are 12 pairs of cranial nerves and 31 pairs of spinal nerves. Of the three types of nerves, the cranial nerves are the most directly involved in speech, language, and hearing.

Cranial Nerves

- The cranial nerves emerge from the brain stem and are attached to the base of the brain. They are part of the lower motor neuron system of the corticobulbar tract of the pyramidal system (discussed later in more detail). The cranial nerves exit through *foramina*, or holes, in the base of the skull. They exit at different levels of the brain stem and the top portion of the spinal cord.
- The cranial nerves are numbered according to the vertical order in which they exit from the skull. They go out to connect to various sense organs and muscles of the neck and head. Table 1.1 lists the cranial nerves and their numbers and basic functions. Some students remember the cranial nerves by the following mnemonic: *On old Olympus' towering top, a Finn and German viewed some hops.*
- *Sensory nerves* are those cranial nerves that carry sensory information from a sense organ (e.g., the nose) to the brain. *Motor* (movement-related) *nerves* carry impulses from the brain to the muscles that make those muscles move. Several cranial nerves are *mixed nerves* because they carry both sensory and motor impulses.
- There are 12 pairs of cranial nerves. The first two cranial nerves are related to the cerebral cortex. Cranial nerves III–XII originate from the brain stem and innervate the muscles of the pharynx, tongue, larynx, head, neck, and face. Figure 1.20 illustrates an inferior view of the brain showing cranial nerves as well as other cerebral structures (described later).
- Cranial nerves I, II, III, IV, and VI are not concerned with speech, language, or hearing:

    - *Cranial nerve I (the olfactory nerve)* is a sensory nerve originating in the nasal cavity. It is involved with smell.

Table 1.1   CRANIAL NERVES

Nerve No.	Name	Function
I	Olfactory	Sense of smell (sensory)
II	Optic	Vision (motor)
III	Oculomotor	Eye movement (motor)
IV	Trochlear	Eye movement (motor)
V	Trigeminal	Face (sensory); jaw (motor)
VI	Abducens	Eye movement (motor)
VII	Facial	Tongue (sensory); face (motor)
VIII	Acoustic	Hearing and balance (sensory)
IX	Glossopharyngeal	Tongue and pharynx (sensory); pharynx only (motor)
X	Vagus	Larynx, respiratory, cardiac, and gastrointestinal systems (sensory and motor)
XI	Spinal Accessory	Shoulder, arm, and throat movements (motor)
XII	Hypoglossal	Mostly tongue movements (motor)

Note. From *Introduction to Communicative Disorders,* 3rd ed. (p. 77), by M. N. Hegde, 2001, Austin, TX: PRO-ED. Copyright 2001 by PRO-ED, Inc. Reprinted with permission.

- *Cranial nerve II (the optic nerve)* is a sensory nerve originating in the retina of the eye.
- *Cranial nerve III (the oculomotor nerve)* and *cranial nerve IV (the trochlear nerve)* are motor nerves that originate in the midbrain area and innervate muscles corresponding to eye movement.
- *Cranial nerve VI (the abducens nerve)* is a motor nerve that controls eye movement.

- Cranial nerves V and VII–XII are involved with speech, language, and hearing and, as such, are described in more detail below.
- *Cranial nerve V, or the trigeminal nerve,* is a mixed (both motor and sensory) nerve (see Figure 1.21).

  - Its *sensory fibers* are composed of three branches: opthalmic, maxillary, and mandibular branches. The opthalmic nerve has sensory branches to the nose, eyes, and forehead. The maxillary branch has sensory branches to the upper lip, maxilla, upper cheek area, upper

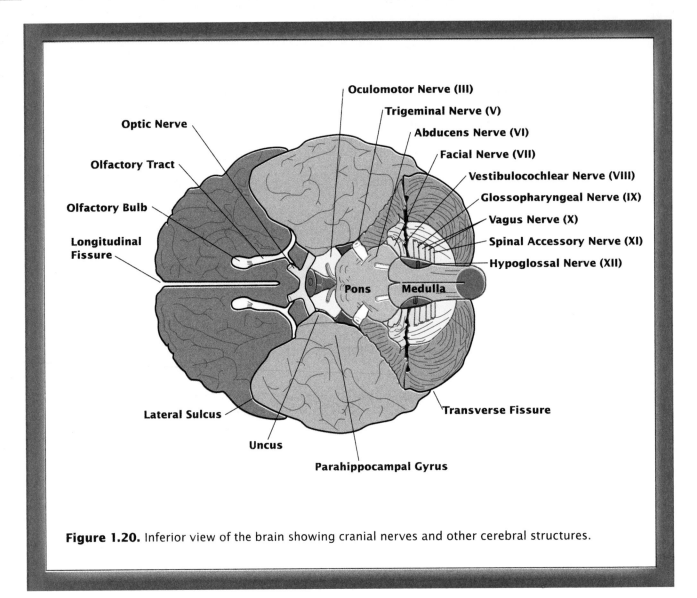

Figure 1.20. Inferior view of the brain showing cranial nerves and other cerebral structures.

teeth, maxillary sinus, and palate. The mandibular branch has sensory branches to the mandible, lower teeth, lower lip, tongue, part of the cheek, and part of the external ear.

- The *motor fibers* of cranial nerve V innervate various jaw muscles, including the temporalis, lateral and medial pterygoids, masseter, tensor veli palatini, tensor tympani, mylohyoid, and anterior belly of the digastric muscle.
- Damage to cranial nerve V may result in an inability to close the mouth, difficulty in chewing, and *trigeminal neuralgia* (sharp pain in the facial area) (Newman & Ramadan, 1998; Zemlin, 1998).

- *Cranial nerve VII, the facial nerve,* is also a mixed nerve (see Figure 1.22).

  - The sensory fibers of the facial nerve are responsible for taste sensations on the anterior two thirds of the tongue.
  - None of the motor fibers of the facial nerve has branches (Figure 1.22) that innervate muscles important to facial expression and speech. These muscles include the buccinator, zygomatic, orbicularis oris, orbicularis oculi, platysma, stapedius, stylohyoid, frontalis,

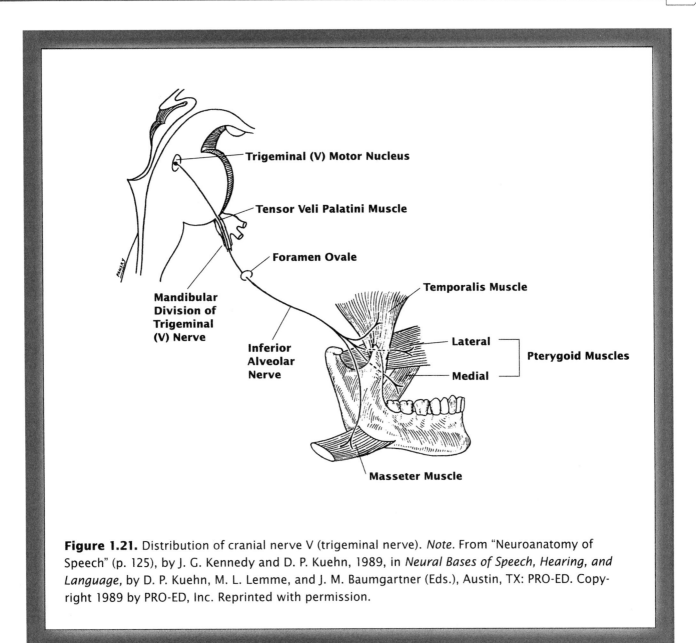

Figure 1.21. Distribution of cranial nerve V (trigeminal nerve). *Note.* From "Neuroanatomy of Speech" (p. 125), by J. G. Kennedy and D. P. Kuehn, 1989, in *Neural Bases of Speech, Hearing, and Language,* by D. P. Kuehn, M. L. Lemme, and J. M. Baumgartner (Eds.), Austin, TX: PRO-ED. Copyright 1989 by PRO-ED, Inc. Reprinted with permission.

procerus, nasalis, depressor labii inferioris, depressor anguli oris, auricular muscles, various labial muscles, and the posterior belly of the digastric muscle.

- A person with damage to the facial nerve often has a masklike appearance with minimal or no facial expression.

- *Cranial nerve VIII, the acoustic (or vestibulocochlear) nerve,* is a sensory nerve for balance and hearing. It has two branches (described further in Chapter 10).

  - The *vestibular branch* is primarily responsible for maintenance of equilibrium or balance.
  - The *acoustic branch* transmits sensory information from the cochlea of the inner ear to the primary auditory cortex of the brain, where it is interpreted.
  - Damage to the vestibular branch of the acoustic nerve results in a hearing loss, problems with balance, or both.

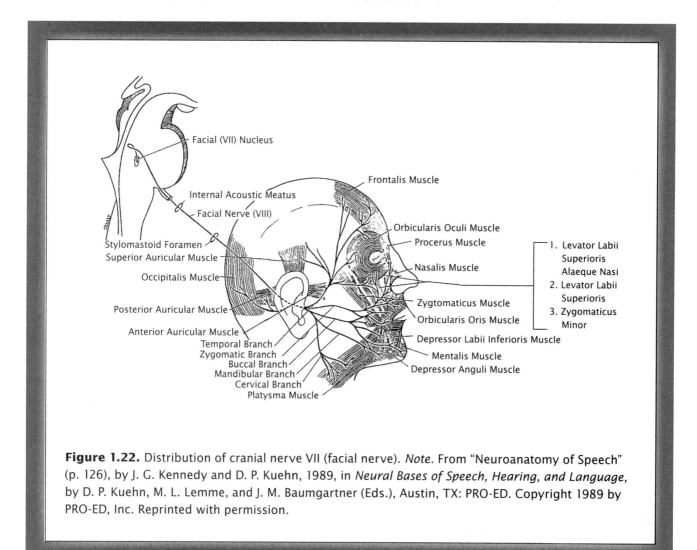

Figure 1.22. Distribution of cranial nerve VII (facial nerve). *Note.* From "Neuroanatomy of Speech" (p. 126), by J. G. Kennedy and D. P. Kuehn, 1989, in *Neural Bases of Speech, Hearing, and Language,* by D. P. Kuehn, M. L. Lemme, and J. M. Baumgartner (Eds.), Austin, TX: PRO-ED. Copyright 1989 by PRO-ED, Inc. Reprinted with permission.

- *Cranial nerve IX, the glossopharyngeal nerve,* is a mixed nerve. It has sensory, motor, and autonomic components.

  - The *sensory* component of the glossopharyngeal nerve assists in processing taste sensations from the posterior third of the tongue. This component also provides general sensation for the tympanic cavity, ear canal, eustachian tube, faucial pillars, tonsils, soft palate, and pharynx.
  - The *motor* fibers of the glossopharyngeal nerve innervate the stylopharyngeus, a muscle that raises and dilates the pharynx.
  - Experts differ on whether the motor fibers of the glossopharyngeal nerve also innervate the superior pharyngeal constrictor (Newman & Ramadan, 1998; Seikel et al., 2000). According to Zemlin (1998), the glossopharyngeal nerve, along with fibers of the vagus nerve (X), supplies motor fibers to the *pharyngeal plexus,* which innervates the upper pharyngeal constrictor muscles.
  - Lesions of the glossopharyngeal nerve may create difficulty in swallowing, unilateral loss of the gag reflex, and loss of taste and sensation from the posterior third of the tongue.

- *Cranial nerve X, the vagus nerve,* is a mixed nerve containing motor, sensory, and autonomic fibers (see Figure 1.23). It is called a wandering ("vagus") nerve because it extends into the chest and the stomach.

- The *motor* fibers of the vagus nerve supply the digestive system, heart, and lungs.
- The *sensory* fibers convey information from the digestive system, heart, trachea, pharynx, and larynx.
- The *recurrent laryngeal nerve* (RLN), a branch of the vagus nerve, regulates the intrinsic muscles of the larynx, excluding the cricothyroid, which is supplied by the superior laryngeal nerve branch. The RLN may be damaged during thyroid surgery, resulting in total or partial paralysis of the vocal folds.
- The *pharyngeal branch* of the vagus nerve supplies the pharyngeal constrictors. It also supplies all the muscles of the velum except the tensor tympani, which is innervated by the

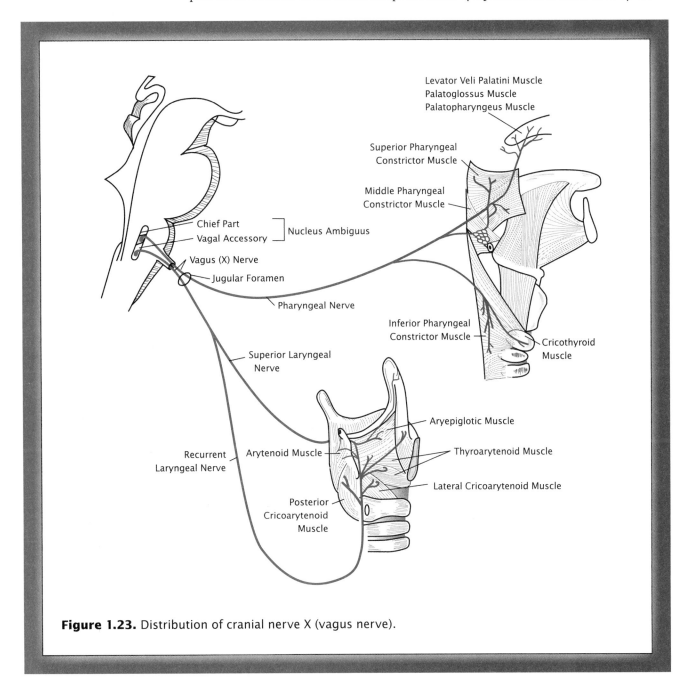

Figure 1.23. Distribution of cranial nerve X (vagus nerve).

trigeminal nerve.

- Damage to the vagus nerve includes a variety of sequelae such as difficulty swallowing, paralysis of the velum, and voice problems if the RLN is damaged.

- *Cranial nerve XI, the spinal accessory nerve,* is a motor nerve (see Figure 1.24). It is both a cranial and spinal nerve because of its cranial and spinal origin.

  - The spinal root supplies the trapezius and sternocleidomastoid muscles, which assist in head and shoulder movements.
  - In concert with the vagus nerve, the cranial fibers of the accessory nerve innervate the uvula and levator veli palatini muscles of the soft palate.
  - Lesions of the spinal accessory nerve may result in neck weakness, paralysis of the sternocleidomastoid, and consequent inability to turn the head, as well as an inability to shrug the shoulders or raise the arm above shoulder level (Zemlin, 1998).

- *Cranial nerve XII, the hypoglossal nerve,* is a motor nerve that runs under the tongue (see Figure 1.25).

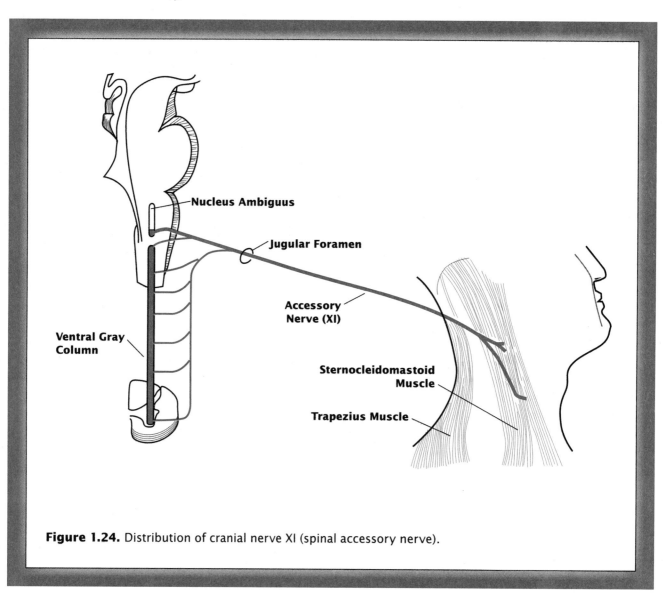

Figure 1.24. Distribution of cranial nerve XI (spinal accessory nerve).

- This nerve supplies three extrinsic tongue muscles: the styloglossus, hyoglossus, and genioglossus.
- The hypoglossal nerve also supplies all the intrinsic muscles of the tongue.
- Lesions to the hypoglossal nerve can result in tongue paralysis, diminished intelligibility, and swallowing problems.

Spinal Nerves

- The spinal nerves of the PNS are closely related to the autonomic nervous system. Together, they control various bodily activities that are executed with little conscious effort or knowledge.
- The spinal nerves can be motor, sensory, or mixed. They transmit motor information from the central nervous system, or CNS, to the muscles, and carry sensory information from peripheral receptors to the CNS.
- Not all the spinal nerves are directly involved with speech production. However, some nerves contribute to speech through innervation of the respiratory musculature. For example, the internal and external intercostals are innervated by the thoracic spinal nerves. The diaphragm is innervated by the motor branches of the C3–C5 spinal nerves (Peña-Brooks & Hegde, 2000).
- There are 31 pairs of spinal nerves. These nerves are attached to the spinal cord through two roots: one is efferent and ventral (toward the front), and the other is afferent and dorsal (toward the back).

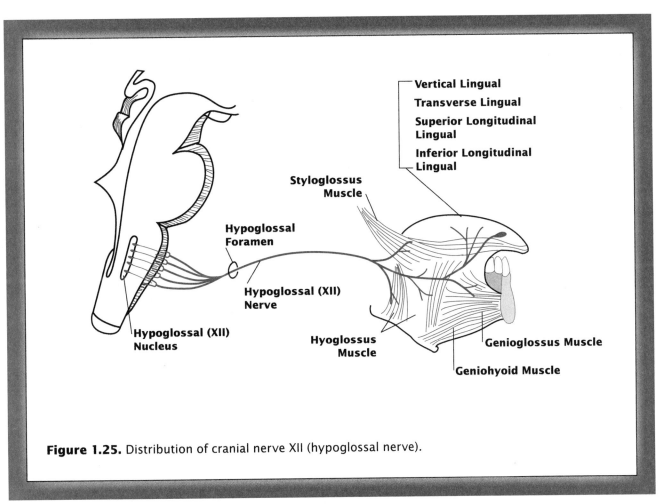

Figure 1.25. Distribution of cranial nerve XII (hypoglossal nerve).

- The 31 pairs of spinal nerves are divided into segments. They are named after the region of the spinal cord to which they are attached (cervical, thoracic, lumbar, sacral, and coccygeal; see Figure 1.26):

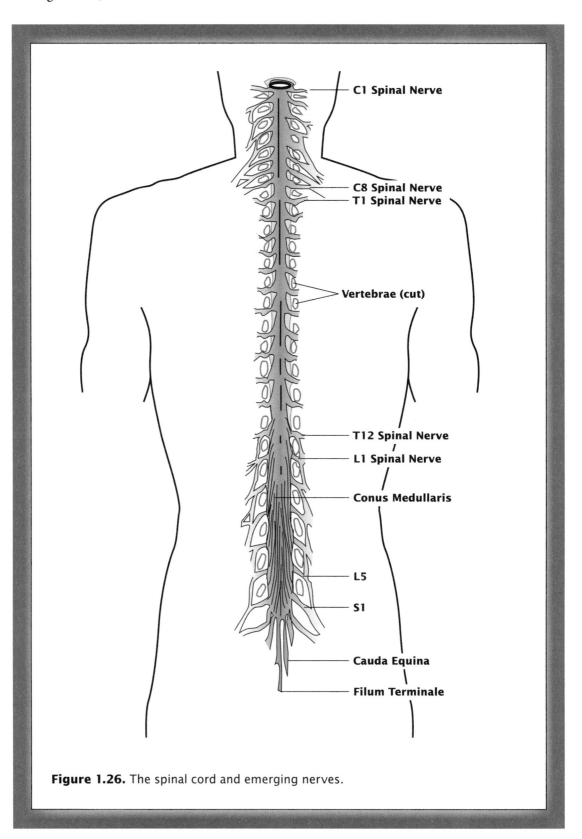

Figure 1.26. The spinal cord and emerging nerves.

C1–C8 = 8 pairs of cervical spinal nerves
T1–T12 = 12 pairs of thoracic spinal nerves
L1–L5 = 5 pairs of lumbar spinal nerves
S1–S5 = 5 pairs of sacral spinal nerves
C1 = 1 pair of coccygeal spinal nerves

- There are several other important spinal cord structures. One is the *conus medullaris,* where the spinal cord ends at the L1 vertebra level. The lowermost nerves are described as the *cauda equina* (horse's tail), which is beneath the *filum terminale,* where there are no spinal cord segments (Seikel et al., 2000).

CONCEPTS TO CONSIDER

Compare the cranial nerves and the spinal nerves. What is the role of each type of nerve in speech and language?

_____
_____
_____
_____
_____

Autonomic Nervous System

- *The autonomic nervous system* (ANS) is generally viewed as part of the peripheral nervous system (Zemlin, 1998). Here, it is artificially presented separately for purposes of simplifying the following information.

- The ANS controls and regulates the internal environment of our bodies; for example, heartbeat is controlled by the ANS. The heartbeat is controlled through the sympathetic and parasympathetic divisions of the ANS, which supply the body's smooth muscles and various glands that secrete hormones.

- The *sympathetic* branch of the ANS mobilizes the body for "fight-or-flight" situations. Activation of the sympathetic branch accelerates the heart rate, dilates the pupils, raises the blood pressure, and increases the blood flow to the peripheral body structures (e.g., the legs, which run from danger). Humans feel emotionally aroused when the sympathetic branch of the ANS is activated.

- The *parasympathetic* branch of the ANS helps bring the body back to a state of relaxation. After the body has mobilized for highly charged situations, the parasympathetic branch lowers blood pressure, slows the heart rate, increases activity within the stomach, and generally relaxes the body. Humans feel relaxed and calm during activation of the parasympathetic branch of the ANS.

- The ANS does not have a direct effect upon speech, language, or hearing. However, the emotionally relaxed and aroused states created by ANS actions may have some effect on various parameters of communication.

- For example, people who stutter may become more dysfluent when the sympathetic branch is aroused. In another example, people who habitually speak too quickly and loudly with consequent trauma to the vocal folds might benefit from the feelings of relaxation provided from activation of the parasympathetic branch.

SUMMARY

✓ The most important part of the peripheral nervous system in relationship to communication is the cranial nerves. Cranial nerves V, VII, VIII, IX, X, XI, and XII are the cranial nerves most directly connected with speech, language, and hearing.

✓ The spinal nerves of the peripheral nervous system control automatic functions such as breathing.

✓ The sympathetic and parasympathetic branches of the autonomic nervous system have an indirect effect on speech when they cause speakers to feel emotionally relaxed or aroused.

THE NERVOUS SYSTEM

Peripheral Nervous System	Central Nervous System
cranial nerves	spinal cord
spinal nerves	brain
autonomic nervous system	
• sympathetic branch	
• parasympathetic branch	

THE CENTRAL NERVOUS SYSTEM

INTRODUCTION

The central nervous system is composed of the spinal cord and the brain. Key structures of the brain include the brain stem, the reticular activating system, the diencephalon, the basal ganglia, the cerebellum, and the cerebrum. Other key structures and systems include the pyramidal and extrapyramidal systems, connecting fibers within the brain, the cerebral ventricles, the protective layers of the brain, and structures that provide the cerebral blood supply. (As noted earlier, the extrapyramidal system is technically not part of the CNS but is included here as it is highly related and interconnected to CNS structures.)

Basic Principles

- The brain gathers information about the environment from the PNS and then sends impulses that lead to actions. The peripheral systems and organs send and receive various kinds of information and possibly demand directions for action.

- The brain acts as a "central station" that coordinates this activity, integrates information, and issues commands.

- The central nervous system is composed of the brain and the spinal cord, as depicted in Figure 1.27. The CNS acts as a *motor command center* for planning, originating, and carrying out the transmission of messages.

- The CNS is enclosed within the vertebral column and the cranial structure. The spinal cord is an elongated structure within the spinal canal of the vertebral columns.

- Pairs of spinal nerves branch out on either side of the vertebral column and reach most parts of the body. The upper portion of the spinal cord is continuous with the lower portion of the brain.

- The brain is the most important structure in the body for language, speech, and hearing. It is housed in and protected by the cranial cavity of the *skull*. The skull is not a single structure, but is made up of separate pieces of bone that eventually become a unified structure.

- Because the brain is so much more related to speech and language than the spinal cord, the rest of this section is devoted to a description of the structures and processes of the brain. Information about the spinal cord is integrated as necessary.

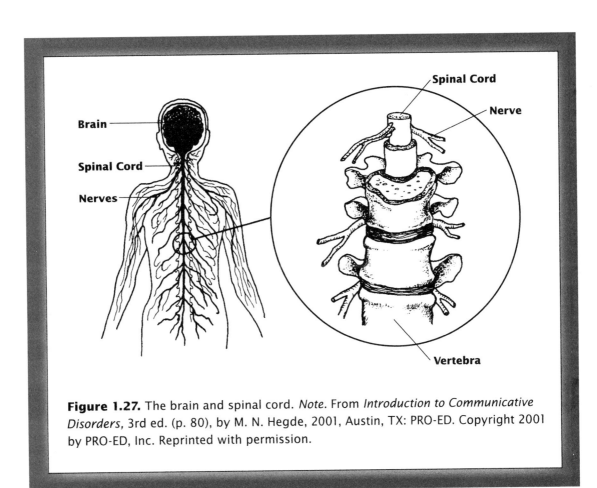

Figure 1.27. The brain and spinal cord. *Note.* From *Introduction to Communicative Disorders,* 3rd ed. (p. 80), by M. N. Hegde, 2001, Austin, TX: PRO-ED. Copyright 2001 by PRO-ED, Inc. Reprinted with permission.

The Brain Stem

■ The *brain stem* is said to be the oldest part of the brain. It connects the spinal cord with the brain via the diencephalon. It also serves as a bridge between the cerebellum and all other CNS structures, including the spinal cord, the thalamus, the basal ganglia, and the cerebrum.

■ Internally, the brain stem consists of *longitudinal fiber tracts, cranial nerve nuclei,* and the *reticular formation.* Outwardly, one sees the key structures of the brain stem as illustrated in Figure 1.28: the midbrain, the pons, and the medulla.

Midbrain

• The *midbrain,* also called the *mesencephalon,* is a narrow structure that lies superior to the pons and inferior to the diencephalon. The midbrain's *superior peduncles* help connect the

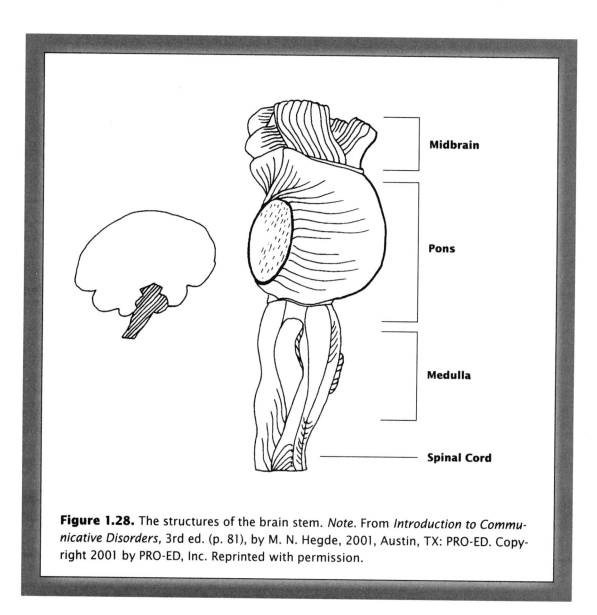

Figure 1.28. The structures of the brain stem. *Note.* From *Introduction to Communicative Disorders,* 3rd ed. (p. 81), by M. N. Hegde, 2001, Austin, TX: PRO-ED. Copyright 2001 by PRO-ED, Inc. Reprinted with permission.

brain stem and the cerebellum. The *substantia nigra* (described later) runs the vertical length of the midbrain at the level of the peduncles.

- The midbrain contains structures that control many motor and sensory functions, including postural reflexes, visual reflexes, eye movements, and coordination of vestibular-generated eye and head movements.
- The midbrain contains the cranial nerve nuclei for the trochlear (IV) and oculomotor (III) nerves. These nerves are not involved in speech production.

Pons

- The *pons*, also called the *metencephalon*, is a roundish, bulging structure that bridges the two halves of the cerebellum. It is located directly inferior to the midbrain.
- The pons and the midbrain together serve as a connection point between the cerebellum and various cerebral structures through the *inferior* and *middle peduncles*. The pons transmits information relative to movement from the cerebral hemispheres to the cerebellum.
- The pons contains many descending motor fibers and is involved with hearing and balance. It also houses the nuclei for the trigeminal (V) and facial (VII) nerves, which are important for speech production.

Medulla

- The *medulla*, also called the *myelencephalon*, is inferior to the midbrain and the pons. It is the uppermost portion of the spinal cord, which enters the cranial cavity through the *foramen magnum* at the base of the skull.
- The medulla contains all the fibers that originate in the cerebellum and cerebrum and move downward to form the spinal cord. It includes several centers that control vital, automatic bodily functions such as breathing, digestion, heart rate, and blood pressure.
- The medulla is very important for speech production because it contains descending fibers that transmit motor information to several cranial nerve nuclei.
- Cranial nerves whose nuclei are housed within the medulla include the vestibulocochlear (VIII), glossopharyngeal (IX), vagus (X), accessory (XI), and hypoglossal (XII) nerves.
- The medulla contains nerve fibers that carry commands from the motor center of the brain to various muscles. These fibers are called *pyramidal tracts*. The pyramidal tracts, described in more detail later, control many movements and supply some of the muscles that are involved in speech.
- At the level of the medulla, many of the pyramidal tracts from the left and right sides of the brains *decussate,* or cross over, to the other side. Thus, the right side of the body is primarily controlled by the left side of the brain and vice versa.

Reticular Activating System

- The *reticular activating system* (RAS) is a structure within the midbrain, brain stem, and upper portion of the spinal cord. It integrates motor impulses flowing out of the brain with sensory impulses flowing into it.

- Thus, the RAS plays a role in the execution of motor activity. It sends diffuse impulses to various regions of the cortex and alerts the cortex to incoming impulses.

- The RAS is the primary mechanism of attention and consciousness. It is important in controlling sleep-wake cycles. It plays a critical role in states of consciousness, in whether a person is asleep, drowsy, alert, or very excited. Generally, the RAS may be viewed as the part of the CNS that responds to incoming information by affecting the state of a person's alertness and consciousness.

Diencephalon

- The *diencephalon* lies above the midbrain and between the brain stem and the cerebral hemispheres. (*Note:* Some experts, such as Zemlin [1998], consider the diencephalon to be part of the brain stem.)

- The diencephalon contains the *third ventricle,* a tall and narrow space filled with cerebrospinal fluid. The diencephalon also contains the thalamus and the hypothalamus.

- The *thalamus* is the largest structure in the diencephalon. It regulates the sensory information that flows into the brain and relays sensory impulses to various portions of the cerebral cortex.

- The thalamus also receives information about motor impulses from the cerebellum and the basal ganglia and relays this information to motor areas of the cerebral cortex.

- The thalamus is critical for maintenance of consciousness and alertness. The exact role of the thalamus in speech and language is unclear.

- The *hypothalamus,* which lies inferior to the thalamus, helps integrate the actions of the ANS. The hypothalamus also controls emotions.

Basal Ganglia

- The *basal ganglia,* illustrated in Figure 1.29, are structures deep within the brain that are located near the thalamus and lateral ventricles. They are primarily composed of gray matter.

- The basal ganglia are a highly complex system of neural pathways that have connections with many subcortical and cortical areas. The basal ganglia receive input primarily from the frontal lobe and relay information back to the higher centers of the brain via the thalamus.

- Experts differ on the exact structure of the basal ganglia, but most agree that they consist of at least three nuclear masses: the globus pallidus, the putamen, and the caudate nucleus. *Corpus striatum* is the collective term for these structures.

- The basal ganglia are part of the extrapyramidal system. The *extrapyramidal system* helps regulate and modify cortically initiated motor movements, including speech. The *substantia nigra,* which is functionally related to (but not a part of) the basal ganglia, is an important part of the extrapyramidal system (Peña-Brooks & Hegde, 2000).

- The extrapyramidal system, described in more detail later, is considered an indirect activation system because motor movements are not directly controlled in the basal ganglia. The extrapyramidal system primarily affects motor movements by communicating with the cerebral cortex via other subcortical structures such as the thalamus.

Caudate Nucleus

Lenticular Nucleus

Figure 1.29. The location of the basal ganglia within the brain. *Note.* From *Introduction to Communicative Disorders,* 3rd ed. (p. 82), by M. N. Hegde, 2001, Austin, TX: PRO-ED. Copyright 2001 by PRO-ED, Inc. Reprinted with permission.

■ Lesions in the basal ganglia can result in unusual body postures, dysarthria (described in Chapter 8), changes in body tone, and involuntary and uncontrolled movements (dyskinesias) that interfere with a person's voluntary attempts to walk, speak, or do many other activities (Freed, 2000).

CONCEPTS TO CONSIDER

Describe one way that the brain stem, the RAS, and the basal ganglia are involved in speech and language functioning.

The Cerebellum

■ The cerebellum, illustrated in Figure 1.30, lies just below the cerebrum and behind the brain stem. Also called the "little brain," the cerebellum consists of two hemispheres (which are different from the cerebral hemispheres).

■ Three primary fiber bundles serve as connections between the brain stem and the cerebellum. These are the *superior, middle,* and *inferior cerebellar peduncles,* which connect with the midbrain, the pons, and the medulla, respectively. All efferent and afferent fibers going to and from the cerebellum pass through these peduncles.

■ Afferent fibers originate from the motor cortex, temporal lobes, cranial nerve VIII, spinal cord, and brain stem. They travel through the middle and inferior cerebellar peduncles and mediate almost all sensorimotor information to the cerebellum.

■ Efferent fibers travel through the superior cerebellar peduncle. These fibers transmit cerebellar outputs to the brain stem and then to the thalamus, motor cortex, and spinal cord.

■ The cerebellum is not a primary motor integration or initiation center. It receives neural impulses from other brain centers and helps coordinate and regulate those impulses. Therefore, it acts as a "modulator" of neuronal activity through its efferent and afferent circuits.

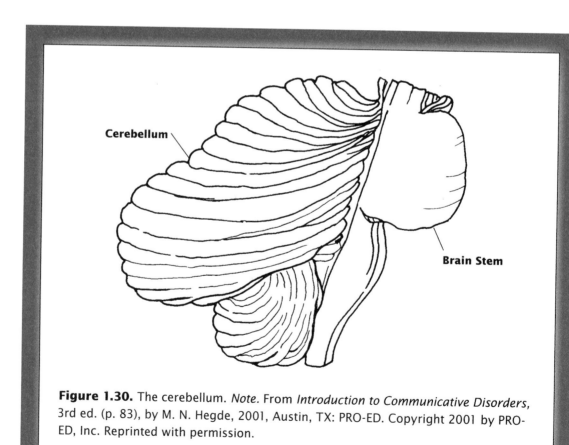

Figure 1.30. The cerebellum. *Note.* From *Introduction to Communicative Disorders,* 3rd ed. (p. 83), by M. N. Hegde, 2001, Austin, TX: PRO-ED. Copyright 2001 by PRO-ED, Inc. Reprinted with permission.

- The cerebellum regulates equilibrium (balance), body posture, and coordinated fine-motor movements. Because these movements are necessary for rapid speech, cerebellar intactness is very important to speech production.

- Damage to the cerebellum results in a neurological disorder called *ataxia,* found in some people with cerebral palsy and in people who have suffered cerebellar damage. These individuals are likely to show abnormal gait, disturbed balance, and a speech disorder called *ataxic dysarthria* (described in Chapter 8). Damage to the cerebellum also creates other problems described in Chapter 8.

The Cerebrum

Basic Facts

- The cerebrum, or *cerebral cortex* (the terms are used interchangeably here), is the biggest and most important CNS structure for language, speech, and hearing. It is a complex structure of intricate neural connections that contains approximately 10–15 billion neurons and weighs about 3 pounds.
- The brain is often referred to as gray matter because the cerebrum has gray cells on top. This differs from the spinal cord and the brain stem, which have gray cells inside.
- The cortex includes the topmost portion of the brain but is actually arranged in six layers. Each layer consists of a different type of cell.
- The surface of the cerebrum appears wrinkled because it is folded to accommodate as much tissue as possible in a small space. Billions of neural cells are packed into this structure and folded into ridges and valleys.
- A *gyrus* is a ridge on the cortex, and the cortex has many gyri (plural). A shallow valley is a *sulcus,* and there are many sulci on the surface of the brain. Deeper valleys are called fissures; there are fewer fissures than sulci. The fissures are the boundaries between the broad divisions of the cerebrum.
- The *longitudinal fissure* courses along the middle of the brain from front to back, and divides the cerebrum into the left and right hemispheres. The *fissure of Rolando,* or *central sulcus,* is a major fissure, which runs laterally, downward, and forward, and arbitrarily divides the anterior from the posterior half of the brain.
- The *Sylvian fissure,* or *lateral cerebral fissure* (sulcus), starts at the inferior portion of the frontal lobe at the base of the brain and moves laterally and upward. The areas of the brain surrounding the Sylvian fissure are especially critical in language, speech, and hearing.
- There are four lobes in the right hemisphere and four lobes in the left hemisphere of the cerebrum. The names of these lobes are based on the cranial bones with which they are in contact, not on function. The four lobes each have their own function, but they work interconnectedly. These cortical lobes are the frontal, parietal, occipital, and temporal lobes. They are illustrated in Figure 1.31.

Frontal Lobe

- The frontal lobe is located on the anterior portion of the cerebrum in front of the central fissure and above the lateral fissure. It makes up approximately one third of the surface area of the cerebrum.
- Intact frontal lobe functioning is critical to the deliberate formation of plans and intentions that dictate a person's conscious behavior. People with damage to the frontal lobe thus have

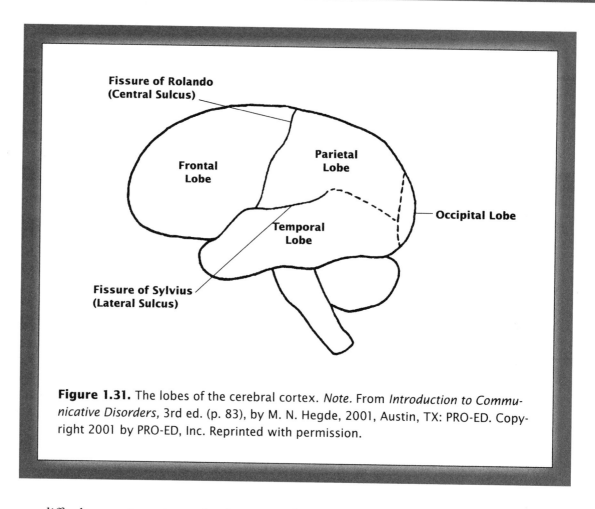

Figure 1.31. The lobes of the cerebral cortex. *Note.* From *Introduction to Communicative Disorders,* 3rd ed. (p. 83), by M. N. Hegde, 2001, Austin, TX: PRO-ED. Copyright 2001 by PRO-ED, Inc. Reprinted with permission.

difficulty carrying out consciously organized activity (Luria, 1973).

- The frontal lobe contains areas that are especially critical to speech production. These include the primary motor cortex containing the precentral gyrus, a supplementary motor cortex, and Broca's area. The major areas pertinent to speech, language, and hearing are illustrated in Figure 1.32.

- The *primary motor cortex,* or *motor strip,* is located on the *precentral gyrus,* a large ridge that lies anterior to the central sulcus. This area controls voluntary movements of skeletal muscles on the opposite side of the body. This demonstrates the neurological principle of *contralateral motor control,* which means that each cerebral hemisphere controls the opposite side of the body.

- All muscles of the body, including those for speech production, are connected to the primary motor cortex through descending motor nerve cells. Figure 1.33 shows regions of the motor cortex that govern motor activation of specific body regions.

- When specific areas of the primary motor cortex are stimulated, corresponding motor responses (e.g., movement of the hand or lip) occur. A large area represents the larynx, jaw, tongue, and lips; this suggests the importance of cortical control of structures involved in speech.

- The motor strip controls muscle movements through a neural pathway called the pyramidal system, mentioned earlier. The motor impulses are modified by the extrapyramidal system with its indirect and complex relay stations (Hegde, 1998).

- The *supplementary motor cortex* of the frontal lobe is believed to be involved in the motor planning of speech. It also plays a secondary role in regulating muscle movements.

- An important motor speech center is *Broca's area,* which is named after the 19th-century

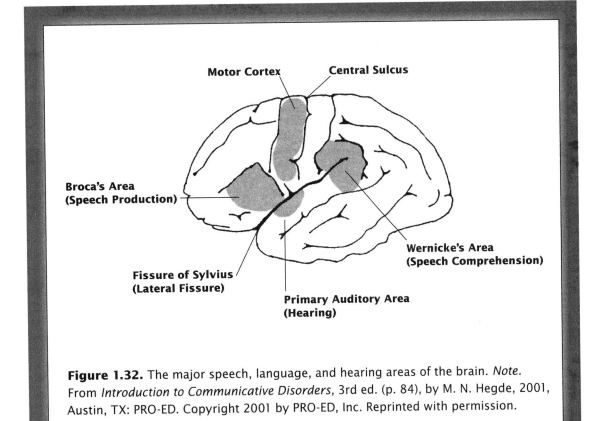

Figure 1.32. The major speech, language, and hearing areas of the brain. *Note.* From *Introduction to Communicative Disorders,* 3rd ed. (p. 84), by M. N. Hegde, 2001, Austin, TX: PRO-ED. Copyright 2001 by PRO-ED, Inc. Reprinted with permission.

French anthropologist and neurosurgeon who "discovered" it during a brain autopsy of a patient with aphasia.

- Broca's area is located in the third convolution of the left cerebral hemisphere. It is anterior to the portion of the primary motor cortex that controls lip, tongue, jaw, and laryngeal movements.
- Broca's area is also called the motor speech area because it controls motor movements involved in speech production. An intact Broca's area is important for production of well-articulated, fluent speech. Lesions in Broca's area cause motor speech problems, which are further described in Chapter 8.

Parietal Lobe

- The parietal lobe is located on the upper sides of the cerebrum behind the frontal lobe and is considered to be the primary somatic sensory area. It integrates contralateral *somesthetic* sensations such as pressure, pain, temperature, and touch.
- The *postcentral gyrus,* also called the *sensory cortex* or *sensory strip,* lies just behind the central sulcus. It is the primary sensory area that integrates and controls somesthetic sensory impulses.
- Two specific areas of the parietal lobe are important for speech and language. These are the areas including and surrounding the supramarginal gyrus and the angular gyrus.
- The *supramarginal gyrus* lies superior to the lateral fissure in the inferior portion of the parietal lobe. Its posterior portion curves around the lateral fissure. Damage to the supramarginal gyrus can cause conduction aphasia (described in Chapter 8) and agraphia, a writing disorder.

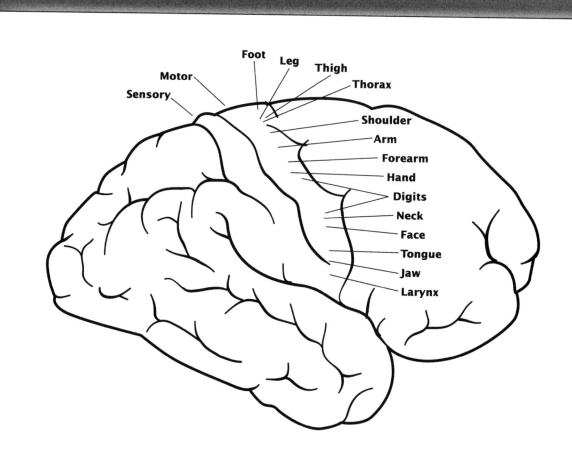

Figure 1.33. The right hemisphere showing regions of the motor cortex that govern motor activation of specific body regions.

- The *angular gyrus* lies posterior to the supramarginal gyrus. Damage to this area can cause writing, reading, and naming difficulties and, in some cases, transcortical sensory aphasia (described in Chapter 8).

Occipital Lobe

- The occipital lobe lies behind the parietal lobe at the lower posterior portion of the head, just above the cerebellum. It is not very relevant to speech and hearing because it is primarily concerned with vision.
- The major structure of the occipital lobe is the *primary visual cortex.* The remainder of the occipital lobe is composed of association visual cortices.

Temporal Lobe

- The temporal lobe is the lowest one third of the cerebrum (see Figure 1.34). It lies inferior to

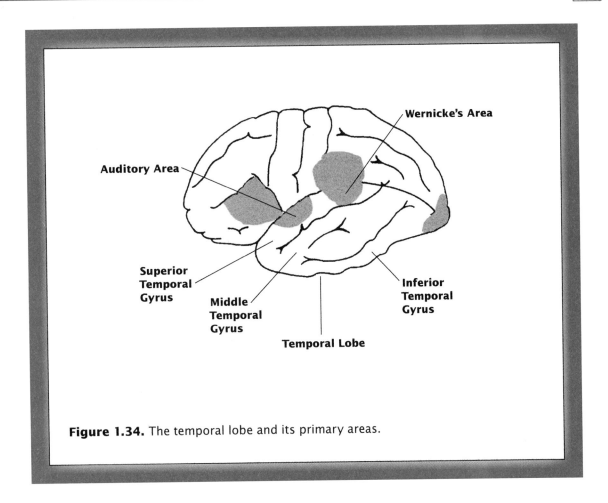

Figure 1.34. The temporal lobe and its primary areas.

the frontal and parietal lobes and in front of the occipital lobe. There are three major gyri in the temporal lobe: the *superior temporal gyrus*, the *middle temporal gyrus*, and the *lower temporal gyrus.*

- The temporal lobe contains two general areas that are critical to adequate hearing and speech. The first critical area is the *primary auditory cortex,* located on the superior temporal gyrus.
- The second critical area, the *auditory association area,* lies posterior to the primary auditory cortex. *Heschl's gyri* is a term sometimes used in reference to the transverse convolutions that make up the auditory association cortex and the primary auditory cortex (Kuehn, Lemme, & Baumgartner, 1989).
- The primary auditory cortex receives sound stimuli from the acoustic nerve (cranial nerve VIII) bilaterally. The auditory association area then synthesizes that information so that it can be recognized as whole units.
- In the dominant hemisphere (left hemisphere for most people), the auditory association area generally analyzes speech sounds so that the person recognizes words and sentences. In the nondominant hemisphere (right hemisphere for most people), the auditory association area generally analyzes nonverbal sound stimuli like environmental noises and music.
- The second critical area within the temporal lobe is *Wernicke's area,* named for Carl Wernicke, a famous neurologist. Wernicke's area is the posterior two thirds of the superior temporal gyrus in the left hemisphere. It is close to the intersection of the parietal, occipital, and temporal lobes.
- Wernicke's area is critical to the comprehension of spoken and written language. It is connected to Broca's area through the arcuate fasciculus (described later in this chapter).
- A lesion in the posterior portion of the superior temporal gyrus causes *Wernicke's aphasia*

(described in Chapter 8), in which the patient demonstrates fluent, meaningless speech and significant language comprehension problems.

> ## CONCEPTS TO CONSIDER
>
> List and briefly describe two important speech- and language-related structures in the frontal lobe and the temporal lobe.
>
> _____
>
> _____
>
> _____
>
> _____
>
> _____

Pyramidal System

Basic Facts

- The *pyramidal system,* as previously stated, is the direct motor activation pathway that is primarily responsible for facilitating voluntary muscle movement (including speech).
- The nerve fiber tract of the pyramidal system comes from the cerebral cortex to the spinal cord and brain stem to ultimately supply the muscles of the head, neck, and limbs. Voluntary movements needed to produce speech are initiated in the primary motor cortex.
- The pyramidal system is composed of the corticobulbar and the corticospinal tracts. Because tracts are bundles of nerve fibers coursing through the CNS, one can imagine the pyramidal system and its two tracts as a group of myelinated nerve fibers carrying crucial neural impulses (Peña-Brooks & Hegde, 2000).
- The projection fibers of both the corticospinal and the corticobulbar tracts originate in the cerebral cortex, and the tracts are part of one unified system. However, these tracts are often discussed separately, if somewhat artificially, for purposes of simplification.

Corticospinal Tract

- The *corticospinal tract* (see Figure 1.35) has nerve fibers that descend from the motor cortex of each hemisphere through the internal capsule. These fibers continue to course vertically through the midbrain and the pons. At the level of the medulla, approximately 80–85% of the fibers decussate.
- The decussated fibers of the corticospinal tract synapse in the anterior horn (motor gray matter) of the spinal cord and communicate with the spinal nerves at different levels. Finally, the spinal nerves exit through the *vertebrae foramina* along the spinal column to innervate the muscles of the limbs and trunk.

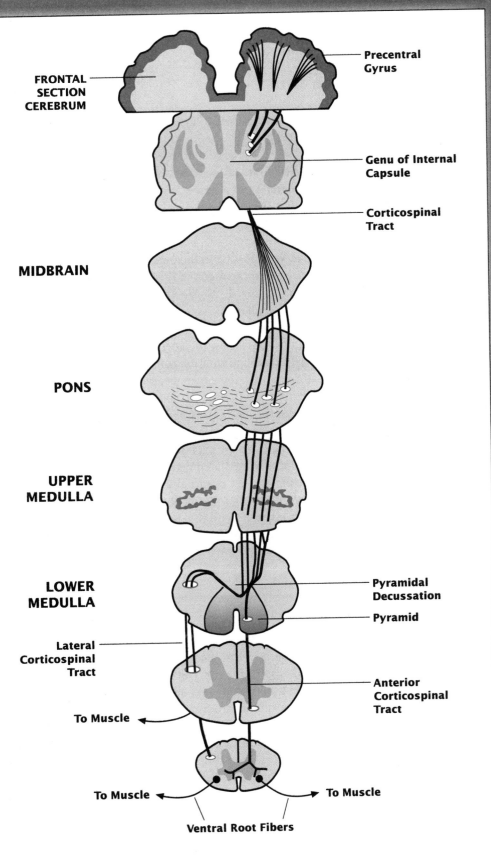

Figure 1.35. The corticospinal pathway as traced from the cerebral cortex to the spinal cord.

- Because of the decussation of fibers at the medullary level, the right side of the body is generally controlled by nerve fibers that originate in the left cerebral cortex, and vice versa. Many stroke patients, for example, have had left-hemisphere strokes and have consequent weakness on the right side of the body.

Corticobulbar Tract

- The *corticobulbar tract* is critical to speech production. The fibers of this tract control all the voluntary movements of the speech muscles (except the respiratory muscles).
- As stated, the fibers of the corticobulbar tract originate in the cerebral cortex—primarily the motor cortex. They course downward vertically through the internal capsule and run along with the corticospinal tract fibers.
- A difference is that the corticobulbar tract fibers terminate in the brain stem at the motor nuclei of cranial nerves III–XII (see Figure 1.36). These fibers then decussate at the level of the brain stem where they terminate. For example, the fibers that terminate at the motor nuclei of the trigeminal nerve decussate in the pons. The fibers that terminate at the motor nuclei of the facial nerve decussate in the medulla (Peña-Brooks & Hegde, 2000).
- The cranial nerves involved in speech exit the skull via small foramina and innervate the muscles of the larynx, pharynx, soft palate, tongue, face, and lips. This innervation allows the muscles to function for production of speech.
- For practical clinical purposes, the corticospinal and corticobulbar tracts are further subdivided into lower and upper motor neurons. This division is clinically helpful in classifying the symptoms associated with lower versus upper motor neuron damage.
- *Lower motor neurons* are the motor neurons in the spinal and cranial nerves. They include nerve fibers that exit the neuraxis (spinal cord or brain) and communicate with the peripheral (cranial and spinal) nerves for innervation of muscles.
- Thus, lower motor neurons are part of the peripheral nervous system and as such are the final route by which centrally mediated neural impulses are communicated to peripheral muscles. Lower motor neuron activity eventually results in muscular movement.
- *Upper motor neurons* are the motor fibers within the central nervous system. Upper motor neurons can be thought of as all the descending motor fibers that course through the central nervous system. As such, upper motor neurons include the pathways of both the pyramidal and the extrapyramidal systems.

Extrapyramidal System

- A general distinction between the pyramidal and the extrapyramidal systems is that the pyramidal system is responsible for carrying the impulses that control voluntary, fine-motor movements. The extrapyramidal system transmits impulses that control the postural support needed by those fine-motor movements (Freed, 2000).

- The extrapyramidal system ("extra" referring to the motor tracts that are not part of the pyramidal system) is important in motor speech production. It is composed of different subcortical nuclei, including the red nucleus, the substantia nigra, the subthalamus, the basal ganglia, and the pathways that connect these structures to one another.

- Whereas the pyramidal system has a direct connection with lower motor neurons, the extrapyramidal system is considered a more indirect activation system that interacts with various motor systems in the nervous system.

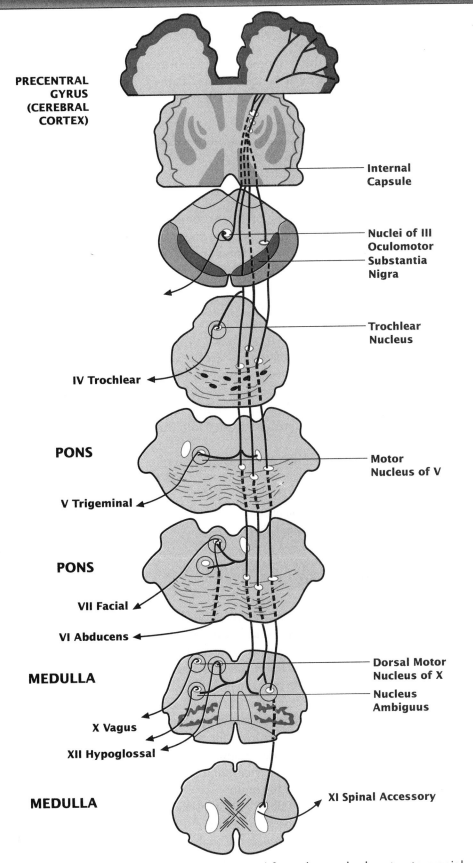

Figure 1.36. The corticobulbar tract as traced from the cerebral cortex to cranial nerve nuclei.

■ The neuronal activity of the extrapyramidal system begins in the cerebral cortex and ultimately influences lower motor neurons. The extrapyramidal system helps maintain posture and tone and helps regulate the movement that results from lower motor neuron activity.

■ Damage to the extrapyramidal system creates motor disturbances that fall under the rubric of "involuntary movement disorders." Patients may show unusual movement patterns of various muscles (including facial muscles) and bizarre postures.

Connecting Fibers in the Brain

■ The structures of the brain are connected with one another through specialized bundles of nerve fibers. These connecting fibers keep information flowing throughout the brain. This alerts various brain structures about sensory stimuli that have been received and actions that are planned and performed.

■ Connecting fibers differ in length. Adjacent areas are connected by shorter fibers; distant areas are connected by longer fibers called *fasciculi* (singular = fasciculus).

■ *Intrahemispheric fibers* allow areas within each hemisphere to communicate with each other. *Interhemispheric fibers* permit communication between hemispheres and are composed mostly of myelinated axonal fibers, or white matter. Interhemispheric fibers form the medullary center of the brain. Depending upon the nature of their connections, the nerve fibers of the medullary center are divided into three types.

■ The three types of connecting fibers are:

- projection fibers
- association fibers
- commissural fibers

Projection Fibers

- *Projection fibers* create connections between the cortex and subcortical structures like the cerebellum, basal ganglia, brain stem, and spinal cord.
- Some fibers transmit motor information to the glands and muscles. Other fibers carry sensory information to the brain. The *internal capsule* contains the concentrated and compact projection fibers near the brain stem.
- The motor projection fibers originate primarily in the premotor and primary motor areas in the frontal lobe. They form the upper motor neuron system of the pyramidal tract, which is the direct activation pathway for voluntary motor movements.
- As projection fibers move upward toward the upper regions of the brain, they fan out in a structure called the *corona radiata*. Through the corona radiata, information is transmitted to other portions of the brain.
- Afferent projection fibers relay sensory information (such as smell) from the peripheral sense organs (e.g., the nose) to the brain. Efferent projection fibers come together in the internal capsule and pass through the thalamus and basal ganglia. These efferent fibers relay motor commands to glands and muscles.

Association Fibers

- *Association fibers* may be long or short; whatever their length, they connect areas within a hemisphere. Association fibers assist in maintaining communication between the structures in a hemisphere.
- The most important of the association fibers is the bundle of *superior longitudinal fibers,* also called *arcuate fasciculus,* that lies just below the surface of the cortex. The arcuate fasciculus arches backward from the lower part of the frontal lobe to the posterior superior part of the temporal lobe.
- The arcuate fasciculus connects Broca's area with Wernicke's area. It is important for verbal memory, language acquisition, and meaningful language production.

Commissural Fibers

- The left and right hemispheres are divided by the medial longitudinal fissure. The *commissural fibers* are interhemispheric connectors; they run horizontally and connect the corresponding areas of the two hemispheres.
- The most important of the commissural fibers, the *corpus callosum,* is a thick, broad band of myelinated fibers that connects the two hemispheres at their base (Nicolosi et al., 2004) (see Figure 1.37).
- Damage to the corpus callosum disconnects the two hemispheres, resulting in *disconnection syndromes* characterized by problems in naming, reading, movement, and other functions.

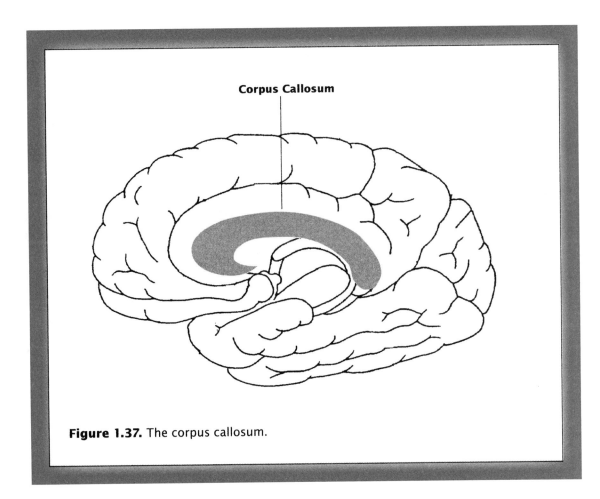

Corpus Callosum

Figure 1.37. The corpus callosum.

The Cerebral Ventricles

■ The term *cerebral ventricles* refers to a system of cavities deep within the brain. These interconnected cavities are filled with cerebrospinal fluid.

■ This fluid is produced by the *choroid plexus,* which is composed of vascular membranous materials. The cerebrospinal fluid circulates throughout the nervous system and nourishes the neural tissues, removes waste products, cushions the brain, and regulates intracranial pressure (Hegde, 1998).

■ There are four cerebral ventricles. The largest of the four ventricles are the two *lateral ventricles* (one in each hemisphere). Located immediately inferior to the corpus callosum, the lateral ventricles are C-shaped and course through the lobes of the cortex.

■ The *third ventricle* is behind the lateral ventricles at the top of the brain stem. It looks like a broad disk and is connected with the lateral ventricles by the *foramen of Munro.*

■ The *fourth ventricle* is located between the cerebellum and the pons. This ventricle is continuous with the central canal of the spinal cord below and the *cerebral aqueduct* above. The cerebral aqueduct connects the fourth and the third ventricles.

Protective Layers of the Brain

■ The spinal cord of the CNS is protected by the vertebral column. The brain is protected by three structures: a layer of skin, skull bones, and layers of tissue called the meninges.

■ The *meninges* contain three layers of membranes that cover the brain and spinal cord (see Figure 1.38):

- The *dura mater* ("tough mother") is the thick, tough, outermost membrane whose one side adheres to the skull and whose other side adheres to the arachnoid.

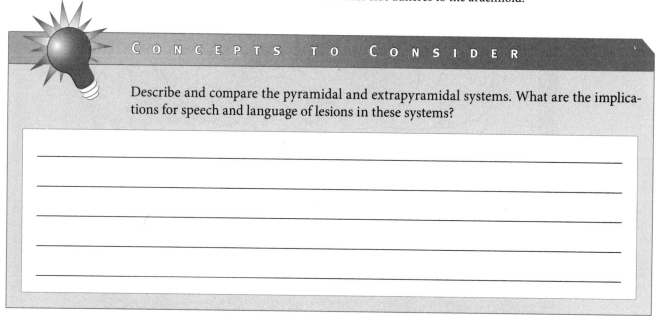

CONCEPTS TO CONSIDER

Describe and compare the pyramidal and extrapyramidal systems. What are the implications for speech and language of lesions in these systems?

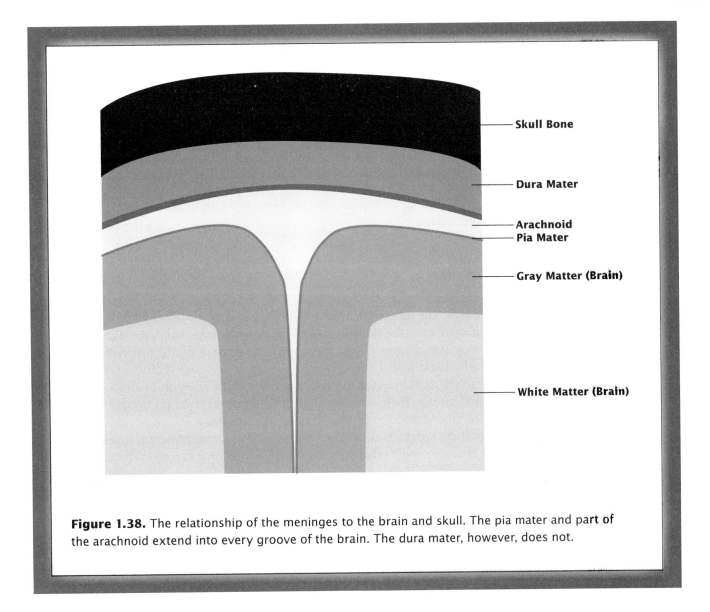

- Skull Bone
- Dura Mater
- Arachnoid
- Pia Mater
- Gray Matter (Brain)
- White Matter (Brain)

Figure 1.38. The relationship of the meninges to the brain and skull. The pia mater and part of the arachnoid extend into every groove of the brain. The dura mater, however, does not.

- The *arachnoid* ("spider web") is the semitransparent, thin, vascular, delicate, and weblike middle membrane; cerebrospinal fluid fills the subarachnoid space between the arachnoid and the pia mater.
- The *pia mater* ("tender mother") is the delicate, thin, transparent membrane that adheres to the brain surface and closely follows its gyri and sulci; many blood vessels penetrate the pia mater to enter the brain.

Cerebral Blood Supply

- The brain makes up approximately 2% of the body's weight; however, it consumes 25% of the body's oxygen and requires 20% of the body's blood.

- The wonderfully complex and intricate brain is a highly vulnerable structure. If its blood supply is interrupted, consciousness may be lost within 10 seconds, electrical activity ceases after 20 seconds, and the brain is permanently damaged within 4–6 minutes.

- The blood supplies oxygen and other nutrients required by the brain. The major structures that supply blood to the brain are the aorta, the vertebral arteries, the carotid arteries, and the circle of Willis.

Aorta

- The *aorta* is the main artery of the heart. It carries blood from the left ventricle to all parts of the body except the lungs.
- Just above the heart, the aortic arch divides into four branches. These branches are the two carotid arteries and the two subclavian arteries. Figure 1.39 illustrates the major vascular supply of the cerebral cortex.

Vertebral Arteries

- The right and left *vertebral arteries* branch out from the two subclavian arteries that emerge from the aortic arch. The subclavian arteries supply primarily the upper extremities.
- The vertebral arteries enter the skull and then branch out to supply the spinal cord and many organs of the body. As they move up to the lower level of the pons, the two vertebral arteries join to form the *basilar artery*.
- As the basilar artery moves toward the upper portion of the pons, it divides again into two *posterior cerebral arteries*. These arteries supply the lateral and lower portions of the temporal lobes and the lateral and middle portions of the occipital lobes.
- Several other branches of the basilar artery, such as the anterior, posterior, superior, and inferior cerebellar arteries, supply other structures such as the inner ear, cerebellum, and pons.

Carotid Arteries

- As the left and right *carotid arteries* (one on each side of the neck) enter the neck, each branches out into an internal carotid artery and an external carotid artery. The arteries enter the brain through the base of the skull and go through the dura mater and subarachnoid space.
- The *external carotid artery* moves toward the face and branches into smaller arteries. It supplies blood to the muscles of the mouth, nose, forehead, and face.
- The *internal carotid artery* is the major supplier of blood to the brain. This artery branches into several smaller blood vessels that supply different parts of the brain. Two key branches of the internal carotid artery are the middle cerebral artery and the anterior cerebral artery.
- The *middle cerebral artery* is the biggest branch of the internal carotid artery, and it supplies the entire lateral surface of the cortex, including the major regions of the frontal lobe.
- The middle cerebral artery supplies blood to major areas involved with motor and sensory functions and language, speech, and hearing functions.
- The areas supplied by the middle cerebral artery include the motor cortex in the precentral gyrus, Broca's area, the primary auditory cortex, Wernicke's area, the supramarginal gyrus, the angular gyrus, and the somatosensory cortex.
- Damage to the middle cerebral artery may result in strokes, aphasia, reading and writing deficits, contralateral hemiplegia, and an impaired sense of pain, temperature, touch, and position.
- The *anterior cerebral artery* supplies primarily the middle portion of the parietal and frontal lobes. It also supplies blood to the corpus callosum and basal ganglia. Branches of the anterior cerebral artery join with the posterior cerebral artery in the posterior medial areas of the brain.

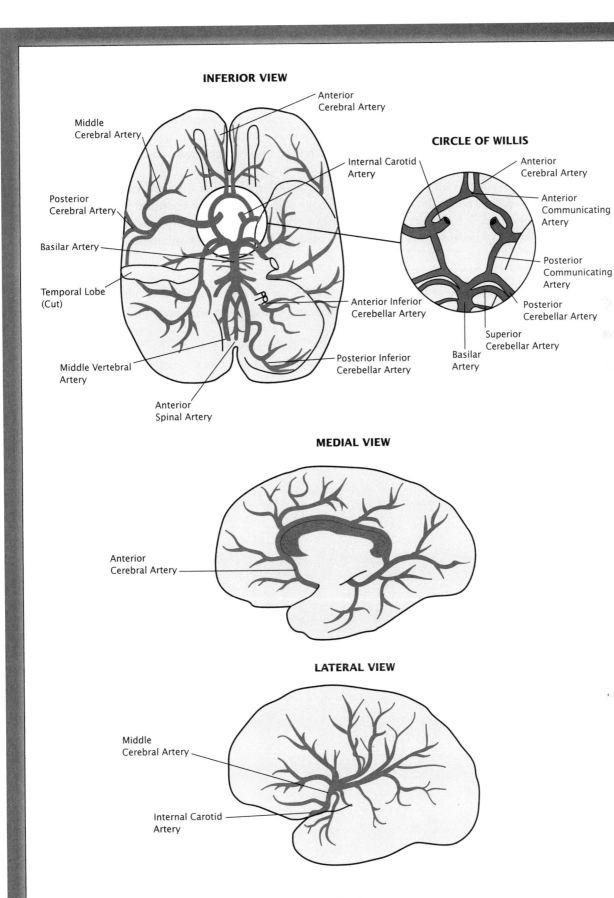

INFERIOR VIEW

Anterior
Cerebral Artery

Middle
Cerebral Artery

Internal Carotid
Artery

Posterior
Cerebral Artery

Basilar Artery

Temporal Lobe
(Cut)

Anterior Inferior
Cerebellar Artery

Middle Vertebral
Artery

Posterior Inferior
Cerebellar Artery

Anterior
Spinal Artery

CIRCLE OF WILLIS

Anterior
Cerebral Artery

Anterior
Communicating
Artery

Posterior
Communicating
Artery

Posterior
Cerebellar Artery

Superior
Cerebellar Artery

Basilar
Artery

MEDIAL VIEW

Anterior
Cerebral Artery

LATERAL VIEW

Middle
Cerebral Artery

Internal Carotid
Artery

Figure 1.39. The major vascular supply of the cerebral cortex.

- Damage to the anterior cerebral artery can cause cognitive deficits such as impaired judgment, concentration, and reasoning. Damage can also cause paralysis of the feet and legs.

Circle of Willis

- The *circle of Willis (circulus arteriosus)* is formed at the base of the brain where the two carotid and the two vertebral arteries join. The circle is completed by the anterior and posterior communicating arteries. The posterior cerebral, anterior cerebral, and middle cerebral arteries branch out from the circle of Willis.
- The circle of Willis provides a common blood supply to various cerebral branches. If an artery is blocked above the circle, brain damage will occur because the brain has no alternate source of blood. If an artery is blocked below the circle of Willis, however, brain damage may be minimal because alternate channels of blood flow may be maintained.

SUMMARY

✓ The central nervous system, composed of the brain and the spinal cord, is a complex and intricate system that depends upon the intact functioning of and interconnections between many structures.

✓ These structures include the brain stem, the reticular activating system, the diencephalon, the basal ganglia, the cerebellum, and the cerebrum with its frontal, parietal, occipital, and temporal lobes.

✓ The pyramidal and extrapyramidal systems are concerned with movement. Projection, association, and commissural fibers connect key brain structures.

✓ Other critical components of the brain include the cerebral ventricles, meninges, and various arteries that supply blood to the brain and its structures.

◆ **RESPIRATION, OR BREATHING, CONSISTS** of a rhythmic cycle of inhalation and exhalation. Respiration provides the energy for voicing and ultimately for speech. The process of respiration relies upon the integrity of many structures. These include the lungs, bronchi, trachea, spinal column, sternum, rib cage, and muscles of inspiration and expiration.

◆ **VOICE IS USUALLY PRODUCED** as exhaled air comes from the lungs through the trachea to the larynx. The larynx houses the vocal folds, which vibrate to produce voice. Optimal voicing relies upon key laryngeal cartilages and structures as well as the functioning of the intrinsic and extrinsic laryngeal muscles. The myoelastic–aerodynamic theory helps explain the physiology of phonation. Cranial nerves VII (facial nerve) and X (vagus nerve) are key in the phonation process.

◆ **THE VOCAL FOLDS VIBRATE** to produce voice, and the voice travels upward to be modified or resonated by the pharynx and the oral and nasal cavities. English sounds have primarily oral or nasal resonance. The source-filter theory explains how speech sounds are ultimately produced through modification of the oral cavity and adjacent structures.

◆ **ARTICULATION FOR SPEECH INVOLVES** movements that produce particular sounds. Key structures for articulation in the oral cavity include the pharynx, soft palate, hard palate, mandible, teeth, tongue, lips, and cheeks. Cranial nerves primarily responsible for innervation of articulatory structures include V (trigeminal nerve), VII (facial nerve), IX (glossopharyngeal nerve), X (vagus nerve), XI (spinal accessory nerve), and XII (hypoglossal nerve).

◆ **THE NERVOUS SYSTEM, COMPOSED** of neurons and other specialized cells, can be divided into two basic parts: the peripheral and central nervous systems. The peripheral nervous system is composed of the spinal nerves and the cranial nerves. Cranial nerves most critical to speech, language, and hearing include trigeminal nerve V, facial nerve VII, vestibulocochlear nerve VIII, glossopharyngeal nerve IX, vagus nerve X, spinal accessory nerve XI, and hypoglossal nerve XII.

◆ **THE CENTRAL NERVOUS SYSTEM** is composed of the brain and the spinal cord. The brain contains many structures, including the brain stem, reticular activating system, diencephalon, basal ganglia, cerebellum, and cerebrum. The brain stem, composed of the midbrain, pons, and medulla, connects the spinal cord with the brain via the diencephalon.

CHAPTER HIGHLIGHTS

◆ **THE CEREBELLUM HELPS COORDINATE** and regulate neural impulses going to and from the brain. It regulates equilibrium, body posture, and coordinated fine-motor movements. An intact cerebellum is critical to speech production, and people with cerebellar damage may show ataxia and dysarthria.

◆ **THE CEREBRUM, OR CEREBRAL** cortex, has four lobes: the occipital, frontal, parietal, and temporal lobes. The occipital lobe is primarily concerned with vision. The frontal lobe contains motor areas, such as Broca's area, that are critical to speech production. The parietal lobe, which integrates sensations such as pain, temperature, and touch, contains the angular gyrus and the supramarginal gyrus, which are critical to speech. The temporal lobe contains the key structures of the primary auditory cortex, the auditory association area, and Wernicke's area.

◆ **THE PYRAMIDAL AND EXTRAPYRAMIDAL** systems are involved in motor movement. The pyramidal system, consisting of the corticospinal and corticobulbar tracts, is primarily responsible for facilitating voluntary movements of muscles, including speech muscles. The extrapyramidal system is a more indirect activation system, which helps maintain posture and tone as well as regulating movement.

◆ **IMPORTANT CONNECTING FIBERS IN** the brain include projection fibers, association fibers, and commissural fibers. The corpus callosum, a critical commissural fiber, connects the two hemispheres. Other important brain structures include the cerebral ventricles, meninges, and structures that supply blood to the brain.

✎ **ADD YOUR OWN CHAPTER HIGHLIGHTS HERE:**

_____

_____

_____

_____

_____

Study & Review Questions

Essay

1. Describe the myoelastic–aerodynamic theory of phonation.

2. What are the key anatomical structures involved in respiration? How do they relate to one another?

3. What are the major cranial nerves involved in articulation? How are they involved?

4. Briefly describe the functions of the cerebellum and the cerebrum.

5. Describe how blood is supplied to the brain. What are some key structures involved?

Multiple Choice

6. Respiration relies on the muscles of inspiration and expiration. The thick, dome-shaped muscle that separates the abdomen from the thorax is called the:

   A. sternocleidomastoid.
   B. levator costarum longis.
   C. serratus posterior superior.
   D. pectoralis major.
   E. diaphragm.

7. Most pharyngeal muscles are innervated by cranial nerves:

   A. V, VII
   B. XI, XII
   C. X, XI
   D. IX, X
   E. VIII, X

8. The primary muscle of the lips is the:

   A. orbicularis oris.
   B. buccinator.
   C. risorius.
   D. levator labii superioris.
   E. zygomatic major.

9. The neurons that transmit information away from the brain are called:

   A. afferent neurons.
   B. efferent neurons.
   C. primary neurons.
   D. secondary neurons.
   E. peripheral neurons.

10. An important structure adjacent to the brainstem that contains the hypothalamus (which controls emotions) and the thalamus (which relays sensory impulses to various portions of the cerebral cortex) is called the:

A. mesencephalon.
B. diencephalon.
C. inferior cerebellar peduncle.
D. superior cerebellar peduncle.
E. postcentral gyrus.

11. The corpus striatum is composed of three nuclear masses, which are the:

A. globus pallidus, caudate nucleus, and putamen.
B. putamen, caudate nucleus, and basal ganglia.
C. supramarginal gyrus, angular gyrus, and putamen.
D. substantia nigra, angular gyrus, and globus pallidus.
E. metencephalon, reticular activating system, and caudate nucleus.

12. The structure that regulates body posture, equilibrium, and coordinated fine-motor movements is the:

A. angular gyrus.
B. corticospinal tract.
C. circle of Willis.
D. cerebellum.
E. supramarginal gyrus.

13. The anterior cerebral artery supplies blood to the:

A. corpus callosum and basal ganglia.
B. corpus striatum.
C. caudate nucleus and globus pallidus.
D. substantia nigra.
E. lateral surface of the cortex.

14. The laryngopharynx and the oropharynx add resonance to sounds produced by the larynx. The nasopharynx adds noticeable resonance to which sounds?

A. k, g, t, d
B. r, l, y
C. f, sh, s
D. m, n, ng
E. w, y, r

15. These are composed of a ring of connective tissue and muscle extending from the tips of the arytenoid cartilages to the larynx. They separate the laryngeal vestibule from the pharynx and help preserve the airway.

A. ventricular folds
B. true vocal folds
C. lamina propria
D. infrahyoids
E. aryepiglottic folds

16. The cranial nerve that innervates the larynx and also innervates the levator veli palatini, palatoglossus, and palatopharyngeus muscles is:

A. cranial nerve X, the vagus nerve.
B. cranial nerve V, the trigeminal nerve.
C. cranial nerve XI, the spinal accessory nerve.
D. cranial nerve VII, the facial nerve.
E. cranial nerve XII, the hypoglossal nerve.

17. Muscles that contribute to velopharyngeal closure through tensing or elevating the velum are the:

A.   tensor veli palatini, levator veli palatini, and salpingopharyngeus.
B.   stylopharyngeus, salpingopharyngeus, and levator veli palatini.
C.   levator veli palatini, genioglossus, and salpingopharyngeus.
D.   palatoglossus, tensor veli palatini, and levator veli palatini.
E.   tensor veli palatini and levator veli palatini.

18. The structure at the inferior portion of the tongue that connects the tongue with the mandible is called the:

A.   dorsum.
B.   root.
C.   blade.
D.   tip.
E.   lingual frenum.

19. When a person is producing voiced and voiceless /th/, the muscle that is most involved is the:

A.   palatopharyngeus.
B.   sternocleidomastoid.
C.   genioglossus.
D.   styloglossus.
E.   buccinator.

20. When a person is adducting and abducting the vocal folds, which muscles from the list below are the most involved with that process?

I. thyroarytenoids
II. digastrics
III. lateral cricoarytenoids
IV. transverse arytenoids
V. sternothyroids

A.   I, III, V
B.   II, III, IV
C.   I, IV, V
D.   I, III, IV
E.   II, III, IV, V

21. The cerebral hemispheres are connected by:

A.   projection fibers.
B.   association fibers.
C.   commissural fibers.
D.   cerebrocortical fibers.
E.   extrapyramidal fibers.

22. The central nervous system's primary mechanism of attention, alertness, and consciousness, which is also related to sleep-wake cycles, is the:

A.   diencephalon.
B.   mesencephalon.
C.   reticular activating system.
D.   corticobulbar tract.
E.   circle of Willis.

23. The primary motor cortex in the frontal lobe is located on the:

A.   precentral gyrus.
B.   homunculus.
C.   supramarginal gyrus.
D.   angular gyrus.
E.   middle temporal gyrus.

24. Which one of the following is FALSE?

    A. Wernicke's area in the temporal lobe is critical to the comprehension of spoken language.

    B. Wernicke's area is connected to Broca's area in the frontal lobe through the arcuate fasciculus.

    C. The occipital lobe contains the primary visual cortex.

    D. The angular gyrus in the occipital lobe is important for interpretation of somesthetic sensations such as pain, touch, and temperature.

    E. The pyramidal system consists of the corticospinal and corticobulbar tracts.

25. Which of the following are TRUE?

    I. The cerebral ventricles are interconnected cavities filled with fluid produced by the dura mater.

    II. The meninges of the brain consist of the dura mater, the pia mater, and the arachnoid.

    III. The basilar artery eventually divides into the two posterior cerebral arteries.

    IV. The external carotid artery is the major supplier of blood to the brain.

    V. The circle of Willis is formed at the base of the brain where the two carotid and two vertebral arteries join.

    A. II, III, IV, V   D. II, IV, V

    B. All Of The Above   E. II, III, V

    C. I, III, IV

REFERENCES AND RECOMMENDED READINGS

Davenport, P., & Sapienza, C. M. (2004). Pulmonary function and breathing for speech. In C. M. Sapienza & J. Casper (Eds.), *Vocal rehabilitation for medical speech–language pathology* (pp. 331-364). Austin, TX: PRO-ED.

Freed, D. B. (2000). *Motor speech disorders: Diagnosis and treatment.* San Diego: Delmar/Singular Publishing Group.

Hegde, M. N. (1998). *A coursebook on aphasia and other neurogenic language disorders* (2nd ed.). San Diego, CA: Delmar/Singular Publishing Group.

Hegde, M. N. (2001). *Introduction to communicative disorders* (3rd ed.). Austin, TX: PRO-ED.

Kent, R. (1997). *The speech sciences.* San Diego, CA: Singular Publishing Group.

Kuehn, D. P., Lemme, M. L., & Baumgartner, J. M. (Eds.). (1989). *Neural bases of speech, hearing, and language.* Austin, TX: PRO-ED.

Luria, A. R. (1973). *The working brain: An introduction to neuropsychology.* New York: Basic Books.

Newman, D., & Ramadan, N. (1998). Neurologic disorders: An orientation and overview. In A. F. Johnson & B. H. Jacobson (Eds.), *Medical speech–language pathology: A practitioner's guide* (pp. 211–242). New York: Thieme.

Nicolosi, L., Harryman, E., & Kresheck, J. (2004). *Terminology of communication disorders: Speech-language-hearing* (5th ed.). Baltimore: Lippincott Williams & Wilkins.

Peña-Brooks, A., & Hegde, M. N. (2000). *Articulatory and phonological disorders in children: A dual level text.* Austin, TX: PRO-ED.

Seikel, J. A., King, D. W., & Drumright, D. G. (2000). *Anatomy and physiology for speech, language, and hearing* (2nd ed.). San Diego, CA: Singular/Thomson.

Zemlin, W. R. (1998). *Speech and hearing science: Anatomy and physiology* (4th ed.). Needham Heights, MA: Allyn & Bacon.

Study & Review
Answers

6. E. The thick, dome-shaped muscle that separates the abdomen from the thorax is called the diaphragm.

7. C. Most pharyngeal muscles are innervated by cranial nerves X, XI.

8. A. The primary muscle of the lips is the orbicularis oris.

9. B. The type of neurons that transmit information away from the brain are called efferent neurons.

10. B. An important structure adjacent to the brainstem that contains the hypothalamus (which controls emotions) and the thalamus (which relays sensory impulses to various portions of the cerebral cortex) is called the diencephalon.

11. A. The corpus striatum is composed of three nuclear masses, which are the globus pallidus, caudate nucleus, and putamen.

12. D. The structure that regulates body posture, equilibrium, and coordinated fine-motor movements is the cerebellum.

13. A. The anterior cerebral artery supplies blood to the corpus callosum and the basal ganglia.

14. D. The laryngopharynx and the oropharynx add resonance to sounds produced by the larynx. The nasopharynx adds noticeable resonance to /m/, /n/, /ng/.

15. E. The aryepiglottic folds are composed of a ring of connective tissue and muscle extending from the tips of the arytenoid cartilages to the larynx. They separate the laryngeal vestibule from the pharynx and help preserve the airway.

16. A. The cranial nerve that innervates the larynx and also innervates the levator veli palatini, palatoglossus, and palatopharyngeus muscles is cranial nerve X, the vagus nerve.

17. D. Muscles that contribute to velopharyngeal closure through tensing or elevating the velum are the palatoglossus, tensor veli palatini, and levator veli palatini.

18. E. The structure at the inferior portion of the tongue that connects the tongue with the mandible is called the lingual frenum.

19. C. When a person is producing voiced and voiceless /th/, the muscle that is most involved is the genioglossus.

20. D. When a person is adducting and abducting the vocal folds, the muscles most involved with this process are the thyroarytenoids, lateral cricoarytenoids, and transverse arytenoids.

21. C. The cerebral hemispheres are connected by the commissural fibers.

22. C. The central nervous system's primary mechanism of attention, alertness, and consciousness, which is also related to sleep-wake cycles, is the reticular activating system.

23. A. The primary motor cortex in the frontal lobe is located on the precentral gyrus.

24. D. The angular gyrus is in the parietal lobe.

25. E. The meninges of the brain consist of the dura mater, the pia mater, and the arachnoid; the basilar artery eventually divides into the two posterior cerebral arteries; and the circle of Willis is formed at the base of the brain where the two carotid and two vertebral arteries join.

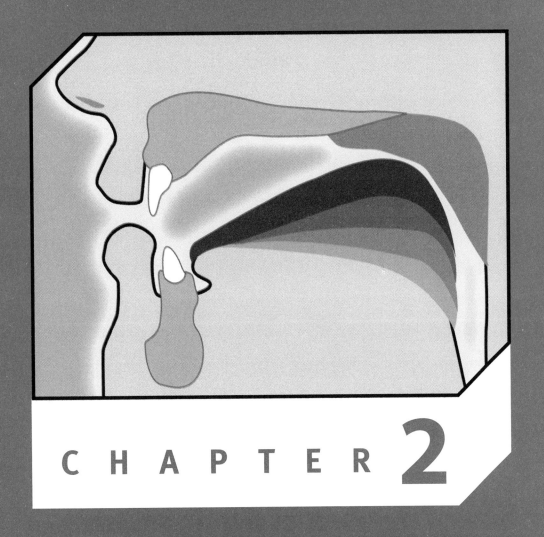

CHAPTER 2

PHYSIOLOGICAL AND

ACOUSTIC PHONETICS:

A SPEECH SCIENCE

FOUNDATION

Speech science is a broad term that includes

several specific fields of study; all are concerned with the study of speech production at both the acoustic and physiologic levels. Speech science provides the foundation for analyzing normal and disordered speech production. Speech sounds can be very broadly categorized into two key areas: production and perception. The *production* of sounds is generally concerned with articulatory physiology; that is, how sounds are produced. The *perception* of sounds is generally concerned with the relationship between sound production and the acoustic signal of speech. *Phonetics*, a branch of speech science, is the study of speech sounds, their production and perception in terms of their articulatory and physical characteristics (Kent, 1998; Kent & Read, 2002; Yavas, 1998). Because much research effort in the speech sciences relates to issues in phonetics, phonetics is a central aspect of speech science (Kent, 1998). Thus, in this chapter, we integrate information in phonetics and speech science by describing *physiological phonetics,* which focuses on speech sound production, and *acoustic phonetics,* which focuses on the acoustic properties of sound waves that result when sounds are produced (Speaks, 1999). Our discussion focuses on the production and perception of Standard American English.

BASIC PRINCIPLES AND DEFINITIONS

INTRODUCTION

Linguists describe language as a system with organized components. *Phonetics,* the study of speech sounds, organizes these sounds into systematic categories according to their perception and production. Speakers of any language need adequate respiration, phonation, resonation, and articulation to produce sounds for speech.

Definitions

■ Linguistically, *language* is a code or system of symbols used to express concepts formed through exposure and experience (Bloom & Lahey, 1978). Behaviorally, language (as well as speech) is verbal behavior. *Speech* is the production of language.

■ *Phonology* is the scientific study of the sound systems and patterns used to create the sounds and words of a language.

■ *Phonemes* are the smallest units of sound that can affect meaning. For example, *man* and *fan* mean different things because of the different initial phonemes /m/ and /f/. Phonemes are families of sounds; the listener perceives members of a family as belonging to the same phoneme. Phonemes are represented by other families or categories of sounds called allophones (Lowe, 1994).

■ *Allophones* are variations of phonemes. Allophones do not change word meanings, and listeners do not perceive them as different from one another. The individual sound /r/ is a phoneme, but it sounds slightly different when it is produced differently by different speakers in different contexts.

■ For instance, the /r/ in *green* would be produced with more tongue retraction than the /r/ in *red*, which would be produced slightly more toward the front of the mouth. A speaker from New York would produce /r/ differently than a speaker from California. These different productions are allophonic variations of the /r/ phoneme.

■ The term *phonemic* refers to the abstract system of sounds; for example, the idealized and abstract description of /s/ is phonemic. Slash marks indicate phonemic representation of a sound, or a general and abstract class of sounds.

■ The term *phonetic* refers to concrete productions of specific sounds. Phonetic productions are enclosed in square brackets [ ], indicating specific sound productions by given speakers.

■ The term *phonetics* is derived from the word phone. A *phone* may or may not be a speech sound; the term refers generically to any sound that can be produced by the vocal tract (Edwards, 2003). Usually, a phone is a single speech sound. *Phonetics* is the study of speech sounds.

■ Researchers have divided phonetics into different categories. A synthesis of these categories follows (Borden, Harris, & Raphael, 2003; Edwards, 2003; Kent, 1998; Kent & Reed, 2002; Yavas, 1998):

  ▪ *Acoustic phonetics* examines the relationship between articulation and the acoustic signal of speech. The concern is the acoustic properties of sound waves (e.g., periodicity and aperiodicity).
  ▪ *Auditory phonetics* is the study of hearing, perception, and the brain's processing of speech.
  ▪ *Articulatory* or *physiological phonetics* is the study of speech sound production; emphasis is on how the articulators produce individual sounds.
  ▪ *Applied phonetics* is the study of the practical application of research in articulatory, perceptual, acoustic, and experimental phonetics.

- *Experimental phonetics* involves the use of objective laboratory techniques to scientifically analyze speech sounds.
- *Descriptive phonetics* refers to the study and explanation of the unique sound properties of various dialects and languages.

Anatomy and Physiology: A Brief Review

■ To produce sounds intelligibly, the speaker needs adequate respiration, phonation, articulation, and resonation. These processes work together synergistically. See Chapter 1 for details.

Respiration

- The respiratory system consists of the lungs, diaphragm, rib cage, airway, and related structures.
- Inhalation and exhalation are necessary components of breathing for speech. They create the rhythmic cycle of respiration. The process of respiration supplies the air necessary for speech production.

Phonation

- As air travels upward from the lungs and through the airway, it reaches the vocal folds housed within the larynx.
- Vocal fold vibrations create phonation, which is necessary for all voiced sounds (described in more detail later). Sounds cannot be properly voiced without adequate phonation.

Resonation

- The air continues to travel upward past the level of the vocal folds and enters cavities above the larynx. In these nasal, pharyngeal, and oral cavities, the air is modified. *Resonance* is the modification of sound by structures or cavities through which the sound passes.
- Resonating bodies do not produce sound; rather, they modify sound produced by another source (e.g., the vocal folds).

Articulation

- *Articulation* is the production of speech sounds.
- The articulators, or primary structures involved in the process of articulation, are the lips, mandible, pharynx, velum, hard palate, tongue, and teeth.

SUMMARY

✓ Every language has a system of sounds that are used to create words in that language. Phonetics is the study of speech sounds.

✓ When speakers produce speech sounds, they need adequate respiration, phonation, resonation, and articulation.

✓ Phonetics can be divided into six specific categories; in this chapter, we focus on physiological and acoustic phonetics.

PHONETIC TRANSCRIPTION

INTRODUCTION

Recording the sounds of the language as spoken by its people has always been a challenge for linguists and phoneticians. Many languages have written symbols for their sounds. A problem for many languages, including English, is that the same sound can be written, or spelled, in many different ways. To deal with this challenge and to provide consistency across languages, the International Phonetic Alphabet was developed. In this section, we describe this alphabet and its broad and narrow symbols.

The International Phonetic Alphabet

- The International Phonetic Alphabet (IPA) was developed to deal with the challenges of *orthographic symbols,* or written representations of sounds. Different orthographic symbols can be used to denote the same sound. For example, the letters *ough* are pronounced differently in the words *through, tough, bough, trough,* and *though.*

- Developed in 1888, the IPA is used internationally today. It was most recently revised in 1989. The IPA provides a set of phonetic symbols that represents sounds accurately and consistently.

CONCEPTS TO CONSIDER

What is the IPA? Why was it developed?

_____

_____

_____

_____

_____

Broad Phonetic Transcription

- When professionals use IPA symbols to transcribe words or sounds, they use *phonemic transcriptions,* which are indicated by enclosing phonemes between slash marks, as /s/. These transcriptions are phonemic because variations in phoneme production are not depicted.

- In *phonetic transcription,* allophones are indicated by placing them in brackets, as [s].

■ Table 2.1 lists and gives examples of speech sound symbols in the IPA. These symbols fall into three basic categories: consonants, vowels, and diphthongs.

Narrow Phonetic Transcription

■ Professionals use narrow phonetic transcription to record more detail about how a speaker produces a sound. Narrow phonetic transcription is especially important when clinicians are assessing speakers with challenges such as a cleft palate, a severe phonological disorder, or hearing loss.

■ *Diacritical markers* are special symbols used in narrow phonetic transcription. Table 2.2 shows the most widely used diacritical markers in the profession of speech pathology.

SUMMARY

✓ The International Phonetic Alphabet is an internationally recognized system of representing speech sounds consistently and accurately.

✓ Speech–language pathologists can transcribe speech using broad phonetic symbols and narrow phonetic symbols. Narrow phonetic symbols give increased detail about how individual speakers produce sounds.

PRODUCTION OF SEGMENTALS: CONSONANTS AND VOWELS

INTRODUCTION

Speech sounds can be broadly classified into two categories: consonants and vowels. Consonants and vowels are often described by their role in the production and perception of syllables. In speech–language pathology, it is useful to further divide consonants and vowels into categories or classification systems. The two most widely used classification systems are (a) the distinctive feature approach and (b) the place-voice-manner approach. (*Note:* Some of this information is also contained in Chapter 5, on articulatory and phonological disorders. In chapter 5, the information is more detailed.)

Consonants and Vowels: The Syllable as a Unit

■ Consonants and vowels may be defined by their role in speech production of syllables. The *syllable* is defined as the smallest phonetic unit.

■ Yavas (1998) describes syllables as motor units composed of three parts:

1. *onset,* or the initial consonant or consonant cluster of the syllable, created by release of the syllable pulse through articulatory movements or action of the chest muscles;
2. *nucleus,* or a vowel or dipthong in the middle of the syllable, created by vowel-shaping movements of the vocal tract; and
3. *coda,* the consonant at the end of the syllable, created by arrest of the syllable pulse through articulatory movements, action of the chest muscles, or both.

Table 2.1 THE INTERNATIONAL PHONETIC ALPHABET (IPA)

IPA Symbol	Examples	IPA Symbol	Examples
/p/	pot	/ʃ/	shine
/b/	bat	/ʒ/	vision
/m/	mat	/θ/	thin
/n/	net	/ð/	then
/ŋ/	sing	/tʃ/	chin
/d/	dime	/dʒ/	Jane
/t/	time	/v/	van
/g/	gum	/w/	wine
/k/	Kim	/l/	lean
/f/	fun	/j/	yawn
/s/	sun	/h/	hen
/z/	Zen	/r/	run
/ɑ/	fall	/ɛ/	bet
/æ/	fat	/e/	late
/ɔ/	fought	/o/	overcoat
/ə/	atop	/ʊ/	put
/ʌ/	fun	/u/	boot
/ɪ/	infect	/ɝ/	shirt
/i/	eat	/ɚ/	later
/eɪ/	main		
/ɑɪ/	lime		
/oʊ/	dome		
/ɑʊ/	how		
/ɔɪ/	boy		
/ɪʊ/	fuse		

Note. From *Introduction to Communicative Disorders,* 3rd ed. (p. 98), by M. N. Hegde, 2001, Austin, TX: PRO-ED. Copyright 2001 by PRO-ED, Inc. Reprinted with permission.

Table 2.2 DIACRITIC MARKERS

[ː] full lengthening. This mark, when placed to the right of a phoneme, indicates that the duration of the phoneme has been increased considerably (almost doubled); e.g., /ɛg/ becomes [ɛːg].

[·] half lengthening. This mark, when placed to the right of a phoneme, indicates that the duration of the phoneme has been somewhat increased (not as much as for full lengthening); e.g., /tɔk/ becomes [tɔ·k].

[˜] nasalization. This mark, when placed above a phoneme, indicates that the phoneme, usually non-nasal, has become nasalized; e.g., /tɔp/ becomes [tɔ̃p].

[ˌ] devoicing. This mark, when placed below a phoneme, indicates that the phoneme, usually voiced, has become devoiced; e.g., /beɪbɪ/ becomes [be̥ɪb̥ɪ].

[ˌ] voicing. This mark, when placed below a phoneme, indicates that the phoneme, usually voiceless, has become voiced; e.g., /sup/ becomes [s̬up].

[ʰ] or ['] aspiration. This mark, when placed at the top right side of a phoneme, indicates that the phoneme, usually unaspirated, becomes aspirated; e.g., /tek/ becomes [tek'].

['] unaspiration. In American English, this mark, placed at the top left side of phoneme /p, t, k/ in the word-initial position, indicates that the phoneme, usually aspirated, becomes unaspirated; e.g., /pat/ becomes ['pat].

[ˌ] labialization. This mark, placed directly below the phoneme, indicates that the phoneme, usually nonlabial, becomes labialized; e.g., /nouz/ becomes [n̫ouz].

[ₘ] nonlabialization. This mark, placed directly below the phoneme, indicates that the phoneme, usually labial, becomes nonlabial; e.g., /wɪθ/ becomes [w̟ɪθ].

[ˌ] dentalization. This mark, placed directly below the phoneme, indicates that the phoneme, usually not linguadental, is produced at the linguadental place of articulation; e.g., /titʃ/ becomes [t̪itʃ].

[˙] palatalization. This mark, placed directly above the phoneme, indicates that the phoneme, usually non-palatal, becomes palatalized; e.g., /zu/ becomes [ż u].

[] closing of vowel. This mark, placed directly below the vowel phoneme, indicates that the phoneme is produced with greater closing than normally required for its production; e.g., /edʒ/ becomes [e̝dʒ].

[ˌ] opening of vowel. This mark, when placed directly below the vowel phoneme, indicates that the phoneme is produced with greater opening than normally required for its production; e.g., /ˈeɪnˌdʒəl/ becomes [ˈe̞ɪnˌdʒəl].

[ˌ] tongue raising. This mark, when placed to the right of the vowel phoneme, indicates that the phoneme is produced with more than usual tongue raising; e.g., /ðe/ becomes [ðe˔].

[ˌ] tongue lowering. This mark, when placed to the right of the vowel phoneme, indicates that the phoneme is produced with more than usual tongue lowering; e.g., /blu/ becomes [blu˕].

[+] or [ɨ] tongue advancement. This mark, when placed to the right of the vowel phoneme, indicates that the phoneme is produced with more than usual tongue advancement; e.g., /tu/ becomes [tu+].

[−] or [ɨ] tongue retraction. This mark, when placed to the right of the vowel phoneme, indicates that the phoneme is produced with more than usual tongue retraction; e.g., /tʃik/ becomes [tʃi−k].

['] lip rounding. This mark, when placed at the top right side of the vowel phoneme, indicates that the phoneme is produced with more than usual lip rounding; e.g., /ʃit/ becomes [ʃi't].

['] lip spreading. This mark, when placed at the top right side of the vowel phoneme, indicates that the phoneme is produced with more than usual lip spreading; e.g., /sun/ becomes [su'n].

[-] vowel centralization. This mark, when placed across the vowel phoneme, indicates that the phoneme, usually noncentral, becomes centralized; e.g., /it/ becomes[ɨt].

[] consonant syllabification. In American English, this mark is placed below the consonants /m, n, ŋ, l/ when these consonants perform the function of the nucleus in a syllable; e.g., /batəl/ becomes [batl̩].

Note. From *Phonetics: Principles and Practices,* 2nd ed. (pp. 227-229), by S. Singh & K. S. Singh, 1982, Austin, TX: PRO-ED. Copyright 1982 by PRO-ED, Inc. Reprinted with permission of the authors.

■ Thus, vowels form the nucleus of syllables; consonants release and arrest syllables. Vowels may also stand alone to form syllables. For example, utterances such as *ah, oh,* and *I* are vowels and may stand alone. Consonants may not stand alone; they function only with vowels. Table 2.3 illustrates basic comparisons between vowels and consonants; these comparisons will be described in more detail later.

■ Vowels may also be termed *syllabics* because they carry syllables. A few consonants have a syllabic nature in that they also can form the nucleus of a syllable (Creaghead, Newman, & Secord, 1989). These syllabic consonants are /l/, /n/, and /m/. The diacritic marker /ˌ/ is used to indicate the syllabic nature of these consonants. Examples follow:

> /m̩/: love '<u>em</u>, leave '<u>em</u>
> /n̩/: butto<u>n</u>, more '<u>n</u>' more
> /l̩/: bott<u>le</u>, midd<u>le</u>

■ Syllables may be open or closed. *Open syllables* end in vowels; *my, hey,* and *ski* are open syllables. *Closed syllables* end in consonants; *cook, lip,* and *hiss* are closed syllables.

■ *Syllabification* is the skill involved in identifying the number of syllables in words. Speakers using syllabification would know, for example, that *categorize* has four syllables whereas *dog* has one syllable.

Classification Systems

Distinctive Feature Approach

• The distinctive feature approach to classification was created by linguists to describe the languages of the world. Linguists believe that each phoneme is a collection of independent fea-

Table 2.3 COMPARISONS OF VOWELS AND CONSONANTS

Vowels	Consonants
Always voiced	May be voiced or voiceless
May stand alone	Always combined with vowel
Velum always elevated	Velum elevated or lowered
Vocal tract open	Vocal tract modified or constricted
Airflow continuous	Airflow modified or stopped
May be described by: • distinctive features • tongue and lip position • tension vs. laxness	May be described by: • distinctive features • place-voice-manner

tures. A distinctive feature is a unique characteristic of a phoneme that distinguishes one phoneme from another (Chomsky & Halle, 1968; Jakobson, Fant, & Halle, 1952).

- Each phoneme (consonant or vowel) is described according to a cluster of features that are either present or absent in that phoneme. The binary system of plus or minus a feature is a hallmark of the distinctive feature approach.
- If a feature is present, a phoneme is given a plus (+) for that feature. If a feature is absent, a phoneme is given a minus (–) for that feature. For example, according to the distinctive feature classification system, /s/ would be described as follows: –vocalic, +consonantal, +anterior, +coronal, +continuant, –high, –low, –back, –nasal, +strident.
- Although phonemes may share certain features, each phoneme has a unique set of features that distinguishes it from all the other phonemes. Table 2.4 lists each phoneme according to the distinctive feature model.

Place-Voice-Manner Approach

- The place-voice-manner approach to classification categorizes consonants in terms of three parameters: place, voice, and manner of production. *Place of articulation* refers to the location of the sound's production, indicating the primary articulators that shape the sounds. For example, /p/ is termed a *bilabial* because it is produced by putting the lips together.
- *Voicing* refers to vocal fold vibration during production of sounds. Voiced sounds are those produced while the vocal folds are vibrating. Voiceless sounds are those produced while the vocal folds are not vibrating. The /p/ is a voiceless sound.

Table 2.4 THE CHOMSKY-HALLE DISTINCTIVE FEATURES OF ENGLISH CONSONANTS

	w	f	v	θ	ð	t	d	s	z	n	l	ʃ	ʒ	j	r	tʃ	dʒ	k	g	ŋ	h	p	b	m
Voiced	+	-	+	-	+	-	+	-	+	+	+	-	+	+	+	-	+	-	+	+	-	-	+	+
Consonantal	-	+	+	+	+	+	+	+	+	+	+	+	+	-	+	+	+	+	+	+	-	+	+	+
Anterior	+	+	+	+	+	+	+	+	+	+	+	-	-	-	-	-	-	-	-	-	-	+	+	+
Coronal	-	-	-	+	+	+	+	+	+	+	+	+	+	-	+	+	+	-	-	-	-	-	-	-
Continuant	+	+	+	+	+	-	-	+	+	-	+	+	+	+	+	-	-	-	-	-	+	-	-	-
High	-	-	-	-	-	-	-	-	-	-	-	+	+	+	-	+	+	+	+	+	-	-	-	-
Low	-	-	-	-	-	-	-	-	-	-	-	-	-	-	-	-	-	-	-	-	+	-	-	-
Back	-	-	-	-	-	-	-	-	-	-	-	-	-	-	-	-	-	+	+	+	-	-	-	-
Nasal	-	-	-	-	-	-	-	-	-	+	-	-	-	-	-	-	-	-	-	+	-	-	-	+
Strident	-	+	+	-	-	-	-	+	+	-	-	+	+	-	-	+	+	-	-	-	-	-	-	-
Vocalic	-	-	-	-	-	-	-	-	-	-	+	-	-	-	+	-	-	-	-	-	-	-	-	-

Note. From *Introduction to Communicative Disorders,* 3rd ed. (p. 104), by M. N. Hegde, 2001, Austin, TX: PRO-ED. Copyright 2001 by PRO-ED, Inc. Reprinted with permission.

- *Manner of articulation* refers to the degree or type of constriction of the vocal tract during consonant production. For example, /p/ is termed a *stop* because it is produced by putting the lips together and completely stopping the airflow. Table 2.5 illustrates how English consonants may be classified according to the place-voice-manner approach.

CONCEPTS TO CONSIDER

Compare and contrast the distinctive feature and place-voice-manner approaches to categorizing phonemes.

_____

_____

_____

_____

_____

Consonants

Basic Principles

- Consonants are speech sounds produced by movements of articulatory muscles. These movements modify the airstream in some manner by interrupting it, stopping it, or creating a narrow opening through which it must pass. Consonants may be voiced or voiceless.
- Consonants may be described according to distinctive features and their place, voice, and manner of production. In this section, we describe these parameters and provide a summary of them for each consonant either singly or as a member of a cognate pair (defined later).

Distinctive Feature Approach

When a person produces /ə/, the tongue is neutral and at rest. For production of many consonants, the tongue moves to a different position. In the distinctive feature system, many sounds are described according to where and how the tongue moves away from the neutral resting position /ə/. The following descriptions are summarized from Peña-Brooks and Hegde (2000); Kent (1998); Creaghead et al. (1989); Yavas (1998); and Borden et al. (2003):

- *Vocalic* sounds include all vowels and the consonants /r/ and /l/. They have little constriction and are associated with spontaneous voicing.
- *Consonantal* sounds include /m/, /b/, /p/, /ŋ/, /g/, /k/, /dʒ/, /tʃ/, /ʒ/, /ʃ/, /r/, /l/, /n/, /s/, /z/, /d/, /t/, /ð/, /θ/, /v/, /f/. These sounds have marked constriction along the midline region of the vocal tract.

Table 2.5 MANNER OF PRODUCTION

Place of Articulation	Nasals	Stops	Fricatives	Affricates	Liquids	Glides	Laterals
Bilabial	ⓜ	p ⓑ				ⓦ	
Labiodental			f ⓥ				
Linguadental			θ ⓓ̵				
Lingua-alveolar	ⓝ	t ⓓ	s ⓩ		ⓛ		Ⓘ
Linguapalatal			ʃ ③	ⓣʃⓓʒ	ⓡ	ⓙ	
Linguavelar	ⓝ̍	k ⓖ					
Glottal			h				

Note. Voiced sounds are circled. Place-Voice-Manner Classification of English Consonants. From *Introduction to Communicative Disorders,* 3rd ed. (p. 101), by M. N. Hegde, 2001, Austin, TX: PRO-ED. Copyright 2001 by PRO-ED, Inc. Reprinted with permission.

- *Lateral* sound includes /l/ only. The /l/ is produced by placing the front of the tongue against the alveolar ridge (midline closure) and lowering the midsection of the tongue bilaterally (lateral opening).
- *Voiced* sounds include /m/, /n/, /ŋ/, /b/, /g/, /l/, /r/, /z/, /d/, /v/, /w/, /dʒ/, /j/, /ʒ/, /ð/. When these sounds are produced, the vocal folds vibrate.
- *Back* sound includes (+) back consonants /k/, /g/, /ŋ/. These sounds are produced with the tongue retracted from the neutral schwa position.
- *Low* sounds include only (+) low /h/. The tongue is lowered from the neutral schwa position.
- *Continuant* sounds include /h/, /r/, /l/, /s/, /z/, /f/, /v/, /w/, /j/, /ʒ/, /ʃ/ ,/ð/, /θ/. These sounds are produced with an incomplete point of constriction. For this reason, the airflow is not entirely stopped at any time and the sounds may be produced continuously until the person runs out of breath.
- *Nasal* sounds include /m/, /n/, /ŋ/. These sounds are produced by lowering the velum so that there is coupling of the oral and nasal cavities and sounds are resonated in the oral cavity.
- *Anterior* sounds include /m/, /p/, /b/, /l/, /n/, /s/, /z/, /t/, /d/, /v/, /f/, /w/, /ð/, /θ/. These sounds are produced with a point of constriction located more anteriorly than that of /ʃ/. The production of /ʃ/ defines the boundary between anterior and nonanterior sounds.
- *Coronal* sounds include /r/, /l/, /n/, /s/, /z/, /t/, /d/, /dʒ/, /tʃ/, /ʒ/, /ʃ/, /ð/, /θ/. These sounds are produced with the tongue blade raised above the neutral schwa position.
- *Round* sounds include /r/ and /w/. These sounds are produced with the lips protruded or rounded.
- *Tense* sounds include /l/, /s/, /f/, /k/, /t/, /p/, /ʃ/, /ð/, /θ/, /dʒ/, /tʃ/. All these consonants are voiceless except /dʒ/ and /l/. These sounds are produced with a relatively greater degree of contraction or muscle tension at the root of the tongue.
- *High* sounds include (+) high consonants /k/, /g/, /ŋ/, /ʃ/, /ʒ/, /j/, /tʃ/, /dʒ/. These sounds are produced with the tongue elevated above the neutral /ə/ position.
- *Strident* sounds include /tʃ/, /dʒ/, /ʒ/, /ʃ/, /s/, /z/, /f/, /v/. These sounds are produced by forcing

the airstream through a small, constricted opening. The result is strident or intense noise.

- *Sonorant* sounds include /n/, /m/, /ŋ/, /l/, /r/, /w/, /j/. These sounds are produced by allowing the airstream to pass relatively uninterrupted through the nasal or oral cavity. There is no stoppage or point of constriction.
- *Interrupted* sounds include /tʃ/, /dʒ/, /t/, /d/, /k/, /g/, /p/, /b/. These sounds may be thought of as the opposites of sonorants because the interrupted sounds are produced by complete blockage of the airstream at the point of constriction.

This list comprises the primary distinctive feature categories used by speech–language pathologists, but there are other categories of distinctive features that have some clinical utility (Bleile, 1996; Ohde & Sharf, 1992; Peña-Brooks & Hegde, 2000; Shriberg & Kent, 2003; Yavas, 1998). These categories are:

- *Syllabics* include liquids /r/, /l/ and nasals /m/, /n/, /ŋ/. All vowels are syllabics, and most consonants are not. Syllabics serve as the nucleus for a syllable.
- *Obstruents* include affricates /tʃ/, /dʒ/, fricatives /f/, /v/, /ð/, /θ/, /s/, /z/, /h/, /ʃ/, /ʒ/, and stops /p/, /b/, /t/, /d/, /k/, /g/. They are made with a notable amount of air obstruction in the vocal tract. Obstruents are made with a narrow constriction or complete closure of the oral cavity so a friction noise is produced or the airstream is stopped completely.
- *Sibilants* include affricates /tʃ/ and /dʒ/ and fricatives /s/, /z/, /ʃ/, /ʒ/. Sibilants are high-frequency sounds that have longer duration and more stridency than most other consonants.
- *Approximants* include glides /w/ and /j/ and liquids /r/ and /l/. Approximants are named as such because of the approximating nature of the contact between the two articulators that help form them. That is, the degree of contact is approximate, not nearly as firm or closed as it is for fricatives, affricates, and stops.
- *Rhotic* is a term sometimes used to describe /r/ and its allophonic variations.

Place-Voice-Manner Approach

Consonants can be described according to place-voice-manner of production as well as distinctive features. The following descriptions of place-voice-manner are summarized from Peña-Brooks & Hegde (2000), Kent (1998), Creaghead et al. (1989), Yavas (1998), and Borden et al. (2003).

Place of Articulation

- *Linguavelars* (also called *velars*) are produced when the dorsum of the tongue contacts the velum. Linguavelars are /g/, /j/, /ŋ/.
- *Linguapalatals* are produced when the tongue blade is pressed against the hard palate to form the point of constriction just posterior to the alveolar ridge. Linguapalatals are /j/, /r/, /dʒ/, /tʃ/, /ʒ/, and /ʃ/.
- *Lingua-alveolars* are produced by contact of the tip of tongue with the alveolar ridge. Lingua-alveolars are /s/, /z/, /n/, /l/, /t/, and /d/.
- *Linguadentals,* also called *interdentals,* are produced by protruding the tongue tip slightly between the cutting edge of the lower and upper front teeth, forming a narrow constriction. Airflow is directed through this constriction, and contact between the tongue and teeth is light. The sounds /θ/ and /ð/ are linguadental.
- *Bilabials* are produced by mutual contact of the upper and lower lips. Bilabials are /w/, /m/, /p/, /b/.
- *Labiodentals* are produced by placing the lower edge of the upper central incisors on the upper portion of the lower lip. A narrow point of constriction is formed from this light contact of the incisors and lip. The sounds /f/ and /v/ are labiodentals.

- *Glottals* are produced at the level of the glottis. The vocal folds are open, and the air passes through them. The only glottal in American English is /h/.

Voicing

- The characteristic of voicing refers to whether the vocal folds are vibrating when a consonant is produced. Sounds such as /r/, /g/, and /z/ are *voiced*. Sounds such as /k/, /t/, and /s/ are *voiceless*.
- *Cognate pairs* are sounds that are identical in every way except voicing. Place and manner of production are the same, but the feature of voicing is different. For example, /p-b/ and /k-g/ are cognate pairs.

Manner of Articulation

- The following information about manner of articulation is summarized from Peña-Brooks & Hegde (2000), Kent (1998), Creaghead et al. (1989), Yavas (1998), and Borden et al. (2003). All sounds in each manner-of-articulation category are described according to place, voice, and manner of articulation as well as distinctive features. Though redundant, this brief description is intended to help the reader quickly remember key attributes of each consonant.

Nasals: /m/, /n/, /ŋ/
- Nasals are produced by lowering the velum to keep the velopharyngeal port open. The open velopharyngeal port allows the sound produced by the vibrating vocal folds to pass through the nasal cavity.
- The vocal tract is lengthened, and there is an overall increase in the area for resonance. Thus, the resonance characteristic is changed by low-frequency components being added to the sounds.

> /m/: place = bilabial
> voice = voiced
> manner = nasal
> distinctive features = +voiced, +consonantal, +anterior, +nasal
>
> /n/: place = lingua-alveolar
> voice = voiced
> manner = nasal
> distinctive features = +voiced, +consonantal, +anterior, +coronal, +nasal
>
> /ŋ/: place = linguavelar
> voice = voiced
> manner = nasal
> distinctive features = +voiced, +consonantal, +high, +back, +nasal

Fricatives: /h/, /ʒ/, /ʃ/, /s/, /z/, /ð/, /θ/, /f/, /v/
- Fricatives derive their name from the friction, the hissing-type quality that results from the continuous forcing of air through a narrow constriction.
- The constrictions in the vocal tract generate aperiodic noise as the airflow passes through them. The constrictions must be narrow enough and the airflow strong enough to create a turbulent airflow. This turbulent airflow creates noisy random vibrations, or frication. Two closely approximating articulators form the constriction through which a continuous airstream must pass. Firm velopharyngeal closure is necessary.

/h/: place = glottal
voice = voiceless
manner = fricative
distinctive features = +continuant, +low

/ʒ-ʃ/: place = linguapalatal
voice = /ʒ/ voiced, /ʃ/ voiceless
manner = fricative
distinctive features = +consonantal, +coronal, +continuant, +high, +strident

/s-z/: place = lingua-alveolar
voice = /s/ voiceless, /z/ voiced
manner = fricative
distinctive features = +consonantal, +anterior, +coronal, +continuant, +strident

/ð-θ/: place = lingua-dental
voice = /ð/ voiced, /θ/ voiceless
manner = fricative
distinctive features = +consonantal, +coronal, +anterior, +continuant

/f-v/: place = labiodental
voice = /f/ voiceless, /v/ voiced
manner = fricative
distinctive features = +consonantal, +anterior, +continuant, +strident

Affricates: /tʃ/, /dʒ/

- The affricates /tʃ/ and /dʒ/ have both a fricative and a stop component. These sounds begin as stops and are released as fricatives. The speaker makes alveolar closure for /d/ or /t/; when the closure is released, the tongue is retracted and shaped for production of /tʃ/ or /dʒ/.
- Usually, the lips are slightly rounded as the fricative portion of the affricate sound is produced.

/tʃ-dʒ/: place = lingua-alveolar
voice = /tʃ/ voiceless, /dʒ/ voiced
manner = affricate
distinctive features = +consonantal, +coronal, +strident

Stops: /p/, /b/, /t/, /d/, /k/, /g/

- The stops are produced by complete constriction or closure of the vocal tract at some point so the airflow is totally stopped. Stops are formed at three basic places: *alveolar* (closure between the tip of the tongue and the alveolar ridge), *velar* (closure between the tongue blade and roof of the mouth), and *labial* (closure of the lips) (Kent, 1998).
- When the airflow is stopped, pressure builds up behind the point of contact; when the built-up air is released, there is a short audible burst of noise. Consequently, stops may also be called *stop-plosives*.

/p-b/: place = bilabial
voice = /p/ voiceless, /b/ voiced

manner = stop
distinctive features = +consonantal, +anterior

/t↓d/: place = lingua-alveolar
voice = /t/ voiceless, /d/ voiced
manner = stop
distinctive features = +consonantal, +anterior, +coronal

/k↓g/: place = lingua-velar
voice = /k/ voiceless, /g/ voiced
manner = stop
distinctive features = +consonantal, +high, +back

Glides: /w/, /j/

- The glides, also called *semivowels* and *sonorants,* are produced by a quick transition of the articulators as they move from a partially constricted state to a more open state for the vowels that follow them. The term *onglide* is used to describe this movement (Edwards, 2003). In comparison to stops, fricatives, and affricates, glides are formed by a relatively transitory and unrestricted point of constriction.

/w/: place = bilabial
voice = voiced
manner = glide
distinctive features = +anterior, +continuant

/j/: place = linguapalatal
voice = voiced
manner = glide
distinctive features = +continuant, +high

Liquids: /r/, /l/

- The liquids are produced with the least oral cavity restriction of all the consonants. The vocal tract is obstructed only slightly more than for vowels.
- The /r/ is also called a *rhotic,* and is commonly produced in two ways. One way is as a *retroflex,* made with the tongue tip retracted and approximating the hard palate; a second way is as a *bunched* /r/, where the dorsum of the tongue is "bunched" or retracted and elevated toward the hard palate.
- The /l/ is also called a *lateral* because when the /l/ is produced, the midsection portion of the tongue is relaxed and open, and thus air is directed through the sides of the tongue.

/r/: place = linguapalatal
voice = voiced
manner = liquid
distinctive features = +consonantal, +coronal, +continuant, +vocalic

/l/: place = lingua-alveolar
voice = voiced
manner = liquid
distinctive features = +consonantal, +anterior, +coronal, +continuant, +vocalic

CONCEPTS TO CONSIDER

Describe /m/ and /s/ in terms of place-voice-manner of articulation and distinctive features.

_____

_____

_____

_____

_____

Consonant Clusters

- While many consonants are produced alone or adjacent to vowels, others are produced adjacent to some consonants. These *consonant clusters,* also known as *blends,* may occur in the initial, medial, or final position of words.
- Most consonant clusters in American English consist of two consonants. However, some three-consonant clusters also occur. Examples of two-consonant clusters are: *mosquito, bless, silk.* Examples of three-consonant clusters are *burst, squirrel, burnt.*

Vowels

Basic Principles

- Unlike consonants, which are mostly produced with some constriction of the vocal tract, vowels are produced with an open vocal tract. The vocal tract is open from the vocal folds to the lips, with no points of constriction.
- Because all vowels are voiced, the sound source for vowels is the vocal folds. Resonance patterns for the vowels are shaped by the vocal tract. The distinctive resonance features for each vowel sound are produced by changing the size and shape of the oral cavity.

Distinctive Feature Approach

Like consonants, vowels can be described according to their distinctive features. The following descriptions are summarized from Peña-Brooks & Hegde (2000), Kent (1998), Creaghead et al. (1989), Yavas (1998), and Borden et al. (2003).

- *Vocalics* include all vowels. These sounds are produced without a marked constriction in the vocal tract.
- *Sonorants* include all vowels. Sonorants are produced by an airstream that passes uncon-

stricted through the oral or nasal cavity.

- *Voiced* vowels include all vowels. All vowels are produced with vocal fold vibration.
- *Rounded* vowels are /o/, /u/, /ʊ/, and /ɔ/. These sounds are produced with the lips protruded or rounded.
- *Tense* vowels are /e/, /ɪ/, /ʌ/, /ɝ/, /o/, and /u/. These sounds are produced with muscle contraction or tension at the root of the tongue.
- *Front* vowels include /ɪ/, /i/, /e/, /ɛ/, and /æ/. The tongue is in a position anterior to the neutral schwa position.
- *Back* vowels are /ɑ/, /ɔ/, /o/, /ʊ/, and /u/. These sounds are made with the tongue retracted from the neutral schwa position.
- *High* vowels include /i/, /ɪ/, /ʊ/, and /u/. These sounds are made with the tongue elevated above the neutral schwa position.
- *Low* vowels include /æ/ and /ɑ/. These vowels are made with the tongue lowered from the neutral schwa position.
- *Rhotic* refers to sounds made with an /r/ coloring. These sounds include the mid-central vowels /ɚ/ and /ɝ/.

Vowel Position Characteristics

- While it is helpful to describe vowels according to their distinctive features, it is also useful to describe vowel production from a position of physiologic rest—that is, what amount of mandibular, tongue, and lip movement away from physiologic rest is necessary for production of each vowel? Figure 2.1 demonstrates the tongue positions with which vowels are typically produced.
- Using this concept, vowels can be characterized according to four dimensions:

    - *lip position,* which causes vowels to be categorized as *rounded* or *unrounded.* For rounded vowels, the lips are protruded. For unrounded vowels, the lips are in a neutral or slightly retracted position.
    - *tense/lax qualities.* Tense vowels have longer duration and are produced with increased tension, while lax vowels are of shorter duration and are produced with relatively less muscular tension.
    - *tongue height,* which causes vowels to be categorized as *high, mid,* or *low* in terms of production within the oral cavity.
    - *tongue forwardness* or *retraction,* which causes vowels to be categorized as front, central, or back in terms of production within the oral cavity.

- In the following section, vowels are described according to these dimensions. Key words containing each vowel serve as examples.

Front Vowels: /ɪ/, /i/, /e/, /ɛ/, /æ/.

- *High* front vowels /ɪ/ and /i/

    /i/: tense, unround; tongue is in a high and forward position. Key words: *heat, meeting, see.*

    /ɪ/ : lax, unround; tongue is slightly lower and more posterior than for /i/. Key words: *bit, sick, tin.*

- *Mid* front vowels /e/ and /ɛ/

    /e/: tense, unround; compared to production of /ɪ/, /e/ involves keeping the tongue lower

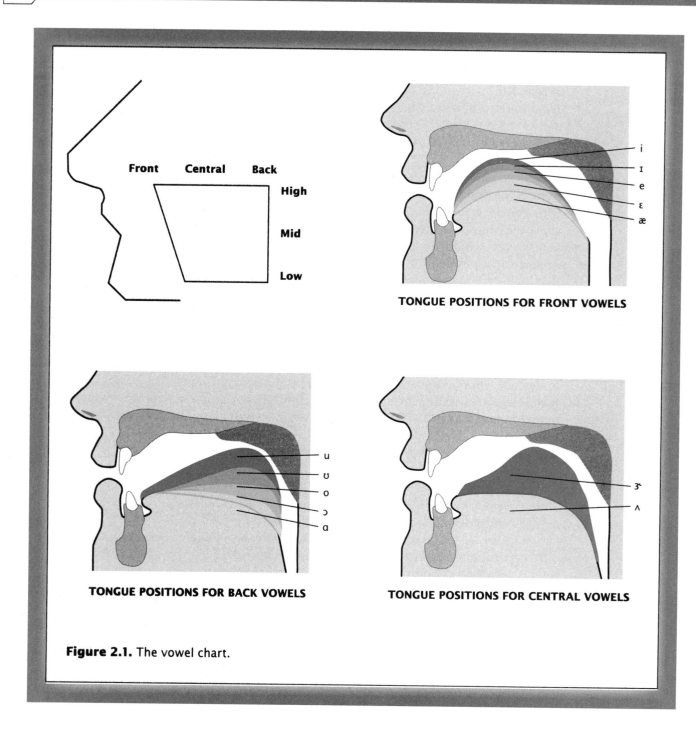

Figure 2.1. The vowel chart.

and slightly more retracted. Key words: *make, later, fate.*

/ɛ/: lax, unround; the /ɛ/ vowel is produced slightly lower than /e/. Key words: *let, ten, sent.*

- *Low* front vowel /æ/
    /æ/: lax, unround; one of the lowest vowels in English, /æ/ is produced with the tongue lower and more retracted than required for production of /ɛ/. Key words: *tan, matter, sat.*

Central Vowels: /ɝ/, /ɚ/, /ə/, /ʌ/.

- The place of production varies for each of the central vowels, also called mid central vowels.
- /ɝ/ and /ɚ/

    /ɝ/: tense, half-round, retroflexed; the tongue blade is bunched and elevated toward the hard palate. The tongue is retracted toward /o/, and tongue height is approximately equivalent to /ɪ/ and /e/. The /ɝ/ is transcribed to represent /r/ production in syllables receiving primary stress (e.g., *certain*). Key words: *curtain, hurt, dirty.*

    /ɚ/: lax, half-round, and retroflexed. The /ɚ/, called *schwar*, is produced in the same manner as /ɝ/. However, schwar is transcribed to represent /r/ production in unstressed syllables such as that in *butter*. Key words: *letter, color, ladder.*

- /ə/ and /ʌ/

    /ə/: lax, unround; the tongue blade is lowered in relation to /ɝ/. The unstressed /ə/ occurs in unstressed syllables such as a̲bove. Key words: a̲ttempt, a̲head, pizz̲a̲.

    /ʌ/: lax, unround; the /ʌ/ vowel is produced in a manner similar to that for /ə/, but the tongue is slightly more retracted toward /ɑ/. The /ʌ/ occurs in stressed syllables. Key words: *m̲o̲ney, fl̲o̲o̲d, u̲p.*

Back Vowels: /u/, /ʊ/, /o/, /ɔ/, /ɑ/.

- *High* back vowels /u/ and /ʊ/

    /u/: tense, round; the tongue is in the highest, most retracted position when a speaker is producing /ʊ/. Key words: *spoon, fruit, bruise.*

    /ʊ/: lax, round; the /ʊ/ vowel is produced in a slightly lower and more forward manner than /u/. Key words: *took, put, foot.*

- *Mid* back vowels /o/ and /ɔ/

    /ɔ/: lax, round; the /ɔ/ vowel is produced a little lower than /u/. Key words: *fought, caught, shawl.*

    /o/: tense, round; in comparison to /u/, /o/ is produced slightly lower in the oral cavity. Key words: *coat, lower, soapy.*

- *Low* back vowel /ɑ/

    /ɑ/: lax, unround; the /ɑ/ vowel is produced with the lowest, most retracted tongue position of all the vowels. Key words: *calm, pocket, father.*

Diphthongs

- Diphthongs are produced as a slow gliding movement from one vowel (the *onglide*) to the adjacent vowel (the *offglide*) (Kent, 1998). For example, in the diphthong /ɑɪ/, /ɑ/ is the onglide vowel, and /ɪ/ is the offglide vowel. Diphthongs contain both an initial and a final segment.
- Diphthongs are represented phonetically by digraph symbols that highlight the initial and final segments (Peña-Brooks & Hegde, 2000). The diphthongs are:

    - /ɑɪ/ (e.g., *mi̲ght, sky, Ty̲ler*)

- /aʊ/ (e.g., cl<u>ou</u>d, h<u>ow</u>)
- /ɔɪ/ (e.g., h<u>oi</u>st, t<u>oy</u>)
- /eɪ/ (e.g., w<u>eigh</u>, h<u>ay</u>)

- *Phonemic* diphthongs /aɪ/, /ɔɪ/, and /aʊ/ cannot be reduced to pure vowels without changing word meaning. For example, /taɪp/ and /tap/ represent two different meanings. *Nonphonemic* diphthongs /oʊ/ and /eɪ/ do not change word meanings. For example, the listener perceives /soʊp/ and /sop/ as the same words.

SUMMARY

✓ Consonants and vowels may be defined by their role in the production of syllables, the smallest phonetic unit.

✓ Two classification systems frequently used to describe consonants and vowels are distinctive features and place-voice-manner of articulation.

✓ Vowels may also be described according to lip position, tense-lax qualities, and tongue height and position within the oral cavity.

THE EFFECTS OF CONTEXT IN SPEECH SOUND PRODUCTION

INTRODUCTION

The sounds of a language may be produced in isolation. Typically, however, they are produced within a context of some kind. Because of the context in which the sounds are produced, they are are influenced by one another in running speech. Sounds as parts of words and ultimately conversational speech are also influenced by suprasegmental parameters, which add variety and expression to speech.

Dynamics of Speech Production

- In most cases, sounds are produced as part of connected speech. Sounds may influence each other in three ways: through adaptation, assimilation, and coarticulation.

- Phonetic *adaptations* comprise two types of variations according to preceding and following sounds: (a) variations in the way the articulators move and (b) the extent to which vocal tract configurations change shape (Creaghead et al., 1989).

- For example, the /m/ in *meek* is produced with more lip retraction than the /m/ in *moo,* which is produced with slight lip protrusion. The adjacent vowels influence the production of /m/.

- In *assimilation,* speech sounds are modified due to the influence of adjacent sounds. Modifications are so extensive that there are perceptible changes in sounds. For example, in the phrase "great zoo," the /z/ in *zoo* is devoiced because of the voiceless /t/ in the preceding word.

- *Coarticulation* refers to the influence of one phoneme upon another phoneme in production or perception. In coarticulation, two different articulators move simultaneously to produce two different speech sounds. Coarticulation creates both adaptation and assimilation.

Suprasegmentals

- *Suprasegmentals,* also referred to as features of *prosody,* add meaning, variety, and color to running speech. They involve larger units than individual units or segmentals do, such as syllables, words, phrases, and sentences.

- Suprasegmentals are affected by a number of variables. These include a person's cultural and linguistic background, emotional state, gender, and age. The most commonly described suprasegmentals or prosodic features that affect speech production are length, stress, rate, pitch, volume, and juncture.

CONCEPTS TO CONSIDER

What is meant by the term *suprasegmentals*? List two suprasegmentals that impact speech production.

_____

_____

_____

_____

_____

- *Length* of vowels and consonants is related to syllable perception and production. If syllables have long vowels, they tend to have short consonants. If syllables have short vowels, they tend to have long consonants.

- *Stress* is an important characteristic of syllables, for it can change the meanings of words. Stressed syllables are often called syllables containing *primary stress,* while unstressed syllables are referred to as those with *secondary* or *weak* stress.

- Stressed and unstressed syllables differ in four ways relative to each other:

Stressed Syllable	Unstressed Syllable
loud	soft
longer	shorter
higher in pitch	lower in pitch
greater muscular effort	less muscular effort

- Syllable stress is especially important in differentiating noun and verb pairs that have identical sounds. For example, the words *object, permit, insult,* and *import* become nouns or verbs depending upon which syllables are stressed (Yavas, 1998).

■ *Rate* of speech refers to the speed with which a person speaks. When people are speaking rapidly, they tend to reduce duration of vowels and to produce consonants with less articulatory effort. Rate reflects the phonetic duration of both sound and silence and may be affected by the speaker's emotion.

■ *Pitch* is the *perception* of the frequency with which the vocal folds vibrate, whereas frequency is a *physical property* of the actual sound waves. Pitch is determined by mass, tension, and elasticity of the vocal folds. In English, pitch can be used to indicate different meanings of spoken units. For example, "We are having fun reading this book" can be a statement if the pitch falls at the end. A rising pitch at the end of this statement turns it into a question.

■ *Volume* is the perception of a speaker's intensity of speech. This perception is related to amplitude, a *physical property* of the actual sound waves. A speaker's loudness may be influenced by many variables, including the amount of background noise in the situation, the speaker's feelings at the moment, and the speaker's or listener's ability to hear.

■ *Juncture,* also called *vocal punctuation,* is a combination of suprasegmentals such as intonation and pausing, that mark special distinctions or grammatical divisions in speech. These distinctions affect the meaning of an utterance. For example, one would say "*What* did you eat?" differently than one would say "*What,* did you *eat?*" Or, one might use juncture to make distinctions between similar-sounding words like *night rate* and *nitrate,* or *I scream* and *ice cream* (Kent, 1998).

SUMMARY

✓ Speech sounds are generally produced within a context where they are influenced by one another.

✓ Suprasegmentals such as juncture, pitch, and stress add meaning and variety to speech as part of human interaction.

SPEECH SCIENCE: PHYSIOLOGICAL PHONETICS, ACOUSTIC PHONETICS, AND SPEECH PERCEPTION

INTRODUCTION

Acoustics is the study of sound as a physical phenomenon. Sound is an audible vibration or disturbance in the air that creates sound waves. These waves, which are disturbances of molecules, are periodic or aperiodic. Vibratory motion may be characterized according to two properties: intensity and frequency.

Acoustics: Basic Definitions

■ *Acoustics,* a branch of physics, is the study of the physical properties of sound and how sound is generated and propagated.

■ *Psychoacoustics* is a study of how humans respond to sound as a physical phenomenon; it is a branch of both psychology and acoustics.

■ *Sound* may be defined both physically and psychologically (perceptually). Physically defined, sound is the result of vibration or disturbance in the air. Psychologically defined, sound is *audible* vibration or disturbance in the air (Borden et al., 2003). Sound waves are movements of particles in a medium containing expansions and contractions of molecules.

■ *Compression*, or *condensation*, is a phase of sound in which the vibratory movements of an object (e.g., the tines of a tuning fork) increase the density of air molecules because the molecules are compressed or condensed; it is the opposite of rarefaction (see below).

■ *Rarefaction* is the thinning of air molecules when the vibrating object returns to equilibrium; it is the opposite of condensation.

■ *Simple harmonic motion* refers to the back-and-forth movement of particles when the movement is symmetrical and periodic; it is also known as a sine wave.

■ *Sinusoidal motion* or *wave* is a wave with horizontal and vertical symmetry because it contains one peak or crest and one valley or trough; a sinusoidal wave contains a single frequency; it is a result of simple harmonic motion.

■ *Aperiodic waves* are those that do not repeat themselves at regular intervals; their vibratory patterns are random and difficult to predict from one time interval to the next. *Periodic waves* are sound waves that repeat themselves at regular intervals.

■ *Amplitude* is one of two characteristics of vibratory motion and is the magnitude and direction of displacement. In acoustics, it is the strength or magnitude of a sound signal; the greater the amplitude, the louder the sound signal.

■ *Intensity* is the quality of sound that creates the sensation of loudness; physically, intensity is the amount of energy transmitted per second over an area of one square meter; it is measured in terms of watt per square meter; it is also expressed in decibels.

■ *Bel* is a logarithmic unit of measure of sound intensity; it is a basic and relative reference measure; it helps express the wide range of sound intensities to which the human ear is sensitive by means of a compressed, logarithmic scale. *Decibel* (dB) is a measure of sound intensity; it equals one tenth of a bel.

■ *csg system* is a metric system of measuring length in centimeters (cm), time in seconds (sec), and mass in grams (g); it can be contrasted with the MKS system. The *MKS system* is a metric system of measuring length in meters (m), mass in kilograms (kg), and time in seconds.

■ *Dyne* is a measure of force in the cgs metric system; 1 dyne is the force required to accelerate a mass of 1 gram from a velocity of 0 cm per second to a velocity of 1 cm per second in 1 second.

■ *Density* is the amount of mass per unit volume. Density of matter that serves as a medium for sound affects sound transmission.

■ *Displacement* is change in position; air molecules are said to be displaced because of the vibratory action of an object. *Oscillation* refers to the to-and-fro movement of the air molecules because of a vibrating object.

■ *Force* is a vector quantity that tends to produce an acceleration of a body in the direction of its application; it is also defined as the product of mass and acceleration. Force is measured in terms of Nt (newton); 1 newton equals the force required to accelerate a mass of 1 kg from a velocity of 0 m (meter) per second to a velocity of 1 m per second in 1 second.

■ *Elasticity* is a property that makes it possible for matter (that helps transmit sound) to recover its form and volume when subjected to distortion; all matter is subjected to distortion when force is applied to it.

■ *Velocity* is a change in position of, for example, air molecules when an object is set to vibration. Velocity is measured in terms of the distance an object moves per the time and the direction it takes as it moves.

■ *Frequency* is one of the two characteristics of vibratory motion and is the rate of vibratory motion that is measured in terms of the number of cycles completed per second or, more recently, in terms of hertz (Hz). *Hertz* is the unit of measure for frequency; it is the same as the cycle per second; 1 cycle per second is 1 Hz.

■ *Natural frequency* is the frequency with which a source of sound normally vibrates. It is determined by the source's mass and stiffness. *Mass* is the quantity of matter, and is not to be confused with *weight,* which is gravitational force exerted on mass. The mass of a medium of sound affects its transmission. Increased mass results in decreased frequency, and increased stiffness results in increased frequency.

■ *Formant frequency* is a frequency region with concentrated acoustic energy; it is the center frequency of a formant, which is a resonance. *Fundamental frequency* is the lowest frequency of a periodic wave; it is the first harmonic.

CONCEPTS TO CONSIDER

Define the terms *sound* and *acoustics.*

_____

_____

_____

_____

_____

■ An *octave* is an indication of the interval between two frequencies. The intervals always maintain a ratio of 1:2; thus, each octave doubles a particular frequency (e.g., 200 Hz is one octave above 100 Hz, and 2,000 Hz is one octave above 1,000 Hz).

■ *Impedance* is acoustic, mechanical, or electrical resistance to motion or sound transmission.

- *Newton's laws of motion* explain motion and its characteristics. Basically, sound involves motion; the law of inertia states that all bodies remain at rest or in a state of uniform motion unless another force acts in opposition. In other words, a body in motion tends to remain in motion and a body at rest tends to stay at rest. The law of reaction forces states that every force is associated with a reaction force of opposite direction.

- *Pressure* is the amount of force per unit area. Force is measured either as dynes or as newtons and is important in understanding the amount of force sound waves exert on the eardrum.

- *Reflection* refers to the phenomenon of sound waves traveling back after hitting an obstacle with no change in the speed of propagation. *Refraction* is the bending of the sound wave due to change in its speed of propagation; this happens, for example, when sound waves move from one medium (e.g., air) to another (e.g., water).

- *Resonance* is the modification of sound by other sources; in speech acoustics, resonance refers to modification of the laryngeal tone predominantly by the nasal and oral cavities.

- A *transmitting medium* is any matter that carries or transmits sound; air, liquids, and solids can all transmit sound; *mass* and *elasticity* of transmitting media affect sound (see the next section).

SUMMARY

- ✓ Acoustics, the study of sound, defines sound as an audible vibration or disturbance in the air that creates sound waves. These waves may be periodic or aperiodic.

- ✓ Vibratory motion can be characterized according to intensity and frequency. Intensity is measured in decibels, and frequency is measured in hertz.

- ✓ Sound may be resonated for speech by the nasal and oral cavities.

INTRODUCTION TO THE STUDY OF SOUND AND ACOUSTIC ANALYSIS OF SPEECH

INTRODUCTION

Sound is the result of vibrations of an elastic object. Physically, sound is a compressional wave; psychologically, it is a compressional wave that produces a sensation. Sound exists both as a physical phenomenon and as a sensory experience (Borden et al., 2003; Kent, 1998, 2004; Speaks, 1999). It is perceived in terms of pitch and loudness. The acoustic analysis of speech is generally conducted through use of a sound spectrograph, which produces a spectrogram. The spectrogram displays various components such as fundamental frequency and many other characteristics of vowels and consonants.

Sound Wave Generation and Propagation

- Sound or vibration propagation needs a medium. Air, liquid, or gas can serve as such a medium. The two main properties of the medium that affect the transmission of sound are the mass (density) and the elasticity.

■ More massive objects (sound media) require greater force to set them into vibratory motion because of their higher inertia. Vibratory motion is possible partly because of the elasticity of objects.

■ For example, the tines of a tuning fork can be set into a to-and-fro motion by striking them because of their elasticity. Elastic objects get distorted when a force is applied to them and in due course recover their original form or position. As they change these, they create waves of molecular disturbances (vibratory motion).

■ Vibrations repeat themselves in *cycles* or *hertz*. The number of times a cycle of vibration repeats itself within a second is the frequency of vibration. When a tone contains a single frequency, it is called a *pure tone*.

■ *Simple harmonic motion* results in a tone of single frequency that repeats itself. Simple harmonic motion also is called *sinusoidal motion*. A graphical representation of a sinusoidal motion is called a *sine wave*.

■ A *complex tone* is created when two or more sounds of differing frequencies are added. The vibrations that make up a complex tone are *periodic* or *aperiodic*. When waves repeat themselves at regular and predictable intervals, they are said to be periodic. When the vibratory patterns are random and the next pattern cannot be predicted from the previous pattern, they are said to be aperiodic. Although it is not always the case, aperiodic waves are equated with noise.

■ It is important to realize that sound waves only imply motion; there is no physical movement of matter. What moves (actually, gets transferred) is energy. Sound is propagated because of the to-and-fro movements of molecules. During these movements, there is a time when the molecules are pressed together *(compression)* and a time when they move apart *(rarefaction)*. Thus, only the molecules swing back and forth to create a wave of disturbance the human ear may detect as sound.

■ The amount of molecular displacement per unit of time is measured in terms of *velocity*. A change in velocity is described as *acceleration* or *deceleration*. Acceleration also is related to direction of movement; when direction changes, velocity also changes.

■ Vibratory motion has two important but independent characteristics that create distinctly different auditory sensation: frequency and amplitude.

Frequency and Pitch

■ *Frequency* is a measure of the number of cycles per second or Hz. A single cycle (or 1 Hz) consists of one instance of compression and one instance of rarefaction within a second.

■ A related measure is called a *period*, which is the amount of time needed for a cycle to be completed. The frequency of vibration is a function of the properties of the vibrating object. For instance, the frequency of vibration of a tuning fork is determined by its metallic density and length. The air molecules vibrate at the same rate as the vibrating object (Speaks, 1999).

■ The medium that transmits the sound does not affect the frequency of sound. However, it does affect the speed of sound. A more dense medium will retard the speed of sound transmission more than a less dense medium, which will propagate sound faster.

- However, a more elastic medium (even if it is more dense) will propagate sound faster than a less elastic (even if it is less dense) medium. Therefore, steel, which is more dense but also more elastic than air, will transmit sound faster than air, which is less dense but also much less elastic than steel.

- Variations in the frequency of vibration create variations in sensation we call pitch. Thus, *pitch* is a sensory (perceptual) experience related to changes in frequency, a physical event. A sound of higher frequency is perceived as a sound of higher pitch than a sound of lower frequency.

- The human ear is not sensitive to all frequencies of sound. The normal ear of a young adult can respond to 20 Hz to 20,000 Hz. The human ear is more sensitive to changes in lower frequencies (below 1,000 Hz) than in higher frequencies.

Amplitude and Loudness

- *Amplitude,* the second important characteristic of vibratory motion, is a measure of the *magnitude* (intensity, strength) of the sound signal. In most cases, a measure of amplitude refers to sound pressure.

- Measured in dynes or newtons, sound pressure is the amount of force per unit area. Amplitude is the extent of molecular displacement; the greater the degree of molecular displacement, the higher the amplitude or intensity of sound.

- While amplitude, intensity, magnitude, and strength of a sound signal are physical concepts, loudness is a sensory concept. *Loudness* is a sensation related to physical amplitude or intensity of the sound. The higher the amplitude of a sound, the greater the perceived loudness of that sound.

- The human ear is sensitive to a wide range of sound intensity, perhaps 10 trillion units of intensity on a linear scale. Measuring this wide range presents a cumbersome problem; therefore, a logarithmic scale is used to express the intensity range to which the human ear is sensitive. On this scale, the ear is sensitive to 130 units called *decibels* (dB). As mentioned earlier, a decibel is one tenth of a *bel,* a unit of measure named after Alexander Graham Bell.

C O N C E P T S   T O   C O N S I D E R

Distinguish between the concepts of *frequency* and *amplitude* as physical phenomena. Relate them to their corresponding psychological or perceptual experiences.

_____

_____

_____

_____

_____

Sound Pressure Level and Hearing Level

■ Instead of describing intensity, one can measure the pressure of sound. Therefore, intensity of a sound is expressed in terms of decibels at a certain *sound pressure level* (dB SPL). Sound pressure is the square root of *power*, which is measured in *watts*. The pressure itself is measured in terms of *pascals* (pa).

■ Sound should reach a certain minimum intensity to stimulate the human auditory system. This minimum level is called the *hearing level* (HL). Sounds of different frequencies need to reach different minimum levels before they stimulate the human ear.

■ For example, sounds of 1,000 to 4,000 Hz can stimulate the auditory system at lower intensities than those at other frequencies. This differential sensitivity of the ear to different frequencies creates problems in the measurement of hearing and hearing loss. This problem has been solved by arbitrarily setting the minimum sound pressure level required to stimulate the auditory system at zero for all frequencies. This minimum level is known as the 0 dB hearing level.

■ Loudness or intensity of speech also is measured in terms of dB SPL. Intensity of normal conversational speech varies between 50 and 70 dB SPL. Very intense sounds exceed 100 dB SPL and may induce pain.

Introduction to the Acoustic Analysis of Speech

The following information is adapted from Case (2002), Nicolosi, Harryman, and Kresheck (2004), Martin and Clark (2003), and Kent and Read (2002).

■ There are several basic techniques for acoustic recording and analysis of speech. Older methods include nondigital or analog methods. Newer methods include DSP (digital signal processing) techniques.

■ The *sound spectrograph* is an electronic instrument that graphically records the changing intensity levels of the frequency components in a complex sound wave. The display of the running short-term spectrum is referred to as a *spectrogram*.

■ When a sound spectrograph is used to create a spectrogram, the complete process happens as follows (Kent & Read, 2002, pp. 58–59):

1. The person speaks into a microphone, which transduces the speech sample so that air pressure variations of the acoustic signal are put into the form of voltage variations
⬇
2. Then, the electrical signal is converted to an electromagnetic signal for storage on the magnetic drum of the spectrograph
⬇
3. The stored magnetic pattern is converted back into an electrical signal for analysis as a spectrogram
⬇
4. The signal is then filtered so that one can determine energy in various frequency regions
⬇

5. The current of the electrical signal is amplified and fed to a marking stylus

⬇

6. As the current flows from the stylus to the paper, there is localized burning of the paper. The burning produces a blackening of the paper in proportion to the current which is flowing through the stylus

■ The resulting spectrogram is a 3-dimensional display of time, intensity, and frequency. Frequency is plotted on the vertical axis, increasing from bottom to top. Intensity is represented on the "gray scale," or the blackness of the pattern. Time appears on the horizontal axis and proceeds from left to right.

■ Today, spectrograms are useful as a fundamental form of speech analysis; contemporary spectrograms are usually generated by computers. A powerful spectrographic instrument produced by Kay Elemetrics Corporation is the Digital Sona-Graph 5500, a DC-16 kHz Spectrum Analyzer that produces waveform displays of amplitude and frequency, spectrograms, fast Fourier transforms, and other analysis displays in real time. The same acoustic analyses are possible on the CSL (Computer Speech Laboratory), also manufactured by Kay Elemetrics Coporation; this has generally replaced the freestanding sonograph.

■ One component of speech displayed on a spectrogram is fundamental frequency. *Fundamental frequency,* mentioned earlier, can be defined as the lowest component frequency of a periodic wave; it is the principal component of a sound wave, and has the greatest wavelength. Fundamental frequency can further be defined as the tone produced by the vibration of the vocal folds before the air reaches any cavities. It is the first harmonic.

■ In a periodic complex sound, all frequencies are can be characterized as whole-number multiples of the fundamental frequency. These tones, called *harmonics* or overtones, occur over the fundamental frequency.

■ In terms of acoustic analysis, vowels are generally easier to analyze acoustically than consonants. In a normal speaker who has no vocal pathology, vowels are associated with a steady-state acoustic pattern and a steady-state articulatory configuration. In addition, vowels are often described very simply according to the frequencies of the first three formants (F1, F2, and F3 frequencies).

■ When extraneous factors such as suprasegmentals are controlled, the fundamental frequency of vowels varies with their height. On average, high vowels have a higher fundamental frequency than low vowels. For example, /i/ has a higher fundamental frequency than /ɑ/.

■ A very general rule in relating vowel articulation to vowel formant frequencies is that F1 varies mostly as a result of tongue height, and F2 varies mostly as a result of tongue advancement (variation in the anterior-to-posterior position of the tongue in the oral cavity).

■ All vowels can be described with basically the same acoustic characteristics, such as formant pattern or duration. Consonants are more complex. They are analyzed according to parameters such as voice onset time, formant transition (when a vowel follows the consonant), turbulent airflow (in the case of fricatives), and others.

■ *Voice onset time* refers to the time between the release of the stop consonant (e.g., /k/) and the beginning of the vowel. It can be further described as the time required to initiate sound at the vocal fold level. *Voice termination time* refers to the time required to cease vocal activity.

SUMMARY

✓ Sound, the result of vibrations of an elastic object, exists both as a physical phenomenon and as a sensory experience.

✓ Physically, sound is a compressional wave; psychologically, it is a compressional wave that produces a sensation.

✓ The frequency of sound is measured by the number of cycles per second or Hz. The intensity of sound is expressed in units called decibels.

✓ The acoustic analysis of speech is generally conducted through use of a sound spectrograph, which produces a spectrogram. The spectrogram displays various components such as fundamental frequency and many other characteristics of vowels and consonants.

◆ **PHONETICS IS THE STUDY** of speech sounds. The key categories of phonetics include acoustic, articulatory/physiological, auditory, applied, experimental, and descriptive phonetics. This chapter focuses on acoustic and articulatory/physiological phonetics.

◆ **BECAUSE A SOUND CAN** be represented visually in many different ways, the International Phonetic Alphabet, or IPA, was developed. The IPA is a set of internationally used phonetic symbols of vowels and consonants. Phonetic transcription of sounds can be broad, reflecting only vowels and consonants, or narrow, reflecting more detail about an individual speaker's sound production.

◆ **SPEECH SOUNDS CAN BE** broadly classified as consonants or vowels, which are described by their role in the production and perception of syllables. Syllables are motor units composed of an onset, a nucleus, and a coda.

◆ **SPEECH SOUNDS CAN BE** more narrowly classified according to two major approaches. The distinctive feature approach describes each phoneme according to a cluster of features that are either present (+) or absent (–) in that phoneme. The place-voice-manner approach describes consonants according to place and manner of articulation as well as voicing.

◆ **SOUNDS, OR PHONEMES, ARE** usually produced within the context of conversational speech. Within that context, sounds influence each other through adaptation, assimilation, and co-articulation. Running speech is given variety and meaning through suprasegmentals such as length of sounds, stress, rate of speech, pitch, loudness, and juncture.

◆ **ACOUSTICS, A BRANCH OF** physics, is the study of sound as a physical phenomenon. Psycho-acoustics is the study of how humans respond to sound as a physical phenomenon. Physically, sound is a compressional wave; psychologically, it is a compressional wave that produces a sensation. Sound exists both as a physical phenomenon and as a sensory experience.

◆ **SOUND IS THE RESULT** of vibrations of an elastic object. It is propagated through waves of disturbances in molecules. A vibrating object is the source of sound, and media such as air, gas, water, and metal can transmit sound. Mass (density) and elasticity are two main properties of the medium that affect the transmission of sound.

CHAPTER HIGHLIGHTS

◆ **VIBRATIONS REPEAT THEMSELVES** (in frequencies, cycles, or hertz). Pure tones contain a single frequency and are the result of simple harmonic motion, also known as a sine wave or sinusoidal motion. Complex tones are a combination of two or more sounds of differing frequencies.

◆ **PITCH IS A SENSORY** (perceptual) experience related to physical changes in frequency. The normal ear of a young adult can respond to frequencies within the range of 20 Hz to 20,000 Hz. Loudness is a sensation related to physical amplitude or intensity of sound. Amplitude is measured in dynes or newtons. Intensity is often expressed in terms of decibels at a certain sound pressure level. A decibel is one tenth of a bel, a basic unit of measure.

◆ **THE MINIMUM INTENSITY OF** sound needed to stimulate the human auditory system, called the hearing level, differs for different frequencies. However, on all audiometers, the minimum required to stimulate the human ear is arbitrarily set at 0 dB for all frequencies. The intensity of normal conversational speech varies between 50 and 70 dB SPL.

✎ **ADD YOUR OWN CHAPTER HIGHLIGHTS HERE:**

Study & Review Questions

Essay

1. Compare and contrast the distinctive feature approach and the place-voice-manner approach to classifying sounds. How do the two approaches differ?

2. Briefly define the terms *stress, pitch, volume,* and *juncture.*

3. Describe /m/, /s/, and /l/ according to the place-voice-manner approach.

4. Describe /r/, /g/, and /n/ according to the distinctive feature approach.

5. Define the term *fundamental frequency.*

Multiple Choice

6. The "typical" speaker of Standard American English would produce the word *emancipation* as:

   A. /ɪmɑnsʌpeʃʌn/
   B. /imɑnsʌpeɪʃən/
   C. /imænsəpeɪʃən/
   D. /ɪmʌnsʌpeʃʌn/
   E. /ɪmænsʌpʃən/

7. The /r/ and /l/ sounds may both be categorized as:

   A. rhotics.
   B. glides.
   C. laterals.
   D. liquids.
   E. retroflexes.

8. A semivowel that can be categorized as a voiced bilabial glide that is +anterior and +continuant is the:

   A. /j/
   B. /w/
   C. /ʃ/
   D. /r/
   E. /h/

9. The term *coarticulation* refers to:

   A. speech sounds being modified due to the influence of adjacent sounds to the point that there are perceptible changes in sounds.
   B. the extent to which vocal tract configurations change shape during the production of consonants and vowels in running speech.

C.   vocal punctuation, or a combination of suprasegmentals such as intonation and pausing.

D.   the influence of various syllables upon one another when a client recites a phonetically balanced list of words.

E.   the influence of one phoneme upon another in production and perception wherein two different articulators move simultaneously to produce two different speech sounds.

10. Broad phonemic transcription involves:

A.   the use of IPA symbols to transcribe phonemes by enclosing them within slash marks (e.g., /f/).

B.   the use of diacritical markers to transcribe phonemes by enclosing them within slash marks (e.g., /f/).

C.   the transcription of allophones by placing them within brackets (e.g., [f]).

D.   the transcription of allophones by the use of diacritical markers.

E.   the use of orthographic symbols to transcribe phonemes by enclosing them within slash marks (e.g., /r/).

11. If a speaker said, "I just love 'em and leave 'em," the phrase "leave 'em" could be transcribed as:

A.   [liv um]

B.   [lev] [em]

C.   /liv uhm/

D.   /liv m̩/

E.   /lev m/

12. The two properties of a medium that affect sound transmission are:

A.   amplitude and intensity.

B.   mass and elasticity.

C.   compression and rarefaction.

D.   pressure and force.

E.   elasticity and compression.

13. A sinusoidal wave is a sound wave:

A.   with horizontal and vertical symmetry.

B.   with one peak and one valley.

C.   with a single frequency.

D.   that is a result of simple harmonic motion.

E.   all of the above.

14. A natural frequency is a frequency:

I. with which a source of sound vibrates naturally.

II. that is affected by the mass and stiffness of the vibrating body.

III. that is the center frequency of a formant.

IV. that is the first harmonic.

V. that is the lowest frequency of a periodic wave.

A.   I, II

B.   I, III, V

C.   I, IV, V

D.   II, III

E.   All of the above

15. An octave is:

A.   the amount of molecular displacement per unit of time.

B.   the amount of time between cycles.

C. an indication of interval between two frequencies.
D. a measure of the magnitude (intensity, strength) of the sound signal.
E. the unit of measure for frequency; it is the same as the cycle per second.

16. The to-and-fro movement of air molecules because of a vibrating object is referred to as:

A. oscillation.
B. amplitude.
C. velocity.
D. displacement.
E. rarefaction.

17. The lowest frequency of a periodic wave is also known as:

A. the fundamental frequency or second harmonic.
B. the fundamental frequency or first harmonic.
C. the formant frequency or first harmonic.
D. the first octave or the fundamental frequency.
E. the second octave or the first harmonic.

18. When two or more sounds of differing frequencies are added, the result is a:

A. complex tone; the vibrations that make up this complex tone may be said to be periodic or aperiodic.
B. complex tone; the vibrations are always periodic, where waves repeat themselves at regular intervals.
C. pure tone, where the vibrations are usually periodic.
D. pure tone, where the vibrations are always aperiodic.
E. complex tone; the vibrations are usually aperiodic, where the vibratory patterns are random and the next pattern cannot be predicted from the previous pattern.

19. When a speaker is producing a vowel and the vowel is being acoustically analyzed, one can state as a general rule that:

A. F2 varies mostly as a result of tongue height, and F1 varies mostly as a result of tongue advancement (variation in the anterior-to-posterior position of the tongue in the oral cavity).
B. F2 varies mostly as a result of tongue height, and F3 varies mostly as a result of tongue advancement (variation in the anterior-to-posterior position of the tongue in the oral cavity).
C. F1 varies mostly as a result of tongue height, and F3 varies mostly as a result of tongue advancement (variation in the anterior-to-posterior position of the tongue in the oral cavity).
D. F1 varies mostly as a result of tongue height, and F2 varies mostly as a result of tongue advancement (variation in the anterior-to-posterior position of the tongue in the oral cavity).
E. F3 varies mostly as a result of tongue height, and F2 varies mostly as a result of tongue advancement (variation in the anterior-to-posterior position of the tongue in the oral cavity).

20. In a periodic complex sound, tones that occur over the fundamental frequency and can be characterized as whole-number multiples of the fundamental frequency are called:

A. complex sinusoidal wave forms.
B. autocorrelational periodic wave forms.
C. multiple bandwidths.
D. tonal configuration forms.
E. harmonics.

REFERENCES AND RECOMMENDED READINGS

Bleile, K. M. (1996). *Articulation and phonological disorders: A book of exercises* (2nd ed.). San Diego, CA: Singular Publishing Group.

Bloom, L., & Lahey, M. (1978). *Language development and disorders.* New York: Macmillan.

Borden, G. J., Harris, K. S., & Raphael, L. J. (2003). *Speech science primer: Physiology, acoustics, and perception of speech* (4th ed.). Baltimore: Lippincott Williams & Wilkins.

Case, J. L. (2002). *Clinical management of voice disorders* (4th ed.). Austin, TX: PRO-ED.

Chomsky, N., & Halle, M. (1968). *The sound pattern of English.* New York: Harper & Row.

Creaghead, N. A., Newman, P. W., & Secord, W. A. (1989). *Assessment and remediation of articulatory and phonological disorders* (2nd ed.). Columbus, OH: Merrill Publishing Company.

Decker, T. N., & Carrell, T. (2004). *Instrumentation: An introduction for students in the speech and hearing sciences* (3rd ed.). Mahwah, NJ: Lawrence Erlbaum Associates.

Edwards, H. T. (2003). *Applied phonetics: The sounds of American English* (3rd ed.). Albany, NY: Delmar Learning.

Jakobson, R., Fant, G., & Halle, M. (1952). *Preliminaries to speech analysis* (2nd ed.). Cambridge, MA: MIT Press.

Kent, R. (1998). *The speech sciences.* Albany, NY: Delmar Learning.

Kent, R. (2004). Normal aspects of articulation. In J. E. Bernthal & N. W. Bankson, *Articulation and phonological disorders* (5th ed.,pp. 1–62). Boston: Allyn & Bacon.

Kent, R. D., & Read, C. (2002). *Acoustic analysis of speech* (2nd ed.). Albany, NY: Delmar Learning.

Lowe, R. J. (1994). *Phonology: Assessment and intervention applications in speech pathology.* Baltimore: Williams & Wilkins.

Martin, F. N., & Clark, J. G. (2003). *Introduction to audiology* (8th ed.). Boston: Allyn & Bacon.

Mullin, W. J., Gerace, W. J., Mestre, J. P., & Velleman, S. L. (2003). *Fundamentals of sound with applications to speech and hearing.* Boston: Allyn & Bacon.

Nicolosi, L., Harryman, E., & Kresheck, J. (2004). *Terminology of communication disorders: Speech-language-hearing* (5th ed.). Baltimore: Lippincott Williams & Wilkins.

Ohde, R. N., & Sharf, D. J. (1992). *Phonetic analysis of normal and abnormal speech.* New York: Merrill.

Peña-Brooks, A., & Hegde, M. N. (2000). *Articulatory and phonological disorders in children: A dual level text.* Austin, TX: PRO-ED.

Pickett, J. M. (1999). *The acoustics of speech communication: Fundamentals, speech perception theory, and technology.* Boston: Allyn & Bacon.

Shriberg, L. D., & Kent, R. D. (2003). *Clinical phonetics* (3rd ed.). Boston: Allyn & Bacon.

Small, L. H. (2005). *Fundamentals of phonetics: A practical guide for students* (2nd ed.). Boston: Allyn & Bacon.

Speaks, C. E. (1999). *Introduction to sound* (3rd ed.). Albany, NY: Delmar Learning.

Yavas, M. (1998). *Phonology: Development and disorders.* San Diego, CA: Singular Publishing Group.

Study & Review
Answers

6. C. The "typical" speaker of Standard American English would produce the word "emancipation" as: /imænsəpeɪʃən/

7. D. The /r/ and /l/ sounds may both be categorized as liquids.

8. B. The /w/ sound is a semivowel that can be categorized as a voiced bilabial glide that is +anterior and +continuant.

9. E. Coarticulation is specifically defined as the influence of one phoneme upon another in production and perception, wherein two different articulators move simultaneously to produce two different speech sounds.

10. A. Broad phonemic transcription involves use of IPA symbols to transcribe phonemes by enclosing them within slash marks.

11. D. If a speaker said, "I just love 'em and leave 'em," the phrase "leave 'em" could be transcribed as /liv m̩/.

12. B. The two properties of a medium that affect sound transmission are mass and elasticity.

13. E. A sinusoidal wave is a sound wave with horizontal and vertical symmetry. It contains one peak or crest and one valley or trough. It contains a single frequency and is a result of simple harmonic motion.

14. A. A natural frequency is a frequency with which a source of sound vibrates naturally and that is affected by the mass and stiffness of the vibrating body.

15. C. An octave is an indication of the interval between two frequencies.

16. A. The to-and-fro movement of air molecules because of a vibrating object is referred to as oscillation.

17. B. The lowest frequency of a periodic wave is also known as the fundamental frequency or first harmonic.

18. A. When two or more sounds of differing frequencies are added, the result is a complex tone; the vibrations that make up this complex tone may be said to be periodic or aperiodic.

19. D. F1 varies mostly as a result of tongue height, and F2 varies mostly as a result of tongue advancement (variation in the anterior-to-posterior position of the tongue in the oral cavity).

20. E. In a periodic complex sound, tones that occur over the fundamental frequency and can be characterized as whole-number multiples of the fundamental frequency are called harmonics.

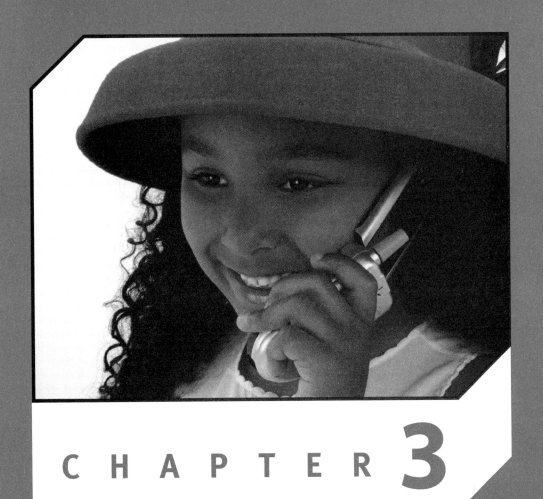

CHAPTER 3

LANGUAGE

DEVELOPMENT

IN CHILDREN

It is language that makes people so efficient

at communication. It is language that provides people with a mechanism for social interaction and communication with one another. As societies have become more complex, organized, and interrelated, the ability to communicate effectively through language has become increasingly important. Good language skills are now crucial for even mundane occupational success or survival as vocations have become more sophisticated and interrelated.

A *language* can be defined as a form of social behavior shaped and maintained by a verbal community. It can also be viewed as a system of symbols used to represent concepts that are formed through exposure and experience (Bloom & Lahey, 1978). Reed (2005) says that "language is a code in which we make specific symbols stand for something else" (p. 2). For example, the word "cookie" is a symbol for something sweet, small, and usually round that children and adults like to eat for dessert. When children learn language, they learn words, or symbols that represent concepts.

In order to understand what constitutes language disorders in children, it is necessary to first understand normal language development. In this chapter, we discuss (a) basic definitions of aspects of language, (b) normal language development milestones, and (c) theories of language development.

TERMS AND DEFINITIONS

INTRODUCTION

There are various approaches to the study of language. The behavioral approach, which will be described in a later section, views language as verbal behavior. The linguistic approach describes different components of language.

Linguistics is the study of language, its structure, and the rules that govern its structure. Linguists, specialists in linguistics, have traditionally described several components of language. These include morphology, syntax, semantics, pragmatics, and phonology. Phonology is described in Chapter 5.

Morphology

- *Morphology* is the study of word structure. It describes how words are formed out of more basic elements of language called morphemes.

- A *morpheme* is the smallest meaningful unit of a language. Morphemes are considered minimal because if they were subdivided any further, they would become meaningless. Each morpheme is different from the others because each signals a distinct meaning. Morphemes are used to form words.

- *Base, root,* or *free* morphemes are words that have meaning, cannot be broken down into smaller parts, and can have other morphemes added to them. Examples of free morphemes are: *ocean, establish, book, color, connect,* and *hinge.* These words mean something, can stand by themselves, and cannot be broken down into smaller units.

- These words can have other morphemes added to them. *Bound* or *grammatic morphemes,* which cannot convey meaning by themselves, must be joined with free morphemes in order to have meaning.

- In the following examples, the free morphemes are underlined; the bound morphemes are in capital letters:

  <u>ocean</u>S   <u>establish</u>MENT   DIS<u>connect</u>   <u>color</u>FUL   UN<u>hinge</u>

- Common bound or grammatic morphemes include the following:

  –ing, the present progressive (cook*ing,* writ*ing*)
  –s, the regular plural morpheme (cat*s,* basket*s*)
  –s, the possessive inflection (man*'s,* lady*'s*)
  –ed, the regular past tense (comb*ed,* wash*ed*)

- Bound morphemes can be divided into the subcategories of prefixes and suffixes. A *prefix* is added at the beginning of a base morpheme; a *suffix* is added at the end of a base morpheme. For example:

Whole Word	Prefix	Base Word	Suffix
prearranged	pre	arrange	ed
disestablishment	dis	establish	ment
misunderstanding	mis	understand	ing

- *Allomorphs* are variations of morphemes; they do not alter the original meaning of the morpheme. For example, the plural morpheme can be denoted by the following allomorphs (with their sounds in parentheses): box*es* (ez), leav*es* (z), cat*s* (s).

- Morphemes are a means of modifying word structures to change meaning. The morphology of a given language describes the rules of such modifications. It describes what kinds of morphemic combinations are permissible in a given language.

- Speakers arrange morphemes so that they can change the m
  one can change "He cooks a meal" to "He cooked a meal"
  pheme and omitting the third-person singular -s, the sp

- Sentence meaning is also conveyed by the order of th
  tated by the rules of syntax.

Syntax

- Syntax and morphology constitute the two major categories of langu
  ogy is the study of word structure; syntax is the study of sentence structure.
  of the word *syntax* is to join, to put together.

- In the study of language, syntax involves:

  - the arrangement of words to form meaningful sentences
  - word order and overall structure of a sentence
  - a collection of rules that specify the ways and order in which words may be combined to
    form sentences in a particular language

- The syntactic rules of languages differ from one another. For example, in English, one might
  use the phrase "the new car." In Spanish, one might say *"el carro nuevo"* ("the car new"). All
  languages are creative, and speakers can generate an infinite variety of structures.

- Structures, however, are governed by rules of syntax. Normal speakers of a language do
  not produce structures with random and meaningless word order. For example, an English
  speaker could say, "He said he was going to come but didn't." Due to syntactic rules, a speaker
  could not say, "He going to was said he didn't but come."

- Sentences can be classified according to their functions. For example:

  - *passive* sentences, in which the subject receives the action of the verb ("The puppy was pet-
    ted by Mike.")
  - *active* sentences, in which the subject performs the actions of the verb ("Mike petted the
    puppy.")
  - *interrogatives* or questions ("Did you see that gorgeous sunset?")
  - *declaratives,* which make statements ("The sunset was gorgeous.")
  - *imperatives,* which state commands ("Shut the door.")
  - *exclamatory* sentences, which express strong feeling ("I never said that!")

- As they mature in syntactic development, children begin to use *compound* and *complex* sentences, which can be defined as follows:

  - A *compound sentence* contains two or more *independent clauses* joined by a comma and a
    conjunction or by a semicolon. There are no subordinate clauses in a compound sentence.
    A *clause* contains a subject and a predicate. An *independent* or *main clause* has a subject
    and predicate and can stand alone. For example:

The officer waved his hands,	and	the cars stopped.
(independent clause)	*(conjunction)*	*(independent clause)*

The bird sang in the tree;   later it flew away.
(independent clause + semicolon)   *(independent clause)*

- A *complex sentence* contains one independent clause and one or more *dependent* or *subordinate clauses*. A dependent or subordinate clause has a subject and predicate but cannot stand alone. For example:

I will be at the station   if it doesn't rain.
(independent clause)   *(dependent clause)*

You can have the lollipop   after you take a bath.
(independent clause)   *(dependent clause)*

- Languages have different syntactic structures. In English, the basic syntactic structure is subject + verb + object. This structure, usually called the *kernel sentence,* can also be called the *phrase structure* or *base structure.*

CONCEPTS TO CONSIDER

Briefly define the terms *morphology* and *syntax*. What do these terms mean?

_____

_____

_____

_____

_____

Semantics

- Semantics is the study of *meaning* in a language. The semantic component is the meaning conveyed by words, phrases, and sentences.

- Semantics involves a person's *vocabulary* or lexicon. Vocabulary development depends heavily upon environmental exposure as well as the individual capacity each child brings to the learning situation.

- Important aspects of vocabulary development include knowledge of:

    - antonyms or opposites (e.g., *big–little*)
    - synonyms or words that mean similar things (e.g., *attractive–pretty; clear–transparent*)
    - multiple meanings of words (e.g., *rock, pound*)
    - humor (e.g., riddles, puns, jokes)

- figurative language, including
  — metaphors (*He's drowning in money.*)
  — idioms (*It's raining cats and dogs; She kicked the bucket.*)
  — proverbs (*Don't put all your eggs in one basket.*)

- deictic words, or words whose referents change depending on who is speaking (e.g., *this, here, that, come, go*)

■ *Semantic categories* are used to sort words. Examples of a few of these categories are *recurrence* (concept of *more*), *rejection* (*no*), and *causality* (*cause and effect*). A child using recurrence might say, "More milk"; if that child didn't want any more, she might show rejection by saying, "No milk."

■ Most words in a child's first 50 spoken words refer to things that the child can act upon (e.g., toys, objects). Young children may use *overextension* (e.g., all round items are balls; all tall men with glasses are Daddy). They may also use *underextension* (e.g., only an Oreo is a cookie; only the family poodle is a dog while a neighbor's German shepherd is not a dog).

■ Word knowledge and world knowledge are components of semantics. *World knowledge* involves a person's autobiographical and experiential memory and understanding of particular events. For example, a child might be able to discuss an aquarium because he has been to several and has been exposed to marine life. Such a child could use words such as *octopus, jellyfish, seaweed,* and others because he has seen them and experienced them personally. He has world knowledge of these words.

■ *Word knowlege* is primarily verbal and contains word and symbol definitions. For example, the child mentioned above might be able to name the planets in the solar system because he has learned them in kindergarten. He has not visited these planets, obviously, but he has seen pictures of them and has memorized their names. He has word knowledge of the planets.

■ A child's word knowledge depends heavily upon his or her world knowledge. For example, a child who has never visited a zoo or been exposed to books about a zoo (world knowledge) might have difficulty understanding and using the word *zoo* (word knowledge).

■ An important concept emphasized today in semantics is called *quick incidental learning* or *fast mapping.* This refers to children's ability to learn a new word on the basis of just a few exposures to it. Normal children use fast mapping to rapidly expand their vocabularies.

■ Another important semantic aspect of children's language development is developing the ability to categorize words. For example, children must learn that *tiger, lion, dog, cat, pig,* and *horse* fall under the category of *animals.*

■ The use of categories helps bring order to the child's experiences. The child who successfully categorizes does not need to treat each experience as a totally new one. New experiences may be "filed" under preexisting categories, or under mental constructs of the child that allow him or her to group similar items together.

Pragmatics

■ *Pragmatics* is the study of rules that govern the use of language in social situations. In pragmatics, one focuses on use of language in context. Pragmatics places greater emphasis on *functions,* or uses of language, than on structure.

■ One can view pragmatics as the dimension of language that considers the *context* of the utterance (i.e., the situation, the listener-speaker relationship) and the *function* of the utterance (i.e., its purpose or goal).

■ *Functions of language* (described in more detail later) include:

- *labeling* (naming something; e.g., a child is playing with a puppy and says "tail")
- *protesting* (objecting to something; e.g., "Don't do that!")
- *commenting* (describing or identifying objects; e.g., "That's a cookie.")

■ Important functions of utterances include:

- providing listeners with adequate information without redundancy
- making the sequence of statements coherent and logical
- taking turns with other speakers
- maintaining a topic
- repairing communication breakdowns

■ Language context involves:

- where the utterance takes place
- to whom the utterance is directed
- what and who are present at the time

■ Children with effective pragmatic skills display adequate *cohesion,* or the ability to order and organize utterances in a message so that they build logically on one another.

■ As they get older, children with effective pragmatic skills distinguish between and appropriately use *direct* and *indirect speech acts or requests.* For example, as a direct speech act or request, a child could say, "Bring me the ball." As an indirect speech act or request, the child could say, "Will you bring me the ball?" Or the child might say "Wouldn't it be nice if I had the ball?"

■ Indirect speech acts or requests are used to convey politeness. By the time a child is 6 years old, she can respond to many forms of indirect requests (Hulit & Howard, 2002). She can also use indirect requests if she chooses to.

■ Pragmatic skills also involve the appropriate knowledge and use of discourse. *Discourse* refers to how utterances are related to one another; it has to do with the connected flow of language. Discourse can involve a monologue, a dialogue, or even conversational exchange in a small group. When people talk with one another, they are engaging in discourse.

■ *Narratives* are a form of discourse in which the speaker tells a story. The speaker talks about a logical sequence of events. This sequence can involve an actual episode from the speaker's life, such as a trip he or she took; or it can involve a story about an event (such as a fairy tale or movie) that did not happen to the speaker directly.

■ Pragmatics is heavily influenced by culture (Roseberry-McKibbin, 2007). For example, in Japanese culture, the use of indirect speech acts is believed to convey speaker sophistication and sensitivity. In American culture, people who use many indirect speech acts may be viewed as weak, unassertive, and unsure of themselves.

■ Pragmatic skills are increasingly recognized as important for social, academic, and vocational success. Effective pragmatic skills enable speakers to relate successfully to others within their linguistic and cultural milieu.

SUMMARY

✓ The linguistic approach analyzes language according to five components: morphology, syntax, semantics, pragmatics, and phonology. In this section, we have discussed the first four components.

✓ Morphology involves the study of word structure. Syntax includes rules for word order and rules for combining words into sentences.

✓ Semantics involves word meanings. A child's semantic skills refer to his vocabulary skills, which are influenced by word and world knowledge.

✓ Pragmatics are the social skills of language—how, where, when, and with whom language is used.

NORMAL LANGUAGE DEVELOPMENT: DEVELOPMENTAL MILESTONES

INTRODUCTION

The development of language rests upon several major variables that interact with one another. First, the individual child brings innate characteristics to the situation. Such characteristics may include a high IQ or a limited attention span. Second, the child's environment, including the caregivers in that environment, plays a major role. The more stimulating the environment, the better and faster children develop language skills. Language development also depends on cultural expectations. In some cultures, children are to be seen and not heard; those children may develop good visual skills, but their verbal skills may not develop at a rate expected by mainstream American professionals.

In this section, we describe language development milestones that represent a range of expectations for when children may develop certain language structures. These milestones depend heavily on the child's linguistic and cultural background; cultures differ in their expectations for children's language development. This section focuses on the role of the caretaker and on semantic, syntactic, morphological, and pragmatic development as consistent with general mainstream American social expectations. Development in the school years is briefly addressed. Chapter 5 contains detailed information about phonological development.

Role of the Caregiver in Language Development

■ Experts consistently cite the crucial role of a child's caregiver in language development, particularly in the early years before school (Bernstein & Levey, 2002; Hulit & Howard, 2002; Owens, 2005; Reed, 2005). Caregivers can be persons such as the child's mother, father, grandparents, older siblings, day care providers, and others. In the United States, in a child's very early months, often the primary caregiver is the mother.

- Ideally, a baby's mother or primary caregiver specifically gears communication for him by use of motherese. *Motherese* refers to speech that includes several characteristics that help babies attend and respond to what they are hearing.

- First, in motherese, utterances are produced with a higher pitch and greater pitch fluctuations. Babies tend to pay more attention to utterances that are higher pitched and that show variation. Utterances are also produced at a slower rate than normal speech, and are usually clear and fluent.

- In addition, motherese is characterized by simpler utterances, longer pauses between utterances, and shorter utterances. Words used generally refer to events or objects in the here and now (McLaughlin, 1998).

- Infants and young children also learn early turn-taking skills through interactions with their caregivers. Games such as peek-a-boo and pat-a-cake help infants learn rudimentary turn-taking skills that serve as the foundation of later conversational turn-taking. Even babies who are only 3 months old begin to produce more speechlike sounds if an adult responds to their vocalizations (Sachs, 2001).

- Eye contact is another important form of communication that begins in infancy. Research documents that parents have more difficulty relating to children who are blind or who have autism, and thus avoid eye contact.

- If a baby cries and the caretaker responds immediately, this increases the baby's motivation to communicate. Motivated babies attempt more varied and frequent interactions (Berko Gleason, 2005).

- A child's language development is highly dependent on the quality of her interaction with her caregivers. High-quality interaction that begins in infancy helps children to develop language faster; frequently these children's language shows early signs of sophistication. Conversely, children who are ignored or punished when they attempt to communicate may show delays, or slowness in developing language skills.

Birth to 1 Year

The following developmental milestones are observed in normally developing children from birth to 1 year of age.

Birth to 3 Months

The child:

- displays startle response to loud sound.
- visually tracks, or moves eyes, to source of sound.
- attends to and turns head toward voice; turns toward sound source.
- smiles reflexively.
- quiets when picked up.
- ceases activity or coos back when person talks (by 2 months).

4–6 Months

The child:

- responds by raising arms when mother says, "Come here," and reaches toward child (by 6 months).
- moves or looks toward family members when they are named (e.g., "Where's Daddy?").
- explores the vocal mechanism through vocal play such as growling, squealing, yelling, making "raspberries" (bilabial trills).
- begins to produce adult-like vowels.
- begins marginal babbling; produces double syllables (e.g., "baba"), puts lips together for /m/.

7–9 Months

The child:

- looks at some common objects when their names are spoken.
- comprehends "no."
- begins to use some gestural language; plays pat-a-cake, peek-a-boo; shakes head for "no."
- uses a wide variety of sound combinations.
- uses inflected vocal play, intonation patterns.
- imitates intonation and speech sounds of others (by 9 months).
- begins variegated babbling (e.g., "mabamaba") (at approximately 9 months).
- uncovers hidden toy (beginning of object permanence).

10–12 Months

The child:

- understands up to 10 words, such as *no, bye-bye, pat-a-cake, hot*; understands one simple direction like "sit down," especially when command is accompanied by gesture.
- begins to relate symbol and object; uses first true word.
- gives block, toy, or object upon request.
- understands and follows simple directions regarding body action.
- looks in correct place for hidden toys (object permanence).
- turns head instantly to own name.
- gestures or vocalizes to indicate wants and needs.
- jabbers loudly; uses wide variety of sounds and intonations; varies pitch when vocalizing.
- uses all consonant and vowel sounds in vocal play.

Pragmatics

As infants develop pragmatics skills, they typically go through the following stages:

- uses *perlocutionary behavior,* in which child's "signals" have an effect on the listener or observer but lack communicative intent. For example, if a child smiles reflexively, an observer may smile back or laugh, even though the child didn't intend to express pleasure or joy.
- at 9–10 months, uses *illocutionary behavior*—signals to carry out some socially organized action such as pointing and laughing; uses intentional communicaton.
- at approximately 12 months, enters *locutionary stage*—begins to use words.

- establishes *joint reference,* or the ability to focus attention on an event or object as directed by another person. (Caretakers begin by establishing eye contact in the early months; later, they point to or name objects that both they and the child can focus on.)

1–2 Years

The following developmental milestones are observed in normally developing children between 1 and 2 years of age.

Syntax

- The child uses one-word sentences, and is in the *holophrastic* single-word phase—one word represents a complex idea. For example, "Up" might mean "Please pick me up because I don't want to sit here playing with the dog anymore." Average MLU (mean length of utterance) is 1.0–2.0.
- The child uses sentence-like words; communicates relationships by using one word plus vocal and bodily cues. The sentence-like word can serve several basic functions:

  - The emphatic or imperative statement ("Car!") (child telling you to look at a car)
  - The question ("Car?") (child asking if that's a car)
  - The declarative statement ("Car.") (child saying it's a car and not something else)

- At approximately 18 months, some children begin to put two words together.
- The child may use three- or four-word responses at 2 years.
- Approximately 51% of the child's utterances consist of nouns.

Semantics

- As mentioned, the child uses *holophrastic* speech—one word is used to communicate a variety of meanings. The child uses 3–20 words and uses gestures. Around 18 months, the child produces 10–50 words.
- The child shows understanding of some words and simple commands; understands "no." Around 18 months, child understands about 200 words.
- The child's most frequent lexical categories are nominals (e.g., *ball, Mommy*) and verbs (e.g., *drink, run*).
- The child uses *semantic relations,* or utterances that reflect meaning based on relationships between different words (e.g., cause–effect relationships). The child begins with one-word utterances and gradually progresses to two-word utterances (see Table 3.1 and Table 3.2).
- The child also exhibits the following during this period:

  - Uses overextensions. For example, all brown-eyed, slender women are "Mommy."
  - Answers the question "What's this?" Responds to yes/no questions by nodding or shaking head.
  - Says "All gone" (emerging negation).
  - Follows one-step commands or simple directions accompanied by gestures (e.g., "Give Mommy the spoon.").
  - Follows directions using one or two spatial concepts such as *in* or *on* (19–24 months).

Table 3.1 RELATIONS EXPRESSED BY SINGLE-WORD UTTERANCES

Before children reach the two-word utterance stage, they typically use single words to express themselves. The relations expressed by single words are as follows:

Relation	Definition	Example
Attribution	An adjective; a property or characteristic of an event, person, or object	*Big* doggy *Clean* dolly Face *dirty*
Action	Child requests or labels an action; indicates movement relationships between objects and people	*Open* box Kitty *run* *Close* door
Locative action	Child refers to a change in an object's location	*There* doggy Ball *up*
Existence	Child is attending to item or object present in the immediate environment, especially a novel one	What's *that?* *This* kitty
Nonexistence or disappearance	An action or object is expected to be present but is not; something was present but disappeared	*All gone* juice *Bye bye* Mom *No* doggy
Denial	Child denies a statement or previous utterance (e.g., in response to a parent saying "Is this a kitty?")	*No* kitty
Rejection	Child does not want something to happen; child refuses an object or action	*No* bath *No* beans
Recurrence	An event happens again; an object reappears or replaces another	*More* cookie *Another* doggie
Possession	Child identifies something as belonging to him or her, or to another person	*His* block Doll *mine*

Note. Adapted from *An Introduction to Children with Language Disorders,* 3rd ed., by V. A. Reed, 2005, Boston: Allyn and Bacon. Adapted with permission.

- Points to one to five body parts on command; points to recognized objects (emerging nomination).
- Listens to simple stories; especially likes to hear stories repeated (19–24 months).
- Asks for "more."
- Refers to self with pronoun and name ("Me Johnny") (19–24 months).
- Verbalizes immediate experiences (e.g., "Bath hot!").
- Begins to use some verbs and adjectives.

Table 3.2 SEMANTIC RELATIONS EXPRESSED BY TWO-WORD UTTERANCES

Semantic Relation	Structure	Example
Notice	Hi + noun	Hi doggy
Nomination	Demonstrative + noun	That chair
Instrumental	Verb + noun	Cut [with scissors]
Conjunction	Noun + noun	Knife spoon
Recurrence	More + noun	More juice
Action-object	Verb + noun	Pet kitty
Action-indirect object	Verb + noun	Give [to] Mommy
Agent-action	Noun (agent) + verb	Doggy bark
Agent-object	Noun (agent) + noun	Baby [drink] juice
Possessor-possession	Noun (possessor) + noun	Mommy sock
Attribute-entity	Adjective/ attributive + noun	Red ball
Entity + locative	Noun + locative	Juice [in] glass
Action + locative	Verb + noun	Jump [on] bed

Pragmatics

- *Presuppositions* emerge. Between 1 and 2 years of age, the child uses expressions that have shared meaning for the listener and speaker.
- The child begins to understand some rules of dialogue (e.g., "When someone talks, you need to listen."). The child is able to take the role of both speaker and listener.
- The child uses nonverbal as well as verbal communication to signal intent. Halliday (1975) considered the listener's responses in describing the following seven functions of communicative intent that develop between 9 and 18 months of age:

  - *Imaginative.* Children pretend or do play-acting; they use language to create an environment; there is a communicative function ("Let's pretend"; child may vocalize to herself while playing with dolls).
  - *Heuristic.* Children attempt to have their environment and events in their environment explained to them; they organize and investigate the environment ("Tell me why." "What that?").
  - *Regulatory.* Children attempt to control the behavior of others ("Do as I tell you to do.").
  - *Personal.* Children express own feelings and attitudes (e.g., child says "yummy" as she licks a lollipop); self-awareness.

- *Informative.* Children can tell someone something, communicate experiences ("I have something to tell you.").
- *Instrumental.* Children attempt to get assistance, material things from others ("I want ball.").
- *Interactional.* Children initiate interactions with others ("Hi, Daddy.").

- Dore (1975) focused on the 12–24 month period in which children use early words to signal communicative intent, focusing more on children's intentions and less on listeners' reactions:

  - Practicing (language)
  - Protesting ("no" and resisting)
  - Greeting ("Hi, Grandma" as Grandma comes in door)
  - Calling/addressing ("Mommy")
  - Requesting action (says "juice" to get juice)
  - Requesting an answer ("Cow?")
  - Labeling (points out and names "hair," "eyes," etc., of a doll)
  - Repeating/imitating (overhears and repeats the word *cat*)
  - Answering (adult: "What's this?" child: "bottle")

2–3 Years

The following developmental milestones are observed in normally developing children between 2 and 3 years of age.

Syntax

The child:

- uses word combinations, has beginning phrase and sentence structure.
- has an average MLU of 2.0–4.0; at 36 months, sentences often average 3–4 words.
- combines 3–4 words in subject-verb-object format (e.g., "Daddy throw ball.").
- uses telegraphic speech; word order is often object-verb (e.g., "doggy sit"), verb-object (e.g., "push Barbie"), subject-verb. Most sentences are incomplete.
- asks wh- questions (e.g., "*What's* that?" "*When* go home?"), yes–no questions.
- expresses negation by adding "no" or "not" in front of verbs (e.g., "Me not do it," or "He no bite.").

Semantics

- Comprehension usually precedes production. At 30 months, the child comprehends up to 2,400 words.
- At 36 months, the child comprehends up to 3,600 words.
- Expressive vocabulary is 200–600 words; average is 425 words at 30 months.
- Meanings seem to be learned in sequence: objects, events, actions, adjectives, adverbs, spatial concepts, temporal (time) concepts.
- First pronouns used are self-referents such as *I* and *me*.

The child:

- answers simple wh- questions (e.g., "What runs?"); generally understands questions; begins asking wh- questions of adults (30 months).
- can identify simple body parts.
- carries out one- and two-part commands such as "Pick up the sock and give it to Mommy."
- understands plurals.
- can give simple account of experiences and tell understandable stories (36 months).

Morphology

The child's use of bound morphemes expands greatly between 2 and 3 years of age. The child:

- develops inflections such as -ing, spatial prepositions in and on, plurals, possessives, articles, and pronouns (see Table 3.3).
- develops simple, irregular past tense (e.g., went).
- develops copular were.
- develops is plus adjective (e.g., "That is pretty.").
- develops regular past-tense verbs (e.g., walked).
- overregularizes past-tense inflections (e.g., goed, throwed, falled).
- overgeneralizes plural morphemes (e.g., feets, mouses).
- uses some memorized contractions, such as don't, can't, it's, that's.

Pragmatics

- The child's utterances, although occasionally egocentric, generally have a communicative intent.
- The child demonstrates rapid topic shifts; a 3-year-old can sustain topic of conversation only about 20% of the time.
- Communication includes criticism, commands, requests, threats, questions, and answers.
- Interpersonal communication expands; the child learns to adopt a role to express his own opinions and personality.

3–4 Years

The following developmental milestones are observed in normally developing children between 3 and 4 years of age.

Syntax

The child:

- learns set of clause-connecting devices, including coordination (e.g., "and") and subordination (e.g., "because"), and uses them in sentences.
- begins using complex verb phrases (e.g., "I should have been able to do it.").
- begins using modal verbs (e.g., could, should, would).
- begins using tag questions (e.g., "You want to go, don't you?").

Table 3.3   AVERAGE ORDER OF ACQUISITION OF 14 GRAMMATIC MORPHEMES IN THREE CHILDREN

	Morphemes	Examples	Average MLU	Stage	Age of Mastery (months)
1	Present progressive –*ing*	Mom com*ing*, Dog bark*ing*	2.25	II	19–28
2/3	Prepositions *in, on*	Toy *in* box, Book *on* table	2.25	II	27–30
4	Regular plural inflection –*s*	My crayon*s*, Dog bone*s*	2.25	II	24–33
5	Irregular past-tense verbs	*Came, ran, sat, broke*	2.75	III	25–46
6	Possessive –*s*	Daddy'*s* hat, Baby'*s* bottle	2.75	III	26–40
7	Uncontractible copula	Here *it is*, There *I am*	2.75	III	27–39
8	Articles	I want *a* cookie, Give me *the* ball	3.50	IV	28–46
9	Past-tense regular –*ed*	Mom pour*ed* juice, I color*ed* pictures	3.50	IV	26–48
10	Regular third-person –*s*	Daddy cook*s*, Kitty meow*s*	3.50	IV	26–46
11	Irregular third person	*Does, has*	4.00	V	28–50
12	Uncontractible auxiliary	She *was* working	4.00	V	29–48
13	Contractible copula	He *is* nice or He'*s* nice	4.00	V	29–49
14	Contractible auxiliary	Mom *is* coming, or Mom'*s* coming	4.00	V	30–50

Note. Adapted from *A First Language: Early Stages*, by R. Brown, 1973, Cambridge, MA: Harvard University Press. Adapted with permission.

- begins using *embedded* forms, which rearrange or add elements within sentences (e.g., "The man *who came to dinner* stayed a week.").
- begins using passive voice (e.g., "She's been bitten by a dog.").
- uses mostly complete sentences; at 48 months, sentences average 5–5 1/2 words per utterance. MLU is approximately 3.0–5.0.
- uses mostly nouns, verbs, and personal pronouns.

- acquires do-insertions and ability to make transformations (e.g., "Does the kitty run around?").
- uses negation in speech (e.g., "Timmy can't swim.").
- begins using complex and compound sentences (e.g., "I can sing and dance."). Seven percent of sentences are compound or complex.

Semantics

The child:

- comprehends up to 4,200 words (by 42 months; at 48 months, comprehends up to 5,600 words).
- uses 900–1000 words expressively.
- asks how, why, and when questions.
- understands some common opposites (e.g., *day–night, little–big, fast–slow*).
- knows full name, name of street, several nursery rhymes.
- labels most things in the environment.
- relates experiences and tells about activities in sequential order.
- can recite a poem from memory or sing a song (by 48 months).
- answers appropriately questions such as "Which is the boy?" "Where is the dress?" "What toys do you have?" (by 42 months).
- can complete opposite analogies such as "Daddy is a man; Mommy is a _____." (by 48 months).
- understands most preschool children's stories (by 48 months).
- uses pronouns *you, they, us,* and *them,* as well as others such as *I, me.*
- understands concepts such as heavy–light, empty–full, more–less, around, in front of–in back of, next to, big–little, hard–soft, rough–smooth (by 42 months).
- understands agent-action (e.g., "Tell me what flies, swims, bites").
- supplies last word of sentence (e.g., "The apple is on the _____.") (closure).
- appropriately answers "what if" questions (e.g., "What would you do if you fell down?") (by 43–48 months).

Morphology

The child:

- uses irregular plural forms (e.g., *children, mice, feet*).
- uses third-person singular, present tense (e.g., "he runs.").
- consistently uses simple (regular) past and present progressives (e.g., *is running*) and negatives (e.g., *not*).
- uses inflection to convert adjective to causative (e.g., *sharp, sharpen*).
- uses simple (regular) plural forms correctly (e.g., *boys, houses, lights*).
- begins to use *is* at beginning of questions.
- uses contracted forms of modals (e.g., *can't, won't*).
- uses *and* as a conjunction.
- uses *is, are,* and *am* in sentences.
- uses possessive markers consistently (e.g., *the boy's clothes*) (by 43–48 months).

- begins to use reflexive pronoun *myself* (by 43–48 months).
- begins to use conjunction *because* (by 43–48 months).

Pragmatics (adapted from Reed, 2005; Shulman, 1983)

The child:

- can maintain conversation without losing track of topic.
- begins to modify speech to age of listener (e.g., uses simplified language with a younger child).
- begins to produce indirectives (e.g., "Are the cookies done?" meaning "I want a cookie.").
- uses requesting (e.g., yes-no questions, wh- questions).
- responds with structures such as *yes, no, because*; expresses agreement or denial (e.g., "That's not really her dress"), compliance or refusal (e.g., "I won't take a bath!").
- uses conversational devices:

    - boundary markers such as *hi, bye* (indicate beginning, end of communication)
    - calls such as "Hey, Mommy!"
    - accompaniments such as "Here you are"
    - politeness markers such as *please, thanks*

- uses communicative functions:

    - role-playing, fantasies
    - protests/objections such as "Don't touch that!"
    - jokes such as "I threw the juice in the ceiling!"
    - game markers such as "You have to catch me!"
    - claims such as "I'm first!"
    - warnings such as "Look out or you'll fall!"
    - teases such as "You can't have this!"

CONCEPTS TO CONSIDER

Briefly describe the syntactic development of a normally developing child between 3 and 4 years of age. What forms is the child using at this stage?

_____

_____

_____

_____

_____

4–5 Years

The following developmental milestones are observed in normally developing children between 4 and 5 years of age.

Syntax

The child:

- averages 6–6.5 words per sentence (by 5 years); has an average MLU of 4.5–7.0.
- speaks in complete sentences.
- uses complex sentences; interprets complex sentences correctly. By 4¹/₂, only about 8% of sentences are incomplete.
- uses future tense (e.g., "She will go to the store.").
- uses *if, so* in sentences.
- begins to use passive voice (some children) (e.g., "The cat was fed by the man.").

Semantics

The child:

- uses concrete meanings and words, but responds to some abstract ideas appropriately.
- has an expressive range of approximately 1,500–2,000 words.
- comprehends about 5,600 words at 48 months; by 54 months, comprehends approximately 6,500 words; by 60 months, comprehends up to 9,600 words.
- can name items in a category (e.g., food, animals). Able to point to categorical item (e.g., fruit).
- uses most pronouns, including possessives (e.g., *mine, his, her*).
- uses *why* and *how.*
- understands time concepts such as *early in the morning, tomorrow, after.*
- uses *what do, does, did* in questions.
- answers simple "when" questions like "When do you sleep?" (55–60 months).
- responds appropriately to "how often, how long" questions (55–60 months).
- asks meaning of words.
- tells long stories accurately.
- can give whole name (first, middle, last).
- begins to understand right and left (5 years).
- can define 10 common words (4¹/₂ years).
- shows objects by use and function (e.g., if directed, "Show me what tells time," "Show me which one gives us milk").
- identifies past and future verbs ("Show me the man who kicked the ball," "Who will kick the ball?").
- demands explanations with frequent use of *why.*

Morphology

The child:

- uses comparatives (e.g., *bigger, nicer, taller*).

- uses *could, would* in sentences.
- uses irregular plurals (e.g., *mice, teeth*) fairly consistently.

Pragmatics

The child:

- modifies speech as a function of listener age (beginning at 4 years).
- begins to judge grammatical correctness and appropriateness of sentences.
- can maintain topic over successive utterances.
- uses egocentric monologue about a third of the time (this monologue does not communicate information to the listener).
- uses indirect speech acts, softens speech (e.g., "I think that goes in there" rather than "Put that in there.").
- begins to tell jokes and riddles (around 5 years).

5–6 Years

The following developmental milestones are observed in normally developing children between 5 and 6 years of age.

Syntax

The child:

- has an average MLU of 6.0–8.0.
- uses present, past, and future tenses consistently.
- uses conjunctions to string words together (e.g., "A bear and a wolf and a fox").
- asks "how" questions.
- uses auxiliary *have* correctly at times.
- uses "if" sentences (e.g., "If I had a cookie, I'd eat it.").
- increases understanding and use of complex sentences; decreases grammatical errors as sentences and vocabulary become more sophisticated.
- comprehends verb tenses in the passive voice (e.g., "The bus was hit by the car," "The cat was fed by the man.").
- uses a language form that approximates the adult model.

Semantics

The child:

- knows spatial relations and prepositions such as *on top, behind, far, near.*
- can distinguish *alike, same, different.*
- distinguishes right and left in self, not in others.
- knows complete address.
- knows most common opposites (e.g., *hard–soft, fat–thin, high–low*); understands "opposite of" (e.g., "What's the opposite of cold?").
- defines objects by use, composition (e.g., "Napkins are made of paper; you wipe your mouth with them").

- tells long stories; retells tales of past and present events.
- comprehends 13,000–15,000 words (by age 6).
- can answer "What happens if … ?" questions.
- understands concepts such as yesterday–tomorrow, more–less, some–many, several–few, most–least, before–after, now–later.
- can state similarities and differences of objects.
- can name position of objects: first, second, third.
- can name days of week in order.
- comprehends *first, last.*
- knows functions of body parts.

Morphology

The child:

- knows passive forms of main verbs.
- knows indefinite pronouns—*any, anything, anybody, every, both, few, many, each,* and others.
- uses irregular plurals with general consistency.
- uses possessives and negatives consistently.
- uses all pronouns consistently.
- uses superlative *-est* (e.g., *smartest*).
- begins to use adverbial word endings (e.g., *-ly*).

Pragmatics

The child:

- understands humor, surprise.
- corrects potential errors by modifying the message.
- can recognize a socially offensive message and reword it in polite form.
- modifies speech according to listener's needs.
- begins to use and understand formal levels of address (e.g., *Mr., Mrs.*).
- gains greater facility with indirect requests (e.g., "I would like a sticker" instead of "Gimme a sticker").
- can differentiate 80% of the time between polite and impolite utterances.
- uses expressions such as "thank you" and "I'm sorry."
- often asks permission to use objects belonging to others.
- contributes to adult conversation.

6–7 Years

The following developmental milestones are observed in normally developing children between 6 and 7 years of age.

Syntax

The child:

- uses *if* and *so.*

- uses reflexive pronouns (e.g., *himself, myself).*
- begins to use perfect tense forms (e.g., *have, had).*
- has full use of passive voice.
- has an average MLU of 7.3 words.
- uses embedding more frequently (e.g., "The girl *who bought the dress* went to the party.").

Semantics

The child:

- comprehends 20,000–26,000 words.
- understands the seasons of the year and knows what you do in each.
- forms letters left to right (reversals and inversions are common).
- prints alphabet and numerals from previously printed model.
- recites the alphabet sequentially, names capital letters, matches lower to upper case letters.
- rote counts to 100.
- tells time related to specific daily schedule.

Morphology

The child:

- uses most morphological markers fairly consistently.
- uses irregular comparatives (*good, better, best*) more correctly.
- continues to improve in correct use of irregular past tense and plurals.
- begins to produce *gerunds* (a noun form produced by adding *-ing* to a verb infinitive, e.g., *fish, fishing*).
- acquires use of *derivational morphemes,* in which verbs are changed into nouns (e.g., *catch* becomes *catcher*).

Pragmatics

The child:

- becomes aware of mistakes in other people's speech.
- is apt to use slang and mild profanity.

7–8 Years

The following developmental milestones are observed in normally developing children between 7 and 8 years of age.

Syntax

The child:

- has an MLU of approximately 7.0–9.0.
- uses predominantly complex sentence forms.

Semantics

The child:

- interprets jokes and riddles literally.
- anticipates story endings.
- uses some figurative language.
- uses details in description.
- creates conversation suggested by a picture.
- enjoys telling stories and anecdotes.
- retells a story, keeping main ideas in correct sequence.

Morphology

The child:

- uses most irregular verb forms, although with some mistakes in irregular past tense.
- uses superlatives (*biggest, prettiest*).
- uses adverbs regularly.

Pragmatics

The child:

- initiates, maintains conversation in small groups.
- is able to role-play, to take the listener's point of view.
- determines and uses appropriate discourse codes and styles (e.g., informal with friends, formal with adults).
- uses nonlinguistic and nonverbal behaviors—posture, gestures—appropriately.
- takes more care in communicating with unfamiliar people; announces topic shifts.
- can sustain a topic through a number of conversational turns, but topics tend to be concrete (by 8 years; after age 11, discussions involving abstract topics can be sustained).

Education, Language, and Literacy Development in the School-Age Years

When children enter school, they grow and change in a number of areas. Some of the major changes children undergo include the following (McLaughlin, 1998; Morrison, 2003; Owens, 2005; Reed, 2005; Roseberry-McKibbin, 2007; Woolfolk, 2004).

- When a normally developing child enters kindergarten, she should have solid speaking and listening (*auditory-oral*) skills. Good auditory-oral skills are strongly related to learning to read and write. Research shows that children who have poor auditory-oral skills often have more difficulty learning to read and write.

- Hopefully, during the preschool years, children have had good exposure to prereading and prewriting skills and activities (e.g., coloring, being read to). Such exposure impacts a child's development of *emergent literacy* or *preliteracy skills,* which are foundational to later reading and writing in school. In the last decade in the United States, there has been a much greater emphasis on literacy skills at the preschool level. Some preschools now actively teach the alphabet, for example.

■ In kindergarten, teachers work on strengthening children's oral language skills. They also address basic reading and writing. In some states, such as California, children are expected to be able to write short paragraphs and read simple books by the end of kindergarten. In other states, reading and writing are postponed until first grade. In many states, kindergarteners are asked to learn basic computer skills.

■ In first grade, teachers focus more heavily on reading and writing, although they still work on oral language skills as well. Children are expected to do math problems involving addition and subtraction, and some teachers also introduce two-digit numbers at this time. Research shows that first grade is a critical time; children who have difficulty in first grade usually have difficulty in the later grades also. Early intervention is critical for children who are struggling in first grade (Woolfolk, 2004).

■ Second-grade teachers emphasize increased skill in reading and writing, and independent reading is encouraged. Children also learn to spell. They are expected to comprehend more abstract language and to develop independent word-recognition skills.

■ Third grade is a transition grade, where children are expected to read longer, more complex stories and write longer, more complex paragraphs. They are also asked to proofread and correct their written work as well as spell more complicated words. Most children learn cursive writing in third grade.

■ In grades four through six, children go from "learning to read and write" to "reading and writing to learn." That is, the emphasis shifts from a focus on how to read and write to using reading and writing as tools for learning more about content areas such as science and social studies. Students often have to write reports. By sixth grade, a child should understand about 50,000 words.

■ It is in grades four through six that children with language disorders are often identified. This is because their weak auditory-oral and written language skills are not strong enough to help them learn information in content areas such as social studies. For example, if a child is struggling with the skills of listening, speaking, reading, and writing, she will have difficulty reading about Antarctica, writing a report on it, and presenting her report to the class.

■ In junior high and high school, teachers generally lecture and students must take notes on what they hear. There may be a different teacher for each subject. Students are tested frequently. Written language becomes extremely important. A high school student should understand about 80,000 words.

SUMMARY

✓ **Children develop language based on their innate characteristics, the environment they are exposed to, and the expectations of their cultures.**

✓ **Children's caregivers play an important role in language development. Ideally, a baby's caregivers use motherese, or speech geared specifically to help babies attend and respond to what they hear.**

✓ The development of syntactic, semantic, morphological, and pragmatic skills depends in large part on those factors. Each child develops at his or her own rate, and variation among children is to be expected.

✓ When a child enters school, she ideally has well developed auditory-oral skills and preliteracy skills. These are critical to later success in reading and writing. In fourth grade, children stop learning to read and write and begin writing and reading to learn. Children with language disorders are often identified between fourth and sixth grade.

THEORIES OF LANGUAGE DEVELOPMENT

INTRODUCTION

Theory drives practice. The way clinicians conduct assessment and treatment depends greatly on their theoretical viewpoints. Some clinicians are eclectic in their approach; that is, they blend aspects of several theories to achieve what they see as a balanced approach to language assessment and treatment. Other clinicians depend primarily on and operate from one theory.

In this section, we describe five major theories of language development: behavioral, nativist, cognitive, information-processing, and social interactionism. These theories differ in describing how language is developed and in their implications for (a) areas that clinicians should target in assessment and intervention, and (b) what procedures should be used to facilitate language learning.

Behavioral Theory

■ The behavioral theory does not explain the acquisition of language, because language often is described by linguists and others as a mental system. Behavioral psychologist B. F. Skinner did not describe language as a mental or cognitive system, because he thought that such a view would preclude an experimental study of language.

■ Skinner's (1957) system of behavioral analysis explains the acquisition of *verbal behavior.* Verbal behavior is considered to be a form of social behavior maintained by the actions of a verbal community. Verbal behaviors are acquired under appropriate conditions of stimulation, response, and reinforcement.

■ Behavioral scientists suggest that learning, not innate mechanisms, plays a major role in the acquisition of verbal behaviors. They do not believe, as nativists do (see below), that a child has an innate knowledge of the universal rules of grammar. Behaviorists focus on the *measurable* and *observable* aspects of language behavior and emphasize performance over competence (Bohannon & Bonvillian, 2005).

■ To behaviorists, the events in the child's *environment* are important. Children learn only the language they are exposed to; severe social deprivation results in language deprivation as well.

■ Verbal behavior is characteristically produced under social stimulation. An audience is necessary; the audience, or person(s) interacting with the speaker, sets the stage for speech. Put differently, verbal behavior is a form of social behavior shaped and maintained by the members of a verbal community.

■ Practically all forms of verbal behaviors can be increased or decreased experimentally. Social reinforcement, for example, can increase babbling, word and phrase responses, and the production of grammatic features.

■ For example, if a child says something like "want bath," the caregiver might say "You want a bath! Good girl! Let's have a bath right now." The caregiver has reinforced the statement by responding verbally and then starting to run the bath water. But if the caregiver ignores or punishes the child, the child is much less likely to express this request again.

■ Thus, behaviorists question the nativist assumption that the environment offers little assistance to the child in acquiring language. In treatment, behaviorists teach verbal behavior to children by modeling correct responses and reinforcing children's correct productions.

■ Verbal behavior is broken down into cause–effect (functional) units, not structures of language. These *functional units* include:

  ▪ *Mands.* Derived from related traditional terms such as *demands* and *commands,* mands involve requests (McLaughlin, 1998). In some cases, a physiological need such as thirst or hunger stimulates speech ("Do you have something to eat?"). Needs of this sort cause various kinds of requests, commands, and demands. These mands are caused by states of motivation and are reinforced by food and other biologically satisfying events.
  ▪ *Tacts.* Sometimes physical objects and events stimulate speaking; verbal responses to this kind of stimulation are called tacts. A tact is a group of verbal responses that describe and comment on the things and events around us. For example, a child is using a tact when she says, "This car is big and red." Tacts are reinforced socially; a smile, a nod of approval, and similar statements by a listener may all reinforce a tact.
  ▪ *Echoics.* Echoics are imitative verbal responses whose stimuli are the speech of another person. Reinforcement for an echoic is based on a close resemblance between the stimulus and the response. Thus, a clinician models target responses, which a child imitates. The clinician reinforces only when the child's imitations at least approximate the clinician's modeled response.

■ Clinicians who conduct language treatment according to principles of the behavioral theory believe that one can teach language by targeting any observable behavior and manipulating the elements of a stimulus, a response, and some type of reinforcement.

■ In treatment, the clinician selects specific target responses, creates appropriate antecedent events, and reinforces correct responses (Fey, 1986). There is a clearly established criterion for success (e.g., 8 out of 10 responses produced accurately).

■ For example, a clinician teaching a child to use plural -*s* might create a game using toy cars. If the clinician points to the cars and asks, "What are these?" and the child says, "Cars," the clinician might respond with "Good job!"

■ Most language development experts believe that a strict behavioral theory of language acquisition is inadequate, especially because behaviorists generally do not account for the abilities that the child brings to the learning task (Owens, 2005).

Nativist Theory

■ The nativist theory is an influential theory of syntax proposed by Noam Chomsky in the late 1950s. This theory has had a significant impact on the fields of linguistics and speech–language pathology.

■ Chomsky stated that syntactic structures are the essence of language and that language is a product of the unique human mind. He said that there are universal rules of grammar that apply to all languages.

■ The nativist theory states that children are born with a *language acquisition device* (LAD). The LAD is assumed to be a specialized language processor that is a physiological part of the brain (Bohannon & Bonvillian, 2005). The LAD knows about languages in general, because it contains the universal rules of language.

■ The child's environment provides information about the unique rules of the language the child is exposed to. The LAD then integrates the universal rules and the unique rules of that language, and thus helps the child learn language in a relatively short time.

■ Nativists believe that children are born with an innate capacity to learn language and that because the basic knowledge necessary to acquire language is already present at birth, language is not learned through environmental stimulation, reinforcement, or teaching.

■ Chomsky described language *competence* and language *performance*. Competence, the knowledge of the rules of universal grammar, is innate. Thus, the child learns language relatively independently of the environment. Performance, the actual production of language, is imperfect because of such factors as fatigue and distraction.

■ Chomsky introduced the ideas of *surface* structure and *deep* structure. Surface structure is the actual arrangement of words in a syntactic order. It is the phrase or sentence that one hears. Underlying this surface structure is the abstract deep structure, which primarily contains the rules of sentence formation.

■ Chomsky stated that surface and deep structures are related through grammatic transformations. A *transformation* is an operation that relates the deep and surface structures and yields different forms of sentences.

■ A transformation can further be viewed as a process by which one arranges and rearranges words to change sentences. Grammatic transformations involve deleting, adding, substituting, and rearranging words to change meaning. Consider the following examples:

  - The girl kicked the ball.
  - Who kicked the ball? (a question transformation)
  - Did the girl kick the ball? (another question transformation)
  - The ball was not kicked by the girl. (a negative transformation)
  - The ball was kicked by the girl. (a passive transformation)

■ Each of these examples involves a transformation of adding, deleting, substituting, or rearranging words to form a different kind of sentence. These transformations account for the creative nature of language.

■ Because Chomsky believed that such creative transformation of sentence forms is the essence of language, his theory is often called the *transformational generative theory of grammar*. According to Chomsky, with knowledge of the rules of grammar and the use of transformations, speakers can generate an endless variety of sentences.

■ A revision of Chomsky's theory was proposed in the early 1980s. The *government binding theory* attempts to describe the way the mind represents the autonomous system of language.

■ Chomsky wanted to present a theory that accounted for the variety in human languages and that explained the development of grammars on the basis of limited input (Owens, 2005). According to Owens, too few child studies have been performed to make a definite statement about the contribution of government-binding theory to our understanding of language development.

■ The nativist theory and its variants lead to few specific implications for assessment and treatment of children who have language disorders. However, Chomskyan theorists believe that in therapy, it is necessary to focus heavily on syntax in selecting treatment goals.

■ Reinforcement, however, is unnecessary. Because language knowledge is innate, reinforcing a child for talking would be tantamount to reinforcing a child for walking. Manipulating the child's environment, as the behaviorist does, is unlikely to be successful, according to this theory.

CONCEPTS TO CONSIDER

Compare and contrast the nativist and behavioral theories. What are the main points of difference between the two?

_____

_____

_____

_____

_____

Cognitive Theory

■ Described as a variant of the nativist theory, the cognitive theory emphasizes *cognition,* or knowledge and mental processes such as memory, attention, and visual and auditory perception. Cognitivists focus on the child's regulation of learning and on internal aspects of behavior (Klein & Moses, 1999).

Table 3.4 PIAGET'S STAGES OF COGNITIVE DEVELOPMENT

SENSORIMOTOR (0–2 YEARS)

Usually divided into six substages:

Substage 1: Birth–2 months:
- Child displays reflexive vocal behavior
- Child displays reflexive sensorimotor behavior

Substage 2: 2–4 months:
- Child makes coordinated eye-hand movements
- Child makes coordinated hand-mouth movements

Substage 3: 4–8 months:
- Child acts on objects and begins to search for objects
- Child imitates some sounds and babbles

Substage 4: 8–12 months:
- Child starts walking
- First word is used
- Child searches for objects based on her memory of where she last saw them
- Child begins to recognize that he has the ability to cause objects to move

Substage 5: 12–18 months:
- Object permanence becomes evident
- Child walks with confidence
- Child may imitate another person's behavior when that person is present (e.g., claps hands or plays peek-a-boo)
- Child experiments with the properties and functions of objects (e.g., uses a spoon to eat cereal, to bang on the table, to drop in front of the dog, etc.)

Substage 6: 18–24 months:
- Child uses words when referents are not present (e.g., says "Mommy" even when Mommy is not in the room)
- Child uses thought to solve problems
- Basic cause-and-effect relations are acquired
- Child uses symbolic play, using one item to represent another (for example, using a Kleenex as a doll's blanket, using a stick as a gun)

PREOPERATIONAL (2–7 YEARS)

Frequently divided into two stages: preconceptual (2–4 years) and intuitive (4–7 years)

Preconceptual (2–4 years):
- Child is egocentric; has difficulty taking perspective of others
- Child overextends word meanings (all men are "Daddy")
- Child underextends word meanings (only the family pet, Rover, is a "dog")

Intuitive (4–7 years):
- Egocentrism continues
- Child displays concreteness of thought (e.g., in Monopoly, has a hard time recognizing that five $100 bills represent the same amount as one $500 bill)
- Perceptions guide thoughts
- Child deals with only one variable at a time
- Classification skills have improved but are still inadequate
- Child displays lack of conservation (e.g., lack of ability to see that a ball of clay can be rolled into a snake shape and still be the same amount of clay)

(continues)

Table 3.4 *Continued.* **PIAGET'S STAGES OF COGNITIVE DEVELOPMENT**

CONCRETE OPERATIONS (7–11 YEARS)

- Child is less egocentric, has increasing ability to see others' points of view
- Child aquires seriation and conservation skills
- Child employs logical causality
- Child uses effective classification skills

FORMAL OPERATIONS (MORE THAN 11 YEARS)

- Child displays lack of egocentricity, is able to see others' point of view
- Child displays ability to think and speak in the abstract
- Child can use inductive and deductive thought processes
- Child can use verbal reasoning and make "if...then" statements
- Child is able to use hypothetical reasoning

Note. Adapted from *An Introduction to Children with Language Disorders,* 3rd ed., by V. Reed, 2005, Boston: Allyn & Bacon. Adapted with permission.

- According to cognitive theory, language acquisition is made possible by cognition and general intellectual processes. Language is only one expression of a more general set of cognitive activities, and proper development of the cognitive system is a necessary precursor of linguistic expression (Bohannon & Bonvillian, 2005).

- Thus, a child must first acquire concepts before producing words. For example, a child who has not been exposed to a *dog* or a *triangle* is not likely to say those words.

- Proponents of the *strong cognition hypothesis* believe in cognitive precursors to language. They state that there are cognitive abilities that are essential prerequisites to language skills. Without these prerequisite cognitive abilities, language skills will not be optimally developed. Language development is dependent on cognitive development.

- Piaget, a supporter of the strong cognition hypothesis, described four stages of cognitive development that children must go through (see Table 3.4). He believed that children successively acquire the necessary cognitive operations that, in turn, lead to higher levels of language development. Children must master the features of one stage in order to progress to the next.

- Children pass through each cognitive stage in the order given but may show variation in the *rate* at which they progress through the stages.

- Although researchers have not proven that there is a causal relationship between cognitive and language skills, it has been observed that certain language skills develop at about the same time as certain cognitive skills. For example, children's use of "all gone" (a disappearance phrase) is associated with the emerging understanding of object permanence.

- The *weak cognition hypothesis* states that while cognition accounts for some of a child's language abilities, it cannot account for all of them; some aspects of language do not develop directly as a result of underlying cognitive skills.

- Cognitive theorists believe that while nonlinguistic, cognitive precursors are innate, language is not. Thus, because they believe that language is neither innate (nativist view) nor learned (behaviorist view), they view language as emerging as a result of cognitive growth.

- A clinical implication of the cognitive theory is that clinicians must assess cognitive precursors to language and facilitate the development of those precursors before working on language itself. Language will not improve until cognitive precursors are developed.

- For example, a young child may not have developed object permanence, or the ability to know that an item exists even when it goes out of sight. Therefore, before teaching that child to say words, the clinician would teach object permanence. When object permanence was firmly established, the clinician would teach the child to say words.

Information-Processing Theory

- Proponents of the information-processing theory are mostly concerned with cognitive *functioning*, not cognitive structures or concepts. In other words, information processing theorists are interested in *how* language is learned.

- Information-processing theorists view the human information-processing system as a mechanism which encodes stimuli from the environment, operates on interpretations of those stimuli, stores the results in memory, and permits retrieval of previously stored information (Nelson, 1998; Owens, 2005).

- Of primary concern are the steps involved in handling or processing incoming and outgoing information. These steps include organization, memory, transfer, attention, and discrimination. Long- and short-term memory are especially important (Owens, 2005).

- Recent literature has included a great deal of discussion about the relationship between information processing and language disorders. Specifically, researchers have been interested in whether or not children with language disorders have concomitant information-processing problems (e.g., Conti-Ramsden, 2003; Hoffman & Gillam, 2004; Montgomery, 2002).

- Ellis Weismer and Evans (2002) suggest that there are two broad categories of information processing related to children's language disorders. The first category or aspect discussed is phonological processing.

- *Phonological processing* deals with the processes involved in the ability to mentally manipulate phonological aspects of language such as word rhyming, word segmentation, syllabication, and others. A child who has difficulty rhyming words or knowing that "c-a-t" means "cat" has phonological processing problems.

- The second category or aspect of information processing discussed by Ellis Weismer and Evans is *temporal auditory processing*. This deals with the ability to perceive the brief acoustic events that comprise speech sounds and track changes in these events as they happen quickly in the speech of other people (Reed, 2005).

- In research on the temporal auditory processing skills of children, researchers have been interested in children's (a) overall processing capacity and (b) speed of processing. In a simple example, researchers might ask if a child with a language disorder is able to listen to someone quickly say "5-9-3-6-2," remember this digit string, and repeat it back immediately and accurately. The child may have difficulty with the length of the digit string, the speed with which the string was said, or both.

■ Children with difficulties in temporal auditory processing often have difficulty with other tasks as well. These include remembering and following long and complex directions, repeating back sentences verbatim, repeating lists of real and nonsense words, and other tasks that tap the ability to hear, remember, and give back information that they have heard—especially if the information was given rapidly.

■ The role of information processing, sometimes called *auditory processing,* in language learning has continued to be highly controversial. Yet, many speech–language pathologists provide treatment for "auditory-processing problems," believing that such treatment will result in enhanced language skills (Gillam, 1999).

■ Foundational to adequate auditory processing is normal auditory sensitivity. When normal auditory sensitivity is established, some clinicians address components of auditory processing in their treatment programs (Mokhemar, 1999).

- *Auditory discrimination.* These skills enable children to identify differences between sound stimuli. Popular available tests ask children, for example, "Listen: cat–bat. Are these words the same or different?" The validity of these tests has been questioned by many professionals. Although the role of auditory discrimination in language development is heavily debated, researchers have found that children with language impairments have poorer auditory discrimination skills than their normally developing peers.
- *Auditory attention.* This is the ability to ignore irrelevant acoustic stimuli and focus on important information. Children with poor auditory attention have difficulty filtering relevant and irrelevant stimuli. Without appropriate auditory attention, children focus equally on all incoming stimuli, thus experiencing sensory overload. Optimal language learning cannot take place under such conditions, as children cannot sort out and attend to the important aspects of speech.
- *Auditory memory.* This refers to the ability to mentally store speech stimuli, or remember what one has heard. Many clinicians and researchers have found that children with language impairments have difficulty with auditory memory. Yet research suggests that while auditory memory may be a factor that exists *concomitantly* with language impairment, there is insufficient evidence to demonstrate that auditory memory problems are a *cause of* language impairment.
- *Auditory rate.* This refers to the ability to process acoustic stimuli that are presented at different rates or speeds. Much research has suggested that children with language impairments have difficulty processing incoming stimuli presented at rapid rates and that if the rate of incoming information is slowed down, they can process it more easily.
- *Auditory sequencing.* This is the ability to identify the temporal order in which auditory stimuli occur. Although the role of auditory sequencing in language development has been debated, it has been found that children with language disorders do more poorly on auditory-sequencing tasks than children who are developing normally.

■ Many researchers would argue that there is insufficient evidence to support the idea that speech–language pathologists should target auditory-processing skills as a part of language therapy. Because auditory-processing skills have not been conclusively demonstrated to be causally related to language impairment, many believe that addressing these skills as part of treatment is a waste of time.

■ However, recent research with small numbers of children with language impairments has shown that directly targeting auditory-processing skills leads to direct improvement in language skills (Miller, Merzenich, Saunders, Jenkins, & Tallal, 1997; Tallal, Miller, Bedi, Wang, Nagarajan, Schreiner, Jenkins, & Merzenich, 1996). More research, with larger numbers of subjects, needs to be conducted in this area.

Social Interactionism Theory

■ The social interactionism theory does not focus on innate linguistic competence (nativism) or specific reinforcement principles (behaviorism). Rather, this theory stipulates that the structure of human language has possibly arisen from language's social-communicative function in human relations (Bohannon & Bonvillian, 2005).

■ Proponents of social interactionism emphasize language *function,* not *structure.* They give credence to the situations in which social interactions occur, believing that interactions vary depending on the situation (Nelson, 1998).

■ Social interactionists believe that language develops because people are motivated to interact socially with others around them. For example, infants seek out human faces and respond to them (Bruner, 1968, cited in Nelson, 1998). Thus, the environment and its inherent social experiences are crucial to the emergence of language (Bohannon & Bonvillian, 2005).

■ Proponents of social interactionism believe that the *child,* as well as his or her caretakers and the environment, plays an active role in language acquisition.

■ Lev Vygotsky (1962), a Russian psychologist, believed that language is a tool for social interaction. He saw language as being intrinsically linked with the social-interactive context.

■ According to Vygotsky, language knowledge is acquired through social interaction with more competent and experienced members of the child's culture. Therefore, Vygotsky emphasized the importance of verbal guidance and adult modeling.

■ Vygotsky stated that a child's conversational partners, including the parents, are significant contributors to the language acquisition process. These partners contribute by *scaffolding,* or by supplying the necessary communicative structure that allows the child to communicate despite limited communication skills.

■ Unlike Piaget, who believed that cognitive development preceded language development, Vygotsky thought that children first learned language in interpersonal interactions and then used that language to structure thought.

■ Vygotsky further believed that as children's language develops, they increasingly use language internally to structure their actions and direct their thoughts. For example, small children playing house by themselves may be observed talking to themselves as they play. Eventually, as they mature, children use language silently internally to mediate thought.

■ According to Vygotsky, cultural tools play a critical role in children's language development. For example, in a culture that only uses Roman numerals, certain ways of thinking mathematically are not possible. But in a culture where people have ready access to calculators and computers, various high levels of mathematical thinking are possible. Children's learning is guided by the cultural tools available and social interactions around these tools (Woolfolk, 2004).

- Social interactionism theorists believe that language, both oral and written, continues to develop across the span of a person's life. Adolescents, for example, continue to refine their skills in figurative language and pragmatics as they mature. Adults who change jobs or vocations must learn the vocabulary relevant to their new station in life.

- Clinicians whose practice is driven by social interactionist theory focus on children's *motivation* for communication. In other words, treatment sessions are built around increasing children's motivation to communicate.

- To motivate children to use language, clinicians supply external situations and contexts, both verbal and nonverbal, that encourage the child to use language to meet his or her needs. For example, a clinician might withhold an attractive bottle of bubbles until the child says, "I want bubbles."

SUMMARY

✓ The nativist, cognitive, behavioral, information-processing, and social interactionism theories have been briefly described. Although other models of language development exist, these five theories have greatly influenced research and practice.

✓ Most speech–language pathologists, rather than allowing their practice to be driven by a single theory, incorporate aspects of all five theories to allow an eclectic blend to serve as a foundation for optimal assessment and treatment of language-impaired children.

CHAPTER HIGHLIGHTS

◆ **LANGUAGE IS A FORM** of social behavior that is shaped and maintained by a verbal community. Language can also be defined as a system of symbols used to represent concepts that are formed through exposure and experience.

◆ **LINGUISTS HAVE TRADITIONALLY DESCRIBED** several components of language: morphology (the study of word structure), syntax (rules specifying how words may be combined to form meaningful sentences), semantics (the study of meaning), and pragmatics (the study of rules that govern language use in various social situations). (Phonology, frequently studied under the aegis of language, is defined and discussed in Chapter 5).

◆ **LANGUAGE DEVELOPMENT IN CHILDREN** depends on several factors: the innate characteristics the individual child brings to the situation (e.g., a high IQ, a limited attention span); the child's environment; and cultural expectations. High-quality interaction with caretakers is critical to optimal language acquisition, and this type of interaction should begin in infancy.

◆ **CLINICIANS USE LANGUAGE DEVELOPMENTAL** milestones to guide their expectations about the language characteristics of children at certain chronological ages. However, a great deal of individual variability exists among children, so developmental milestones can serve only as a *general* guide and frame of reference. Most schools have a set of expectations for students to demonstrate increasingly sophisticated language skills as they progress through the grades.

◆ **THEORIES OF LANGUAGE DEVELOPMENT** provide the foundational underpinnings for assessment and treatment of children with language problems. Key theories that have impacted clinical practice include the behavioral theory (Skinner), the nativist theory (Chomsky), the cognitive theory (Piaget), the information-processing theory, and the social interactionism theory (Vygotsky).

◆ **THE BEHAVIORAL THEORY WAS** proposed by Skinner, who explained language acquisition as the development of verbal behavior. He suggested that learning, not an innate and unmeasurable mechanism such as the language acquisition device, plays a major role in language development. He emphasized the importance of the environment in language learning.

CHAPTER HIGHLIGHTS

◆ **ACCORDING TO THE NATIVIST** theory, proposed by Chomsky, children are born with a language acquisition device that contains the universal rules of language. Chomsky has described the concepts of deep and surface structures as well as the concepts of language competence and language performance.

◆ **PROPONENTS OF THE COGNITIVE** theory state that cognition and intellectual processes make language acquisition possible. Piaget, a supporter of the strong cognition hypothesis, stated that children pass through four overlapping developmental cognitive stages: the sensorimotor, preoperational, concrete operations, and formal operations stages.

◆ **THE INFORMATION-PROCESSING THEORY FOCUSES** on *how* language is learned; that is, on what types of cognitive functioning are necessary for language learning. A strong emphasis of this theory is auditory processing, composed of the components of auditory discrimination, attention, memory, rate, and sequencing. Recent research has also proposed the categories of phonological processing and temporal auditory processing.

◆ **PROPONENTS OF THE SOCIAL** interactionism theory, influenced by Vygotsky, emphasize language function over language structure. Social interactionists believe that language develops as a function of social interaction between a child and his environment (including significant others in that environment). Motivation is key in using language.

✎ **ADD YOUR OWN CHAPTER HIGHLIGHTS HERE:**

_____

_____

_____

_____

_____

_____

Study & Review Questions

Essay

1. Briefly describe the terms *morphology*, *semantics*, *pragmatics*, and *syntax*.

2. What is the role of the caregiver in a child's language development? Why is it important for caregivers to provide high-quality interaction for children as young as infancy?

3. A parent comes to you and asks you what kind of language skills her 2½-year-old child should be demonstrating. What would you tell her?

4. Describe two theories of child language development that especially make sense to you. What are the clinical implications (Monday morning applications) of these theories?

5. Briefly describe a child's educational journey from kindergarten through high school. What does a child need to be successful in school? How do educational and language demands differ from grade to grade?

Multiple Choice   40 | 20

6. A child says "red crayon." This is an example of which type of semantic relations?

   A. attribute + entity   D. attribute + locative
   B. action + locative   E. possession + attribute
   C. agent + action

7. You have been asked to give a workshop to a group of parents of infants who attend a developmental nursery. The parents are interested in what they can do to communicate more successfully with their infants. Most of the infants are between 1 and 10 months of age. Most of the parents do not have much money or access to toys and objects, but you are told that they do spend plenty of time with their babies. You are asked to speak about what specifically these parents can do to successfully interact with their infants in daily routines such as bathing, dressing, and eating. You will tell these parents:

   A. When your baby starts to cry, let him do so for 5–10 minutes before you respond; this will teach the baby independence and motivate him to express himself in words later on (instead of crying).
   B. Ideally, speak to the baby in utterances that are higher pitched and have greater pitch fluctuations than ordinary speech.
   C. Increase the baby's rudimentary turn-taking skills by responding to his vocalizations and playing games such as peek-a-boo.

D. A, B, C

E. B, C

8. A child using *recurrence* would say:

A. "Face dirty."

B. "All gone juice."

C. "More cookie."

D. "Doll mine."

E. "Close door."

9. An example of a sentence using an *embedded form* would be:

A. I saw the squirrel climbing the tree.

B. The girl ate a cookie, three crackers, and some fruit.

C. Mom and Dad are going to the store to buy some groceries.

D. Because he was on time, they were happy with him.

E. The boy who got a haircut looks nice.

10. A mother comes to you, concerned because her son Jake was born prematurely and had to spend the first few months of his life in a neonatal intensive care unit. Now Jake is 9 months old, and his mother wants to make sure that his language development is "on target for his age." You go to Jake's home to observe him, and you also ask his mother to give you a detailed description of his communication patterns. As you evaluate Jake's language development, you need to remember that one of the following does NOT occur between 8 and 10 months of age in the normally developing child. Which one is it?

A. comprehension of *no*

B. using the phrase "all gone" to express emerging negation

C. using variegated babbling (e.g., "madamada")

D. uncovering a hidden toy (beginning of object permanence)

E. use of gestural language such as shaking head no, playing peek-a-boo

11. Which of the following statements is/are true with regard to Brown's morphemes?

A. Children may vary in terms of the *rate* with which they develop the morphemes, but children usually develop them in the same sequence.

B. One of the last morphemes to develop, in Stage V, is uncontractible copula (e.g., "There *it is*").

C. The first morpheme to develop is present progressive *-ing* (e.g., "Dad cook*ing*").

D. A, B

E. A, C

12. A 7-year-old girl, Ashton, is referred to you by her second-grade classroom teacher, Mr. Alvarez. Mr. Alvarez says that Ashton "doesn't always get along with her peers" and "doesn't know how to hold a decent conversation." You assess Ashton personally, and also observe her on the playground during recess and in the cafeteria at lunchtime. You see that Mr. Alvarez is right. Ashton has difficulties in conversational exchanges with her peers, and they frequently ignore her. You notice that when talking to you, Ashton seems uncomfortable and doesn't say much, even when you use a variety of interesting games and toys. In therapy, your first priority with Ashton will be to:

A. teach her the appropriate use of compound and complex sentences in appropriate contexts.

B. teach her the appropriate use of allomorphs when presented with pictures of different people and activities.

C. increase her skills in quick incidental learning so that she can expand her vocabulary.

D. increase her skills in discourse.

E. work on developing her literacy skills so that she will be successful with the second grade curriculum.

13. Pragmatic skills involve:

    A. understanding words with multiple meanings (e.g., *rock*)
    B. use of narratives, a form of discourse in which a speaker tells a story
    C. use of appropriate cohesion, or the logical order and organization of utterances in a message
    D. B, C
    E. A, B, C

14. A 5-year-old child has been referred to you for a language assessment. There is a concern about his expressive language skills, and you decide to gather a language sample to assess expressive morphology and syntax. At one point, when looking at a book, the child points to a book character and says "Him no eat cookies." This is an example of:

    A. 4 words, 5 morphemes, personal pronoun + negative + verb + plural noun
    B. 4 words, 6 morphemes, modal + negative + verb + auxiliary
    C. 4 words, 4 morphemes, personal pronoun + copula + negative + noun
    D. 4 words, 5 morphemes, negative + personal pronoun + copula
    E. 4 words, 5 morphemes, personal pronoun + auxiliary + negative + plural noun

15. Which one of the following Piagetian stages, which includes object permanence, corresponds with the emergence of a normally developing child's first word?

    A. preoperational   **D.** concrete operations
    B. formal operations   **E.** none of the above
    C. sensorimotor

16. Halliday described seven functions of communicative intent that develop between 9 and 18 months of age. You are working in an early intervention program, where you must frequently evaluate very young children's language development, especially communicative intent. One day, you are observing a child who has been in the program for slightly over a year. She was brought to the program upon the advice of her pediatrician, who recommended a language stimulation program to increase her expressive language skills. As you observe this child and look for her to express varying communicative intents, she says, "Why doggy bark?" This is an example of which one of Halliday's intents?

    A. heuristic   **D.** informative
    B. instrumental   **E.** imaginative
    C. regulatory

17. A fourth-grade child, Alex, has been referred to you for language testing by his teacher. His parents are concerned and upset with the teacher because they feel that Alex needs more help in reading and writing skills than he is receiving. They tell you that the math and science homework assignments are too difficult for him, and that they feel that the fourth-grade teacher is making unreasonable demands. You find out that Alex did not attend preschool, and even in kindergarten, the teacher wrote on his first trimester progress report that Alex "began school not knowing basic concepts; he didn't talk as much as the other children either." You will tell Alex's parents that:

    A. the teacher really is being unreasonable, and that in fourth grade, time should definitely be spent on developing foundational reading and writing skills.
    B. Alex definitely has a language delay and needs therapy.
    C. the teacher is making reasonable demands that are consistent with fourth-grade curriculum standards.

D. you would like to conduct an assessment of Alex's language skills in a variety of domains to see if he needs support services in oral and written language.

E. C, D

18. You are asked to assess Tina, a girl who has Down Syndrome. She is 4 years and 10 months old, and her parents tell you that they wish for her to begin kindergarten in the fall (it is July, and school begins in September). You assess Tina's receptive and expressive language skills, and find that she has an average MLU of 3.0 and an expressive vocabulary of 350 words. Tina sustains a topic of conversation about 20% of the time, and overregularizes past tense inflections. You tell Tina's parents that:

A. Tina's overall language skills are very generally within normal limits for her age.

B. though Tina's language skills are approximately 6 months delayed for her age, Tina will be able to participate in a regular kindergarten classroom.

C. Tina's language skills are generally commensurate with those of a 2- to 3-year-old child, and starting kindergarten in the fall would probably be difficult for her.

D. Tina's language skills are generally commensurate with those of a 1-year-old and, thus, Tina needs to be in a preschool setting with very young children.

E. Tina's skills are not like those of any normally developing child, but rather are deviant, and she needs to go to a special school for children with Down Syndrome.

19. You are observing a clinician in a private practice setting. He specializes in child language disorders, and serves elementary-age children from a variety of local public schools. When you observe this clinician doing therapy, you see that he has a well-structured reward system for each child. Some children receive a fruit loop for each correct response they make; others work to earn stickers and even small toys. This clinician has written down each specific behavior that he wishes to elicit from each child, with a percentage of accuracy attached. For example, an objective for one child reads, "When presented with a picture of two or more objects, Jimmy will label the picture using plural –s 80% of the time." This clinician probably subscribes to which theory of child language development?

A. information processing
B. nativist
C. social interactionist

D. government binding
E. behaviorist

20. You are asked to work with a 3½-year-old child whose language has been somewhat slow to develop. Matthew is the youngest of four children, and his parents tell you that his older siblings often talk for him. After assessing Matthew's language, you find that he consistently uses the following morphemes: present progressive -ing, prepositions in and on, and regular plural –s. Matthew's parents would like to enroll him for therapy because they want him to go to a local preschool, and they want him to "sound like the other kids and have good grammar." Which of the following morphemes would you begin with when Matthew starts therapy?

A. possessive –s
B. irregular past tense verbs
C. articles the, a, an

D. contractible auxiliary
E. regular past tense –ed

21. A first-grade teacher refers 6-year-old Mandy to you for an assessment. The teacher is concerned because Mandy has difficulties with rhyming words and sounding out words. The teacher tells you that "For example, if I say c-u-p; what word is that? Mandy is unable to say 'cup.'" Mandy also reportedly has problems with remembering what she hears. The teacher tells you that "sometimes I have to give the children three or four directions, and I have to do it quickly because we have to go somewhere like an assembly. Mandy is

the only one in my class who doesn't remember what I tell the kids to do." Based on this brief description, you suspect that Mandy might have difficulties in which of the following areas?

A. temporal auditory processing
B. divergent semantic production
C. phonological processing
D. A, C
E. A, B, C

22. A young child who says "down" when a cup of juice spills off of the dinner table is using the relation of:

A. action.
B. possession.
C. locative action.
D. attribution.
E. recurrence.

23. A child has been referred to you for an assessment of his pragmatic skills. The chief complaint of adults and children whom he interacts with is that he frequently gives commands and sounds rude and bossy. His classroom teacher says she is "fed up with his bossiness" and peers do not include him in their games. His father tells you that the boy frequently says things like "Take me to Pizza Palace" or "Get me the *Spiderman 2* DVD." The father would like intervention to help his son say things like "I wonder if we could get a *Spiderman 2* DVD at the store?" instead of giving orders. In therapy, you know you will need to work on the boy's facility with:

A. passive sentence transformations.
B. cohesion.
C. narrative skills.
D. indirect requests.
E. didactic monologues.

24. A young child who often says things like "my doggy" or "her ball" is using the single word relation of:

A. recurrence.
B. possession.
C. location.
D. denial.
E. attribution.

25. You have been asked to assess the language skills of 6-year-old Tammieh, who has been referred by her classroom teacher. The teacher says that Tammieh "talks in these really short sentences. I don't know if she is just shy, or if there is more going on." The teacher is concerned because in first grade, she has worked on oral language skills daily with her class. The end of the year is coming soon, and the teacher is concerned about how Tammieh will perform in second grade. You decide to conduct an informal language screening to decide whether or not you need to formally evaluate Tammieh's expressive language skills. You find that she uses many sentences such as "He has a ball" and "I like Pokémon." Tammieh uses few compound or complex sentences. You talk with her parents, and find that this performance is also typical at home. Your next step would be to:

A. tell the teacher and parents that Tammieh is within normal limits for her age, and that a formal language evaluation is unnecessary.
B. inform the teacher and parents that Tammieh may have autistic-like tendencies and that she needs to be formally evaluated by a team of special educators.
C. tell the teacher and parents that you will take a "wait and see" approach. If the second-grade teacher has concerns similar to those of the first-grade teacher, you will follow up with a formal evaluation of Tammieh's language skills.
D. tell the teacher and parents that you would like to formally evaluate Tammieh's language skills because at 6 years of age, she should have an average MLU of 6.0–8.0, and her language should approximate the adult model.
E. immediately place Tammieh into therapy based upon these screening results because she clearly has a language delay and you want to begin therapy immediately.

REFERENCES AND RECOMMENDED READINGS

Berko Gleason, J. (2005). *The development of language* (6th ed.). Boston: Allyn & Bacon.

Bernstein, D. K., & Levey, S. (2002). Language development: A review. In D. K. Bernstein & E. Tiegerman-Farber, *Language and communication disorders in children* (5th ed., pp. 27–94). Boston: Allyn & Bacon.

Bernstein, D. K., & Tiegerman-Farber, E. (2002). *Language and communication disorders in children* (5th ed.). Boston: Allyn & Bacon.

Bloom, L., & Lahey, M. (1978). *Language development and disorders.* New York: Macmillan.

Bohannon, J. N., & Bonvillian, J. D. (2005). Theoretical approaches to language acquisition. In J. Berko Gleason, *The development of language* (5th ed., pp. 230–291). Boston: Allyn & Bacon.

Brown, R. (1973). *A first language: Early stages.* Cambridge, MA: Harvard University Press.

Bruner, J. (1968). *Processes of cognitive growth: Infancy (Vol. III, Heinz Werner Lecture Series).* Worcester, MA: Clark University Press.

Conti-Ramsden, G. (2003). Processing and linguistic markers in young children with specific language impairment (SLI). *Journal of Speech, Language, and Hearing Research, 46*(5), 1029–1037.

Dore, J. (1975). Holophrase, speech acts, and language universals. *Journal of Child Language, 2,* 21–40.

Ellis Weismer, S., & Evans, J. (2002). The role of processing limitations in early identification of specific language impairment. *Topics in Language Disorders, 22*(3), 15-29.

Fey, M. E. (1986). *Language intervention in young children.* Boston: Little, Brown.

Gillam, R. B. (1999). Computer-assisted language intervention using Fast ForWord: Theoretical and empirical considerations for clinical decision-making. *Language, Speech, and Hearing Services in Schools, 24*(1), 2–9.

Halliday, M. (1975). *Learning how to mean: Explorations in the development of language.* London: Edward Arnold.

Hoffman, L. M., & Gillam, R. (2004). Verbal and spatial information processing constraints in children with specific language impairment. *Journal of Speech, Language, and Hearing Research, 47,* 114–125.

Hulit, L. M., & Howard, M. R. (2002). *Born to talk: An introduction to speech and language development* (3rd ed.). Boston: Allyn & Bacon.

Klein, H. B., & Moses, N. (1999). *Intervention planning for children with communication disorders: A guide for clinical practicum and professional practice* (2nd ed.). Boston: Allyn & Bacon.

Kuder, J. (2003). *Teaching students with language and communication disabilities* (2nd ed.). Boston: Allyn & Bacon.

McLaughlin, S. (1998). *Introduction to language development.* San Diego, CA: Singular Publishing Group.

Miller, S., Merzenich, M. M., Saunders, G., Jenkins, W. M., & Tallal, P. (1997). Improvements in language abilities with training of children with both attentional and language impairments. *Society for Neuroscience, 23,* 490–492.

Mokhemar, M. A. (1999). *The central auditory processing kit.* East Moline, IL: Linguisystems, Inc.

Montgomery, J. (2002). Understanding the language difficulties of children with specific language impairments: Does verbal working memory matter? *American Journal of Speech–Language Pathology, 11*(1), 77–91.

Morrisson, G. S. (2003). *Teaching in America* (3rd ed.). Boston: Allyn & Bacon.

Nelson, N. W. (1998). *Childhood language disorders in context: Infancy through adolescence* (2nd ed.). Needham Heights, MA: Allyn & Bacon.

Owens, R.E. (2005). *Language development: An introduction* (6th ed.). Boston: Allyn & Bacon.

Paul, R. (2001). *Language disorders from infancy through adolescence: Assessment and intervention* (2nd ed.). St. Louis, MO: Mosby-Year Book.

Reed, V. A. (2005). *An introduction to children with language disorders* (3rd ed.). Boston: Allyn & Bacon.

Roseberry-McKibbin, C. (2007). *Introduction to language disorders in children: A multicultural approach.* Boston: Allyn & Bacon.

Sachs, J. (2001). Communication development in infancy. In J. Berko Gleason, *The development of language* (5th ed. pp. 40-69). Boston: Allyn & Bacon.

Shulman, B. (1983). *Pragmatic development chart.* San Francisco: Word-Making Productions.

Skinner, B. F. (1957). *Verbal behavior.* Norwalk, CT: Appleton-Century-Crofts.

Tallal, P., Miller, S. L., Bedi, G., Byma, G., Wang, X., Nagarajan, S. S., Schreiner, C., Jenkins, W. M., & Merzenich, M. M. (1996). Language comprehension in language-learning impaired children improved with acoustically modified speech. *Science, 271*, 77–84.

Vygotsky, L. (1962). *Thought and language.* Cambridge: MIT Press.

Woolfolk, A. (2004). *Educational psychology* (9th ed.). Boston: Allyn & Bacon.

Study & Review Answers

6. A. When a child says "red crayon," this is an example of attribute + entity.

7. E. In terms of infant language stimulation, it is best to respond immediately to the baby's crying and to use motherese (characterized by higher pitch and greater pitch fluctuations). It is also helpful to increase the baby's rudimentary turn-taking skills.

8. C. A child using recurrence would say "more cookie."

9. E. Embedding refers to adding or rearranging elements within sentences; in this example, the phrase "who got a haircut" makes the sentence one that uses an embedded form.

10. B. Most children use "all gone" to express emerging negation between 1 and 2 years of age.

11. E. Children tend to develop Brown's morphemes in the same sequence, but the rate of acquisition may vary. The *-ing* morpheme is the first to develop, and the uncontractible copula develops in Stage III.

12. D. Based upon your observations and the teacher's report, your first priority in therapy will be to work on Ashton's discourse skills, or skills in the give-and-take of conversation.

13. D. Pragmatic skills involve the ability to use narratives and to use appropriate cohesion.

14. A. If you are conducting a language sample with a 5-year-old and the child says, "Him no eat cookies," this is an example of 4 words, 5 morphemes, personal pronoun + negative + verb + plural noun.

15. C. Children usually use their first word between 10–14 months of age, which corresponds to the sensorimotor cognitive development stage.

16. A. The heuristic function involves children attempting to have events in their environment explained to them ("Tell me why").

17. E. The teacher is making reasonable demands; in fourth grade, children use reading and writing skills to learn information in content areas such as science and math. It is important for you to evaluate Alex's language skills to see if he needs intervention, because there are several "red flags" such as his difficulties that began in kindergarten and his struggles with the fourth-grade curriculum.

18. C. According to language development milestones, Tina's language skills are commensurate with those of a 2 to 3-year-old; in kindergarten, she will be learning along with children who are 5–6 years of age and are developing normally.

19. E. This clinician bases his therapy on the behaviorist theory, which promotes the concept of stimulus, response, and reinforcement of behaviors that are observable and measurable.

20. B. According to Brown's list of morphemes, irregular past tense verbs would be next to develop; thus, this would be a good starting point for therapy.

21. D. Mandy's difficulties with rhyming and sounding out words indicate a problem with phonological processing. Her difficulties with remembering directions probably indicate problems with temporal auditory processing.

22. C. When the cup of juice spills off the dinner table and the child says "down," she is using the relation of locative action.

23. D. The ability to say something like "I wonder if we could get a *Spiderman 2* DVD at the store?" indicates facility with indirect requests.

24. B. Utterances such as "my doggy" and "her ball" represent the relation of possession.

25. D. Based on your screening results, it will be important to conduct a formal, in-depth assessment of Tammieh's language skills. She definitely should be using longer, more complex utterances that approximate the adult model.

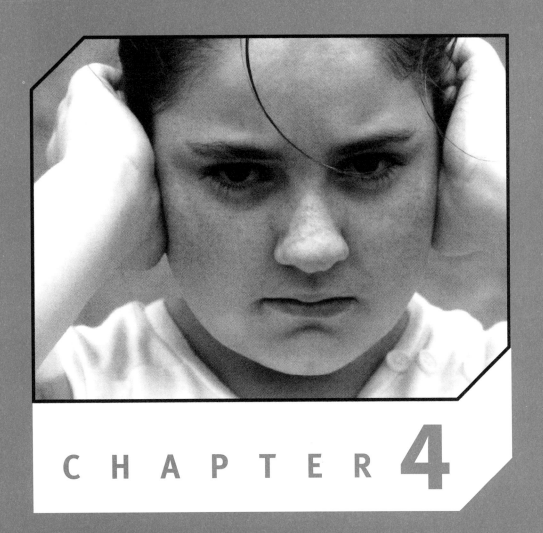

CHAPTER 4

LANGUAGE

DISORDERS

IN CHILDREN

As stated in the previous chapter, language

may be defined as a form of social behavior shaped and maintained by a verbal community. It may also be viewed as a system of symbols used to represent concepts that are formed through exposure and experience (Bloom & Lahey, 1978). Children with disorders of language have limited language skills. Both the ability to understand spoken language and the production of verbal skills may be impaired in these children. Children with these impairments cannot interact, in their families, communities, or cultures, in a manner consistent with that of their peers or with societal expectations. Throughout their lives, children with language disorders find themselves at a disadvantage in personal, academic, and occupational settings (Roseberry-McKibbin, 2007). Roughly 12–14% of school-age children exhibit language disorders. This includes more boys than girls.

Language problems are caused by or associated with several factors. There are many theoretical models from which to view these problems, their causes, and associated factors. In this chapter we discuss three broad categories of children with language problems: (a) children with *specific language impairment* (also known as *language-learning disabilities*); (b) children with *language problems associated with other clinical conditions,* including mental retardation, autism, and acquired brain injury; and (c) children who have language difficulties related to a combination of *physical and social-environmental factors,* including poverty, neglect or abuse, alcohol or drug exposure in utero, and attention-deficit disorder (Hegde & Maul, 2005; Nelson, 1998; Paul, 2001; Reed, 2005). We then discuss assessment and treatment principles and procedures that can be used when serving children with language problems.

INTRODUCTION TO CHILDREN WITH LANGUAGE DISORDERS

Language problems in children are described by many terms: language delay, language disorder, language-learning disability, and specific language impairment. Various early risk factors are known to be associated with later language disorders in children. Children with language problems have certain distinguishing characteristics that clinicians need to be aware of as they provide services to these children.

Description of Language Disorders in Children

Children with language disorders exhibit the following kinds of deficiencies (Hegde & Maul, 2005; Roseberry-McKibbin, 2007):

- *Limited amount of language.* A significant deficiency in the quantity of language learned and understood is a major, general characteristic of children with language disorders or language-learning disabilities.

- *Deficient grammar.* Another major characteristic of children with language disorders is deficient grammar. Both syntactic structures and morphologic features may be difficult for these children to learn under normal conditions.

- *Inadequate or inappropriate social communication.* Deficiencies in social communication, often described as pragmatic aspects of language, also constitute a significant component of language disorders. The social communicative behaviors of children with language disorders may be inadequate or even inappropriate. Failure to initiate conversation and inappropriately interrupting the speakers are examples.

- *Deficient nonverbal communication skills.* Children with language disorders may be deficient in nonverbal communication as well. Their use of gestures, facial expressions, and so forth, may be limited.

- *Deficient literacy skills.* Children with language disorders are known to experience academic problems in school, including difficulties in reading, writing, and spelling.

Risk Factors for Language Disorders in Children

Various early risk factors are known to be associated with later language disorders in children; some important risk factors include the following:

- Prenatal conditions such as maternal drug abuse (including alcohol and nicotine), maternal infections (e.g., rubella, herpes simplex, and HIV)

- Perinatal conditions such as abnormally long labor, precipitated or uncontrolled labor, abnormal presentation of the infant, any condition that causes brain injury during delivery

- Neonatal conditions such as premature birth, low or very high birthweight, poor feeding, infections of the newborn, and the presence of physical and sensory abnormalities

- Presence of any one of many genetic syndromes (e.g., Down syndrome, fetal alcohol syndrome, fragile X syndrome); family history of language disorders

- Environmental factors, including extremely deprived or impoverished home and social environment associated with low socioeconomic status and severe forms of child neglect

- Prelinguistic communication deficits, which include avoidance of eye contact, limited or no babbling, frequent crying, little interest in such gestures as "bye-bye," and showing little or no emotion

- Failure to respond when asked to point to body parts

- Failure to follow such simple instructions as "go get your shoes"

- Delayed production of the first words, including "Mama" and "Dada"

- Lack of social smile and lack of or little interest in social play

- Reduced use of gestures or, conversely, communiating only through gestures

- Impaired learning of speech sounds

CHILDREN WITH SPECIFIC LANGUAGE IMPAIRMENT

As stated, language disorders in children who are otherwise normal are described as *specific language impairment* (SLI), also known as *language-learning disability* (LLD). A majority of children with language disorders exhibit SLI. About 7–8% of kindergarten children exhibit SLI. Children with SLI have certain characteristics that distinguish them from other populations (Casby, 1997; Leonard, 1998; Hegde & Maul, 2005).

Characteristics of Children with Specific Language Impairment

General Characteristics of Children with Specific Language Impairment

- Children with SLI manifest an impairment specific to language. This impairment is not secondary to other developmental disabilities (Hegde & Maul, 2005; Roseberry-McKibbin, 2007).
- Children with SLI have no known etiology or associated condition such as a sensory-motor problem, mental retardation, or significant neurological impairment. Some children with SLI have subtle congitive deficiencies, although general intelligence is within the normal range.
- The sequence of language development in children with SLI is the same as that of normally developing children. However, problems may be seen with various components of language.
- Children with SLI display varied profiles. Some have great difficulty in syntax, with relatively normal pragmatic performance and moderate difficulty with semantic skills, for example. Children with SLI represent a widely varied and heterogeneous group.
- There are two major explanations of SLI. The first is that of *underlying deficits.* In this view,

SLI is due to deficits in cognitive, auditory, perceptual, and intellectual functions that underlie language.

- The second explanation is that SLI reflects the normal variation in linguistic skills, that children with SLI are at the lower end of the normal continuum of language skills. Just as some people have poor math or musical skills, some people have poor linguistic skills (Leonard, 1991, 1998).

Specific Characteristics of Children with Specific Language Impairment

- Children with SLI often have articulatory and phonological problems. They may have poor speech intelligibility and may exhibit *phonological processes* (simplification rules such as final consonant deletion) longer than normal children.
- Children with SLI may manifest less complex syllable structure; for example, they may use more consonant-vowel (CV) combinations than same-age peers who are using CVCV combinations. Children with SLI may also have fewer consonants in their phonetic repertoire.
- Children with SLI are often late in starting to talk. They have a slow rate of word acquisition, especially between 18 and 24 months of age, when children typically show a great vocabulary spurt.
- Children with SLI may either overextend (e.g., calling all adult males Daddy) or underextend words (e.g., a child may call only the family pet "dog" but fail to use the term for other dogs).
- Children with SLI often demonstrate *word-finding* or *word-retrieval problems*. These word-finding problems may result in dysfluencies such as pauses and interjections or fillers (*um, you know*). Word-finding problems may also result in the use of vague or general words (*this, that, thing*) instead of specific referents.
- Learning abstract or figurative words is often hard for children with SLI. They frequently use concrete, not abstract words, to express themselves. For example, a child with SLI might say "I'm mad" instead of "I feel frustrated with this situation."
- The majority of children with SLI have marked morphological problems. Experts believe that these problems may be due to:

    - *perceptual problems;* children do not perceive morphological features as well as they do other features, because those features are produced with less stress and lower intensity;
    - *syntactic problems;* the syntactic complexity involved in sentence comprehension and production may have a negative effect on morphology.

- Morphological problems include omissions of:

    - regular and irregular plural morphemes
    - possessive morphemes
    - present progressive –*ing*
    - third-person singular (e.g., "He plays ball")
    - articles (*a, an, the*)
    - auxiliary and copula verbs (e.g., the auxiliary *is* in "She is running" or the copula *is* in "She is smart")
    - regular past-tense inflections and irregular past-tense words
    - Comparatives and superlatives (e.g., –*er* in smaller and –*est* in smallest)

- Children with SLI may also show confusion with the following structures:

    - singular and plural forms of words

- plural and singular forms of auxiliary and copula verbs (*are, is*)
- subject case markings (*him, he,* or *her, she*)
- regular and irregular forms of plural and past-tense morphemes

- Children with SLI frequently use shorter utterances than normally developing children. That is, their MLU is shorter than that of normal peers.
- Children with SLI use transformations and complex and compound sentences less frequently or not at all; simple, declarative sentences may predominate.
- The speech of some young children with SLI is *telegraphic*. Instead of saying "The cat is eating her food," the child might say, "Cat eat food." The child preserves the meaning of the utterance while omitting the smaller grammatical elements.
- Understanding or comprehending complex sentences is difficult for many children with SLI. This especially presents problems in the classroom setting, where SLI students spend much of their time in large groups of normally developing children who understand complex teacher talk.
- The pragmatic skills of children with SLI vary greatly. While some have fairly normal pragmatic language skills, others have difficulty initiating and sustaining topics of conversation. They may also have difficulty with narrative skills.
- Many children with SLI are passive—that is, unassertive and unresponsive—in communicative interactions (Fey, 1986). Other children with SLI are assertive yet unresponsive; they initiate conversations but are unaware of and unresponsive to their partners' needs.
- Children with SLI may have difficulty with the following aspects of pragmatic skills:

  - topic initiation
  - turn taking
  - topic maintenance
  - appropriate conversational repair strategies (e.g., asking "What do you mean?" when a speaker's utterances are not understood or changing one's own productions when a listener fails to understand)
  - discourse and narrative skills
  - staying relevant during conversation

- Narratives of children with SLI are less complete, contain fewer utterances, and show more communication breakdowns than those of normally developing children.
- Young children with SLI are at risk for later problems with reading and writing.

SUMMARY

✓ Children with SLI manifest an impairment specific to language. This impairment is not due to known etiological factors or associated conditions such as sensory-motor problems or mental retardation. However, certain early risk factors are associated with later language impairment.

✓ Children with SLI generally show specific difficulties in all aspects of language skills: syntax, morphology, phonology, semantics, and pragmatics.

✓ However, there is great heterogeneity in the SLI population, with children manifesting different profiles of problems with various language components.

CHILDREN WITH LANGUAGE PROBLEMS ASSOCIATED WITH PHYSICAL AND SENSORY DISABILITIES

INTRODUCTION

Language disorders in some children are associated with other kinds of disabilities. For instance, mental retardation, autism, hearing loss, traumatic brain injury, and cerebral palsy are associated with language disorders. Language problems coexist with these disabilities.

Mental Retardation

- Mental retardation is defined as a "disability characterized by significant limitations both in intellectual functioning and in adaptive behavior as expressd in conceptual, social, and practical adaptive skills. The disability originates before the age of 18" (American Association on Mental Retardation, 2002, p. xx). Measured in terms of IQ, mental retardation is subaverage intelligence. Limited communication skills is one of the significant features of mental retardation.

- Children with mental retardation (MR), also known as children who are *developmentally disabled or delayed,* are a diverse group. Some are affected by inherited genetic syndromes such as Down syndrome that is due to a chromosomal abnormality; others are affected by environmentally induced genetic abnormalities (e.g., fetal alcohol syndrome).

- A variety of prenatal factors (e.g., rubella, maternal lead poisoning, maternal anoxia, prenatal trauma), natal factors (e.g., fetal anoxia), and postnatal factors (e.g., lead poisoning and rabies vaccine) can cause mental retardation. In addition, traumatic brain injury, low birth weight, endocrine and metabolic disorders (e.g., hypothyroidism and phenylketonuria), cranial abnormalities (e.g., micro- and macrocephaly) cause mental retardation. Consequently, children with MR show a variety of symptoms along with communicative problems.

- The severity of these problems varies with the extent of the retardation. The greater the extent of the retardation, the more severe the communicative problems. The language of children with MR is deficient in phonologic, morphologic, semantic, syntactic, and pragmatic components.

- Most experts agree that the language of children with MR is *delayed* rather than deviant. That is, children with MR show language skills that are commensurate with those of younger normally developing children; they follow the same *sequence* of language development as those children. However, profoundly retarded children may show *echolalia* (parrot-like repetition of what others say), which is uncommon in children who are learning language normally.

- Some children with MR have concomitant problems such as:

  - distractibility and a short attention span
  - congenital microcephaly ("small head")
  - difficulties with gross- and fine-motor skills
  - physical structural deficits such as a cleft palate

■ Cognitively, children with MR tend to have depressed skills. These children are very concrete and have difficulty with abstract concepts. This is thought to affect language skills, particularly semantic skills.

■ Children with MR have semantic difficulties in that they frequently have smaller, more concrete vocabularies than normally developing children. There may also be a gap between comprehension and expression skills, comprehension being superior to expression.

■ Morphologic skills are especially poor in most children with MR. Due to difficulty with the abstract nature of bound morphemes, the speech of many children with MR is telegraphic. Such children tend to omit bound morphemes and *function words,* or the small words that help make up sentences (e.g., instead of saying "The man is going to the store," children with MR might say, "Man go store.").

■ The syntax of children with MR is reduced both expressively and receptively. They master syntactic constructions as normally developing children do but at a slower pace. They frequently use short and simple syntactic structures and have difficulty understanding long and complex sentences.

■ Pragmatically, children with MR may be passive in interacting with others. Or, because of their reduced communication skills, they may be physically aggressive and communicate physically rather than verbally.

■ Because many children with MR have other problems (e.g., medical, gross motor), it is usually necessary to use a multidisciplinary approach to assessment and treatment.

CONCEPTS TO CONSIDER

Many parents believe that SLI and MR are the same thing and think that if their child is diagnosed as SLI, then he or she has mental retardation. Describe how you would explain to a parent the differences between SLI and MR.

_____

_____

_____

_____

_____

Autism Spectrum Disorders

■ Leo Kanner (1943), an Austrian child psychiatrist, originally described autism as a profound emotional disorder of childhood. It was believed for many years that autism was a form of child psychosis. Currently, most experts support genetic or neurophysiological theories of autism, including hypotheses that cortical or subcortical dysfunction, or both, may be involved.

■ In 1944, another Austrian psychiatrist, Hans Asperger, also described a group of children with unusual behaviors and called their condition autistic psychopathy. It is now believed that both Kanner and Asperger described the same clinical condition, except that Kanner's children generally had IQs below 70 and Asperger's children had IQs above 70. The term *Asperger's* is still used, but it represents children who are autistic and are high functioning.

■ Because of the wide variations in the symptom complex of autism, the phenomenon is described as *autism spectrum disorder,* which implies that autism exists on a continuum of severity. *Pervasive developmental disorders* is another term recommended by the American Psychiatric Association (2000) to include children with autism, Asperger's syndrome, Rett's syndrome, and childhood disintegrative disorder. Much of the research is concerned with autism and some lately with Asperger's syndrome. Therefore, we will mostly be concerned with these two syndromes in this section.

■ Autism is diagnosed before age 3. The diagnostic criteria include (a) impaired social interaction, (b) disturbed communication, and (c) stereotypic patterns of behavior, interests, and activities (American Psychiatric Association, 1994).

■ Characteristics of children with autism include:

- generally below-average (IQ 70 or below) intelligence
- a lack of responsiveness to and awareness of other people
- a preference for solitude and objects rather than people
- a lack of interest in nonverbal and verbal communication
- stereotypic body movements such as constant rocking
- insistence on routines; strong dislike of change
- a dislike of being touched or held
- self-injurious behaviors such as head banging (in some children)
- unusual talent in some areas such as arithmetic (in some children)
- seizures in about 25% of children with autism
- hyper- or hyposensitivity to sensory stimulation

■ Language problems associated with autism include:

- inadequate or lack of response to speech
- lack of interest in human voices and a better response to environmental noises; a fascination with mechanical noises
- slow acquisition of speech sound production and language in general
- disinterest in interaction with others
- use of language in a meaningless, stereotypic manner, including echolalia
- perseveration on certain words or phrases
- faster learning of concrete than abstract words, including more ready learning of words that refer to objects as opposed to emotions
- lack of generalization of word meanings
- lack of understanding of the relationships between words
- pronoun reversal (use of *you* for *I* and *I* for *you;* referring to self as *she, him,* or *her*)
- use of short, simple sentences; occasional use of incorrect word order
- omission of grammatic features such as plural inflections, conjunctions

- pragmatic problems such as lack of eye contact and lack of topic maintenance; reduced initiation or lack of assertiveness
- difficulty establishing joint reference

■ Children with autism may have associated problems, such as:

- motor deficits
- central auditory problems
- mental retardation
- evidence of brain injury, especially damage to the left cerebral hemisphere
- abnormal electrical activity of the brain
- seizures
- hearing loss
- hypo- or hypersensitivity to touch

■ Because many children with autism have one or more of these associated problems, it is frequently necessary to use a multidisciplinary team approach to assessment and intervention.

■ Treatment for autism has emphasized social skills training. Systematic and prolonged language training has resulted in meaningful communication patterns in many children. Behavioral management techniques, when combined with behavioral language training, have been shown to be effective. If the autism is severe, the use of alternative, augmentative communication devices may be warranted.

■ Characteristics of children with Asperger's syndrome include (Zager, 2005):

- similar characteristics to those with autism except for communication skills and intellectual levels, which are higher (IQ 70 or above)
- impaired social interactions that are similar to those of children with autism
- repetitive and stereotyped behaviors that are similar to those of children with autism

■ Communication deficits of children with Asperger's syndrome include:

- Some sources claim that children with Asperger's syndrome do not have significant communication disorders (American Psychiatric Association, 1994); this claim is coming under increasing criticism.
- Generally, children with Asperger's syndrome acquire language skills better than those with autism; they may have excellent vocabularies and seemingly normal syntactic skills. However, their social communication is quite atypical (Ozonoff, Dawson, & McPartland, 2002).
- Children with Asperger's syndrome may talk obsessively about their preoccupations; their speech is often more a monologue than a dialogue; they may not allow others to take conversational turns; they may not grasp that their listeners are bored or in a hurry.

■ Communication treatment of children with Asperger's syndrome will be concerned mostly with their pragmatic deficits. These deficits often present significant challenges to children with Asperger's syndrome as they attempt to interact with family, peers, and teachers (Prelock, Beatson, Bitner, Broder, & Ducker, 2003).

■ One popular treatment paradigm is called the SCERTS model (Prizant, 2004). The SCERTS acronym emphasizes the importance of targeting goals in social communication (SC) and emotional regulation (ER) by implementing transactional supports (TS). These transactional supports include visual supports, environmental arrangements, and communication style adjustments.

Brain Injury

Children can have brain injury due to various causes. Brain-injured children may be classified into various subgroups depending on the injury's cause and sequelae. Two major subgroups of brain-injured children include those who sustain injury due to head trauma (with resulting traumatic brain injury) and those who have cerebral palsy. Traumatic brain injury is treated in greater detail in Chapter 8; here we summarize information relevant to children's language disorders.

Traumatic Brain Injury (TBI)

- TBI in children refers to cerebral damage due to external physical force. The injury is not congenital, nor is it a result of a neurological disease. A *focal injury* is restricted to one area of the brain; *diffuse injury* involves multiple areas because damage is widespread (Cooper & Golfinos, 2000; Hux, 2003; Murdoch & Theodoros, 2001). (See Chapter 8 for details about different kinds of injuries associated with head trauma.)
- TBI in children is most frequently caused by vehicular and sports-related accidents, falls, physical abuse, assaults, and gunshot wounds.
- A multidisciplinary team approach to assessment and treatment is always necessary. Medical personnel may be especially involved.
- Immediate effects of TBI include:

  - coma or loss of consciousness
  - confusion and post-traumatic amnesia (memory loss)
  - abnormal behaviors, including aggression, anxiety, irritability, hyperactivity, lethargy, and withdrawal
  - motor dysfunctions, including tremors, rigidity, spasticity, ataxia, and apraxia

- Cognitive and language problems may be associated with TBI. Some of these are observed only initially and may resolve; others may be long term:

  - comprehension problems, especially of sentences
  - word-retrieval problems leading to reduced fluency
  - syntactic problems, including limited MLU, fewer utterances, and difficulty expressing and understanding long, complex sentences
  - reading and writing problems; poor academic performance
  - pragmatic problems such as difficulty with turn taking and topic maintenance (often related to poor inhibition and lack of self-monitoring)
  - difficulty with attention and focus
  - memory problems
  - inability to recognize one's own difficulties
  - reduced speed of information processing
  - difficulties with reasoning and organization

- Children with TBI have unique needs. Frequently, their problems persist over time. A problem in the schools for children with TBI is that traditional, standardized language tests are often not sensitive to the special problems these children manifest (Ylvisaker, 1995).

- Children with TBI need to be assessed regularly in natural settings to determine how they are functioning in those settings. Such children should be served through a comprehensive team approach that helps them integrate back into school and society.

Cerebral Palsy

Cerebral palsy (CP) is a disorder of early childhood in which the immature nervous system is affected. This results in muscular incoordination and associated problems. Cerebral palsy is not a disease; it refers to a group of symptoms associated with brain injury in still developing children (Koman, Smith, & Shilt, 2004; Mecham, 1996). With an incidence rate of 2.5 per 1,000 children, CP is a common childhood disability. Most prenatal, natal, and postnatal factors that affect the brain also are involved in CP.

- Associated problems may include orthopedic abnormalities, seizures, feeding difficulties, hearing loss, perceptual disturbances, and intellectual deficits. However, not all children with CP have all these problems.
- CP is not a progressive disease. It generally occurs for the following reasons:

    - *prenatal brain injury* due to maternal rubella, mumps, accidents, or other factors
    - *perinatal brain injury* due to difficulties in the birth process such as prolonged labor, prematurity, breech delivery
    - *postnatal brain injury* due to anoxia, accidents, infections, and diseases such as scarlet fever and meningitis

- Children with CP can manifest paralysis of various body parts. These may be categorized as follows:

    - *hemiplegia* (one side of the body, the right or left, is paralyzed)
    - *paraplegia* (only the legs and lower trunk are paralyzed)
    - *monoplegia* (only one limb or a part thereof is paralyzed)
    - *diplegia* (either the two legs or the two arms are paralyzed)
    - *quadriplegia* (all four limbs are paralyzed)

- Although many types of CP have been described, most professionals categorize CP into three major types:

    - *ataxic CP*, which involves disturbed balance, awkward gait, and uncoordinated movements (due to cerebellar damage)
    - *athetoid CP*, which is characterized by slow, writhing, involuntary movements (due to damage to the indirect motor pathways, especially the basal ganglia)
    - *spastic CP*, which involves increased spasticity (increased tone, rigidity of the muscles) as well as stiff, abrupt, jerky, slow movements (due to damage to the motor cortex or direct motor pathways)

- Speech and language problems associated with CP depend heavily on the type of CP and the presence of associated problems such as mental retardation. Some children with CP have normal language skills, while others have severe language problems. Dysarthria, described in greater detail in Chapter 8, is common among children with CP.
- Treatment for children with CP should involve a multidisciplinary team approach and the use of alternative, augmentative methods of communication if necessary.

SUMMARY

✓ Children who have physical and sensory disabilities such as mental retardation, autism spectrum disorders, and brain injury manifest unique language characteristics that tend to coexist with the disabilities.

✓ Children whose disabilities are severe may require the use of augmentative, alternative communication devices.

✓ A comprehensive team approach to assessment and treatment is necessary for children whose language problems co-occur with physical and sensory disabilities.

CHILDREN WITH LANGUAGE PROBLEMS RELATED TO PHYSICAL AND SOCIAL-ENVIRONMENTAL FACTORS

INTRODUCTION

Some children manifest language difficulties that are related to a combination of physical and social-environmental factors such as poverty, neglect or abuse, alcohol or drug exposure in utero, and attention deficit hyperactivity disorders. Researchers and clinicians are seeing increasing numbers of children who have a wide variety of language problems that coexist with these factors (Roseberry-McKibbin, 2007).

Language Problems Related to Poverty

■ There is no demonstrated causal relationship between poverty and language-learning difficulties. Professionals should be careful never to equate poverty with dysfunction. Many children from low-income backgrounds have excellent language skills because they have had good stimulation in the home.

■ Other children, however, show problems in language development and learning. Research shows that while not directly causing language problems, limited access to health care and low educational levels of caretakers tend to affect the language skills of children from low-income homes (Roseberry-McKibbin, 2007; Roseberry-McKibbin & Brice, 1998).

■ Socioeconomic status is more critical to language development than ethnic background. The factor most highly related to socioeconomic status is the mother's educational level (Battle & Anderson, 1998).

■ Limited access to health care can affect language skills (O'Hanlon & Roseberry-McKibbin, 2004) because:

- children who are often sick and do not get adequate medical treatment miss much school, thus limiting academic and language exposure;
- children who come to school sick have difficulty concentrating and learning;
- children who do not have access to medical care frequently have untreated ear infections;
- mothers of low-income children often get inadequate prenatal care, which affects the neural development of the fetus; and
- mothers who get inadequate prenatal care tend to have premature or low-birthweight

babies; prematurity and low birth weight are associated with language and cognition problems.

■ Research has documented a strong correlation between education and income levels. For example, long-term welfare dependency is strongly associated with lack of a high school diploma and low literacy levels (Friedlander & Martinson, 1996). This may affect the language development of children from low-income homes because some caretakers who have had limited educational opportunities may not:

- provide adequate oral language stimulation for the children
- provide opportunities for literacy
- have the economic means to expose the children to a variety of enriching experiences (e.g., trips to zoos, museums)
- have the economic means to purchase toys and books that stimulate language development

■ Children from backgrounds of poverty show wide variation in their language skills. Some of these children have excellent language skills. Others show such deficits as the following:

- difficulty in reading and writing
- difficulty referencing time and temporal concepts due to a lack of routine and structure in the home
- lack of familiarity with "school-type" tasks such as reciting the alphabet, singing rhyming songs, reading books
- delayed vocabulary skills due to lack of language stimulation and lack of exposure to a variety of experiences
- delayed morphosyntactic skills
- less verbal elaboration and overall verbalization

Language Problems Related to Neglect or Abuse

■ Statistics indicate that increasing numbers of children come from backgrounds in which they experience neglect, abuse, or both (NA). NA can be found across all socioeconomic levels and ethnic groups.

■ The effect of NA on language depends greatly upon the *extent* and *severity* of the NA. A child who regularly undergoes severe physical, emotional, or verbal abuse, or all of these, will have more severe language problems than a child who experiences neglect without abuse.

■ While it is difficult to make generalizations about this heterogeneous group of children, certain trends have emerged characterizing the effect of NA on language development and skills.

■ Among mother–child pairs in which abuse has been identified, mothers have been observed to be less likely to engage in reciprocal interactions with their infants. In addition, some of these mothers have been found to punish exploration and risk-taking that accompany normal development (Nelson, 1998).

■ Children who undergo abuse tend to have *expressive language delays*. Some of these children are hit or yelled at when they speak; thus, they speak less and therefore do not develop oral language optimally.

■ Children who experience NA are frequently deprived of adequate language stimulation related to *isolation*. Physical or social isolation, or both, reduce the human contacts needed to acquire language optimally. Children's opportunities for hearing and practicing a variety of language structures are reduced. Thus, their expressive and receptive language skills are underdeveloped.

■ Research has shown a relationship between communicative disorders (particularly those associated with physical anomalies and disabilities) and NA. Parents of children with special needs tend to become frustrated more easily than parents of normally developing children. Frustration creates stress, which can lead to NA.

■ To best serve children who experience NA, speech–language pathologists may serve on multidisciplinary teams that address the emotional and physical as well as the language needs presented by these children.

C O N C E P T S T O C O N S I D E R

List two language problems (per area) one might find in children who (a) have autism, (b) have experienced TBI, (c) have cerebral palsy, (d) are from low-income backgrounds, or (e) have experienced neglect or abuse.

_____

_____

_____

_____

_____

Language Problems Related to Parental Drug and Alcohol Abuse

■ Speech–language pathologists participate in multidisciplinary teams to serve increasing numbers of children who have language problems related to maternal alcohol consumption or drug use during pregnancy. Children who have been prenatally exposed to drugs, alcohol, or both, present a wide variety of problems depending on the extent, pattern, and type of exposure to such substances.

■ Recent research has shown that *paternal* alcohol consumption, drug use, smoking, or exposure to environmental toxins can also negatively affect fetal development. Sperm can be damaged by cigarette smoke, marijuana, and alcohol. Men exposed to those teratogens have a greater chance of fathering babies with abnormalities like hydrocephalus, Bell's palsy (paralysis of cranial nerve VII), and mouth cysts.

■ *Fetal alcohol syndrome* (FAS) is a pattern of mental, physical, and behavioral defects that develop in infants born to some women who drink heavily during the pregnancy. FAS is the leading cause of mental retardation in the Western world.

- FAS causes direct language problems and creates difficulties in areas associated with language development. Problems associated with FAS include:

  - pre- and post-natal growth problems; abnormally low birthweight and length; small head size (microcephaly)
  - central nervous system dysfunction: delayed motor development, mild-profound mental retardation or learning disabilities
  - abnormal craniofacial (skull and face) features
  - malformations of major organ systems, especially of the heart; the child may have a small trachea and kidney problems
  - behavior problems, including hyperactivity and attention-deficit disorder
  - poor play and social skills, including poor organizational responses to environmental stimuli
  - learning and academic problems; poor reading, writing
  - speech problems such as articulation delay; may have cleft palate or oral-motor coordination problems
  - swallowing problems, including impaired sucking reflex at birth
  - language delays
  - cognitive problems—reasoning, memory, learning
  - auditory processing problems
  - hearing problems—conductive and sensorineural losses

- *Fetal alcohol effects* (FAE) are signs in babies (e.g., mild physical and cognitive deficits) that have been linked to the mother's drinking during pregnancy. Babies with FAE do not meet the diagnostic criteria for FAS.

- Children who are prenatally exposed to drugs also have difficulties in language and related skills, including:

  - motor/neurological problems:
    — poor visual tracking
    — blanking out, staring spells, bizarre eye movements
    — gross- and fine-motor problems
    — tremors; increased startling
    — decreased awareness of body in space

  - affective/behavioral problems:
    — emotional lability; mood swings from apathy to aggressiveness
    — depressed affect; decreased laughter
    — great difficulty with transitions and changes
    — refusal to comply with simple commands; testing of limits
    — inability to self-regulate, modify own behavior

  - social attachment and related problems:
    — lack of eye contact; gestures to initiate social interaction
    — separation anxiety
    — indiscriminate attachment to new people
    — aggressiveness with peers
    — decreased responsiveness to praise, rewards

- cognitive skill impairments:
  - poor on-task attention
  - increased distractibility to extraneous sounds, movements
  - impulsivity; poor use of trial-and-error strategies
  - difficulty with immediate, short-term, and long-term memory

- language learning problems:
  - fewer spontaneous vocalizations from infancy
  - delayed language acquisition
  - decreased use of words; gesturing to communicate wants and needs
  - word-finding problems
  - prolonged infantile articulatory-phonological disorders
  - difficulty following directions
  - difficulty answering wh- questions
  - difficulty understanding opposites, uses for objects

■ Children prenatally exposed to drugs and alcohol may have language problems that are not readily detected by standardized language measures. Thus, such children may be denied services in the public schools because they do not fit a recognized category such as *learning disabled* or *mentally retarded.*

■ Early intervention is critical for children who are prenatally exposed to drugs and alcohol. These children appear to especially benefit from structure and routine. Caregivers must be involved as much as possible in treatment efforts.

Language Problems Related to Attention Deficit Hyperactivity Disorder

■ Speech–language pathologists are seeing increasing numbers of students with language problems related to *attention deficit hyperactivity disorder* (ADHD). The nature of this relationship is not clear, but many students with ADHD manifest language problems, auditory-processing problems, or both. Thus, speech–language pathologists are increasingly involved on multidisciplinary teams that identify and serve students with ADHD.

■ Students with ADHD are at risk because they frequently experience academic and behavior problems. In some cases, language and auditory-processing difficulties contribute to or co-exist with those problems (Long, 2005). It is important for clinicians to provide intervention in cases where these factors are present.

■ Students with ADHD are described as having chronic difficulties in the areas of impulsivity, attention, and overactivity to a degree inappropriate to their age and developmental level. They are more likely to receive lower grades in academic subjects, and over half of children with ADHD will fail at least one grade by adolescence (Westby & Cutler, 1994).

■ The American Psychiatric Association (2000) divides symptoms of ADHD into two categories: (a) inattention and (b) hyperactivity-impulsivity. Children may have a combination of characteristics in one or both of these categories, and subclassifications are made on the basis of the combination of characteristics presented by the individual child.

- Behavioral characteristics of ADHD students include:

  - frequent fidgeting with hands or feet or squirming in seats
  - difficulty remaining seated when required to do so
  - high distractibility by extraneous stimuli
  - difficulty sustaining attention in tasks or activities
  - difficulty waiting turns in games or group situations
  - frequent loss of things necessary for tasks or activities at school or at home
  - frequent participation in physically dangerous activities without considering the possible consequences

- Research and clinical experience indicate that students with ADHD tend to manifest the greatest amount of difficulty in auditory processing and social interaction skills. Specifically, ADHD students (American Psychatric Association, 2000; England, 1994; Westby & Cutler, 1994):

  - often blurt out answers to questions before the questions have been completed;
  - have difficulty following through on instructions;
  - often do not seem to be listening;
  - often talk excessively;
  - often interrupt or intrude on others;
  - use non sequiturs during discourse;
  - have poor turn-taking skills;
  - frequently manifest false starts because they change their minds while structuring a response;
  - use an excessive number of fillers and pauses because verbal expression occurs with minimal preplanning;
  - have difficulty describing things in an organized, coherent manner—have general difficulty with expressive language organization;
  - do not tell stories or use narrative skills effectively due to disorganization and impulsivity of thought;
  - have difficulty with social entry (limited knowledge of how to successfully initiate or join ongoing interactions);
  - experience problems with verbal reciprocity, tend to be less talkative and responsive when others initiate interactions;
  - use inappropriate register; for example, use the same interactive style with adults and peers;
  - do not perceive or act appropriately upon interlocutors' nonverbal cues; and
  - do not use comprehension monitoring strategies; for example, do not request a repetition of information when they experience a comprehension breakdown.

- Speech–language pathologists must become actively involved in interdisciplinary, collaborative teams that create effective service delivery models for students with ADHD. Goals of treatment may include work on auditory processing skills, pragmatics, and expressive language organization.

SUMMARY

✓ **Increasing numbers of children have language problems related to physical and social-environmental factors such as poverty, neglect or abuse, alcohol or drug exposure in utero, and attention deficit hyperactivity disorders.**

✓ Speech–language pathologists are increasingly serving on multidisciplinary teams that address the comprehensive profile of needs presented by these children.

ASSESSMENT PRINCIPLES AND PROCEDURES

INTRODUCTION

Language assessment is a process of observation and measurement of a child's language behaviors to determine (a) whether a clinically significant problem exists, (b) the nature and extent of the problem, and (c) the course of action that must be taken to help the child and the family. In this section, we discuss common procedures and principles that can be applied to children of any age, use of standardized and non-standardized forms of assessment, and specific recommendations for preschool children, elementary-age children, and adolescents.

Language Assessment: General Principles and Procedures

■ Whatever the age of the child being assessed, clinicians typically follow a set of common procedures that serve as the foundation for the assessment (Hegde, 2001a). Procedures common to assessing any disorder in clients of any age are described in Chapter 11. Here, we will summarize what is especially relevant to assessing language disorders in children. Typically, clinicians need to:

- obtain results of visual or audiological evaluations;
- obtain any available relevant medical data that might be important;
- obtain psychological data, including the results of cognitive functioning and intelligence testing; and
- interview the family members (especially the parents or other primary caregivers) to better understand the problem as they see it, obtain information about the child's language development, assess family communication patterns, and ascertain caregiver preferences about treatment targets.
- for elementary-age and adolescent students:
  — obtain assessment data on educational achievement that might suggest learning disabilities;
  — obtain samples of the student's writing from his or her teachers;
  — examine classroom textbooks to select words, phrases, and sentences that could be included in the assessment; and
  — talk to the teacher about the academic demands the child faces in the classroom and select potential treatment targets based on the teacher's recommendations.

■ Language assessment generally falls into three broad categories: screening, standardized assessment, and nonstandardized or informal assessment.

Screening

- Screening refers to the process of quickly obtaining a general overview of a child's language skills.

- Most clinicians use screening initially to decide whether further assessment is necessary. Screening usually indicates one of two things: (a) there is not a clinically significant language problem, and no further assessment needs to be completed; or (b) there is a possible language problem and further assessment is needed.
- Many clinicians use informal measures to screen language. These are often constructed by individual clinicians and consist of simple activities such as conversational samples that quickly sample children's expressive and receptive language skills. Published screening tests are also available.

Standardized Assessment

- Standardized tests provide clinicians with a quantitative means of comparing the child's performance to the performance of large groups of children in a similar age category.
- Standardized tests are preferred by many clinicians because they yield quantitative, psychometrically based measures such as language age, percentile rank, and standard deviation. Federal or state laws may require the use of these normatively based quantitative measures for placement of a child into special education services within the public school system (Klein & Moses, 1999).
- When using standardized tests, clinicians must consider *participant (subject) sampling.* All standardized tests sample participants, and few or no tests sample all segments of the population. Therefore, many tests are not applicable across all population groups. This is especially true of culturally and linguistically diverse populations because of their underrepresentation in the normative samples.
- It is important to avoid using a test whose normative sample does not include subjects who represent the child being tested. Clinicians must consider all relevant variables: socioeconomic class, urban or rural environment, and ethnocultural and linguistic background (Roseberry-McKibbin, 2002, 2007).
- Standardized tests, even when they sample subjects adequately, tend to sample behaviors inadequately. For example, a behavior tested, such as use of a regular plural, is tested only in one or two contexts. This is inadequate behavior sampling (Hegde, 1998). Clinicians must follow up standardized tests with extended, informal sampling of behaviors targeted on items a child has missed on a standardized test.
- Clinicians must avoid using a standardized test as the sole measure for making clinical judgments about a child's language skills and the presence of a language-learning disability. Standardized tests should be supplemented with language samples and other informal measures.

Nonstandardized, Informal Assessment

- Although widespread use of standardized language tests continues in the United States, many researchers and clinicians are increasingly turning to nonstandardized measures of language. There are several reasons for this.
- One major reason is that the use of standardized tests is often biased and inappropriate with the increasing number of linguistically and culturally diverse students in the United States (Roseberry-McKibbin, 2003).
- Another reason is that many standardized tests do not reflect children's day-to-day lives and functional communication skills and needs. Some professionals view standardized tests as artificial measures of formal, noncontextual language that is not reflective of children's language interaction in daily life. Thus, clinicians are increasingly using several current major alternatives to standardized tests.

Individualized (Client-Specific) Assessment

- *Individualized* or *client-specific procedures* are a preferred alternative to standardized tests. Client-specific procedures form a valid basis for developing client-specific treatments. These procedures use the evocation of language samples over time, by means of culturally appropriate client-specific materials instead of standard stimuli. Baselines before starting treatment are another valid pretreatment measure of language skills.
- *Baselines* can be used as *extended measurements.* Baselines are measures of target behaviors in the absence of planned treatment (Hegde, 1998). Clinicians can establish baselines of communicative behaviors targeted for treatment. Because they are extended and repeated, baselines provide more reliable assessment data than tests and other procedures.

Authentic Assessment

- *Dynamic assessment,* a form of authentic assessment, looks at learner modifiability, or a child's ability to learn when provided with instruction. It often takes place in a test-teach-retest paradigm, in which the child is tested, taught new material, and then retested to see how well and quickly he or she learned the material. A major advantage of dynamic assessment is that a child is not penalized for a lack of experiences assumed by many standardized tests (Roseberry-McKibbin, 2003).
- *Portfolio assessment,* another form of authentic assessment that is popular in many public schools, involves collecting samples of a child's work or performance over a period of time and observing the growth that occurs when instruction is provided.

Social Assessment Methods (Gallagher, 1991)

- *Peer assessment.* Peers can be interviewed as to their perceptions of the child as an interlocutor, classmate, or friend.
- *Teacher and parent assessment.* Interviews and rating instruments can be filled out by teachers and parents indicating their perceptions of the student's language skills.
- *Self-assessment.* The student can fill out a rating scale, complete an interview, or use a combination of these to assess his or her own language skills and language needs.

Language Sampling

- *Language sampling* is a measure of language vital to a diagnosis of language disorders in children. This is a procedure of recording a student's language under relatively typical conditions, which usually involve conversation.
- The clinician's main task in obtaining a language sample is to stimulate the child to speak as freely and naturally as possible. This can be accomplished through the use of a variety of toys, books, stories, pictures, and games. Other conversation partners, such as peers and family members, may interact with the child.
- Clinicians must remember that a single language sample is not sufficient; additional samples must be obtained. Brief language samples should be recorded subsequent to the first sample.
- Clinicians may informally analyze a language sample or use a number of published protocols that are available. These include *Language Assessment, Remediation, and Screening Procedure* (LARSP; Crystal, Fletcher, & Garman, 1976); *Developmental Sentence Scoring* (Lee, 1974); and *Language Sampling, Analysis, and Training Procedure* (LSAT; Tyack & Gottsleben, 1974).
- Some language sampling programs are available as computer software; these include *Computerized Profiling* (Long & Fey, 1993); *Lingquest 1* (Mordecai & Palin, 1982); and *Systematic Analysis of Language Transcripts* (SALT; Miller & Chapman, 1983).

- Many clinicians use a language sample to obtain a measure of a child's *mean length of utterance* (MLU), which is usually calculated in morphemes through the following method:

$$MLU = \frac{number\ of\ morphemes}{number\ of\ utterances}$$

- Clinicians can analyze not only the child's MLU, but also the presence or absence of Brown's 14 grammatical morphemes (see Chapter 3, Table 3.3). There is a set of generally accepted rules for counting morphemes; these are summarized in Table 4.1.
- Language samples can also be analyzed through a *type-token ratio* (TTR), which is calculated as follows:

$$TTR = \frac{number\ of\ different\ words\ in\ sample}{number\ of\ words\ in\ sample}$$

- TTR represents the variety of different words the child uses expressively, thus assessing the child's semantic or lexical skills. To calculate TTR as shown above, the clinician first counts all the words in the sample (even if they are repeated). These words become the denominator. The clinician then counts each different word in the sample—for example, if "dog" occurs 10 times, it is only counted once. The number of different words the child uses becomes the numerator. For children 3–8 years of age, the TTR is typically 1:2, or .5. In other words, the total number of words spoken by the child during the language sample is usually about twice the number of different words in the sample (Johnson, 1996).

CONCEPTS TO CONSIDER

Briefly compare and contrast standardized, formal language assessment and nonstandardized, informal language assessment. In what situations would you want to use each type of assessment?

_____

_____

_____

_____

_____

Assessment of Infants and Toddlers

- The assessment and treatment of infants and toddlers has taken on increasing visibility in past years. There are several reasons for this. First, laws such as P.L. 99-457, Preschool Amendments to the Education of the Handicapped Act, 1986, have provided incentives at the state and federal levels for speech–language pathologists to identify and treat infants and toddlers with established risk of language disorders or who experience conditions that put them at risk for developing language disorders.

Table 4.1   RULES FOR COUNTING MORPHEMES

COUNT AS 2 MORPHEMES

Structure	Examples
Regular past tense –*ed*	wash*ed*, wav*ed*, look*ed*
Present progressive –*ing*	writ*ing*, decorat*ing*, runn*ing*
Possessive marker –*'s*	Mommy*'s*, teacher*'s*, friend*'s*
Plural marker –*s*	cookie*s*, present*s*, glass*es*
Third person singular present tense marker	swim*s*, flie*s*, drink*s*

COUNT AS 1 MORPHEME

Structure	Examples
Compound words (2 or more free morphemes)	birthday, hotdog, railroad
Proper names	Dr. Cho, Mr. Cook, Uncle Ed, Wiley E. Coyote
Each recurrence of a word for emphasis	no, no, no; awesome, awesome, awesome!
Ritualized reduplications	night-night; choo-choo
Contracted negatives	won't, can't, don't
Diminutives	dolly, horsie, kitty
Irregular past-tense verbs	swam, ate, wrote
Auxiliary verbs	*is* or *will*
Catenatives	gotta, hafta, wanna

DO NOT COUNT

Structure	Examples
Fillers	um, ah, er, uh
Dysfluencies, except the one complete form	l-l-l-lollipop

Note. Adapted from *A First Language: The Early Stages*, by R. Brown, 1973, Cambridge, MA: Harvard University Press; and *Language Disorders: A Functional Approach to Assessment and Intervention*, 4th ed., by R. E. Owens, 2004, Boston: Allyn & Bacon. Adapted with permission.

- Second, due to advances in medical science, many more medically fragile pre-term infants are surviving; these infants often have needs in multiple areas such as speech and language, motor skills, and others. The assessment of infants and toddlers holds special challenges for clinicians, who must account for risk factors as well as overt language problems.

Risk Factors for Language Disorders in Infants and Toddlers

- As mentioned, infants and toddlers may fall into one of two categories: those with an *established risk* of developing language disorders, and those who experience conditions that put them *at risk* of developing language disorders.
- Factors involving an *established risk* of developing language disorders are mostly biological or disease related. These factors include (Rossetti, 2001):

    - congenital malformations (e.g., cleft palate, spina bifida)
    - genetic syndromes (e.g., Down syndrome)
    - atypical developmental disorders (e.g., autism)
    - sensory disorders (e.g., hearing loss, visual impairment)
    - neurologic disorders (e.g., cerebral palsy, muscular dystrophy)
    - metabolic disorders (e.g., Tay-Sachs disease, pituitary diseases)
    - chronic illnesses (e.g., diabetes, cystic fibrosis)
    - severe infectious diseases (e.g., HIV, encephalitis)
    - severe toxic exposure (e.g., lead poisoning, fetal alcohol syndrome)

- Conditions that place children *at risk* for developing language disorders include environmental factors, genetic background, and some disease-related conditions (Rossetti, 2001):

    - serious prenatal and natal complications, including low birthweight (< 1,500 g), child being small for gestation age (< 10th percentile), and anoxia
    - early signs of behavior disorders (e.g., irritability, withdrawal)
    - child's tendency toward frequent and unusual accidents
    - chronic middle ear infections (otitis media)
    - family history of predisposing genetic or medical conditions
    - chronic or severe physical illness, mental illness, or mental retardation in the primary caregiver or one or both parents
    - serious questions raised by a professional, a parent, or a caregiver about the child's development
    - chronically dysfunctional interaction between members of the family
    - caregiver or parental substance abuse; caregiver or parental history of abuse
    - parental education below ninth grade, parental unemployment, or chronic welfare dependency
    - isolation of the child or separation of the child from the primary caretaker or parent
    - unstable or dangerous living conditions (e.g., homelessness)
    - lack of health insurance; poor family health care; inadequate prenatal care

Prelinguistic Behavioral Deficiencies in Infants and Toddlers

- Although language problems in infants and toddlers may be caused by or associated with many factors, such as those listed, some infants who later exhibit SLI may not show primary impairment. Several characteristics distinguish such infants:

- difficulty establishing eye contact, mutual gaze, and joint reference
- communication of needs through greater use of gestures and vocalizations than words and phrases; frequent delays in onset of first word and onset of two-word combinations
- reduced amount of babbling, fewer consonants in babbling, and less complex babbling

General Assessment Guidelines and Procedures for Infants and Toddlers

- Make a family-centered communication assessment of infants and toddlers in both home and clinic settings (Hegde, 2001a; Rosetti, 2001).
- Begin assessment as early as possible and repeat assessments throughout the childhood period. Assess the family constellation, family resources, family strengths and limitations, and family communication patterns.
- Work on a team with other professionals. Make interdisciplinary decisions regarding what assessment materials and methods to use and how assessment results will be used.
- Conduct interviews and gather an extensive case history, including maternal health during pregnancy, circumstances of the birth, and early development patterns of the infant (e.g., fine and gross motor, speech and language).
- Take into consideration the cultural practices in family communication patterns, child rearing, caretaker–child interactions, and accepted roles for children in adult–child interactions (Weitzner-Lin, 2004).

Specific Assessment Guidelines and Procedures for Infants and Toddlers

- With infants and toddlers (depending upon the age), clinicians generally need to assess language-related areas such as hearing and infant readiness for communication as well as language comprehension, verbal communication, infant–caregiver interaction, and play activities.

Language-Related Skills

- Assess the infant's attentional and physiological state (including alertness, drowsiness, light or deep sleep states, eye opening, crying, toleration of handling, etc.).
- Assess the infant's readiness for communication (e.g., whether the baby shows reciprocal interaction with the environment).
- If necessary, refer the infant to an audiologist.

Language Comprehension and Verbal Communication

- Use language development milestones (see Chapter 3) to assess the presence or absence of verbal communication behaviors as well as language comprehension skills. This can be done through direct observation, parent report, or both.

Infant–Caregiver Interaction

- Use instruments such as the *Mother-Infant Play Interaction Scale* by Walker and Thompson (1982) and the *Observation of Communication Interaction* by Klein and Briggs (1986). These instruments offer suggestions for how to observe the baby and the mother or another caregiver, preferably in the home setting or in a natural interactive clinical situation. These instruments help assess:

- the infant's mood and affect, responsiveness or lack thereof
- how the caregiver modifies the interaction when the infant gives negative cues (e.g., when the infant is tired of peek-a-boo and averts her gaze, the caregiver changes activities)
- how the caregiver visually focuses on the baby (e.g., the caregiver holds or places the infant at his or her eye level and maintains eye contact)
- how the caregiver stimulates and handles the baby (holding, rocking, cuddling, stroking)
- how the caregiver expresses his or her affection for the baby (e.g., smiling and laughing)

Play Activities

- Observe the child engaged in play with one or several other children. Observe the child's pattern of interaction during play and evaluate whether the child:
  - exhibits aggressive or uncooperative behaviors
  - does not share toys
  - talks little during play
  - passively watches others play
  - plays cooperatively with other children
  - engages in isolated or parallel play
  - engages in constructive activities with or alongside other children
  - engages in pretend play and role playing

Published Assessment Instruments for Infants and Toddlers

Few standardized instruments are available to use in the assessment of children under 3 years of age. Most instruments for children age 3 and under are developmental scales that help structure clinicians' or parents' observations of the child to take note of the presence or absence of behaviors of interest. Clinicians may also use the developmental milestones list in Chapter 3 to structure individualized assessments for infants and toddlers. Finally clinicians may consider using the published instruments listed in Table 4.2.

Assessment of Preschool and Elementary-Age Children

- Language problems often become apparent during the elementary school years. They are frequently brought to the surface by reading and writing deficiencies that cause academic problems and even failure. It is when children experience academic difficulties that they are usually referred for speech–language assessment. In ideal circumstances, language problems would be noted and treated when children are in preschool.

Description of Language Disorders in Preschool and Elementary-Age Children

Language problems of preschool and elementary-age children can be associated with a variety of factors such as language-learning disability, mental retardation, environmental factors, and others (Long, 2005). Characteristics of such children with language problems may include the following:

- *Difficulty in comprehending spoken language.* This includes problems with comprehending syntactically longer and more complex productions, as well as difficulty comprehending the meaning of complex words, phrases, sentences, and abstract terms.

Table 4.2   COMMONLY USED PUBLISHED ASSESSMENT INSTRUMENTS FOR INFANTS AND TODDLERS

Assessment Instrument	Description
Preschool Language Scale–3 (I. Zimmerman, V. Steiner, & R. Pond)	Used to assess expressive and receptive language in infants and children through 6-11 years
Birth to 3 Developmental Scale (T. S. Bangs & S. Dodson)	Used to assess developmental delays in multiple areas
Early Language Milestone Scale (2nd ed.) (J. Coplan)	Used to assess speech and language development in children from birth through 3 years
Bayley Scales of Infant Mental Development–Revised (N. Bayley)	Used to assess cognitive, psychomotor, social, visual, and auditory skills in infants
Sequenced Inventory of Communication Development–Revised (D. Hedrick, E. Prather, & A. Tobin)	Used to assess nonverbal and verbal communication in infants and children through 4 years
Receptive-Expressive Emergent Language Test–2 (K. Bzoch & R. League)	Used to interview parents and gain a multidimensional analysis of emergent language in children from birth through 3 years
Battelle Developmental Inventory (J. Newborg, J. Stock, L. Wnek, J. Guidubaldi, & J. Svinicki)	Used to assess the following skills in infants: memory, discrimination, perceptual, conceptual, motor, adaptive, and communication
Rossetti Infant-Toddler Language Scale (L. Rossetti)	Used to assess interaction and communication patterns in infants and toddlers
Communication and Symbolic Behavior Scales (A. M. Wetherby & B. Prizant)	Used to assess nonverbal and verbal communication patterns in infants and children through 6 years
Assessment of Preterm Infant Behavior (H. Als, B. Lester, E. Tronick, & T. Brazelton)	Used with infants in NICU (neonatal intensive care unit); assesses attentional and physiological states
Vineland Adaptive Behavior Scale (S. Sparrow, D. Balla, & D. Cicchetti)	Used to assess daily living, socialization, and motor skills as well as receptive and expressive language in infants and toddlers
Preschool Language Assessment Instrument (M. Blank, S. A. Rose, & L. J. Berlin)	Used from ages 3-0 to 5-11 to assess ability to integrate vocabulary and language structure knowledge to solve problems and follow directions (also available in Spanish)

- *Slow or delayed language onset.* This can include delayed babbling, slower vocabulary growth rate, delayed acquisition of vocabulary, slowness in combining words into phrases and sentences, and overall slower acquisition of language milestones.
- *Limited language output or expressive language.* This includes generally limited verbal repertoire, lack of complex or longer word productions, limited amount of vocabulary produced and comprehended, and lack of abstract words in the child's repertoire.
- *Problematic syntactic skills.* This includes use of shorter instead of longer sentences, simpler instead of more complex sentences, single words or phrases in place of sentences, and a limited variety of syntactic structures.
- *Problematic pragmatic skills.* This includes difficulty with initiating and maintaining conversations, turn taking, using conversational repair strategies, maintaining eye contact, and narrative skills.
- *Problematic learning of grammatic morphemes.* This includes difficulty with comparatives and superlatives (e.g., *small, smaller, smallest*), omission of bound morphemes (e.g., past tense *–ed*, plural *–s*), and incorrect use of learned grammatic morphemes, including overgeneralizations (e.g., *womans/women, goed/went*) past the appropriate developmental point.

General Assessment Guidelines and Procedures for Elementary-Age Children

- Begin by screening language to determine if a more detailed assessment is needed; do this through brief language sampling or through formal screening measures such as those listed in Table 4.3.

Table 4.3 COMMONLY USED STANDARDIZED SCREENING MEASURES

Assessment Instrument	Description
Denver Developmental Screening Test II (W. K. Frankenburg & Associates)	Used from age 2 weeks to 6 years to assess motor, language, and personal-social development
The Communication Screen (N. Striffler & S. Willig)	Used from age 2-10 to 5-9 to assess auditory comprehension and vocabulary skills
Preschool Language Screening Test (E. Hannah & J. Gardner)	Used from age 3 to 5-6 to assess motor, visual, and auditory perceptual concepts
Bankson Language Screening Test–2 (N. W. Bankson)	Used from age 4 to 7 to screen syntactic, semantic, and morphologic skills and visual and auditory perception
Fluharty Preschool Speech and Language Screening Test–3 (N. B. Fluharty)	Used from age 2 to 6 to screen basic language skills

- Obtain a case history.
- Use social assessment methodologies; conduct interviews as appropriate and necessary. Obtain information from parents, teachers, and peers about the child's communication patterns.
- Evaluate semantic, syntactic, morphologic, and pragmatic aspects of both expressive and receptive oral language.
- Evaluate reading and writing skills if relevant, and relate communication skills to academic demands and performance if relevant.
- Assess the family constellation and communication patterns. Consider factors related to bilingualism, second-language acquisition, and use of a social dialect if relevant.
- Suggest treatment targets based on findings generated by use of these assessment procedures.

Specific Assessment Guidelines and Procedures for Elementary-Age Children

Obtain an extended speech and language sample for a typical analysis of language functions. Language samples can be collected on different days with different interlocutors (e.g., peers, teachers, family members) over a period of time in order to obtain the most representative sample of the child's language.

- Language samples can be analyzed and a description given of the child's skills in the areas of semantics, morphology, syntax, and pragmatics. Language comprehension can also be analyzed.
- To assess *syntactic skills,* calculate the child's mean length of utterance (MLU), as well as the complexity of his or her utterances. Evaluate the child's use of:

  - verb phrases (e.g., *he is swimming, that is red*)
  - noun phrases (e.g., *my books, big dress, that crayon*)
  - prepositional phrases (e.g., *the crayons in the box*)
  - sentence types such as simple, declarative, compound, complex, active, questions, negatives, and requests

- To assess *morphologic skills:*

  - use appropriate pictures to assess a child's production of regular and irregular plural nouns as well as present progressive *–ing* (e.g., "What are these things? What is the boy doing?")
  - assess production of comparatives and superlatives by showing three pictures and saying things like, "This man is big; this man is even _____, and this man is the very _____ .")
  - evoke the possessive morpheme by showing pictures and asking questions such as "whose hat is this?"
  - evoke the production of the third-person singular by asking such questions as "What flies?" and "Who cooks?" after showing pictures of a bird flying and a man cooking
  - assess production of adjectives by showing pictures and asking the child to complete such sentences as "This boy is _____" (short); "This car is _____" (green); and so forth
  - evoke past-tense constructions by telling a story, through pictures, and then asking the child to use the pictures to retell the story

- To assess *semantic skills:*

  - ask parents to list words the child uses, especially if the child only produces a few words

- ask parents to describe the types and number of words the child uses at home
- have the child name and describe pictures, toys, and objects as you show them
- have the child tell a story depicted pictorially (e.g., using a book or cards)
- tell the child a short story and then have the child retell the story to you
- note phenomena such as unusual word usage, over- and underextensions of words, signs of misunderstanding words, and the use of general terms (e.g., *this, that, thing*) for more specific ones

- To assess *pragmatic skills,* observe the following parameters:

    - eye contact and other nonverbal behaviors
    - narrative skills
    - topic initiation and maintenance
    - turn-taking skills
    - conversational repair—is the child able to ask questions when messages are not clear, and to respond effectively to listener requests for clarification?

- To assess *language comprehension:*

    - note inappropriate or irrelevant responses that indicate lack of comprehension
    - note the complexity level at which comprehension breaks down (e.g., comprehension of phrases or sentences but not paragraphs)
    - give specific commands that gradually increase in length and complexity (e.g., "Point to the blue square," "Point to the small blue square," "Point to the blue square and the green triangle," "Point to the big blue square and the small green triangle")
    - ask the child to point to correct pictures that help assess comprehension of grammatic morphemes (e.g., "Show *me the dog is barking*" "Show me *the ball is in the bag*" "Show me *three shoes*")
    - assess comprehension of abstract statements by asking the child to explain the meaning of common proverbs (e.g., "Tell me what 'A penny saved is a penny earned' means"). It is important to remember that proverbs and other figurative language expressions are extremely culture bound.

Standardized Tests for Elementary-Age Children

State and federal laws frequently require the use of formal scores, gathered from formal tests, for the diagnosis of a language disorder in a preschool or elementary-age child. Clinicians can choose from the standardized tests listed in Table 4.4.

Assessment of Adolescents

- Language disorders often persist from the early childhood years into adolescence. Research increasingly shows that such language problems, unless treated, usually carry over into adulthood and have an impact upon the person's life in multiple areas: academic, vocational, and social/personal.

- The area of adolescent language is receiving increased attention in speech–language pathology because of its far-reaching effects (Nippold, 1998). (*Note:* In referring to adolescents, the terms *student* and *client* are used interchangeably.)

Table 4.4 COMMONLY USED STANDARDIZED TESTS OF CHILDREN'S LANGUAGE SKILLS

Standardized Test	Description
Assessment of Children's Language Comprehension (R. Foster, J. J. Giddan, & J. Stark)	Used from age 3 to 6-11 to assess receptive syntax and vocabulary
Test of Auditory Comprehension of Language–3 (E. Carrow-Woolfolk)	Used from age 3–9 to assess comprehension of grammatic features, word classes and relations, elaborated sentence constructions
Peabody Picture Vocabulary Test–III (L. M. Dunn & L. M. Dunn)	Used from age 2-6 to adult to assess receptive knowledge of single words
Receptive One-Word Picture Vocabulary Test–Revised (M. F. Gardner)	Used from age 2-11 to 12 to assess comprehension of single words
Expressive One-Word Picture Vocabulary Test–Revised (M. F. Gardner)	Used from age 2 to 11-11 to assess production of single words
Boehm Test of Basic Concepts (A. E. Boehm)	Used from kindergarten to second grade to assess comprehension of basic semantic concepts
Clinical Evaluation of Language Fundamentals–4 (E. Semel, E. Wiig, & W. Secord)	Used from age 6 to 21-11 to assess receptive and expressive syntax, morphology, and semantics
Detroit Test of Learning Aptitude–Primary–4. (D. D. Hammill & B. R. Bryant)	Used from age 3-6 to 9-11 to assess motoric, cognitive, linguistic, attentional domains
Multilevel Informal Language Inventory (C. Goldsworthy & W. Secord)	Used from age 4–12 to assess expressive semantics, morphology, and syntax
Test for Examining Expressive Morphology (K. G. Shipley, T. Stone, & M. Sue)	Used from age 3 to 8-11 to assess production of various morphemes

(continues)

Table 4.4 *Continued.* **COMMONLY USED STANDARDIZED TESTS OF CHILDREN'S LANGUAGE SKILLS**

Standardized Test	Description
Test of Early Language Development–3 (W. P. Hresko, D. K. Reid, & D. D. Hammill)	Used from age 2-7 to 7-11 to assess production and comprehension of syntactic and semantic structures
Test of Language Development–Primary–3 (P. L. Newcomer & D. D. Hammill)	Used from age 4 to 8-11 to assess expressive and receptive semantics, syntax, and morphology
Language Processing Test–Revised (G. J. Richard & M. A. Hanner)	Used from age 5–11 to assess verbal reasoning and expressive vocabulary
Test of Language Development–Intermediate:3 (D. D. Hammill & P. L. Newcomer)	Used from age 8-0 to 12-11 to assess receptive and expressive syntax and semantics and articulation
Test of Word Finding–2 (D. J. German)	Used from age 6-6 to 12-11 to assess single-word retrieval skills
The WORD Test–Elementary–Revised (R. Huisingh, M. Barrett, L. Zachman, C. Bladgen, & J. Orman)	Used from age 7–11 to assess expressive vocabulary and semantic skills
Bankson Language Test–2 (N. W. Bankson)	Used from age 3-0 to 6-11 to assess pragmatics, semantic knowledge, and morphology and syntax
Test of Pragmatic Skills–Revised (B. B. Shulman)	Used from age 3 to 8-11 to assess nonverbal and verbal pragmatic skills
Utah Test of Language Development–4 (M. J. Mecham)	Used from age 3 to 9-11 to assess language expression and comprehension
Token Test for Children (F. DiSimoni)	Used from age 3 to 11-11 to assess auditory comprehension of spatial and temporal concepts
Comprehensive Receptive and Expressive Vocabulary Test (G. Wallace & D. D. Hammill)	Used from age 4 to 17-11 to assess receptive and expressive oral vocabulary

CONCEPTS TO CONSIDER

Briefly describe two guidelines for assessing infants and two guidelines for assessing preschool and elementary-age children.

_____

_____

_____

_____

_____

Description of Language Disorders in Adolescents

- Certain characteristics are commonly found in adolescents with language problems. These characteristics include difficulty in the areas of syntax, semantics, pragmatics, and reading and writing.
- *Syntactic problems:*

  - limited length of sentences; sentences shorter than would be expected
  - difficulty in using complex sentences containing subordinate clauses
  - difficulty using cohesion devices or connectives (e.g., the use of such expressions as *moreover, furthermore, therefore, for example*)
  - lack of agreement (e.g., noun-verb agreement)
  - persistent use of syntactic errors
  - limited use of low-frequency structures (e.g., passive sentences like "The book was written by the author," or such noun phrase postmodifications as "a flower called the tulip" or "Mrs. McKibbin the math teacher")

- *Semantic problems:*

  - word-retrieval problems in conversational speech, resulting in dysfluencies such as repetitions, revisions, and false starts
  - problems with word-definition skills; possibly especially evident in defining scientific and technical words
  - word-relation problems; difficulty understanding and correctly using words that are related by similar or contrastive meanings (synonyms and antonyms)
  - difficulty in understanding and correctly using figurative language (e.g., idioms, metaphors, and proverbs)
  - difficulty in learning and using peer-group slang
  - difficulty in understanding and correctly using words with abstract and multiple meanings (e.g., *rock, pound*)

- difficulty in using precise terms with clear referents (as demonstrated by excessive use of such terms as *this, that, thing, stuff,* etc.)

- *Pragmatic problems:*

  - difficulty modifying statements or adding new information (restatement of the same information without modification for listener)
  - maze behavior (false starts and repeated attempts to express the same idea; e.g., "You know, the um, the, you know, it was the um … the thing")
  - inappropriate use of gestures and other nonverbal cues
  - difficulty maintaining a topic of conversation
  - difficulty distinguishing facts from opinions
  - tactless expressions; difficulty being indirect when necessary (e.g., "You look really bad" rather than "It must have been a difficult night last night")
  - difficulty asking relevant questions and making relevant comments during conversation; may make inappropriate interruptions, and may use non sequiturs
  - difficulty using the correct register (e.g., the use of a more formal register with teachers and other authority figures than with peers)

- *Reading and writing problems:*

  - grammatical errors (e.g., "The whale were in the sea")
  - difficulty comprehending material that is read
  - spelling difficulties
  - use of nontechnical language instead of technical language
  - poor formation of letters (may be related to fine-motor problems)
  - lack of punctuation skills (e.g., misuse or omission of such things as periods and commas)
  - poor organization of narratives and essays, leaving the reader confused
  - sparse information, lack of appropriate detail

General Assessment Guidelines and Procedures for Adolescents

- Begin by screening language to determine if a more detailed assessment is needed; do this through brief language sampling or through formal screening measures such those listed in Table 4.5.
- Obtain a case history.
- Use social assessment methodologies. For example, conduct interviews with parents, teachers, and peers about the adolescent's everyday communication patterns.
- Evaluate syntactic, semantic, morphologic, and pragmatic aspects of both receptive and expressive oral language.
- Evaluate reading and writing skills and assess how those skills relate to the demands of the classroom.
- Relate written and oral communication skills to potential vocational needs and demands.
- Consider factors related to second-language acquisition, bilingualism, and use of a social dialect.
- Create treatment targets based upon test results; ensure that targets will result in improved functional written and oral communication.
- Remember that adolescent language assessment may take more time than assessment of language in a younger child because of the need to obtain extended narratives, writing samples, and interviews with people in the adolescent's environment.

Table 4.5 COMMONLY USED STANDARDIZED SCREENING TESTS FOR ADOLESCENTS

Screening Test	Description
Screening Test of Adolescent Language (E. M. Prather, S. Beecher, M. L. Stafford, & E. Wallace)	Used from age 6–12 to assess vocabulary, language processing, auditory memory, verbal expression
Clinical Evaluation of Language Fundamentals–Revised Screening (E. Semel, E. Wiig, & W. Secord)	Used from age 5–16 to assess auditory comprehension, pragmatics, and expressive and receptive morphology, syntax, and semantics
Classroom Communication Screening Procedure for Early Adolescents (C. S. Simon)	Used from age 9–14 to assess following directions, verbal expression skills, and metalinguistic skills
Adolescent Language Screening Test (D. L. Morgan & A. M. Guilford)	Used from age 11–17 to assess phonology, morphology, pragmatics, semantics, and syntax

Specific Assessment Guidelines and Procedures for Adolescents

- When assessing adolescents, clinicians can use a combination of formal and informal measures to assess syntactic, pragmatic, semantic, and reading and writing problems, which are common in adolescents with language disorders (Reed, 2005).
- Clinicians should obtain an extended speech and language sample in order to analyze language as it occurs naturally in the environment.
- It is necessary to obtain a sample of a conversation between the client and the following interlocutors: a teacher, one or more peers, and a family member or members.
- To assess *syntactic skills:*

  - assess the use of vague, wordy, and roundabout expressions instead of more precise (thus shorter) expressions
  - assess the use of connectives or cohesion devices; note the contexts in which the student should have used such devices but did not
  - assess agreement (e.g., noun-verb agreement) in oral and written language
  - conduct an analysis of syntactic skills through the use of speech and language samples, narratives, and writing samples
  - assess sentence length in *C-units* (communication units) or *T-units* (terminable units) (Both C-units and T-units contain an independent clause and subordinate clauses, but the C-units also may be incomplete sentences produced in response to questions. Count

the number of words per unit and calculate both the mode—the most frequently observed length—and the mean.)

- To assess *semantic skills,* such as:

  - *word definition skills*—obtain a list of words from the student's teachers and textbooks; ask the student to define them
  - *word-retrieval problems* in conversational speech—take note of such dysfluencies as pauses, revisions, false starts, repetitions, and others; notice which words are retrieved with difficulty
  - *word-relation problems*—have the student define and contrast synonyms (e.g., *pretty-beautiful*) and antonyms (*pretty–ugly*)
  - *difficulty in using precise terms* during conversation, narrative tasks, and writing—take note of the frequency with which the student uses such vague expressions as *stuff, thing, this, that, you know*
  - *difficulty in understanding and correctly using figurative language*—make a list of common idioms, proverbs, and metaphors and then ask the student what they mean (e.g., *don't count your chickens before they hatch; fit as a fiddle; kicked the bucket*)

- To assess *pragmatic skills:*

  - assess the frequency with which the client asks you to repeat information, suggesting poor listening skills
  - assess the use of correct register depending on the situation (e.g., use of slang register with peers and more formal register with authority figures)
  - note any inappropriate body language during conversation (e.g., standing too close, using inappropriate gestures)
  - introduce various topics and evaluate the student's ability to maintain those topics over successive utterances
  - ask the student to read a story and then retell it; ask the student to orally narrate a story; evaluate the student's ability to correctly sequence events in a manner understandable to the listener
  - count the frequency of maze behaviors such as false starts and repeated attempts to express the same ideas
  - note interruptions, irrelevant comments, and non sequiturs
  - make vague and nonspecific statements; evaluate whether the student makes requests for clarification

- To analyze *reading and writing skills:*

  - ask the student to read grade-level material; analyze the type and frequency of reading errors made
  - ask questions about the material read to evaluate reading comprehension
  - analyze multiple writing samples for:
    — difficulty forming letters and other handwriting problems
    — spelling errors
    — punctuation errors
    — errors in syntax
    — cohesion and overall organization
    — appropriateness of content, including the adequacy of information offered and details given

Table 4.6 COMMONLY USED STANDARDIZED LANGUAGE TESTS FOR ADOLESCENTS

Standardized Test	Description
Clinical Evaluation of Language Fundamentals–3 (E. Semel, E. Wiig, & W. Secord)	Used from age 6 to 21-11 to assess receptive and expressive syntax, morphology, and semantics
Woodcock Language Proficiency Battery–Revised (R. W. Woodcock)	Used from age 2–95 to assess oral and written language
Bilingual Syntax Measure (M. K. Burt & H. C. Dulay)	Used with 3rd through 12th graders to assess expressive syntax in English and Spanish
Comprehensive Receptive and Expressive Vocabulary Test (G. Wallace & D. D. Hammill)	Used from ages 4 to 17-11 to assess receptive and expressive oral vocabulary
Expressive One-Word Picture Vocabulary Test–Upper Extension (M. Gardner)	Used from age 12 to 15-11 to assess single-word naming skills
Receptive One-Word Picture Vocabulary Test– Upper Extension (M. Gardner & B. Brownell)	Used from age 12-0 to 15-11 to assess single-word receptive vocabulary skills
The Word Test–Adolescent (L. Zachman, M. Barrett, R. Huisingh, J. Orman, & C. Blagden)	Used from age 12-10 to 17-11 to assess expressive semantic skills
Test of Adolescent and Adult Language–3 (D. D. Hammill, V. L. Brown, S. C. Larsen, & J. L. Wiederholt)	Used from age 12-0 to 24-11 to assess auditory comprehnsion and oral and written language skills
Test of Problem Solving–Adolescent (L. Zachman, M. Barrett, R. Huisingh, J. Orman, & C. Blagden)	Used from age 12-0 to 17-11 to assess verbal problem-solving ability and sentence production
Fullerton Language Test for Adolescents (2nd ed.) (A. R. Thorum)	Used from age 11-0 to adult to assess semantic, morphologic, and syntactic skills
Test of Language Development–Intermediate:3 (D. D. Hammill & P. L. Newcomer)	Used from age 8-0 to 12-11 to assess receptive and expressive syntax and semantics
Test of Adolescent/Adult Word Finding (D. J. German)	Used from age 12–80 to assess naming of verbs and nouns, categories, description, and sentence completion

Standardized Tests for Adolescents

- A problem with many formal, published adolescent language tests is that they contain sections that evaluate aspects of language that develop at much younger ages in normal children. For example, some adolescent language tests evaluate students' production of Brown's grammatical morphemes (Nippold, 1998).
- Thus, many clinicians prefer to use nonstandardized procedures to assess langue problems in adolescents. However, state and federal laws frequently require the use of formal scores, gathered from formal tests, for the diagnosis of a language disorder in an adolescent. Some formal tests available on the market are listed in Table 4.6.

SUMMARY

✓ Language assessment is used to observe and measure children's language behaviors. The purpose of assessment is to ascertain whether a clinically significant problem exists and what direction to take in treatment if a problem does exist.

✓ Assessment can involve the use of standardized instruments as well as informal, nonstandardized measures of language.

✓ Children of different age levels require: (a) common foundational assessment procedures such as hearing screening and a case history, and (b) specialized procedures reflecting special needs of children in certain age groups.

TREATMENT PRINCIPLES AND PROCEDURES

INTRODUCTION

A wide variety of programs and procedures is available for serving children with language problems. Clinicians may select from different service delivery models to provide the most cost-effective, comprehensive services possible for children with language problems. These models include individual therapy, therapy in small groups, therapy carried out in the classroom setting with a small group or with the whole class, and therapy carried out by nonprofessional people (e.g., parents, interpreters) who have been trained by the clinician. In this section, we describe: (a) general language treatment principles, (b) specific language intervention techniques and programs that may be modified according to the age and individual needs of the child being served, and (c) augmentative and alternative communication principles for children with severe disorders of language.

General Principles

- It is important to involve the family in therapy as much as possible. Family members should take part in selecting treatment targets for the child and should be educated in the treatment procedures to be used. Family involvement is especially important for the generalized production of language skills in natural settings and maintenance of skills over time in such natural settings as the home and classroom.

- Clinicians must especially target language behaviors that create social penalties for children

(Johnson, 1996). For example, an adolescent who constantly interrupts others will probably be excluded from important peer groups.

■ Clinicians should select treatment procedures that have been experimentally evaluated and shown to be effective. Clinicians have an ethical responsibility of rejecting procedures that are simply advocated by authorities with no evidence of effectiveness.

■ Clinicians should use a multimodal approach to treatment. Most children benefit from hearing, seeing, and touching. Instead of focusing exclusively on the auditory modality, clinicians need to use visual and tactile stimulation to reinforce language targets being taught (Roseberry-McKibbin, 2007).

■ To learn and retain language treatment targets, most children need *multiple exposures to multiple exemplars* of those targets. For instance, instead of the clinician showing a picture of a Labrador and teaching the child the word *dog*, the clinician needs to have many pictures of different dogs and perhaps even some toy dogs for the child to play with.

■ Clinicians should incorporate literacy—reading and writing—activities into therapy when appropriate (Hegde & Maul, 2005). Because literacy skills are language-based, speech–language pathologists have much to contribute to the improvement of reading and writing skills in children (American Speech-Language-Hearing Association, 2001). Various kinds of literacy skills may be taught in the context of speech and language therapy as described in a later section. Children who are regularly introduced to books and reading not only will develop better language skills, but will also perform better in the classroom (Goldsworthy, 2003).

■ Clinicians who provide language treatment must always consider the child's cultural and linguistic background. The child's background affects many variables, including the language used in therapy, and the appropriateness of certain materials and procedures (Roseberry-McKibbin, 2002).

■ Clinicians should focus on *academic* and *social* languages—the language needed for success in school and the language needed to be socially competent.

■ Clinicians must remember that a child's chronological age is not always an indicator of what kind of treatment is appropriate. The child's *developmental level* is a much more reliable indicator of what treatment procedures and goals will be appropriate.

■ Computer-assisted therapy is increasingly being used with children who have language problems. Many companies are publishing software that addresses a variety of language needs. However, clinicians must use caution when selecting such procedures as many may not offer evidence for their effectiveness.

■ Collaboration with the classroom teacher is extremely important in bridging classroom language requirements with treatment targets. Children will experience much better carryover of language targets if those targets are reinforced in the classroom. Clinicians can use classroom materials in therapy, go into the classroom to conduct therapy, and collaborate in many other ways (Klein & Moses, 1999).

■ As mentioned, it is increasingly important to be flexible in selecting a service delivery model. Depending on the child's needs, clinicians can use one or a combination of the following delivery models:

- one-one intervention
- small-group intervention
- whole-classroom intervention, in which the child is worked with as part of his or her class in the classroom setting
- indirect intervention, in which the clinician sets the goals and a peer, parent, teacher's aide, interpreter, or other person carries out the treatment

C O N C E P T S   T O   C O N S I D E R

You are working as a clinician in the public schools. You have been asked to give an in-service to speech–language pathology interns in your district about language therapy for children. Describe three general principles of language therapy that you will share with those interns.

_____

_____

_____

_____

_____

Specific Techniques and Programs

■ The following specific techniques and programs can be modified for both group and individual therapy. They can also be modified based upon the child's developmental level and individual needs (Hegde, 2001b; Hegde & Maul, 2005). We mention several techniques for which there is little or no evidence mainly because they are popular and clinicians need to know them (to critically evaluate them).

Discrete Trial Procedure

- Discrete trials are useful in the initial stages of treatment when the skills have to be shaped or established. However, they are not efficient for ensuring the skill generalizes to the child's natural environment. Therefore, in the later stages of treatment, the clinician should use a more naturalistic method to be described.
- In discrete trial training, the clinician:

    - Places a stimulus picture in front of the child (e.g., the picture of two books)
    - Asks the child a relevant question (e.g., "Antonio, what do you see?")
    - Immediately models the correct response for the child (e.g., "Say *two cups*") and waits for a few seconds for the child to imitate the modeled response
    - Reinforces the child for correct imitation (verbal praise, token, smile, etc.)

- Gives corrective feedback if the child missed the target response (e.g., *two cup*) by saying "No, that is not correct"
- Records the response on a recording sheet
- Waits for a few seconds and initiates the next trial

Basic Behavioral Techniques

- There is a great deal of controlled and replicated experimental evidence for the effectiveness of the following behavioral techniques that may be used as a part of many larger programs of language treatment:

    - *Instructions.* Giving adequate instructions as to what is expected of the child and how a target behavior is perfomed is essential to begin treatment (e.g., "When you see two of these, you say 'cups.' When you see only one, you say 'cup'.").
    - *Modeling.* This is an effective technique to teach a skill that is nonexistent. The clinician's modeling should be followed by the child's imitation and positive reinforcement for imitative behaviors.
    - *Prompting.* Prompts are like hints; when modeling is no longer needed, the child may be prompted by such statements as: "Remember, what you said for this?" "These are two, not one, so what do you say?" "Here is one book, here are two _____?"
    - *Shaping.* This is a procedure in which a complex reponse is broken down into smaller components that are taught sequentially to achieve the final target skill. For example, a child who cannot imitate "Mommy" may be taught to put the lips together, then produce any kind of vocal response, then the initial syllable, and finally the full word.
    - *Manual guidance.* This involves offering physical assistance to produce a response. For instance, after asking the child to point to a picture, the clinician may take the child's hand and point to the correct picture.
    - *Fading.* This minimizes the need for special procedures to evoke language responses. For example, prompts may be faded by a progressively soft voice so the child continues to respond even when the prompts are no longer heard.
    - *Immediate, response-contingent feedback.* Positive reinforcement for correct responses and corrective feedback for incorrect responses are necessary to teach the skills.

- See Chapter 11 for several other basic treatment procedures that may be used during language treatment.

Expansion

- Using expansion, the clinician expands a child's telegraphic or incomplete utterance into a more grammatically complete utterance. For example, the child says, "Doggy bark," and the clinician says, "Yes, look at the doggy barking." It is often more effective to have the child imitate the longer production and reinforce for it than to simply display a longer production for the child. Efficacy data are needed for simply displaying behaviors for the child.

Extension

- The clinician comments on the child's utterances and adds new and relevant information (this may also be called *expatiation*). For example, a child says, "Play ball." The clinician says, "Yes, you are playing with a big, red plastic ball that bounces." There is a need to experimentally support the effectiveness of this procedure.

Focused Stimulation

- The clinician repeatedly models a target structure to stimulate the child to use it. This is usually done during a play activity that the clinician designs to focus on a particular language structure (e.g., the plural morpheme –s).
- The clinician uses various stimulus materials, talks about them, and repeatedly models the plural constructions (e.g., "Look, here are two *pigs*. I see two *pigs* here. Over here are some *boys* playing. The *boys* are drinking from *cups*. The *cups* have *flowers* on them.").
- The clinician does not correct the child's incorrect responses but instead models the correct target (e.g., the child says, "I see two duck swimming." The clinician says, "Yes, *two ducks* are swimming in the pond.").
- The effectiveness of focused stimulation needs to be established.

Milieu Teaching

- This refers to a group of techniques that have been experimentally evaluated and shown to be effective in teaching a variety of language skills to children. This method teaches functional communication skills through the use of typical, everyday verbal interactions that arise naturally. Milieu teaching uses effective behavioral procedures in naturalistic settings. Three specific techniques constitute milieu teaching:

    - *Incidental teaching.* In this method, the adult who waits for the child to initiate a verbal response:
        — pays full joint attention to the stimulus that prompted a response from the child.
        — prompts an elaboration of the response (e.g., "What do you want?") or models an elaboration ("You want that ball! What do you want?"); if the child fails to elaborate, a traditional model ("Say …") may be given.
        — praises the child and hands the desired object when the child elaborates (spontaneously or imitatively).

    - *Mand-model.* This variation of the incidental teaching method teaches language through the use of typical adult–child interactions in a play-oriented setting. The clinician, using attractive stimulus materials, designs a naturalistic interactive situation. He or she then establishes joint clinician–child attention to a particular material such as a set of paints.
        — The clinician then *mands* a response from the child (e.g., "Tell me what you want" or "Tell me what this is"). If the child gives no or a very limited response, the clinician models the complete, correct response.
        — If the child does not imitate the entire modeled sentence, the clinician prompts (e.g., "Tell me the whole sentence"). The child is praised for imitating or for responding correctly without modeling and is given the item he or she wanted.

    - *Delay.* In this procedure, the clinician waits for the child to initiate verbal responses in relation to stimuli spread around.
        — Without prompting a response, the clinician looks at the child expectantly for at least 15 seconds.
        — If the child does not initiate, the clinician prompts a response or models it.
        — The clinician gives the desired object when the child imitates, spontaneously requests, or fails to say anything after three models each separated by 15 seconds.

- The milieu teaching methods can also be used by parents or others who work with the child.

Parents and peers have been effectively trained in the use of milieu teaching.

Joint Routines or Interactions

- These routinized, repetitive activities are frequently used in early language stimulation with young children. Clinicians can use routines such as peek-a-boo to establish interaction with a child.
- The clinician can also design his or her own routines of action (e.g., always starting therapy sessions by telling the same short story, which contains certain target language structures) and encourage the child to use the repetitive words, phrases, and sentences.
- Experimental evidence is needed to support the use of these interactions.

Joint Book Reading

- The clinician stimulates language in children through the use of systematic storybook reading. Joint book reading allows for repetitive use and practice of the same concepts and phrases. It is also helpful for establishing joint attention (in which the clinician and the child are focused on the same thing).
- The clinician selects appropriate storybooks with attractive, colorful, culturally appropriate pictures. He or she reads the same story several times during several sessions so that the children memorize it.
- The clinician uses prosodic features frequently to draw attention to specific language structures. For example, the clinician might emphasize the past-tense *–ed* morpheme through increased emphasis on words containing that morpheme (e.g., "The man *looked* out the window and *opened* his eyes wide when he *viewed* the snowman.")
- When the children are quite familiar with the story, the clinician stops at points containing target language structures and prompts the children to supply the appropriate words, phrases, or sentences (e.g., "The woman was driving her _____"). Clinicians can manipulate the activity by pausing at different junctures so children supply different language structures or produce progressively longer utterances.
- Children can be asked eventually to "read" (recite from memory, but looking at the text and pictures) and pause while other children supply words, phrases, or sentences. Joint book reading helps develop vocabulary acquisition as well as a sense of story grammar in children.
- There is some evidence that joint book reading promotes language and literacy skills in children. It is also helpful if the adult who is reading to the child engages in print referencing, or a strategy which encourages children's attention to and interactions with print. For example, the adult can focus on how various letters are formed, how print moves from left to right, and so on (Justice & Ezell, 2004).

Narrative Skills Training

- *Narratives* are speakers' descriptions of events (episodes, stories) and experiences. Narratives should be produced in a cohesive, logically consistent, temporally sequenced manner. Narratives are part of pragmatic language skills. Several strategies may be used to teach pragmatic narrative skills; of those described, script therapy has been experimentally evaluated and supported; the rest need further evidence for their effectiveness. To teach narrative skills, clinicians can:

    - let the children act out the stories (e.g., stage a drama)
    - use scripts based on such events as grocery shopping, birthday parties, eating in a restaurant, and running an imaginary store; have the children play out the scripts (actions), in-

cluding verbal exchanges; for instance, the children can play the roles of store people and customers and exchange specific verbal responses the clinician models and reinforces
- use video modeling (a technique known to be effective) in which videotape interactions between two or more children with typical language skills and have the child who needs to learn those skills watch and then imitate the actions, including verbal interactions; fade the video modeling
- use the peer-training method to teach advanced language skills, including narrative skills; let the peer model and reinforce language skills in the child; this may be an excellent way of promoting generalized productions and maintenance; this technique is known to be effective
- get children involved in routinized, daily activities (e.g., discussing the calendar and the weather)
- repeatedly tell or read the same stories so that children memorize the characters, events, words, and temporal sequences
- pause before important phrases or descriptions when retelling stories, so that children can supply them
- ask children to tell stories or narrate events with and then without the help of pictures, scripts, or both
- ask children to narrate new events or experiences (not rehearsed or scripted)
- during all such activities and structured situations, use such effective procedures as instructions, modeling, prompting, positive reinforcement, and corrective feedback; merely organizing situations may not be effective

Story Grammar

- Children with language disorders frequently have difficulty with the structure of narratives. Clinicians can teach and model the following elements of story grammars (Larson & McKinley, 1995) within the script therapy format known to be effective:

  - setting statements (the introduction to the story, the physical setting, the characters, the temporal context)
  - initiating events (episodes that begin the story)
  - internal response (the characters' thoughts, emotions, reactions)
  - theme of the story (the main idea)
  - goals of the characters (what the characters are trying to accomplish)
  - attempts (actions the characters take to achieve their objectives)
  - direct consequences (results of actions)
  - conclusion (how everything turns out, lessons or morals learned from the story)

Parallel Talk

- The clinician plays with the child and describes and comments upon what the child is doing and the objects the child is interested in. For example, the clinician says, "You are putting the lady in the truck" or "That cow you have is brown and white." The effectivenss of this procedure needs to be established.

Recasting

- Recasting children's limited productions into longer or syntactically different forms can be useful in teaching complex grammatical forms. The child's own sentence is repeated in modified form, but the clinician changes the modality or voice of the sentence rather than simply adding grammatical or semantic markers (Johnson, 1996).

- For example; the child says, "The baby is hungry"; the clinician says, "Is she hungry?" (Changed to question form.) Child: "The dog chases the cat." Clinician: "The cat is chased by the dog." (Changed to passive voice.)
- The effectiveness of mere recasting needs to be established. However, if the clinician asks the child to imitate the recasted and modeled sentences, reinforces correct imitations, provides corrective feedback for incorrect responses, and fades the modeling, and so forth, the clinician will have used techniques otherwise known to be effective.

Reauditorization

- The clinician repeats what the child says during language stimulation activities. Reauditorization may be combined with other techniques such as modeling (often without requiring imitation).
- For example, the child says, "Am swinging"; the clinician repeats, "Am swinging."
- The effectiveness of this procedure has not been established.

Self-Talk

- The clinician describes her own activity as she plays with the child. Using language structures that are appropriate for that child, the clinician might say something like, "Look, I'm putting the dress on the doll. See, I'm putting the dress on her.").
- The effectiveness of this procedure has not been established.

Whole-Language Approach

- This philosophical approach to language holds that learning written language should be like learning oral language. That is, proponents of the whole-language approach believe that children learn literacy in the same way they learn spoken language: through being immersed in a literate environment, communicating through print, and getting supportive feedback. Therefore, the approach does not involve specific language skill training (Gillam, 1995).
- There is no controlled evidence to support the use of the whole-language approach. Failure to learn language and literacy skills using this approach has been a widespread concern among educators and clinicians.

Teaching Literacy Skills

- Literacy skills may be taught independently or as a part of language treatment. Integrating literacy instruction with language treatment is efficient for speech–language pathologists (Goldsworthy, 2003).
- The clinician should offer effective intervention for oral language disorders to provide a foundation for literacy skills and to prevent reading and writing problems.
- The clinician should select language targets in consultation with the teacher to better integrate language teaching with classroom instruction; target words, phrases, and sentences that are especially used in the classroom and in the books the child is expected to read will be especially useful.
- The clinician should work with the family members to educate them on the importance of a literacy-rich home environment and to provide the child with books, pens, paper, and other literacy-related materials to promote reading and writing at home. The parents should be

asked to provide role models by engaging in literacy activities themselves and to include their children in such activities.

- The parents should be trained to read more to the child and encourage printing of the alphabet and writing simple words at an early age.
- In teaching language targets, the clinician should use printed words that accompany pictorial and other stimuli used in teaching words, phrases, and sentences.
- The clinician may use story books to promote complex language skills as well as print recognition by pointing to words as she reads the stories.
- If time and resources permit, the clinician may teach reading and writing directly.

Augmentative and Alternative Communication

Basic Principles

- *Augmentative and alternative communication* (AAC) methods supplement deficient oral communication or provide alternative means of communication for children with extremely limited oral communication skills. Children with severe physical impairments, autism, and severe mental retardation are often candidates for AAC (Balandin, 2005).
- AAC methods and materials may also benefit adults and children with apraxia, aphasia, cerebral palsy, laryngectomy, glossectomy, tracheostomy, spinal cord injury, and others.
- AAC devices can be *low-technology devices,* such as notepads or message boards, which do not use electronic instruments. *High-technology devices,* or methods that use electronic instruments such as computers, may also be used.
- When AAC users want to communicate messages, they use *displays,* which are systems or devices that show the message to their communication partner. Displays range from communication boards to computer screens.
- Symbols used by AAC users may be iconic or noniconic. *Iconic symbols* look like the object or picture they represent. For example, a hieroglyphic picture of a house is an iconic symbol indicating the word *house.*
- *Noniconic symbols* are arbitrary, abstract, and geometric. They do not resemble the objects they represent and must be specifically taught. Flexible plastic shapes and chips are examples of noniconic symbols.
- Regardless of the type of AAC device used, users of the device send messages through two means: direct selection and scanning. In *direct selection* the user selects a message by touching a key pad, touching an item or object, depressing an electronic key, pointing, or some other direct means.
- In *scanning,* the user is offered available messages by a mechanical device or communication partner. The messages are offered sequentially until the AAC user indicates the messages he or she wants to communicate.
- Speech–language pathologists may, as part of treatment, help children learn to use AAC devices in a variety of settings outside the treatment room. These settings include the home, classroom, and various places in the community (Glennen & DeCoste, 1997).
- In both assessment and treatment of children who use AAC devices, a team approach is extremely important. Team members may include a speech–language pathologist, physical therapist, occupational therapist, psychologist, social worker, engineer, vocational counselor, teacher, and nurse (Balandin, 2005; Glennen & DeCoste, 1997). The team may work with the child to use one of several forms of AAC: gestural (unaided), gestural-assisted (aided), or neuro-assisted (aided) methods (Hegde, 2001b).

Gestural (Unaided) AAC

- In *gestural (unaided)* AAC, no instruments or external aids are used. Rather, the child uses gestures and other patterned movements, which may be accompanied by some speech. Gestures play a major role in communication of messages. Widely used current gestural (unaided) forms of AAC are described as follows:

- *Pantomime* mostly uses gestures and dynamic movements that involve the entire body or parts of the body. The child uses transparent messages, facial expressions, and dramatizations of meanings. *Transparent messages* are those that are likely to be understood with no additional cues by an observer without special training (Glennen & DeCoste, 1997). Balandin (2005). describes transparency as "ease of deciphering what the symbol means" (p. 387). Conversely, a message or symbol that is *opaque* is one which is not easily decipherable.

- *Eye-blink encoding* is a simple system in which the child learns to communicate a message by a specific number of blinks. For example, one blink means no; two blinks means yes.

- *American Indian Hand Talk* (AMER-IND) is a sign language system developed by North American Indians. AMER-IND is not phonetic; rather, gestures and movements are used as pictorial representations of concepts and ideas.

- *American Sign Language* (ASL) consists of manual signs for the 26 letters of the alphabet as well as signs for words and phrases. Recognized as a separate language, ASL may be used alone or with oral speech.

- *Limited manual sign systems* are composed of several different systems with a limited number of gestures and signs. These are often used by patients in medical settings to communicate self-care and other basic needs, and to say *yes* and *no*.

- *Left-Hand Manual Alphabet* is composed of concrete gestures that approximate printed letters of the alphabet. It is most appropriate for people with right-sided paralysis.

Gestural-Assisted (Aided) AAC

- In *gestural-assisted (aided)* AAC, gestures or movements are combined with an instrument or message-display device. Gestures are used: (a) to display messages on a mechanical device such as a computer monitor, or (b) to scan or select messages displayed on a nonmechanical device such as a communication board.

- Mechanical devices tend to involve high technology and sophisticated electronics. These devices are often run by software, and they generate printed messages or speech. Nonmechanical devices use no electronic technology; there is no message storage, speech output, or printed output.

- Messages on both mechanical and nonmechanical devices take various forms. Seven common types of symbols are used:

  - *picsyms,* a set of graphic symbols that represent nouns, verbs, and prepositions
  - *pic symbols* (pictogram ideogram communication), white drawings on a black background
  - *blissymbols,* a set of semi-iconic and abstract symbols that can be taught to speakers of any linguistic and cultural background
  - *sig symbols,* a set of ideographic or pictographic symbols based on ASL and often used in conjunction with ASL
  - *rebuses,* pictures that represent events or objects along with words, grammatic morphemes, or both
  - *Premack-type symbols, or carrier symbols,* abstract plastic shapes; each shape is associated

with a word or phrase, and children may arrange the plastic shapes as one would printed words

- *Picture Exchange Communication System* (PECS) is a low-technology-aided method of communication that is known to be effective. The clinician initially teaches the child to exchange specific pictures to communicate with a partner (e.g., hands the picture of a glass of water to the partner to request water); it is known that PECS eventually promotes spontaneous verbal expressions as well.

Neuro-Assisted (Aided) AAC

- *Neuro-assisted (aided)* AAC is useful for children who have such profound motoric impairments and limited hand mobility that they cannot use a manual switching device. This type of AAC uses bioelectrical signals such as muscle-action potentials to activate and display messages on a computer monitor.
- The electrical activity of the muscles associated with their contraction is used to activate switching mechanisms. Electrodes attached to the child's skin pick up electrical discharges that are then amplified so they can activate special kinds of switches (called *myoswitches*) or specific displays.
- The user receives feedback (e.g., onset of sound or light) when a switch or display is activated. The user then learns, through biofeedback, to use muscle-action potentials for activating messages.
- Equipment for users of neuro-assisted (aided) AAC is expensive and can be challenging to maintain.

Facilitated Communication

- *Facilitated communication* is a technique of language treatment for children with severe impairments such as autism or cerebral palsy. The facilitator uses physical contact with the child's hand, wrist, or elbow to facilitate pointing on a message board, writing, or typing.
- The use of facilitated communication is not recommended because it is known to be ineffective. The messages children type or convey are controlled mostly by the therapist, not the child.

SUMMARY

✓ Clinicians can use many different service delivery models and treatment programs and procedures to serve children with language problems.

✓ Treatment must always be individualized to meet the needs of each child, with family and classroom involvement being an intrinsic part of therapy.

✓ Some children have extremely limited oral communication skills because of conditions such as autism and cerebral palsy. For these children, augmentative and alternative communication methods can supplement oral communication or provide alternative means of communication.

◆ **LANGUAGE PROBLEMS IN CHILDREN** are caused by or associated with a number of factors. Children who demonstrate language-learning disabilities may appear normal except for their language problems, which cannot be associated with any known etiology or condition.

◆ **CHILDREN CAN ALSO HAVE** language problems associated with specific, known, physical and sensory disabilities such as mental retardation, autism, and brain injury. It is important to provide individualized assessment and treatment based on those children's particular needs. A comprehensive team approach is especially critical, because those children often have multiple needs aside from speech and language problems.

◆ **SOME CHILDREN HAVE LANGUAGE** problems related to physical and social-environmental factors. These factors include poverty, neglect and abuse, maternal or paternal drug or alcohol use, and attention-deficit disorder. Speech–language pathologists are seeing increasing numbers of children with language problems related to these factors. Early intervention and prevention are critical components of treatment.

◆ **ASSESSMENT OF LANGUAGE SKILLS** involves observation and measurement of a child's language behaviors to determine whether a clinically significant problem exists. Assessment can involve screening; the use of formal, standardized measures; the use of informal, nonstandardized measures; or a combination of these.

◆ **FORMAL, STANDARDIZED MEASURES PROVIDE** clinicians with a means of quantifiably comparing a child's performance to the performances of large groups of children in a similar age category. Many clinicians rely on these measures because they yield quantitative data (e.g., percentile ranks), which many state laws require before a child can receive treatment in the public school system.

◆ **BECAUSE OF THE PROBLEMS** inherent in using formal, standardized measures, clinicians have increasingly turned to informal, nonstandardized measures. These include client-specific measures, baselines as extended measurements, forms of authentic assessment such as dynamic and portfolio assessment, social assessment methodologies, and language sampling.

◆ **CLINICIANS ARE INCREASINGLY SERVING** infants and toddlers who have an established risk of language disorders or who experience conditions that put them at risk for developing language disorders. Working with families and with interdisciplinary teams is critical in providing comprehensive, appropriate services.

◆ **MANY CHILDREN WITH LANGUAGE** problems are identified in preschool or elementary school. These children usually have difficulties with most or all parameters of language: morphology, syntax, phonology, semantics, and pragmatics. In elementary school, problems in written language and, thus, in academics are usually seen.

◆ **LANGUAGE PROBLEMS FROM CHILDHOOD** frequently carry over into adolescence. Assessment of adolescent language can be challenging because language problems affect all aspects of the adolescent's life: social-personal, academic, and, potentially, vocational.

◆ **TREATMENT OF LANGUAGE DISORDERS** must be individualized to meet children's needs. Many different service delivery models, programs, and procedures exist for meeting those needs. Clinicians are increasingly collaborating with classroom teachers to provide carryover of language treatment targets into classroom settings. Clinicians are increasingly incorporating literacy into speech–language therapy. Children with severe language disorders may use augmentative and alternative communication devices to assist them.

🖊 **ADD YOUR OWN CHAPTER HIGHLIGHTS HERE:**

Study & Review Questions

Essay

1. Describe three specific characteristics of a child who has been diagnosed with specific language impairment (SLI).

2. Compare and contrast the characteristics of children with autism and those with Asperger's syndrome. How are these children different? How are they alike?

3. Discuss the impact of environmental factors such as poverty and maternal drug and alcohol abuse on a child's language development.

4. There is plenty of controlled and replicated experimental evidence for the effectiveness of behavioral techniques that may be used as a part of many larger programs of language treatment. List and briefly describe three of these techniques.

5. Messages on both mechanical and nonmechanical AAC devices take various forms. List three common symbols that might be found on these devices. Define the terms *transparent* and *opaque*.

Multiple Choice

6. A clinician is working with parents on home language stimulation activities for their 3-year-old daughter Hannah, who is language delayed. Among other things, Hannah needs to increase her expressive language skills to a level more commensurate with her chronological age. Her mean length of utterance is restricted and her utterances are more typical of a young 2-year-old child. The clinician has recommended that at home, the parents use a technique in which they play with Hannah and describe and comment upon what she is doing and the objects she is interested in. For example, the parents might say, "You are making the car go fast" or "That pig is pink." The parents are using the technique of:

   A. self-talk.
   B. expansion.
   C. expatiation.
   D. parallel talk.
   E. joint reference.

7. You are seeing a 6-year-old child, Tyler, with a language-learning disability. When you assess Tyler, you find that he has adequate language comprehension. He is able to follow directions, understand vocabulary, and comprehend sentences of appropriate length and complexity for his age. However, Tyler's teacher and parents report that he has "no friends" and that they are concerned about his social skills. When you observe Tyler several times on the school playground and in the classroom and the school cafeteria, you see that while he is well behaved and nondisruptive, he does not initiate interactions with others. Treatment should focus on:

A. increasing mean length of utterance.
B. working on bound morphemes.
C. increasing assertiveness in conversation.
D. increasing sentence complexity.
E. increasing narrative skills.

8. You are seeing a 9-year-old boy, Emile, whose *Peabody Picture Vocabulary Test—3* score is one year above age level. Emile appears to be performing adequately in the classroom. His teacher reports that he is at grade level in most subjects. However, Emile often interrupts others and irritates his listeners; as a result, he is avoided by many peers. His mother reports that he is not invited to other children's birthday parties, and that she has heard that other mothers view him as rude and disrespectful. Treatment should focus on increasing skills in the area of:

A. pragmatics.
B. syntax.
C. morphology.
D. semantics.
E. phonology.

9. You are working with an adolescent, Alyssa, who has receptive and expressive language problems. She is getting D's in most of her classes at the junior high school and has few friends. In therapy, it would be best to focus on:

A. increasing Alyssa's auditory memory skills.
B. increasing her use of complex sentences containing subordinate clauses.
C. increasing her social use of language and collaborating with her classroom teachers.
D. increasing her ability to understand and use figurative language.
E. increasing her word-retrieval and word-definition skills.

10. A child who shows slow, writhing, involuntary movements has which type of cerebral palsy?

A. spastic
B. mixed
C. ataxic
D. hemiplegic
E. athetoid

11. Which one of the following is NOT TRUE?

A. Standardized language tests have the advantage of providing clinicians with a means of quantifiably comparing a child's performance to the performance of large groups of children in a similar age category.
B. Another advantage of standardized language tests is that they sample behaviors adequately, providing multiple contexts for sampling target language behaviors.
C. Authentic assessment can involve both dynamic and portfolio assessments.
D. In language sampling, some clinicians calculate a type-token ratio, which represents the variety of different words a child uses expressively.
E. Clinicians are increasingly turning to informal, nonstandardized measures because many standardized tests are biased against linguistically and culturally diverse children.

12. You are assessing the expressive language skills of a 4-year-old with delayed language. One of the things he says is: "Um, ah, my birthday party fun—we ate cake, cookies!"

This would count as:

A. 10 words, 10 morphemes
B. 10 words, 12 morphemes
C. 10 words, 9 morphemes
D. 10 words, 11 morphemes
E. 10 words, 8 morphemes

13. You move to a new elementary school and begin seeing the children on the caseload at this school. One child, who is being treated to "increase semantic skills," has five goals listed on her IEP. Which one of these goals is inappropriate?

A. increase types and numbers of words the child uses in the classroom
B. increase specific word usage and decrease usage of nonspecific words such as *this, that, thing*
C. decrease overextensions of words
D. increase use of appropriate discourse skills, turn taking, conversational repair strategies
E. increase comprehension of vocabulary words used in the classroom

14. A child with traumatic brain injury would most likely manifest which of the following symptoms?

A. comprehension problems, word-retrieval problems, syntactic problems
B. reading and writing difficulties, difficulties with reasoning and organization
C. hypersensitivity to touch, insistence on routines, lack of interest in human voices, comprehension and word-retrieval problems
D. A, B
E. A, B, C

15. Which of the following is NOT TRUE with regard to treatment of children with language disorders?

A. Because many children with language disorders have difficulties with auditory processing, clinicians should conduct therapy primarily through the auditory modality.
B. Collaboration with classroom teachers is becoming increasingly important in helping children generalize treatment target behaviors.
C. It is helpful, when appropriate, to incorporate reading and writing (literacy) activities into therapy.
D. A child's chronological age is not always the best predictor of the kind of treatment that will be appropriate; developmental level is a more reliable indicator.
E. Service delivery models can be flexible, ranging from one-one intervention with the clinician to indirect intervention in which the clinician trains significant others to carry out language activities with the child.

16. A 3rd-grade teacher refers 8-year-old Allyson to you. The teacher is concerned because he feels that "Allyson's verbal expression skills just are not what they should be. When she talks, she speaks in real simple sentences. Sometimes I feel like I'm dealing with a kindergartener, not a 3rd grader." When you speak with Allyson's parents, they share that "Allyson never was much of a talker. She talked late—later than her brothers and sisters. But Allyson was always real well behaved, and we never thought she had a problem." You decide that as part of your assessment of Allyson's language skills, you will gather and analyze a language sample using type-token ratio (TTR). When you eventually calculate TTR based on a language sample you gathered from Allyson, you find that her TTR is .31. You conclude that:

A. Allyson is developing normally in the area of syntax.
B. Allyson is delayed in the area of pragmatics.
C. Allyson is low in her lexical skills, or the number of words she uses expressively.
D. Allyson has receptive morphological problems.
E. Allyson has receptive phonological problems.

17. A clinician is providing services for a school-age child, Myron, who uses an AAC device. Myron's parents and teacher report that Myron is having trouble with this device; others frequently do not understand what he is trying to communicate. Myron is showing increasing signs of frustration, and the clinician has been asked to help reduce his frustration by facilitating his communication with other people. To help Myron communicate more effectively with others so that they understand his messages better, the clinician needs to make sure that the symbols on Myron's AAC device are:

A. PECS-friendly.
B. opaquely referenced
C. noniconically opaque

D. opaque
E. transparent

18. Justin is a 7-year-old second-grade child who has been diagnosed with Asperger's syndrome. He has a record of language difficulties beginning when he was a toddler. Justin has just transferred to your school district, and speech-language services have been recommended for him. Justin's parents are anxious for him to begin therapy as soon as possible. You read over the file of reports written by personnel from Justin's previous school district, and meet with your school's Student Study Team (SST) to discuss Justin and recommend the best possible program for him in your school district. The report from the previous speech-language pathologist says, among other things, that Justin's language sample results showed that he had difficulty with forms such as *-er* (bigger) and *-est* (biggest). Problems with these forms reflect a difficulty in the area of:

A. morphology.
B. pragmatics.
C. literacy skills.

D. semantics.
E. phonology.

19. Because of his diagnosis of Asperger's syndrome, you can assume that Justin will probably have characteristics such as:

A. generally below average (IQ 70 or below) intelligence, a lack of responsiveness to and awareness of other people, and stereotypic body movements such constant as rocking.
B. a preference for solitude and objects rather than people, a lack of interest in nonverbal and verbal communication, and insistence on routines.
C. seemingly excellent vocabulary, seemingly normal syntactic skills, and speech which often seems to be a "monologue" where Justin does not allow his conversational partner to take turns.
D. an IQ of 70 or below, speech characterized by monologues, and head banging.
E. a strong dislike of change, a dislike of being touched or held, and "monologic" speech where Justin disregards the listener's need for conversational turns.

20. The SST believes that Justin might profit from the SCERTS approach to intervention, which refers to:

A. an emphasis on improving social communication, implementing ongoing evaluation of regulatory behavior, and training syntactic skills for increased communication success.
B. an emphasis on the importance of targeting goals in social communication and emotional regulation by implementing transactional supports such as visual supports, environmental arrangements, and communication style adjustments.
C. an emphasis on improving semantic communicative effectiveness, regulation of emotional state, and transactional environmental supports such as increased auditory cues.
D. a holistic approach that encourages social communication, effectiveness in regulating transactions, and successful dialogue with others in the environment.
E. a dynamic approach to intervention that encompasses successful communication, effective regulatory training of appropriate emotional expression, and social dialogue practice.

REFERENCES AND RECOMMENDED READINGS

American Association on Mental Retardation. (2002). *Mental retardation: Definition, classification, and systems of support.* Annapolis Junction, MD: AAMR Publications.

American Psychiatric Association. (1994). *Diagnostic and statistical manual of mental disorders—DSM IV* (4th ed.). Washington, DC: Author.

American Psychiatric Association. (2000). *Diagnostic and statistical manual of mental disorders* (4th edition, text revision ed.). Washinghton, DC: Author.

American Speech-Language-Hearing Association. (2001). *Roles and responsibilities of speech–language pathologists with respect to reading and writing for children and adolescents: Position statement.* Rockville Pike, MD: Author.

Baker, L. J., & Welkowitz, L. A. (Eds.). (2004). *Asperger's syndrome: Intervening in schools, clinics, and communities.* Mahwah, NJ: Lawrence Erlbaum Associates.

Balandin, S. (2005). Language and augmentative and alternative communication (AAC). In V. A. Reed, (Ed.), *An introduction to children with language disorders* (3rd ed., pp. 384–403). Boston: Allyn & Bacon.

Battle, D. E., & Anderson, N. (1998). Culturally diverse families and the development of language. In D. E. Battle (Ed.), *Communication disorders in multicultural populations* (2nd ed., pp. 213–246). Newton, MA: Butterworth-Heinemann.

Brice, A. E. (2002). *The Hispanic child: Speech, language, culture and education.* Boston: Allyn & Bacon.

Bloom, L., & Lahey, M. (1978). *Language development and language disorders.* New York: Macmillan.

Brown, R. (1973). *A first language: The early stages.* Cambridge, MA: Harvard University Press.

Casby, M. W. (1997). Symbolic play of children with language impairment: A critical review. *Journal of Speech and Hearing Research, 40*(3), 468–479.

Catts, H. W., & Kamhi, A. G. (2005). *Language and reading disabilities* (2nd ed.). Boston: Allyn & Bacon.

Chapman, R. S. (1992). *Processes in language acquisition and disorders.* St. Louis, MO: Mosby-Year Book.

Cooper, P. R., & Golfinos, J. G. (Eds.). (2000). *Head injury* (4th ed.). New York: McGraw-Hill.

Crystal, D., Fletcher, P., & Garman, M. (1976). *The grammatical analysis of language disability: A procedure for assessment and remediation.* London: Edward Arnold.

Duker, P., Didden, R., & Sigafoos, J. (2004). *One-to-one training: Instructional procedures for learners with developmental disabilities.* Austin, TX: PRO-ED.

England, C. A. (1994). Assessing students with attention deficit hyperactivity disorder: Student interactions within social context. *California Speech and Hearing Association, 20*(5), 4–6.

Fey, M. E. (1986). *Language intervention with young children.* Boston: College-Hill Press.

Fey, M. E., Catts, H. W., & Larrivee, L. S. (1995). Preparing preschoolers for the academic and social challenges of school. In M. E. Fey, J. Windsor, & S. F. Warren (Eds.), *Language intervention: Preschool through the elementary years* (Vol. 5, pp. 3–38). Baltimore: Paul H. Brookes.

Fey, M. E., Windsor, J., & Warren, S. F. (1995). *Language intervention: Preschool through the elementary years.* Baltimore: Paul H. Brookes.

Friedlander, D., & Martinson, K. (1996). Effects of mandatory basic education for adult AFDC recipients. *Educational Evaluation and Policy Analysis, 18*(4), 327–337.

Gallagher, T. (Ed.). (1991). *Pragmatics of language: Clinical practice issues.* San Diego, CA: Singular Publishing Group.

Gillam, R. (1995). Whole language principles at work in language intervention. In D. F. Tibbits (Ed.), *Language intervention beyond the primary grades: For clinicians by clinicians* (pp. 219–255). Austin, TX: PRO-ED.

Glennen, S. L., & DeCoste, D. C. (1997). *Handbook of augmentative and alternative communication.* San Diego, CA: Singular Publishing Group.

Goldsworthy, C. L. (2003). *Developmental reading disabilities: A language based treatment approach* (2nd ed.). San Diego, CA: Singular/Delmar Publishing Group.

Hallahan, D. P., Lloyd, J. W., Kauffman, J. M., Weiss, M. P., & Martinez, E. A. (2005). *Learning disabilities: Foundations, characteristics, and effective teaching* (3rd ed.). Boston: Allyn & Bacon.

Hegde, M. N. (1998). *Treatment procedures in communicative disorders* (3rd ed.). Austin, TX: PRO-ED.

Hegde, M. N. (2001a). *Hegde's pocket guide to assessment in speech–language pathology.* San Diego, CA: Singular Publishing Group.

Hegde, M. N. (2001b). *Hegde's pocket guide to treatment in speech–language pathology.* San Diego, CA: Singular Publishing Group.

Hegde, M. N., & Maul, C. M. (2005). *Language disorders in children: An evidence-based approach to assessment and intervention.* Boston: Allyn & Bacon.

Hux, K. (Ed.). (2003). *Assisting survivors of traumatic brain injury.* Austin, TX: PRO-ED.

Johnson, B. A. (1996). *Language disorders in children: An introductory clinical perspective.* Albany, NY: Delmar Publishers.

Justice, L.M., & Ezell, H.K. (2004). Print referencing: An emergent literacy enhancement strategy and its clinical applications. *Language, Speech, and Hearing Services in Schools, 35,* 185–193.

Kanner, L. (1943). Autistic disturbances of affective contact. *Nervous Child, 2,* 217–250.

Klein, D., & Briggs, M. (1986). *Observation of communicative interaction* (DHS Publication No. MCJ 06351-01-0). Washington, DC: U.S. Government Printing Office.

Klein, H. B., & Moses, N. (1999). *Intervention planning for children with communication disorders: A guide for clinical practicum and professional practice* (2nd ed.). Needham Heights, MA: Allyn & Bacon.

Koman, L. A., Smith, B. P., & Shilt, J. S. (2004). Cerebral palsy. *Lancet, 363,* 1619–1631.

Larson, V., & McKinley, N. (1995). *Language disorders in older students: Pre-adolescents and adolescents.* Eau Claire, WI: Thinking Publications.

Lee, L. (1974). *Developmental sentence analysis.* Evanston, IL: Northwestern University Press.

Leonard, L. (1991). Specific language impairment as a clinical category. *Language, Speech, and Hearing Services in Schools, 22,* 66–68.

Leonard, L. (1998). *Children with specific language impairment.* Cambridge, MA: MIT Press.

Light, J. C., Beukelman, D. R., & Reichle, J. (2003). *Communicative competence for individuals who use AAC* (3rd ed.). Baltimore: Paul H. Brookes.

Long, S. L. (2005). Language and children with learning disabilities. In V. A. Reed, *An introduction to children with language disorders* (3rd ed., pp. 132–167). Boston: Allyn & Bacon.

Long, S., & Fey, M. (1993). *Computerized profiling* (Macintosh Version 1.0, MS-DOS Version 7.1). San Antonio, TX: Psychological Corporation.

Maurice, C., Green, G., & Foxx (Eds.). *Making a difference: Behavioral intervention for autism.* Austin, TX: PRO-ED.

Mecham, M. (1996). *Cerebral palsy* (2nd ed.). Austin, TX: PRO-ED.

Miller, J., & Chapman, R. (1983). SALT: *Systematic analysis of language transcripts.* Madison: University of Wisconsin, Language Analysis Laboratory, Waisman Center.

Mordecai, D., & Palin, M. (1982). *Lingquest 1 & 2* [computer software]. Napa, CA: Lingquest Software.

Murdoch, B. E., & Theodoros, D. G. (2001). *Traumatic brain injury: Associated speech, language, and swallowing disorders.* Albany, NY: Thomson Learning.

Myles, B. S., & Simpson, R. L. (2003). *Asperger Syndrome: A guide for educators and parents* (2nd ed.). Austin, TX: PRO-ED.

Nelson, N. W. (1998). *Childhood language disorders in context: Infancy through adolescence* (2nd ed.). Needham Heights, MA: Allyn & Bacon.

Nicolosi, L., Harryman, E., & Kresheck, J. (2004). *Terminology of communication disorders: Speech-language-hearing* (5th ed.). Baltimore: Williams & Wilkins.

Nippold, M. (1998). *Later language development: The school-age and adolescent years* (2nd ed.). Austin, TX: PRO-ED.

O'Hanlon, L., & Roseberry-McKibbin, C. (2004). Strategies for working children from low-income backgrounds. *ADVANCE for Speech–Language Pathologists and Audiologists, 14*(6), 12–20.

Owens, R. E. (2004). *Language disorders: A functional approach to assessment and intervention* (4th ed.). Boston: Allyn & Bacon.

Ozonoff, S., Dawson, G., & McPartland, J. (2002). *A parent's guide to Asperger Syndrome and high-functioning autism: How to meet the challenges and help your child thrive.* New York: The Guilford Press.

Paul, R. (2001). *Language disorders from infancy through adolescence: Assessment and intervention* (2nd ed.). St. Louis, MO: Mosby-Year Book.

Prelock, P. A., Beatson, J., Bitner, B., Broder, C., & Ducker, A. (2003). Interdisciplinary assessment of young children with Autism Spectrum Disorder. *Language, Speech, and Hearing Services in Schools, 34,* 194–202.

Preschool Amendments to the Education of the Handicapped Act, 1986. Act 20 U.S.C. 1471 *et seq.*

Prizant, B. M. (2004). *Autism spectrum disorders and the SCERTS model: A comprehensive educational approach.* Baltimore: Paul H. Brookes.

Rice, M. L., & Warren, S. F. (Eds.). (2004). *Developmental language disorders: From phenotypes to etiologies.* Mahwah, NJ: Lawrence Erlbaum Associates.

Reed, V. A. (2005). *An introduction to children with language disorders* (3rd ed.). Boston: Allyn & Bacon.

Roseberry-McKibbin, C. (2002). *Multicultural students with special language needs: Practical strategies for assessment and intervention* (2nd ed.). Oceanside, CA: Academic Communication Associates.

Roseberry-McKibbin, C. (2003). *Assessment of bilingual learners: Language difference or disorder?* [Video] Rockville Pike, MD: The American Speech-Language-Hearing Association.

Roseberry-McKibbin, C. (2007). *Introduction to language disorders in children: A multicultural approach.* Boston: Allyn & Bacon.

Roseberry-McKibbin, C., & Brice, A. (1998). *Service delivery issues in serving clients from low-income backgrounds.* Paper presented at the national meeting of the American Speech-Language-Hearing Association, San Antonio, TX.

Rossetti, L. M. (2001). *Communication intervention: Birth to three* (2nd ed.). Albany, NY: Thomson Learning.

Sellars, C. W., Vegter, C. H., & Ellerbusch, S. E. (20003). *Pediatric brain injury: A practical resource* (2nd ed.). Austin, TX: PRO-ED.

Silverman, F. H. (1995). *Communication for the speechless* (3rd ed.). Needham Heights, MA: Allyn & Bacon.

Tibbits, D. F. (Ed.). (1995). *Language intervention beyond the primary grades: For clinicians by clinicians.* Austin, TX: PRO-ED.

Tyack, D., & Gottsleben, R. (1974). *Language sampling, analysis, and training.* Palo Alto, CA: Consulting Psychologists Press.

Vargas, C. M., & Prelock, P. A. (2004). *Caring for children with neurodevelopmental disabilities and their families.* Mahwah, NJ: Lawrence Erlbaum Associates.

Verhoeven, L., & von Balkom, H. (2004). *Classification of developmental language disorders.* Mahwah, NJ: Lawrence Erlbaum Associates.

Walker, L., & Thompson, E. (1982). Mother-infant play interaction scale. In S. Humenick-Smith (Ed.), *Analysis of current assessment strategies in the health care of young children and child rearing families* (p. 56). Norwich, CT: Williams & Wilkins.

Weitzner-Lin, B. (2004). *Communication assessment and intervention with infants and toddlers.* Philadelphia: Elsevier.

Westby, C., & Cutler, S. K. (1994). Language and ADHD: Understanding the bases and treatment of self-regulatory deficits. *Topics in Language Disorders, 14*(4), 58–76.

Ylvisaker, M. (1995). Intervention for students with traumatic brain injury. In D. F. Tibbits (Ed.), *Language intervention beyond the primary grades: For clinicians by clinicians* (pp. 313–372). Austin, TX: PRO-ED.

Zager, D. (2005). *Autism spectrum disorders: Identification, education, and treatment* (3rd ed.). Mahwah, NJ: Lawrence Erlbaum Associates.

Study & Review
Answers

6. D. If parents are using a technique in which they play with their child and describe and comment upon what she is doing and the objects she is interested in (e.g., the parents might say, "You are putting the dolly to sleep" or "You have the red dog book"), the parents are using the technique of parallel talk.

7. C. A 6-year-old child with a language-learning disability and adequate language comprehension but difficulty initiating interactions with others would best be served by treatment focusing on increasing assertiveness in conversation.

8. A. Pragmatics, or social language, is the area in which this student needs the most help.

9. C. Adolescence is a time when the use and comprehension of appropriate social language is critical. In addition, collaboration with classroom teachers would yield directions for use of specific classroom materials and ideas that could be used in therapy to target Alyssa's deficient language skills while increasing her academic performance.

10. E. A child who shows slow, writhing, involuntary movements has athetoid cerebral palsy.

11. B. Standardized tests tend to sample language behaviors inadequately, providing only one or two contexts that sample each behavior.

12. C. This utterance would count as 10 words, 9 morphemes.

13. D. Increasing use of appropriate discourse skills, turn taking, and conversational repair strategies would be appropriate targets for a child working on pragmatic skills, not semantic skills.

14. D. Hypersensitivity to touch, insistence on routines, and lack of interest in human voices are generally characteristic of children with autism, not children with traumatic brain injury.

15. A. It is critical to use a multimodal approach to treatment because most children with language disorders will learn more quickly and retain more information this way.

16. C. A TTR of .31 is low—a TTR of .5 is within average range. Thus, this indicates that Allyson is low in her lexical skills, or the number of words she uses expressively.

17. E. To help Myron communicate more effectively with others so that they understand his messages better, the clinician needs to make sure that the symbols on Myron's AAC device are transparent, or easily decipherable by others.

18. A. Problems with forms such as *-er* (bigger) and *-est* (biggest) reflect difficulty in the area of morphology.

19. C. Because Justin has Asperger's syndrome, not autism, the clinician would expect to see seemingly excellent vocabulary skills, seemingly normal syntactic skills, and speech that often appears to be a "monologue," where Justin does not allow his conversational partner to take turns.

20. B. The SCERTS model emphasizes the importance of targeting goals in social communication and emotional regulation by implementing transactional supports, which include visual supports, environmental arrangements, and communication style adjustments.

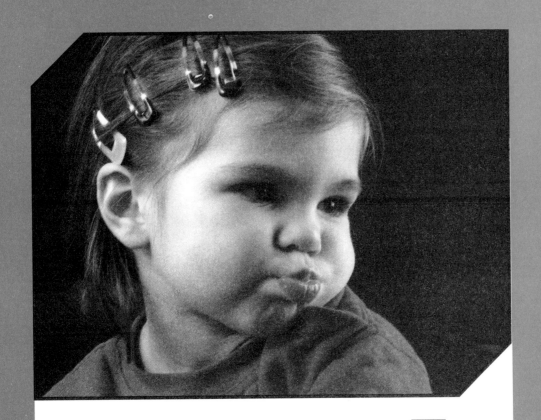

CHAPTER 5

ARTICULATORY-

PHONOLOGICAL

DEVELOPMENT

AND DISORDERS

The ability to communicate clearly is a gift

that most people take for granted. But sometimes clear communication with others is disrupted by one or more variables that cause a child to be misunderstood by members of his or her speech community. In some cases this leads to only minor problems; other children experience emotional, social, and even academic difficulties related to disturbed speech patterns.

To describe these difficulties, many authors use the term *articulation and phonological disorders;* some prefer either *articulation disorder* or *phonological disorder. Articulation disorder* refers to speech-motor-control problems; *phonological disorder* refers to the fact that phonology is a part of the language system, and speech requires language knowledge. For purposes of this chapter, we have used the term *articulatory-phonological disorders* (abbreviated Ar-Ph disorders) to acknowledge that many children present with reduced intelligibility due to a combination of speech-motor and phonological (language knowledge) factors. We describe foundational principles of articulation and phonology, acquisition and typical development of Ar-Ph skills, disorders of Ar-Ph, assessment of Ar-Ph disorders, and finally treatment of children who have Ar-Ph disorders.

FOUNDATIONS OF ARTICULATION AND PHONOLOGY

In order to understand typical development and disorders of Ar-Ph, it is necessary to understand the basic definitions used to describe development and disorders. It is also helpful to understand the place-voice-manner and distinctive feature paradigms, which provide a way to classify the speech sounds of the English language. In this section, definitions and concepts from Chapter 2 are reviewed and summarized as part of the foundation for discussion of Ar-Ph development and disorders.

Basic Definitions

- *Language* is an abstract system of symbols used to communicate meaning; it is larger than speech. Speech is the actual motor production of oral language.

- Experts put forth many explanations of the differences between articulation and phonology. Fundamentally, the *articulation* approach looks at children's acquisition of individual phonemes and emphasizes speech-motor control. The *phonological* approach studies children's acquisition of sound patterns and the processes underlying such patterns. Phonology focuses on the underlying knowledge of the rules of the sound system of a language.

- A *phoneme* is a class of speech sounds; it is an abstract name given to variations of a speech sound. Because they make a difference in meaning, phonemes are often described as the smallest unit of sound that can affect meaning. For example, *rat* and *fat* have different meanings because of the different initial phonemes /r/ and /f/.

- A phoneme is a group, class, or family of sounds whose variations are called *allophones*. For example, although the phoneme /k/ sounds the same perceptually to the listener, it is produced in slightly different manners in the words *kitten, bucket,* and *cook.* These slightly different manners or variations are called allophones.

- The term *phonemic* refers to the abstract system of sounds, whereas the term phonetic refers to concrete productions of specific sounds. Thus, the idealized and abstract description of /t/ is phonemic and is put in slashes. The specific sound production by a speaker would be indicated in brackets [t].

- The English language has 46 speech sounds, which may be classified as vowels or consonants (see Chapter 2 for a more in-depth description). *Vowels* are always voiced, and the mouth is more open in vowel production than it is in consonant production.

- Vowels are classified according to the tongue positions needed to produce them (front, central, back, high, mid, low). Vowels are also classified according to lip position; for instance, the vowels /o/ and /u/ are produced with lip rounding, while the vowel /i/ is produced with slight lip retraction.

- When two vowels are combined, they form *diphthongs,* which are produced by a continuous change in the vocal tract shape (Peña-Brooks & Hegde, 2000). The /eɪ/ sound in *shake* and *lace* is a dipthong, as is the /ɑɪ/ sound in words such as *high* and *why.*

- Vowels may be described according to the *distinctive feature paradigm*. Consonants may be described according to both the distinctive feature paradigm and the *place-voice-manner paradigm.*

Distinctive Features Paradigm

- One method of classifying vowels and consonants is based on distinctive features. Linguists who developed the distinctive features theory wanted to describe all the phonemes used in the languages of the world.

- These linguists believe that the phoneme is not the basic unit of speech. They propose that a phoneme is a *collection of independent features*. A distinctive feature is a unique characteristic of a phoneme that distinguishes one phoneme from another (Chomsky & Halle, 1968).

- Distinctive feature theory uses a binary system; the features are either present or absent (+ or –). For example, *voicing* is a distinctive feature. The phoneme /g/ is assigned a plus value for voicing; the phoneme /t/ is assigned a minus value for voicing. Table 5.1 lists English consonants and their distinctive features.

Place-Voice-Manner Paradigm

- Consonants are produced by constricting the oral cavity. Consonants are traditionally classified according to three parameters: place, voice, and manner (see Table 5.2; Chapter 2 also describes these parameters):

  - *place* of articulation describes the location of the constriction (e.g., bilabial, linguadental)
  - *voicing* describes the presence or absence of vocal fold vibrations in the production of consonants
  - *manner* of articulation describes the degree or type of constriction in the vocal tract

Table 5.1 THE CHOMSKY-HALLE DISTINCTIVE FEATURES OF ENGLISH CONSONANTS

	w	f	v	θ	ð	t	d	s	z	n	l	ʃ	ʒ	j	r	tʃ	dʒ	k	g	ŋ	h	p	b	m
Voiced	+	-	+	-	+	-	+	-	+	+	+	-	+	+	+	-	+	-	+	+	-	-	+	+
Consonantal	-	+	+	+	+	+	+	+	+	+	+	+	+	-	+	+	+	+	+	+	-	+	+	+
Anterior	+	+	+	+	+	+	+	+	+	+	+	-	-	-	-	-	-	-	-	-	-	+	+	+
Coronal	-	-	-	+	+	+	+	+	+	+	+	+	+	-	+	+	+	-	-	-	-	-	-	-
Continuant	+	+	+	+	+	-	-	+	+	-	+	+	+	+	+	-	-	-	-	-	+	-	-	-
High	-	-	-	-	-	-	-	-	-	-	-	+	+	+	-	+	+	+	+	+	-	-	-	-
Low	-	-	-	-	-	-	-	-	-	-	-	-	-	-	-	-	-	-	-	-	+	-	-	-
Back	-	-	-	-	-	-	-	-	-	-	-	-	-	-	-	-	-	+	+	+	-	-	-	-
Nasal	-	-	-	-	-	-	-	-	-	+	-	-	-	-	-	-	-	-	-	+	-	-	-	+
Strident	-	+	+	-	-	-	-	+	+	-	-	+	+	-	-	+	+	-	-	-	-	-	-	-
Vocalic	-	-	-	-	-	-	-	-	-	-	+	-	-	-	+	-	-	-	-	-	-	-	-	-

Note. From *Introduction to Communicative Disorders*, 3rd ed. (p. 104), by M. N. Hegde, 2001, Austin, TX: PRO-ED. Copyright 2001 by PRO-ED, Inc. Reprinted with permission.

Table 5.2   PLACE-VOICE-MANNER CLASSIFICATION OF ENGLISH CONSONANTS

Place of Articulation	MANNER OF PRODUCTION						
	Nasals	Stops	Fricatives	Affricates	Liquids	Glides	Laterals
Bilabial	(m)	p (b)				(w)	
Labiodental			f (v)				
Linguadental			θ (ð)				
Lingua-alveolar	(n)	t (d)	s (z)		(l)		(l)
Linguapalatal			ʃ (ʒ)	(tʃ)(dʒ)	(r)	(j)	
Linguavelar	(ŋ)	k (g)					
Glottal			h				

Note. Voiced sounds are circled. From *Introduction to Communicative Disorders,* 3rd ed. (p. 101), by M. N. Hegde, 2001, Austin, TX: PRO-ED. Copyright 2001 by PRO-ED, Inc. Reprinted with permission.

Manner of Articulation Categories

- *Stops* are produced by completely stopping the airflow. The air pressure is built up in the oral cavity and then released in a manner resembling a small explosion (plosive manner). Thus, stops are also known as stop-plosives and consist of the phonemes /p/, /b/, /t/, /d/, /k/, /g/.
- *Fricatives* are produced by severely constricting the oral cavity and then forcing the air through it, creating a *hissing* or *friction* type of noise. The /f/, /v/, /ð/, /θ/, /s/, /z/, /ʃ/, /ʒ/, /h/. sounds are fricatives.
- *Affricates* are a combination of stops and fricatives. The two English affricates are /tʃ/, /dʒ/.
- *Glides* are produced by gradually changing the shape of the articulators. The two English glides are /w/, /j/.
- *Liquids* are produced with the least restriction of the oral cavity. The two English liquids, /r/ and /l/, are also called semi-vowels. The /l/ sound is also called a *lateral* because in producing this sound, air escapes through the sides of the tongue.
- *Nasals* are produced while keeping the velopharyngeal port open so the sound produced by the larynx passes through the nose. Nasal resonance is thus added to the three nasal sounds of English, /m/, /n/, and /ŋ/.

Place of Articulation Categories

- *bilabials,* produced primarily by the two lips, are /p/, /b/, /m/, /w/
- *labiodentals,* produced by the lips and teeth, are /f/, /v/
- *linguadentals,* produced by the tongue making contact with the upper teeth, are /ð/ and /θ/
- *lingua-alveolars,* produced by raising the tip of the tongue to make contact with the alveolar ridge, are /t/, /d/, /s/, /z/, /n/, /l/

- *linguapalatals,* produced by the tongue coming in contact with the hard palate, are /ʃ/, /ʒ/, /tʃ/, /dʒ/, /r/, /j/
- *linguavelars,* produced by the back of the tongue raising to contact the velum, are /k/, /g/, /ŋ/
- the *glottal* sound, produced by keeping the vocal folds open and letting the air pass through them, is /h/

SUMMARY

- ✓ Speech is the motor production of oral language. The articulation approach to speech looks at children's acquisition of individual phonemes and emphasizes motor control.

- ✓ The phonological approach studies children's acquisition of sound patterns within the language system. Consonants and vowels make up the two major categories of speech sounds.

- ✓ Consonants and vowels can be described according to the distinctive features paradigm, and consonants can also be described according to the place-voice-manner paradigm.

ACQUISITION OF ARTICULATORY AND PHONOLOGICAL SKILLS: TYPICAL DEVELOPMENT

INTRODUCTION

Most people take normal Ar-Ph development for granted. But sometimes children do not develop Ar-Ph skills at the expected pace. In order to understand what Ar-Ph errors are age appropriate and what Ar-Ph errors indicate problematic development, it is necessary to understand theories of development and normal milestones of development in infants and children.

Theories of Development

Early studies of children's articulatory and phonological development consisted mainly of *diary studies,* which described individual children (frequently the children of the researchers). Those early studies focused primarily on environmental influences and on universals of acquisition.

■ Today's theories and models of development account much more for the child as a learner with unique learning strategies and individual patterns of production. The following is a brief summary of major theories or models of children's articulatory and phonological development (Bauman-Waengler, 2004; Kent, 2004; Peña-Brooks & Hegde, 2000; Stoel-Gammon & Dunn, 1985; Vihman, 2004):

Behavioral Theory

- The behavioral explanation of speech sound acquisition is based on conditioning and learning (Mowrer, 1960; Olmsted, 1971). This explanation treats the acquisition of speech like acquisition of any other skill. Thus, it is presumed that the acquisition of speech does not require such special phenomena as innate universals. The behavioral theory prevailed from the 1950s to the early 1970s (Vihman, 2004).

- The behavioral theory emphasizes that the child develops the adultlike speech of his or her community through interactions with the caretaker. The theory holds that the child's babbling is gradually shaped into adult forms through principles of classical conditioning that occur primarily during caretaker–child interactions.
- Some experts argue that this theory does not account for an infant's creativity or capacity to produce new patterns. In addition, the evidence is not compelling that caretakers selectively reinforce the child's sounds in the prelinguistic period.

Structural Theory

- Proponents of the structural theory, such as Jakobson (1968) and Chomsky and Halle (1968), based their assumptions on linguists' structural theory of language.
- According to the structural theory, phonological development follows an innate, universal, and hierarchical order of acquisition of distinctive features. The child begins with the maximal contrasts of /p/ and /ɑ/, and differentiates and fine tunes them into more subtle contrasts.
- Jakobson stated that babbling was not continuous with early speech, thus proposing the hypothesis of *discontinuity* between early babbling and subsequent speech development.
- Currently, there appears to be little support for the idea of discontinuity or for the idea of development of feature contrasts. Further, because of the variability among individual children, the idea of invariable universals of development is not supported.

Biological Theory

- Locke (1983, 1990) stated, in the biological theory, that the foundation of phonological acquisition consists of innate dispositions to certain motor actions. For instance, a babbling child has a universal phonetic repertoire because of motoric constraints and the shape and size of the vocal tract.
- According to the biological theory, the child's environment has an influence only around the time that the first word emerges. But production constraints remain until the child is approximately 18 months old, when he or she begins to produce characteristics of the adult language of the environment.
- A problem with the biological theory is that, according to recent research, infants from a single linguistic background manifest individual differences even in the babbling stage. If universal constraints were so firmly set, this would not occur.

Cognitive Theory

- The cognitive theory or model, developed in the 1970s, was also known as the *problem-solving model.* This model did not apply adult models to the child, but emerged from speech sound acquisition data (Ferguson 1978, 1986; Macken & Ferguson, 1983; Menn, 1983; Waterson, 1971).
- The cognitive theory holds that children face various challenges in their attempts to acquire the adult phonological system, and that each child uses unique strategies in this process. These strategies depend in large part on the child's natural predisposition. Rather than targeting segments, the child appears to be targeting whole words. The child's individual creativity contributes greatly to this process.
- In early life children are believed to have incomplete perception of the phonetic features of adult words. Waterson describes early word groups as schemata that share certain overall features. These features are derived from the adult form and include syllable structure, intonation pattern, nasality, continuance (presence of fricatives), and voicing (Vihman, 2004).

- According to Waterson, children's perception and production are imperfect at first and must undergo development and changes to arrive at an adultlike system.
- Waterson's approach is a useful complement to phonological process-based analysis. It especially captures the "gestalt" underlying certain productions of children that are very irregular when compared in a segment-by-segment fashion with the adult model.
- A major criticism of the cognitive model is that it overemphasizes the individual creative aspects of phonological acquisition. Not enough attention is paid to constraints on learning that may result from psychological and physiological maturation. In addition, there is not enough focus on learning constraints that may result from the language of the child's environment and from the structure of language in general (Vihman, 2004).

Natural Phonology Theory

- In the study of phonology, a topic of great interest is *naturalness*. A natural class, process, property, or rule is one that is preferred or frequently used in phonologic systems. One phonological property is more natural than another if the first is used in a greater number of languages and if it develops before the other property.
- Researchers use the terms *marked* and *unmarked* to describe sounds according to this paradigm. *Unmarked* sounds are ones that appear to be natural; they tend to be easier to acquire, and thus are acquired earlier than marked sounds. Unmarked sounds appear in more different languages than marked sounds. *Marked* sounds are less natural and tend to be acquired later (Kent, 2004).
- For example, /b/ is usually considered an unmarked sound because it is acquired easily and early by most children, and because /b/ occurs in many languages of the world. The /th/ sound is considered by some to be marked, because children acquire it later and this sound is less commonly found in languages around the world.
- Developed by Stampe (1969), the natural phonology theory proposes that natural phonological processes are innate processes that simplify the adult target word. Some experts believe that natural phonological processes are innate or are acquired early in life and fairly easily by children (Kent, 2004).
- Children's task, according to Stampe, is to suppress processes that do not occur in their languages. For example, in German, word-final obstruents (stops, affricates, and fricatives) are devoiced. In German, *Hund (dog)* is pronounced [hunt]. German-speaking children do not need to suppress the process of word-final obstruent devoicing, because that process is compatible with their community language. English-speaking children do need to suppress that process, however, to match the adult pronunciation of their community. Thus, in English, children need to learn to voice word-final /d/ as in the word *glad*.
- Stampe believed that children represent or store speech forms correctly. What leads to the use of phonological processes is *output constraints,* or constraints on production that lead to simplification of the adult model.
- The concept of the universal or innate status of child phonological processes or rules is controversial (Vihman, 2004). Also, there is no empirical evidence that children have full and accurate perception from the earliest stages of speech production.

Generative Phonology Theory

- Smith (1973) developed this model based upon a description of the phonology of his son at 2–4 years. According to Smith, the child does not have a psychologically real, productive system that underlies his or her forms.
- The child's system is viewed in its own right. The child "rewrites" or maps the adult forms onto his or her system. Generative phonology states that people operate on a highly organized

system of phonological rules in putting together the morphemes of language (Yavas, 1998).

- According to Smith, children have a set of ordered universal tendencies that are either innate or learned very early in life. Like the natural phonology theory, the generative phonology theory holds that a child stores speech forms correctly but has production constraints that lead to the use of phonological processes.

- As for the natural phonology theory, there is no empirical evidence that children have full and accurate perception from the earliest stages of speech production. In addition, many researchers do not believe in the innate status of child phonological processes and rules.

Linear vs. Nonlinear Phonology Theories

- The foundational goals of the linear generative phonologies are to: (a) describe phonological patterns that occur in natural languages, (b) create rules that account for these systems, and (c) identify universal principles that apply to various phonological systems. These theories are based on the premise that all speech segments are arranged in a sequential order, that all sound segments have equal value, and that all distinctive features are equal. Thus, no one specific sound segment has control over other segments (Bauman-Waengler, 2004).

- Basically, linear generative phonology is "characterized by rules that operate in a domain of linear strings of segments" (Kent, 2004, p. 52). Linear phonological theories assume that phonological properties are linear strings of segments, and that sound segments are composed of a bundle of independent characteristics or features.

- In the 1980s, nonlinear phonology was developed as an alternative to linear generative phonology and gained attention because linear generative phonology was perceived to have flaws. Linear generative phonology became increasingly viewed as inadequate to account for the effects of stress and other prosodic variables.

- Nonlinear phonology was developed as an alternative to account for the influence of stress and tone features in levels of representation independent of segmental or linear representation. There are various nonlinear phonology theories, and they deemphasize processes or rules and focus on prosodic phenomena (Ball & Kent, 1997; Vihman, 2004). Nonlinear phonological theories assume that there is some sort of hierarchy that helps to organize both segmental and suprasegmental phonological units or properties (Peña-Brooks & Hegde, 2000).

CONCEPTS TO CONSIDER

What is the difference between linear and nonlinear theories of phonology? Explain.

_____

_____

_____

_____

_____

- Nonlinear theories explore the relationships among units of different sizes; for example, they acknowledge the fact that syllable structure could affect the segmental level of a child's production (Bauman-Waengler, 2004). Clinically, one of the biggest contributions of nonlinear phonology has been its attention to multisyllabic words and the way in which therapy is organized (see Bernhardt & Stemberger, 2000; Smit, 2004).

Infant Development: Perception and Production

Perception

- Various types of research methodology have been used to study infant perception. The two major ones are the *high-amplitude sucking paradigm* and the *visually reinforced head turn*. These methodologies observe infants' reactions to changes in their environment (for a further description, see Vihman, 2004).
- Research on infant perception has shown that:

  - 4- to 17-week-old infants can discriminate between the vowels [u] and [i], [ɑ], and [ɪ]
  - 2-month-old infants can discriminate between [bɑ] and [gɑ]
  - 2- to 3-month-old infants can discriminate between [rɑ] and [lɑ]
  - 1- to 4-month-old infants can discriminate between [vɑ] and [sɑ], [sɑ] and [shɑ], and [pɑ] and [bɑ]
  - 6- to 8-month-old infants can discriminate between [sɑ] and [zɑ]

- It has generally been found that infants under one year of age are able to distinguish sounds that are not used in their language. However, this ability begins to decline around 12 months of age. With increasing experience of the sounds of their own language, babies eventually lose their ability to distinguish between sounds that are not used in their language.

Production

- The infant's vocal tract is significantly different from the adult's. Structural differences (e.g., a high larynx, a tongue placed far forward in the oral cavity) constrain an infant's productions especially during the first 4 months of life. Between 4 and 6 months of age, when the epiglottis and velum grow further apart, the infant becomes capable of producing a much greater variety of sounds.
- Oller (1980) proposed approximate, overlapping stages of development of prelinguistic, non-reflexive vocalizations:
  1. *Phonation stage* (birth–1 month). Speechlike sounds are rare, and most vocalizations are reflexive (e.g., burping, coughing, crying). Some nonreflexive vowels or syllabic consonants may occur.
  2. *Cooing or gooing stage* (2–3 months). Most of the infant's productions are acoustically similar to /u/. Some velar consonantlike sounds may occur.
  3. *Expansion stage* (4–6 months). The infant is "playing" with the speech mechanism, exploring his or her capabilities through such productions as growls, squeals, yells, and raspberries (bilabial trills). Some CV-like combinations and vowel-like sounds may be produced.
  4. *Canonical or reduplicated babbling stage* (6–8 months). The infant produces strings of CV syllables, such as [mamamama], [dadadada], or [dedede]. Although the infant does not have sound-meaning correspondence, the timing of the CV syllables approximates

that of adult speech. By about 8 months, children with hearing losses fall behind hearing peers in language development.

5. *Variegated or nonreduplicated babbling stage* (8 months–1 year). The infant continues to use adultlike syllables in CV sequences, but a variety of consonants and vowels appear in a single vocalization (e.g., [duwɑbe]).

- Infants make a gradual progression through these stages and into the production of first words. This process is continuous and represents an important transition from the prelinguistic to the linguistic stage of phonological development, which begins around the first year, when the first meaningful word is produced (Lowe, 1994).
- During the first 3 years of life, a child's vocal tract anatomy and function change. For example, lip closure improves, the larynx moves farther down the vocal tract, tongue muscle tone increases, and tongue movements become dissociated from jaw movements (Hillis & Bahr, 2001). With these changes comes improved ability to articulate.

Typical Articulation Development in Children

- The articulation development approach looks at children's development of single phonemes (Peña-Brooks & Hegde, 2000). For example, one might ask when most children master the /r/ sound. The articulation, or segmental acquisition, approach focuses on the age of mastery for single phonemes of English (Stoel-Gammon & Dunn, 1985) based on speech-motor control.

- To assess when mastery of sounds occurs, researchers have generally used cross-sectional and longitudinal methods.

Research Methods

Cross-Sectional Studies

- *Cross-sectional* research studies are used to establish norms of articulation development.
- *Norms* are the typical behaviors of a representative group of children. The main research question is this: At what age do children master different speech sounds?
- In cross-sectional research, a certain number of children are selected from each age level targeted for the study. The children's speech production is sampled by various test stimuli and by spontaneous conversation.
- At each age level, the specific sounds mastered by a majority of children are determined. The different sets of sounds that are mastered by children of different ages then make up the norms.
- Studies disagree somewhat about the age at which children master speech sounds because of the studies' differences in research methods. For example, some studies consider a sound mastered when 75% of the children produce it correctly, whereas others consider a sound mastered when 90% of the children produce it correctly.
- Norms are based on statistical averages that apply to large groups of children. Thus, norms are useful only as broad guidelines; they are of little help in predicting the performance of an individual child. Individual children vary greatly in their articulatory skills.
- Also, norms are generally based on studies of white, monolingual, English-speaking children. Therefore, they may be invalid for use with linguistically and culturally diverse children.

Longitudinal Studies

- The second type of study, using a *longitudinal method,* observes the process of learning. One or several children are observed for an extended period of time. Speech samples are recorded frequently to trace the development of speech sound learning.
- While longitudinal studies do not yield norms, they help us understand various stages and processes of sound acquisition in greater depth than cross-sectional studies do.

Research Findings: Speech Sound Acquisition

- As stated, norms for speech sound acquisition differ depending on the research methods used as well as the definition of *mastery,* which differs across investigators.
- Table 5.3 summarizes the most commonly reported normative data for mastery of phonemes (these data are based on white, monolingual, English-speaking children).
- The combination of the results of cross-sectional and longitudinal studies in speech sound acquisition have shown us the following:

  - Vowels are acquired before consonants.
  - The nasal consonants /m/, /n/, and /ŋ/ are among the earliest to be acquired. They are usually mastered between 3 and 4 years of age.
  - Stop sounds are mastered earlier than fricatives. Most stops are mastered between 3 and 4.5 years of age. The stop /p/ may be mastered the earliest.
  - Glides /w/ and /j/ are mastered earlier than fricatives. Glides are mastered between 2 and 4 years.
  - The liquids /r/ and /l/ are mastered relatively late (between 3 and 5 years).
  - Fricatives and affricates are mastered later than stops and nasals. The fricative /f/ is mastered earlier than other fricatives (around age 3). Fricatives /ð/, /θ/, /dʒ/, /s/, and /z/ are mastered the last (between 3 and 6 years).
  - Consonant clusters (e.g., *br* in the word *brown*) are acquired later than most other sounds.

Typical Phonological Development in Children

Foundational Concepts

- As stated, the articulation approach to normal development looks at children's acquisition of individual phonemes and emphasizes speech-motor control. The phonological process approach studies children's acquisition of sound *patterns* and *processes* underlying such patterns. The phonological process approach focuses on language knowledge.
- Researchers who utilize the phonological process approach believe that children's errors are a way of simplifying the adult model of correct articulation. Such simplifications are called *phonological processes.*
- Phonological processes are described based on findings of longitudinal as well as large- and small-group studies. The phonological process framework helps us describe the error patterns in the speech of young children (Stoel-Gammon & Dunn, 1985).

Major Categories of Phonological Processes

- Children may use one or more phonological processes when producing a given word. For

Table 5.3   AGE IN YEARS-MONTHS AT WHICH CHILDREN MASTERED PHONEMES: SIX STUDIES

Phonemes	Poole (1934)	Wellman et al. (1931)	Templin (1957)	Sander (1972)	Prather et al. (1975)	Arlt (1976)
m	3-6	3	3	before 2	2	3
n	4-6	3	3	before 2	2	3
p	3-6	4	3	before 2	2	3
h	3-6	3	3	before 2	2	3
w	3-6	3	3	before 2	2-8	3
b	3-6	3	4	before 2	2-8	3
k	4-6	4	4	2	2-4	3
g	4-6	4	4	2	2-4	3
j	4-6	4	3-6	2	2-4	–
ŋ	4-6	–	3	2	2	3
t	4-6	5	6	2	2-8	3
d	4-6	5	4	2	2-4	3
f	5-6	3	3	3	2-4	3
l	6-6	4	6	3	2-4	4
v	6-6	5	6	4	4+	3-6
ʃ	6-6	–	4-6	4	3-8	4-6
ʒ	6-6	6	7	6	4	4
ð	6-6	–	7	5	4	5
θ	7-6	–	6	5	4+	5
r	7-6	5	4	3	3-4	5
s	7-6	5	4-6	3	3	4
z	7-6	5	7	4	4+	4
tʃ	–	5	4-6	4	3-8	4
dʒ	–	–	7	4	4+	4

Note. From *Introduction to Communicative Disorders*, 3rd ed. (p. 107), by M. N. Hegde, 2001, Austin, TX: PRO-ED. Copyright 2001 by PRO-ED, Inc. Reprinted with permission.

example, in the production of "hou" for "house," a child uses the single process of final-consonant deletion. But in saying "Les" instead of "Celeste," a child uses the processes of weak-syllable deletion, consonant-cluster reduction, and stridency deletion.

- Children's phonological processes can be divided into three categories: substitution, assimilation, and syllable structure. Each process is described in the following section (Bleile, 2004; Lowe, 1994; Stoel-Gammon & Dunn, 1985; Peña-Brooks & Hegde, 2000; Vihman, 2004).

Substitution Processes

- This is a group of phonological processes in which one class of sounds is substituted for another:
    - In *vocalization* a vowel (usually /o/ or /u/) is substituted for a syllabic consonant (usually a liquid). For example, a child might say "bado" instead of "bottle," or "noodoo" instead of "noodle."
    - In *gliding* a liquid consonant is produced as a glide. Children frequently make the following substitutions: w/l (wæmp/læmp), j/l (jaɪt/laɪt), w/r (wiŋ/riŋ). Gliding can also occur in consonant clusters (e.g., pwɪti/prɪti).
    - In *velar fronting* an alveolar or a dental replaces a velar; this usually occurs in word-initial position (e.g., ti/ki, doʊt/goʊt).
    - In *stopping* a fricative or affricate is replaced by a stop. For example, a child might make the following substitutions: tu/ʃu, dɪs/ðɪs, bip/bitʃ, noʊd/noʊz.
    - In *depalatization* a child substitutes an alveolar affricate for a palatal affricate (e.g., wats/watʃ, dzoʊk/dʒoʊk), or substitutes an alveolar fricative for a palatal fricative (e.g., wɪs/wɪʃ, sip/ʃip).
    - In *affrication* an affricate is produced in place of a fricative or stop (e.g., tʃʌn/sʌn, tʃu/ʃu, butʃ/buʃ).
    - In *deaffrication* a fricative replaces an affricate (e.g., pez/pedʒ, sɪp/tʃɪp, siz/tʃiz).
    - In *backing* a posteriorly placed consonant is produced instead of an anteriorly placed consonant (velars are substituted for alveolars). For example, a child might make the following substitutions: boʊk/boʊt or gaen/daen.
    - In glottal replacement a glottal stop (ʔ) is produced in place of other consonants (e.g. tuʔ/tuθ, bʔə/batəl).

Assimilation Processes

- In the following assimilation processes, the productions of dissimilar phonemes sound alike:
    - *reduplication,* in which a child repeats a pattern (e.g., wawa/watɚ, baba/batəl)
    - *regressive assimilation* (also called *consonant harmony*), which occurs due to the effect of a later occurring sound on an earlier sound (e.g., gʌk/dʌk, bɪp/zɪp)
    - *progressive assimilation* (also called consonant harmony), in which an earlier occurring sound influences a later occurring sound (e.g., kɪk/kɪs, bup/but)
    - *voicing assimilation,* which can be either *devoicing* (e.g., pɪk/pɪg) or *voicing* (e.g., bad/pad)

Syllable Structure Processes

- The following syllable structure processes affect the structure of entire syllables, not just certain sounds:
    - *unstressed- or weak-syllable deletion,* which involves omission of an unstressed syllable (e.g., -meɪdo/tomeɪto, -haɪnd/bihaɪnd, ɛfʌnt/ɛləfʌnt)
    - *final-consonant deletion,* in which the final consonant is omitted (e.g., bɛ-/bɛd, kae-/kaet)
    - *epenthesis,* in which a schwa vowel is inserted between the consonants in an initial cluster (e.g., təri/tri, bəlaek/blaek) or after a final voiced stop (e.g., stapə/stap, gʊdə/gʊd)
    - *consonant-cluster simplification or reduction,* in which a consonant or consonants in a cluster are deleted (e.g., -pid/spid, sid/spid, bɛs-/bɛst, pun/spun)
    - *diminutization,* or addition of /i/ to the target form (e.g., dagi/dag, ɛgi/ɛd)
    - *metathesis,* or production of sounds in a word in reversed order; also known as a spoonerism (e.g., pik/kip, lɪkstɪp/lɪpstɪk, pɪsgɛti/spʌgɛti)

✓ Understanding typical Ar-Ph development necessitates an understanding of the structural, behavioral, biological, cognitive, prosodic, natural phonology, and generative phonology theories. In addition, it is important to understand the differences between linear and nonlinear theories of phonology.

✓ It is also important to understand the basics of infant perception and production. In the first year of life, infants go through the stages of cooing/gooing, expansion, canonical or reduplicated babbling, and variegated or nonreduplicated babbling. These stages precede the development of the first word.

✓ Typical Ar-Ph development can be studied through the articulation or segmental acquisition approach, or through the phonological process approach. Familiarity with normal development and acquisition of Ar-Ph skills is essential to assessing and diagnosing Ar-Ph disorders.

SUMMARY

ARTICULATORY AND PHONOLOGICAL DISORDERS

INTRODUCTION

Typically-developing children's difficulty in producing certain speech sounds is called a *functional articulation disorder*. A functional disorder (sometimes also described as an *idiopathic disorder*) cannot be explained on the basis of neurological damage, muscle weakness or paralysis, or structural problems such as cleft palate. The term *functional* does not explain the disorder; it implies only that an *organic cause* was not found. Thus, many clinicians believe that the origin of functional articulation disorders is unknown. Though this term has been criticized, it is still used in many circles today (Haynes & Pindzola, 2004). *Organic disorders* are those that arise from various physical anomalies that affect the function or structure of the speech mechanism. For example, there can be physical damage to the central or peripheral nervous system, the oral mechanism, or all of these. Treatment for organically based disorders usually should be multidisciplinary and involve members of the medical community. In this section, we describe general factors related to Ar-Ph disorders, provide a description of articulatory errors, and discuss organically based disorders that occur secondary to oral structural variables, hearing loss, and neuropathologies.

General Factors Related to Articulatory and Phonological Disorders

■ Researchers have discovered several factors that coexist with Ar-Ph disorders. While these factors cannot be said to be causally related to Ar-Ph disorders, they are correlated with Ar-Ph disorders.

Gender

- There is some evidence that female children generally have slightly superior articulatory skills to those of male children. However, the evidence is weak, and the reported sex differences are small or negligible (Bernthal & Bankson, 2004).
- Nonetheless, more boys than girls tend to have articulation and phonological disorders.

Intelligence

- Intelligence has not been shown to be causally related to Ar-Ph disorders. Children of normal intelligence may have difficulty with Ar-Ph skills.

- Intelligence is associated with defective articulation only when intelligence is significantly below normal. Many institutionalized children with mental retardation show disordered articulation.

Birth Order and Sibling Status

- There is some evidence that first-born and only children have better articulation skills than those who have older siblings (Bernthal & Bankson, 2004).
- It has also been suggested that the greater the age difference between the siblings, the better the articulation of the younger child. This is because if siblings are too close to each other in age, the older one may provide a model of inadequate articulation for the younger child.

Socioeconomic Status

- Research has shown that socioeconomic status (SES) is not a strong factor in the etiology of articulation disorders. Thus, there is no evidence that coming from a low-income background causes a child to have articulation disorders.
- However, some studies have shown that children from lower SES backgrounds make more errors of articulation than children from middle- and upper-class backgrounds.
- One might hypothesize that because families of low-income children tend not to have health insurance, these children cannot be readily treated for factors such as middle-ear infections and dental problems that are associated with Ar-Ph errors.

Language Development and Academic Performance

- Research has shown that younger children with severe phonological disorders are more likely to demonstrate language problems than children with mild–moderate language delays (Bernthal & Bankson, 2004).
- Research (e.g., Clarke-Klein & Hodson, 1995; Swank & Catts, 1994) has indicated that young children with phonological disorders may be at risk for problems with reading and spelling in the elementary school years.

Auditory Discrimination Skills

- Researchers used to think that children with Ar-Ph disorders had poor auditory discrimination skills, which caused the disorders. Studies have produced inconsistent results, however; some children have scored poorly on auditory discrimination tests, whereas others have scored within normal limits.
- Because of these equivocal research findings, it is believed that there is not a strong relationship between articulation and auditory discrimination skills. However, many clinicians still conduct intensive work on auditory discrimination, believing that improved auditory discrimination skills lead to improved articulation skills.

Description of Articulatory Errors

- Earlier in this chapter, *phonological error patterns* were described in detail. It was stated that children may manifest error patterns such as final-consonant deletion, consonant-cluster reduction, assimilation, and others. These error patterns underlie lack of intelligibility.

■ The child is often able to physically produce a sound (e.g., /k/ and /g/), but if she displays the phonological pattern of *fronting* (e.g., tæt/kæt, do/go), then she makes errors of the /k/ and /g/ sounds despite the motoric ability to produce the sounds correctly.

■ Children may also make errors that can be categorized as *articulatory errors.* These errors typically involve misproductions of specific phonemes. The child is motorically unable to produce the erred phoneme (e.g., /r/, /s/), so treatment must involve teaching correct production and emphasizing speech-motor control.

■ Children may make the following articulation errors:

- *Substitutions:* Replacements of sounds; an incorrect sound is produced in place of a correct sound (e.g., tink/θink).
- *Omissions or deletions:* Required sounds are omitted in words (e.g., bo-/bot).
- *Labialization:* Sounds are produced with excessive lip rounding.
- *Nasalization:* Oral sounds (especially oral stops like /k/) are produced with inappropriate, usually excessive, nasal resonance.
- *Pharyngeal fricative:* Fricatives such as /h/ are produced in the pharyngeal area.
- *Devoicing:* Voiced sounds are produced with limited vocal fold vibrations or without vocal fold vibrations (e.g., dak/dag).
- *Frontal lisp:* Sibilant consonants are produced with the tongue tip placed too far forward (between or against the teeth); /s/ and /z/ are the sounds most commonly involved.
- *Lateral lisp:* Sibilant sounds such as /s/ and /z/ are produced with air flowing inappropriately over the sides of the tongue.
- *Stridency deletion:* Strident sounds are omitted (e.g., mæ-/mæʃ, -tap/stap); sometimes stridency deletion is described as a phonological process.
- *Unaspirated:* Aspirated sounds (e.g., /k/, /t/) are produced without aspiration.
- *Initial, medial, final position error:* Error in the production of a beginning, medial, or final sound of a word.
- *Prevocalic, intervocalic, postvocalic error:* Errors that occur with reference to consonant position in syllables (e.g., dæbdəlɑɪjən/dændəlɑɪjən would involve a postvocalic error; the substitution of gag/dag would involve a prevocalic error).

CONCEPTS TO CONSIDER

Describe three factors that are related to articulatory-phonological disorders.

Organically Based Disorders

Oral Structural Variables

- Some children with deviations of the oral structure have normal Ar-Ph skills. However, Ar-Ph disorders may also be found in the absence of structural anomalies. Thus, there is no demonstrable causal relationship between structural anomalies and Ar-Ph disorders. Nevertheless, the following oral structural abnormalities have been associated with Ar-Ph disorders in some children.

Ankyloglossia (Tongue-Tie)

- Normally, the free tip of the tongue is mobile and permits the production of tip-alveolar sounds such as /t/, /d/. However, if the *lingual frenum,* which attaches the tongue to the base of the mouth, is too short, tongue tip mobility is reduced.
- When the frenum is thus attached too close to the tip of the tongue, this is diagnosed as a "tongue-tie" or *ankyloglossia.*
- Clipping or cutting the frenum used to be a common surgical procedure; it is more rare nowadays. Research has shown that ankyloglossia is not a frequent cause of misarticulations, and children with short lingual frenums can have normal articulation.

Dental Deviations

- *Malocclusion* refers to deviations in the shape and dimensions of the mandible and maxilla (*skeletal malocclusion*) and the positioning of individual teeth (*dental malocclusion*).
- Most children with malocclusions have a misalignment of the mandible and maxilla and the upper and lower rows of teeth. There are three basic categories of malocclusions, with many more subtypes within categories (see Moller, 1994, for a comprehensive description).
- In *class I malocclusion,* the arches themselves are generally aligned properly, but some individual teeth are misaligned.
- In *class II malocclusion,* the upper jaw or maxilla is protruded and the lower jaw or mandible is receded. This is also referred to as an overbite. *Overjet* occurs when the child has a Class II malocclusion and the upper teeth from the molars forward are positioned excessively anterior to the lower teeth.
- In *class III malocclusion,* the maxilla is receded and the mandible is protruded.

Oral-Motor Coordination Skills

- Oral-motor coordination skills are frequently evaluated through tests of *diadochokinetic rate* (maximum repetition rate of syllables in rapid succession). For example, a child might be asked to say "pʌtʌkʌ" as fast as possible in succession. The goal is to assess the functional and structural integrity of the lips, jaw, and tongue.
- Some clinicians have observed that children who do poorly on diadochokinetic tests also have difficulty with Ar-Ph skills. However, not all children with articulation difficulties do poorly on diadochokinetic tests.
- The relationship between diadochokinesis and speech sound production in conversational speech is unclear (Stoel-Gammon & Dunn, 1985). Research has not substantiated the hypothesis that poor oral motor coordination skills cause articulation problems.

Orofacial Myofunctional Disorders (Tongue Thrust)

- The term *tongue thrust* has recently been expanded to be more inclusive. The current definition of *orofacial myofunctional disorders* (OMD) encompasses any anatomical or physiological characteristic of the orofacial structures (palate, cheeks, tongue, lips, jaw, teeth) that interferes with normal speech, physical, dentofacial, or psychosocial development. This includes swallow, labial and lingual rest, and speech posture differences (Kellum, 1994).
- Usually, a child with OMD exhibits deviant swallows. In a normal swallow, the tongue tip is placed behind the alveolar ridge and the body of the tongue pushes the fluid or solid posteriorly for swallowing.
- In the deviant swallow, the tongue tip pushes against the front teeth (usually the upper central incisors). The tongue tip may protrude between the upper and lower teeth and thus come in contact with the lower lip.
- During speech production, the tongue also may exert some force against the front teeth, and even at rest, the tongue may be carried more forward in the oral cavity. This can contribute to an anterior open bite.
- According to the American Speech-Language-Hearing Association (ASHA) (1996), OMD causes errors in the production of /s/, /z/, /ʃ/, /ʒ/, /tʃ/, and /j/; in addition, tip-dental sounds /t/, /d/, /l/, and /n/ may be misarticulated due to weak tongue tip musculature. (*Note:* Some researchers believe that OMD does not *cause* errors of articulation but exists in a correlational relationship with those errors.) Thus, some clinicians perform *oral myofunctional therapy* to correct the deviant swallow.
- ASHA (1996) has stated that myofunctional therapy is appropriate and within the purview of speech–language pathologists who assess and treat the effects of OMD on swallowing, rest postures, and speech. Such speech–language pathologists traditionally work on a team also composed of a dentist, an orthodontist, and a physician.

Hearing Loss

- Various kinds of articulation problems are frequently seen in individuals with hearing loss. The degree of hearing loss is frequently related to the severity of the Ar-Ph problem.
- Individuals who are born with a profound hearing loss generally have the greatest challenges with articulation, as they cannot monitor their speech production. These individuals may have difficulties with both consonant and vowel productions, making many substitutions, distortions, and omissions of phonemes.
- Children with mild hearing losses (10–30 dB), especially if those losses are secondary to middle-ear fluid and infections, may have Ar-Ph problems. Omissions of high-frequency voiceless sounds (e.g., /s/, /t/) are common. These children may also use the phonological processes of final-consonant deletion, stridency deletion, and fronting.

Neuropathologies

Dysarthria

- Dysarthria is a speech-motor disorder caused by peripheral or central nervous system damage. This damage causes paralysis, weakness, or incoordination of the muscles of speech. In children, dysarthria can be caused by cerebral palsy, head injury, degenerative diseases, tumors, and strokes.
- All the speech production systems are affected: phonation, resonation, respiration, resonance, and articulation. Thus, assessment and treatment must incorporate all of those systems.
- Dysarthric speech usually is associated with monotonous pitch, deviant voice quality, variable

speech rate, and hypernasality. Reduced intelligibility is a key feature of dysarthria, with the child's speech sounding "slurred."

- Children with dysarthria have the following common articulatory error patterns:

  - voicing errors occur, especially those that involve devoicing of voiced sounds
  - bilabial and velar sounds are easier than alveolar fricatives and affricates, labiodental fricatives, and palatal liquids
  - stops, glides, and nasals are easier than fricatives, affricates, and liquids

- Treatment for childhood dysarthria is very repetitive and structured. It involves increasing muscle tone and strength, increasing range and rate of motion, and treating other parameters (e.g., respiration) that affect intelligibility.
- Treatment involves intensive and systematic drill, modeling, phonetic placement, and emphasis on accuracy of sound production.
- For children who cannot be 100% intelligible, compensatory strategies (e.g., prosthetic devices) are often used to assist in communication. For very severely involved children, alternative or augmentative communication devices may be used.

Apraxia

- Apraxia of speech is caused by central nervous system damage. There is no weakness or paralysis of the muscles; however, the central nervous system damage makes it difficult to program the precise movements necessary for smoothly articulated speech. Thus, apraxia of speech is described as a *motor programming disorder.*
- Researchers and clinicians have long debated the existence of *developmental apraxia of speech* (DAS) as a clinical entity (this is also called childhood apraxia of speech, or CAS). Children with DAS are believed to have central neural problems (Hall, Jordan, & Robin, 1993) or a disordered physiological mechanism (Klein, 1996).
- These problems are congenital and lead to difficulties in motor programming, although the child has not experienced frank, overt damage such as a stroke.
- Children who are thought to have DAS demostrate sensorimotor problems in positioning and sequentially moving muscles for the volitional production of speech (Yavas, 1998). They frequently show groping behaviors and poor intelligibility due to inconsistent and multiple articulation errors. Inconsistent errors are a hallmark of DAS.
- Children with DAS usually have the following common characteristics (Bankson & Bernthal, 2004; Smit, 2004):

  - prolongation of speech sounds
  - repetition of sounds and syllables
  - most difficulty with consonant clusters followed by fricatives, affricates, stops, and nasals
  - more frequent occurrence of omissions and substitutions
  - voicing and devoicing errors
  - vowel and diphthong errors
  - unusual errors of articulation including metathesis (e.g., dɛks/dɛsk) and addition of phonemes
  - difficulty with volitional, oral, nonspeech movements
  - deviations in prosody (e.g., rate, stress)
  - resonance problems (possibly due to poor velopharyngeal control)
  - history of feeding problems
  - history of tactile aversions or sensitivities (e.g., very defensive when the clinician attempts to put a tongue depressor into the mouth)

- Research indicates that children with DAS may have deficits in phonological representation;

for example, they often have difficulty with rhyming and with identifying syllables (Marquardt, Sussman, Snow, & Jacks, 2002). They are also at risk for language, reading, and spelling problems (Lewis, Freebairn, Hansen, Ieyngar, & Taylor, 2004).

- Treatment for DAS is similar to treatment for adults with apraxia. It should progress hierarchically from easy to difficult tasks.

- DAS treatment is multimodal, involving extensive drills stressing sequences of movement involved in speech production, imitation, decreased rate of speech, normal prosody, and increased accuracy in the production of individual consonants, vowels, and consonant clusters. Children may also need intervention for oral language, spelling, and reading deficits.

- DAS therapy often produces very slow gains; therefore, treatment should be intensive. Children may need speech therapy for as long as nine years (Lewis et al., 2004). Home practice and self-monitoring are essential components of DAS treatment.

SUMMARY

✓ Articulatory errors involve misproductions of specific phonemes and are usually functionally or organically based although the specific etiology is often unclear.

✓ General factors related to articulation disorders include gender, intelligence, birth order, sibling status, socioeconomic status, language development and academic performance, and auditory discrimination skills.

✓ Organically based disorders have a variety of etiologies that are either correlated with the disorders or cause them. These include tongue-tie, dental deviations, oral motor coordination problems, orofacial myofunctional disorders (tongue thrust), and hearing loss.

✓ Children with articulation disorders based on the neuropathologies of apraxia of speech and dysarthria have unique characteristics that must be addressed in a comprehensive treatment program.

ASSESSMENT OF ARTICULATORY AND PHONOLOGICAL DISORDERS

INTRODUCTION

When a child is referred for an Ar-Ph disorder, the clinician's first job is to determine whether there is a clinical problem. If so, the characteristics of the problem must be described. This process of identifying and describing a clinical problem is *assessment*. In this section, we discuss the components of assessment, which include carrying out general and related assessment objectives, conducting screenings, and conducting in-depth testing. In-depth testing usually involves conversational and evoked speech samples, stimulability assessment, and the administration of standardized tests. Assessment data collected through in-depth testing are scored and analyzed as a foundation for treatment.

General Assessment Objectives

- In most cases, the clinician's general assessment objectives include:

    - case history
    - screening

- oral peripheral examination
- hearing screening
- language assessment, if language problems are suspected

■ Further general assessment objectives include (Peña-Brooks & Hegde, 2000):

- assessing the child's Ar-Ph performance in single-word positions and in conversational speech
- assessing the presence of phonological processes that may help establish patterns in mis-articulations
- evaluating a child's performance based on developmental norms
- evaluating stimulability of speech sounds that are misarticulated
- identifying potential treatment targets

Related Assessment Objectives

■ In certain cases, clinicians may need to obtain data (if relevant) regarding:

- audiological assessment
- physical or neurological disabilities
- dental abnormalities that are negatively impacting intelligibility
- possible influences of another language or dialect (Goldstein & Iglesias, 2004)
- concomitant language problems
- intellectual and behavioral assessment in cases of children with such problems as behavior disorders and mental retardation

Screening

■ A screening is a brief, initial procedure that helps determine whether a child should be assessed further and in more depth. Children who pass a screening procedure are judged to have age-appropriate Ar-Ph skills. Those who fail a screening are scheduled for a comprehensive assessment.

■ Different procedures are available to screen Ar-Ph skills. If the child is willing to talk, a brief conversational sample may suffice. Sometimes clinicians use pictures to test the production of certain speech sounds. Clinicians may also use standardized screening tests or the screening portions of full-length assessment tests of articulation.

Assessment Procedures

Case History

- The first step in a comprehensive evaluation is to take a case history (see Chapter 11 for a detailed description).
- When a child has an Ar-Ph problem, the clinician may probe more deeply into such areas as:

- what the child and family think the problem is

- when the problem was first noted
- whether the problem is stable or changing
- the results of any previous treatment
- the child's general health, including especially the occurrence of ear infections
- any accidents, injuries, and diseases that could have caused brain damage
- the effects of the disorder on the child's academic and social life

- The clinician also must assess the child's possible multilingual/multicultural status. If children speak or are exposed to other languages, the influence of such other languages should be evaluated (Ray, 2002; Roseberry-McKibbin, 2002).
- Lastly, many children with Ar-Ph disorders also have concomitant language problems. Therefore, it is important for the clinician to assess a child's language skills as well (Haynes & Pindzola, 2004; Hoffman & Norris, 2002).

Orofacial Examination

- The clinician examines the client's facial and oral structures to rule out gross organic problems such as cleft palate.
- The clinician notes the general symmetry of facial structures, the shape and mobility of the client's lips and tongue, and any missing teeth or dental malocclusions.
- The clinician examines the client's hard and soft palates, looking for clefts, fistulas, or structural problems such as a high and vaulted hard palate. The client's soft-palate mobility is evaluated to make sure that the soft palate can move back and up to close the velopharyngeal port during the production of non-nasal sounds (for further details, see Chapter 11).
- Many clinicians also perform tests of diadochokinetic skill, which evaluate the child's oral motor coordination as well as the integrity of oral structures and functions.
- The goal of the orofacial examination is to assess the presence of any structural or functional factors that might be contributing to the Ar-Ph disorder. If one or more of these factors are present, the clinician must assess the client's potential for improvement in treatment if the factors are not addressed.
- Despite the presence of abnormal structural or functional factors (e.g., a high and vaulted palate), the child may be stimulable for errored sounds and capable of improving speech.
- However, for some children, abnormal structure, function, or both must be addressed before treatment progress is possible. For example, the first author worked with a second-grade boy who had been in speech therapy for four years (with previous clinicians) with minimal progress on the treatment targets of /s, z, ʃ, ʒ/. It was found that due to the boy's thumb-sucking patterns, he had a marked class II malocclusion with substantial overjet. He was physically unable to produce the target phonemes due to the condition of his dentition. It was determined that probably orthodontia would be required before articulation treatment could be successful.

Hearing Screening

- Generally, the child's hearing is screened by a brief audiological procedure. A hearing screening does not determine actual hearing thresholds but only suggests that hearing is or is not within normal limits.
- A child who fails a hearing screening is referred to an audiologist for a complete hearing evaluation. This evaluation may include pure-tone testing, tympanometry, or both.

Specific Components of an Assessment

Conversational Speech Samples

- It is optimal to collect 50–100 utterances as a representative sample of connected speech. Clinicians can phonetically transcribe all words or just the words that contain errors. It is best to transcribe on the spot if possible.
- It is a good idea to repeat the child's unintelligible words after him or her so that if the sample is tape recorded, the clinician can understand the speech sample at a later time.
- Samples should be tape recorded in a quiet environment with a high-quality recorder and cassette tapes. Noisy toys are not recommended; if they are used, the clinician can use them on the carpet or on a table with a tablecloth to reduce noise.
- Young children might give more representative speech samples if they interact with their family members; in such cases, the clinician can observe the interaction and record notes.
- Clinicians can use broken toys, games, large pictures, storybooks, and open-ended questions to evoke speech. Especially successful topics include pets, TV shows, siblings, movies, favorite stories, and weekend or vacation activities.

Evoked Speech Samples

- Clinicians can collect speech samples not only through spontaneous conversation, but also through evoked samples. Below are three types of evoked samples that may be used to assess a child's production of sounds in single words (Bleile, 2004):

  - *Imitation.* Typically, the child imitates the clinician's model of single words. Imitation can be *immediate* (e.g., clinician: "Say truck." child: "Truck.") or delayed (e.g., clinician: "Truck. This truck is big and yellow. What is this?" child: "Truck."). In delayed imitation, a short phrase is placed between the clinician's model and the child's response.
  - *Naming.* The child names objects or pictures, usually after the clinician asks "What's this?"
  - *Sentence completion.* The child finishes the clinician's sentence. For example, the clinician might say "Look, here's a big, brown, barking _____." The child would fill in the word "dog" to complete the sentence.

- It is best to evoke single-word productions in conjunction with connected speech samples. Some children make more errors in connected speech samples when sounds are produced in a coarticulated context.

Stimulability Assessment

- *Stimulability* refers to the child's ability to imitate the clinician's model. Clinicians should select the sounds the child misarticulates and assess the child's stimulability for those sounds. A stimulable child is generally able to imitate the clinician's modeled productions.
- The clinician should ask the child to watch, listen carefully, and "say what I say." It is best initially to model sounds in isolation. Sounds can later be modeled in words and, if desired, nonsense syllables.
- Researchers disagree about the prognostic value of stimulability. Some believe that a stimulable child will outgrow errors of articulation without therapy; others believe that a child will make faster improvement in therapy. Still other researchers believe that stimulability has

questionable value in predicting improvement with or without therapy.

- Many clinicians believe that stimulable sounds are easier to teach than non-stimulable sounds. Therefore, many clinicians use stimulable sounds as a starting point for treatment.
- Bleile (2002) recommended that clinicians assess a child's ability to produce sounds (a) through imitation, (b) in one or more phonetic environments, (c) in key words, (d) through phonetic placement and shaping, or (e) a combination of these contexts. According to Bleile, in therapy, a child's frustration can be reduced if he has at least some capacity to produce a target sound.

Standardized Tests

- Many standardized tests of articulatory and phonological skills are available. For many clinicians, standardized tests are convenient to give because they know what the target words are. When used to test highly unintelligible children, standardized tests may be more reliable than spontaneous, connected samples.
- Standardized tests also satisfy the requirements of many school districts, which require formal test scores (Tyler & Tolbert, 2002). In such cases, clinicians can supplement standardized test results with conversational speech samples.
- Most standardized tests of articulation skills assess the child's production of all phonemes in the initial, medial, and final positions of words at the single-word level. Usually, each phoneme is sampled only once in each position. Such tests yield information such as, "Johnny made th/s substitutions in the initial, medial, and final positions of words."
- Instruments that measure phonological processes assess a child's production of words in isolation and in connected speech. However, instead of focusing on individual sounds that are misarticulated, phonological process measures assess the child's use of phonological processes and the percentage of the time he or she uses those phonological processes. For example, a test might yield the information that "Johnny used the phonological process of final consonant deletion in 80% of all tested contexts."
- Most tests of Ar-Ph skills use picture stimuli. In addition, computerized measures are increasingly being used (Ingram & Ingram, 2002). Some clinicians in public school settings do not have access to computers; thus, computerized measures are more typically used in university and research settings.

CONCEPTS TO CONSIDER

Briefly describe three major components of an assessment for articulatory-phonological disorders.

_____

_____

_____

_____

_____

Scoring and Analysis of Assessment Data

Independent vs. Relational Analysis

- Clinicians can score and analyze assessment data in two ways: independent analysis or relational analysis. A more complete picture of a child's Ar-Ph skills emerges when both types of analyses are performed.
- In *independent analysis,* a child's speech patterns are described without reference to the adult model of the language of the child's community. For example, an independent analysis might state that a child's speech contains [f, b, s, k], but would not state if these sounds were produced correctly in comparison to the adult community's standard form (Bleile, 2004; Stoel-Gammon & Dunn, 1985).
- In a *relational analysis,* which is more commonly used in clinical settings, a child's speech is compared to the adult model of his or her speech community. For example, a statement in relational analysis might say, "The child produced a w/r substitution." This statement involves an evaluation in relation to acceptable speech in the larger community.

Standard Procedures

- The following procedures should be followed when scoring and analyzing assessment data:

  - Use the International Phonetic Alphabet to transcribe the child's speech. Use diacritics, if possible, to make a more detailed analysis of errors. This is especially critical for children from bilingual backgrounds and children with organically based problems such as cleft palate.
  - Note how consistently the errors are produced and calculate the percentage of misarticulation for each phoneme in error (e.g., /k/ is misarticulated in 80% of contexts).
  - List the phonetic contexts in which any of the misarticulated sounds were produced correctly (e.g., /r/ is produced correctly in word-initial gr-blends).
  - Calculate the percent correct imitated productions on stimulability trials.
  - Analyze the results of any standardized Ar-Ph test according to the manual's prescribed procedures.

- List the sounds in error and classify them according to an acceptable format (e.g., omissions-substitutions-distortions; errors in the pre-, inter-, and postvocalic positions of words).
- If the child has multiple misarticulations and it appears that a pattern analysis will be worthwhile, carry out a phonological analysis. List the phonological processes the child uses and the percentage of time those processes are used (e.g., "Susie used the phonological process of consonant cluster reduction in 60% of the possible contexts.").
- Use published guidelines to decide if the child is using phonological processes that should have disappeared by his or her age. For example, a 4-year-old should not be using the process of reduplication. Table 5.4 summarizes guidelines given by Stoel-Gammon & Dunn (1985).
- Calculate the child's intelligibility (in percent) based on the number of utterances or words that are understood with or without knowledge of the context. For example, the clinician could say, "In the known context of discussing a current movie, Mario's connected speech was 60% intelligible to the examiner."

Table 5.4   PHONOLOGICAL PROCESSES DISAPPEARING BEFORE AND PERSISTING AFTER AGE 3

Disappearing by Age 3	Persisting After Age 3
Reduplication	Final consonant devoicing
Weak/unstressed syllable deletion	Consonant-cluster reduction
Consonant assimilation	Stopping
Prevocalic voicing	Epenthesis
Fronting of velars	Gliding
Final consonant deletion	Depalatization
Diminutization	Vocalization

- Decide whether the child should receive treatment based on the following factors:

  - the child is making Ar-Ph errors at an age when he or she should be producing those patterns and sounds correctly;
  - the child's production differs markedly from that of peers of a similar cultural and linguistic background;
  - the child's speech is so unintelligible that it represents a clinically significant problem (e.g., there are social penalties for the child); and
  - the number of phonemes in error indicates that the child qualifies for treatment in a given clinical setting such as the public school.

- Distinguish Ar-Ph disorders from hearing impairment, DAS, and dysarthria associated with a known neurological condition such as cerebral palsy.
- Distinguish Ar-Ph disorders from normal, predictable errors manifested by a child who speaks a language other than English or who is exposed to models who speak a language other than English.
- Describe associated conditions such as autism, fetal alcohol syndrome, or cleft palate and suggest additional or more intensive evaluation if necessary.
- Make a statement of prognosis, considering whether variables such as hearing impairment, environmental factors, physical disabilities, and mental retardation may affect treatment outcome.

SUMMARY

✓ Assessment serves several purposes. The first is to determine whether the child manifests a clinically significant Ar-Ph problem. The second is to identify and describe the problem if it exists.

✓ Clinicians usually begin by screening to rule out children who do not need in-depth assessments. An in-depth assessment usually begins with a case history, an orofacial examination, and a hearing screening.

✓ Specific assessment components include conversational and evoked speech samples, stimulability assessment, and the administration of standardized tests. Assessment data are then scored and analyzed to provide directions for treatment.

TREATMENT OF ARTICULATORY AND PHONOLOGICAL DISORDERS

INTRODUCTION

Treatment for articulatory and phonological disorders may be organized under two major categories: motor approaches and cognitive-linguistic approaches. Bernthal and Bankson (2004) state that this dichotomy is somewhat artificial because motor and cognitive-linguistic skills are intertwined; thus, these categories are not mutually exclusive. Yet, these two broad categories help clinicians conceptualize the foundation for treatment of children who are unintelligible. Treatment depends very much upon whether the child's errors reflect a lack of linguistic knowledge (phonological errors), a lack of motor skills (articulation errors), or both (Bernthal & Bankson, 2004).

It is generally believed that motor-based approaches are best for children with several sounds in error (e.g., /r/, /s/, /l/), and that cognitive-linguistic approaches are most appropriate for highly unintelligible children with multiple sound errors. But because many children have difficulties in both areas, clinicians frequently use a combination of motor and cognitive-linguistic approaches to remediation. In this section, we describe general considerations in the treatment of children with Ar-Ph disorders. We then elaborate upon motor and cognitive-linguistic approaches and briefly discuss the phenomenon of phonological awareness.

General Considerations in Treatment

- No matter what specific treatment program or combination of programs is used, most clinicians use certain basic procedures in providing treatment for children with Ar-Ph disorders. These steps usually consist of:

    - thorough assessment and analysis of the child's Ar-Ph system
    - determination of any existing patterns
    - selection and prioritization of intervention targets
    - establishment of baselines of target sounds in all contexts: words, phrases, sentences, and conversational speech
    - specific training for target patterns, sounds, or both
    - preparation of generalization and maintenance activities

- Most clinicians use a multimodal approach to treatment. This involves use of auditory, visual, and kinesthetic cues.

- Based on the individual needs of the child, clinicians must decide between training broad and training deep. *Training broad* involves treating several sounds simultaneously. Practice is limited on any specific sound, and the child receives practice on a wide, or broad, range of sounds. *Training deep* involves one or several sounds being treated intensively. Other sounds are selected only when the child has achieved mastery of the initial targets.

- Because the primary goal of treatment is effective communication, clinicians are increasingly using language- and meaning-based activities in therapy for Ar-Ph disorders. While some approaches to treatment necessarily involve drills, and sometimes drills on nonsense syllables, it is important to make activities meaningful to the child's communication in his or her daily environment.

■ The concept of *communicative potency* looks at how functional words are within an individual child's communication environment. Words and phrases such as *stop, yes, give me,* and *some more* allow children greater control over their environments (Lowe & Weitz, 1994).

■ Therefore, treatment should use communicatively potent words as much as possible. Children should be taught that correct production of sounds and patterns results in improved communication with others and increased control over their environments.

■ If a child has a language disorder that accompanies the Ar-Ph disorder, the clinician must integrate language therapy into Ar-Ph therapy. This can be accomplished in many ways, including increasing morphosyntactic skills as well as narrative skills if the child has deficits in these areas (Hoffman & Norris, 2002; Tyler, Lewis, Haskill, & Tolbert, 2002).

■ It is very important to involve caregivers in therapy, especially in the generalization and maintenance stages. In addition, children must be taught self-monitoring skills.

■ Clinicians commonly use standardized tests to assess treatment progress, but this is usually ineffective because tests include only a small number of items to sample each sound or pattern. For example, most standardized tests of articulation test each phoneme only once in each word position. Using a standardized test as a measure of pretreatment skills and posttreatment gains usually fails to show treatment gains.

■ Clinicians must always take the child's cultural and linguistic background into account. It is important to distinguish between Ar-Ph *differences* and *disorders*. Differences usually arise from the influence of the child's first language. Disorders exist when the child makes errors that are not typical for his or her cultural and linguistic speech community.

■ For example, a Spanish-speaking child typically makes b/v and d/ð substitutions. These differences do not constitute disorders and should not be treated as such. A child has a disorder only when his or her Ar-Ph patterns in the primary language or in English differ from those of peers from a similar cultural and linguistic background (Roseberry-McKibbin, 2002).

Motor-Based Approaches

General Principles

■ Articulation errors are viewed as resulting from *motor difficulties,* in which the child is physically unable to produce the sound, and from *faulty perceptual skills.* Thus, motor-based approaches to articulation therapy focus on: (a) establishing correct perception of erred phonemes, and (b) motor production of individual phonemes (e.g., separate work on /r/, /s/, /l/).

■ Those who use motor-based approaches usually describe articulation errors according to the categories of *substitutions, distortions, omissions,* and *additions.* The question asked is: Is the child producing the sound correctly or not? There is no attempt to describe underlying patterns that might be affecting classes of sounds (Klein, 1996).

- *Van Riper's traditional approach,* first published in the mid-1930s, is the foundation for motor approaches to articulation therapy. Van Riper (1978) focused on *phonetic placement, auditory discrimination/perceptual training,* and *drill-like repetition and practice* at increasingly complex motor levels until target phonemes were automatized.
- The underlying assumption is that motor practice leads to automatization and thus to generalization of correct productions to untrained contexts (Bernthal & Bankson, 2004). Practice and drill are critical components of treatment.
- Practice occurs at increasingly complex motor levels until a sound is generalized into conversational speech. Thus, many clinicians who use the Van Riper approach to therapy teach /s/, for example, in the following order: isolation, syllables, words, phrases, sentences, reading (if the child reads), and then conversation.
- *Auditory discrimination/perceptual training* is designed to teach clients to distinguish between correct and incorrect productions of speech sounds. For example, the clinician may say, "Listen. Which is the right way to say this word? *Wabbit* or *rabbit?*" Or the clinician might have the client begin by correctly distinguishing the /w/ from the /r/ sound.
- This is based on the assumption that auditory discrimination training is a precursor to speech sound production training. That assumption is questioned by many researchers and clinicians who believe that production training induces correct discrimination.
- *Phonetic placement* is used when the client cannot imitate the modeled production of a phoneme such as /r/. Phonetic placement begins with having the child produce a sound in isolation. The clinician uses verbal instructions, modeling, physical guidance (e.g., manipulating the client's tongue with a tongue depressor), and visual feedback (e.g., mirrors, drawings) to show the client how target sounds are produced.
- Motor-based approaches are most successful with children who have only several phonemes in error (e.g., /r/, /s/, /l/) and who are not highly unintelligible. Motor approaches work well for children who have physical difficulty producing target phonemes.
- In recent years, some clinicians have begun to incorporate the use of oral motor exercises to help children who have physical difficulty produce target phonemes. While many grass-roots clinicians believe that these exercises are effective, research has not proven that oral motor exercises facilitate changes in speech sound productions (Forrest, 2002; Lof, 2002; Williams, 2002).
- Motor-based approaches can be incorporated into programs that are based on cognitive-linguistic principles (e.g., the phonological process approach) for clients who have a combination of motor-based and cognitive-linguistic-based errors.
- Commonly used motor-based approaches include McCabe and Bradley's multiple phoneme approach (MPA), Baker and Ryan's Monterey Articulation Program, McDonald's sensory-motor approach, and Irwin and Weston's paired stimuli approach (PSA).

McCabe and Bradley's Multiple Phoneme Approach

- This behaviorally oriented treatment method (McCabe & Bradley, 1975) emphasizes that all articulation errors should be treated in all sessions. The MPA is appropriate for children making six or more errors, and focuses on sound production in conversational speech. The MPA, unlike most other motor-based approaches, does not emphasize auditory discrimination training. The MPA consists of three phases.
- *Phase I* consists of two steps: *establishment* (whose goal is the production of consonants in response to a printed letter or phonetic symbol representing it), and a *holding procedure* (designed to maintain correct production of sounds produced in isolation).
- *Phase II* involves five transfer steps of target sounds to: (a) syllables, (b) words, (c) phrases and sentences, (d) reading and storytelling, and (e) conversation.
- *Phase III* has as its goal the maintenance of 90% whole-word accuracy in conversational speech

produced in different speaking situations without treatment or external monitoring.

- This approach provides an organized way of administering treatment and collecting data. Some children improve quickly and become much more intelligible with daily therapy utilizing this approach. However, it might prove difficult for preschoolers who do not recognize printed letters and who might be confused by the presentation of several sounds in each session.

Baker and Ryan's Monterey Articulation Program

- Developed by Baker and Ryan (1971), this motor-based hierarchical and detailed program uses behavioral principles and programmed learning concepts. Imitation is heavily emphasized. There are three phases: an establishment phase, a transfer phase, and a maintenance phase.
- The *establishment phase* includes a basic program of 18 steps, 91 branching steps, and several sound evocation programs. Target sounds are produced in the following order: isolation, nonsense syllables, words, phrases, sentences, contextual reading, story narration, picture description, and finally conversational speech.
- The *transfer phase* consists of 15 steps. These steps encompass home training, clinician training in different settings (e.g., conversations outside the clinic room and on the playground), and training in the classroom.
- The *maintenance phase* is completed subsequent to the transfer phase and consists of five steps that involve periodic rechecks to help the child maintain accuracy in the production of newly acquired sounds.
- Detailed and wide in scope, the Monterey approach is excellent for use with children who need a highly structured motor-articulation treatment approach. Repetition and motor practice are strongly emphasized (Bernthal & Bankson, 2004). However, the detail and technicality of the program might seem overwhelming to some clinicians.

McDonald's Sensory-Motor Approach

- Developed around 1964, McDonald's sensory-motor approach is based on the assumption that the *syllable,* not the isolated phoneme, is the basic unit of speech production. Principles of *coarticulation* are important in this approach.
- This system was unique in the mid-1960s because it disagreed with the established assumptions that (a) perceptual training should precede production training, and (b) treatment should begin with sounds in isolation.
- According to McDonald, *phonetic environment* is very important in treatment; thus, training should begin at the syllable level. The clinician should administer a deep test (e.g., *McDonald's Deep Test of Articulation*) to find phonetic contexts where an otherwise misarticulated sound was produced correctly. For example, a child with an /s/ distortion might produce /s/ correctly in the context of *watch-sun*.
- McDonald's approach includes several basic steps (each step has smaller, more detailed increments; only the basics are presented here):

  - heighten the client's responsiveness to connected motor productions; begin with nonerror sounds in a variety of bi- and trisyllabic contexts (in nonsense syllables) with differing stress patterns
  - train correct production of misarticulated sounds; find a context, for example, in which /s/ is produced correctly (*watch-sun*) and have the child produce *watch-sun* in various syllable stress and phrase and sentence patterns
  - vary the phonetic contexts (e.g., *watch-sit, watch-saw*) and have the child practice correct

production of the targets in different contexts
  - generalize by facilitating transfer to other phonetic contexts and then to natural communication activities

- McDonald's sensory-motor approach may be helpful for children with oral-motor coordination difficulties. However, research does not support the assumption that syllabic production of nonerror productions will facilitate the correction of errored productions (Bernthal & Bankson, 2004).

Irwin and Weston's Paired Stimuli Approach

- Developed by Irwin and Weston (1975), the PSA is based on principles of behavioral psychology and uses *operant reinforcement contingencies*. It depends on identifying a key word in which a target sound appears only once, in either initial or final position, and is produced correctly 9 out of 10 times.
- Key words are used to teach the production of sounds in other contexts. Pictures are used to evoke the target words. A single speech sound is targeted at any one time, as opposed to approaches that target multiple speech sounds simultaneously.
- In the PSA, the clinician would take the following steps at the word level:

  - select a target sound for instruction (e.g., /r/)
  - find or create four key words, two containing the target sound in the initial position and two containing it in the final position
  - select at least 10 training words in which the target sound is misarticulated and in which the sound appears only once in the same position as the key word (e.g., *rock, run, red*)
  - select pictures as stimuli to evoke the word productions
  - put the first key word (e.g., a picture of a ring) in initial position in the center and arrange the 10 training words (pictures) around it; this is known as a *training string*
  - instruct the child to say the key word, name one of the target words, and say the key word again (e.g., *ring–rock–ring*)
  - next, ask the child to name another target word; alternate the key word and all training words in this manner
  - include three training strings in each session
  - reinforce correct productions and adhere to a training criterion of 8–10 correct productions of the training words in two successive training strings without reinforcement

- Word-level training as described above would be followed by training at the sentence and conversational levels.
- The PSA is efficient because it usually builds on behaviors already in the client's repertoire and takes little time to teach the child. The child can practice the sound in a variety of phonetic contexts.

Cognitive-Linguistic Approaches

General Principles

- As previously mentioned, cognitive-linguistic approaches are sometimes used in combination with motor approaches when a child has difficulties with both the motoric and the cognitive-linguistic aspects of speech sound production.

- Cognitive-linguistic approaches assume that the child has a rule-governed system with specific patterns, but that this system differs from that of the adult system in the child's community. Thus, therapy is geared toward modifying the child's underlying rule system so that it matches the adult standard.
- The primary goal of cognitive-linguistic approaches is to establish phonological rules in a client's repertoire. Instead of focusing on individual sounds in treatment, therapy focuses on relationships among sounds (Bernthal & Bankson, 2004).
- Thus, the clinician is attempting to remediate *underlying patterns or rules* instead of discrete phonemes. For example, the clinician might treat the underlying pattern of *stridency deletion* instead of focusing on treating "omission of /s/, /f/, and /ʃ/," as one would if using a motor approach.
- The clinician selects sounds or target behaviors called *exemplars*. The assumption is that treatment of these exemplars will facilitate generalization to a whole class of sounds or other sounds in the same word position. In other words, the goal is to speed remediation through generalization of treatment results from a treated sound to untreated sounds.
- Most cognitive-linguistic treatment programs utilize *minimal pairs*, or pairs of words that differ by one feature (e.g., *shine–pine; bee–beach*). The goal is to show the child that sound production affects meaning.
- The most commonly used cognitive-linguistic approaches are the distinctive features approach (DFA), the minimal pairs contrast approach, the phonological knowledge approach (PKA), and the phonological process approach (PPA).

Distinctive Features Approach

- This goal of this approach is to establish missing distinctive features or feature contrasts by teaching relevant sounds (Lowe, 2002). The DFA assumes that teaching a feature in the context of a few sounds will result in generalized production of other sounds with the same feature or features.
- For example, a child might make the following errors: paɪn/faɪn, beɪs/veɪs, top/sop, and tʌn/sʌn. The target sounds for which the child substituted other sounds all share a common feature: stridency. Thus, the clinician might begin by teaching /f/ in hopes that the feature of stridency would generalize to /v/ and /s/ without direct training of /v/ and /s/.
- Clinicians using the DFA try to find a child's underlying patterns (e.g., problems with the feature of stridency) and train one or several sounds in that pattern in hopes that generalization to other sounds in that pattern will occur.
- In many distinctive features approaches, clinicians use minimal pairs. For example, a child might make a t/s substitution. The /t/ can be categorized as –strident, –continuant whereas the /s/ can be categorized as +strident, +continuant. The clinician might present the child with minimal pairs such as *tea-see, tap-sap,* and others to exemplify the phonemic contrast not recognized by the child (e.g., the /s/ vs. the /t/) (Bauman-Waengler, 2004).
- Early distinctive feature approaches were hybrids of phonological and articulation approaches; the distinctive features used to promote generalization were phonological, and the treatment activities were motor-based. More research is needed to fully support the DFA; currently, it is not widely used by clinicians.

Minimal Pair Contrast Approach

- In the minimal pair contrast approach, the clinician uses pairs of words that differ by only one feature—the feature the clinician is trying to help the child to conceptualize (Klein, 1996). For example, the clinician might contrast the words *see* and *tea*.

- The clinician focuses on these word pairs so that the child learns the *semantic* as well as the *motoric* differences between the phonemes. In other words, the child is taught that different sounds signal different meanings.
- As an example, the clinician might remediate the phonological process of final consonant deletion by using pictures contrasting *boat* and *bow*, *bee* and *bead*, and *tea* and *teeth*. Through use of these minimal pair contrasts, the child learns that the final consonant makes a difference in word meaning.

CONCEPTS TO CONSIDER

Although the dichotomy is artificial, many clinicians and researchers have found it useful to categorize treatment approaches into motor and cognitive-linguistic approaches. For which children might each approach be appropriate?

Phonological Knowledge Approach

- The PKA, proposed by Elbert and Geirut (1986), is an approach to treating phonological disorders in children. It looks at a child's *phonological knowledge,* or knowledge of the phonological organization and rules of his or her language.
- The PKA is based on the assumption that sound productions reflect children's knowledge of phonological rules of the adult system, and it recommends that assessment include procedures (e.g., a continuous, representative, conversational speech sample) to estimate the child's phonological knowledge.
- Those who use the PKA recommend starting treatment with the sounds that reflect the least knowledge, progressing to those reflecting greater degrees of knowledge. Thus, treatment is begun on the sounds that are most consistently misarticulated.
- Specifically, in this *least knowledge method,* treatment targets differ from the client's existing repertoire by multiple features. Thus, treatment targets should allow the child the opportunity to acquire skills needed to produce more than single sounds.
- For example, for a child who produces only /p/ and no fricatives, /z/ might be a treatment target because it teaches many new features: place of production (alveolar vs. bilabial), voicing contrast (voiced vs. voiceless), and manner of production (stop vs. fricative).
- This relatively new approach to treatment of phonological disorders is undergoing more efficacy research. The approach directly contradicts the traditional approach, and there is currently controversy in the literature about which approach is most effective (Klein & Moses, 1999).

Phonological Process Approach

General Tenets

- The PPA is based on the assumption that a child's multiple errors reflect the operation of certain phonological rules and that the problem is essentially phonemic, not phonetic.
- A child's errors are grouped and described as *phonological processes* (e.g., "Johnny manifests the use of consonant-cluster reduction and weak-syllable deletion"), not as *discrete sounds* (e.g., "Johnny makes w/r, θ/s, and w/l substitutions").
- Currently, the phonological process approach to assessment and remediation is receiving most attention in textbooks (Klein & Moses, 1999). Hodson and Paden's cycles approach (see below) is a widely used phonological process approach.

Hodson and Paden's Cycles Approach

- In this phonological pattern approach designed to treat children with multiple misarticulations and highly unintelligible speech, error patterns are targeted for remediation based on stimulability, intelligibility, and percentage of occurrence (40% or greater).
- Because they believe that phonological acquisition is a gradual process, Hodson and Paden (1991) recommend that error patterns not be drilled to a criterion of mastery (e.g., 90% accuracy). Rather, the clinician introduces correct patterns, gives the child limited practice with them, and returns to them at a later date.
- A cycle runs 5–16 weeks, and each child usually requires three–six cycles (30–40 hours at 40–60 minutes per week). Each sound in an error pattern receives 1 hour of treatment per cycle before the clinician proceeds to the next sound in the error pattern. Only one error pattern is treated in each therapy session, but all error patterns are treated in each cycle.
- Thus, for example, cycle 1 might target the phonological processes of final-consonant deletion and fronting. During treatment session one, the clinician would spend the whole hour targeting /p/ in word-final position; during session two, the whole hour would be spent targeting /t/ in word-final position; in session three, the clinician would spend the whole hour targeting /k/ (to address the process of fronting) and so forth. During cycles 2 and 3 (if the child needs three cycles), the clinician would repeat the treatment in the above-described manner.
- Each treatment session consists of the following activities (Hodson & Paden, 1991): (a) review of the previous session's target words, (b) auditory bombardment (listening to target words that are amplified), (c) activities involving new target words, (d) play break, (e) more activities involving new target words, and (f) repeating auditory bombardment and dismissal. Families are also given activities for home practice.
- Because many highly unintelligible children have phonological awareness deficits, metaphonology activities are incorporated into therapy sessions for these children. *Metaphononology* is defined as the ability to reflect on and pay attention to the phonological structure of language (Bauman-Waengler, 2004). Metaphonology activities are designed to increase skills in such areas as rhyming and syllable segmentation and blending (Hodson, Scherz, & Strattman, 2002).

Phonological Awareness Treatment

- Within recent years, the profession of speech–language pathology has begun to focus on the concept of *phonological awareness*. This term refers to the explicit awareness of the sound structure of a language, or attention to the internal structure of words (Owens, 2004).

- Phonological awareness is viewed as a subcategory of *metalinguistic awareness,* which refers to the child's ability to manipulate and think about the structure of language.

- Some researchers have begun to link limited phonological awareness skills with later problems in reading and spelling (e.g., Cassar & Treiman, 2004; Troia, 2004). It is suggested that young children with severe phonological disorders lack, among other things, phonological awareness—and that these children are at risk for reading and spelling problems later in their childhood.

- It is recommended that in early childhood, these children receive explicit training to increase their phonological awareness. It is believed that this training may prevent later problems with reading and writing (Goldsworthy, 2003; Owens, 2004).

- Treatment activities are generally designed to increase children's awareness of the sound structure of language. Thus, treatment can include a variety of activities such as sound-blending, rhyming, alliteration, and others that focus specifically on sound-structure awareness (Justice & Schuele, 2004; Kamhi & Pollock, 2005).

- More research is needed to conclusively demonstrate (a) a causal relationship between decreased phonological awareness and later reading and spelling problems and (b) the efficacy of phonological awareness treatment activities in preventing reading and spelling problems in later childhood.

Metaphon Therapy

- In the 1980s, some researchers and clinicians became dissatisfied with the use of minimal pairs in therapy for children with phonological disorders because the use of these minimal pairs was insufficient to produce the desired changes in the children's phonological systems.
- Eventually the idea of *metaphon therapy* was established. This type of therapy is based on metalinguistic awareness. Metaphon therapy is designed to enhance children's metaphonological skills (mentioned earlier).
- Metaphon therapy assumes that children's difficulties do not necessarily lie in the actual motor production of speech sounds but in the acquisition of the rules of the phonological system. Thus, clinicians operate from the premise that the best way to help children improve their rule systems is to give them information that will encourage them to make their own changes and thus sound more intelligible.
- The metaphon therapy approach is often used with preschool children who have moderate to severe phonological disorders. It focuses on feature differences between sounds to help children develop an awareness that sounds can be classified by characteristics such as place (front–back), duration (long–short), and others (Bankson & Bernthal, 2004). The therapy consists of several phases (Howell & Dean, 1994). Examples of activities are as follows.
- Children might play games in which they match long and short ribbons (to exemplify long and short sounds); they might place blocks at the front or back of a dollhouse (to exemplify front and back sounds). They might play games that describe sounds in general (e.g., noisy vs. quiet sounds); they might play a train game with an engine, middle car, and caboose to signify beginning, middle, and end sounds in a word (Bauman-Waengler, 2004).
- If the children produce sounds or words incorrectly, the clinician talks to them about why they did this. For example, the clinician might say "Here is a picture of a cat. You said 'ca–.' I heard the engine and the middle train car, but the caboose was left out. Can you say the word

again with the caboose too?" More research is needed to explore the efficacy of the metaphon therapy approach.

SUMMARY

✓ Clinicians take certain foundational steps in treating any child with an Ar-Ph disorder. Then, based upon the needs of the individual child, they may use a motor-based approach, a cognitive-linguistic approach, or a combination of those approaches in treatment.

✓ Motor-based approaches, which focus on improving the child's perceptual and motor skills, treat sounds as isolated segments (e.g., treating /l/, /r/, /s/, etc.). Commonly used motor-based approaches include Van Riper's traditional approach, McCabe and Bradley's multiple phoneme approach, Baker and Ryan's Monterey Articulation Program, McDonald's sensory-motor approach, and Irwin and Weston's paired stimuli approach.

✓ Cognitive-linguistic approaches are geared toward finding a highly unintelligible child's underlying patterns and rule system and modifying that rule system to match the adult standard. Common cognitive-linguistic approaches include the distinctive features approach, the minimal pair contrast approach, the phonological knowledge approach, and the phonological process approach.

✓ Last, some researchers and clinicians are beginning to conduct phonological awareness treatment for young children who, it is suspected, have phonological awareness deficiencies that will cause reading and spelling problems in later childhood. Metaphon therapy is also becoming more common.

ADULTS WHO SPEAK ENGLISH AS A FOREIGN LANGUAGE

INTRODUCTION

Clinicians may encounter adults who have learned English as a foreign language (EFL). EFL adults may have learned English as a second, third, fourth, or fifth language. They seek speech-language services because they perceive that their accents reduce their English intelligibilty. Many adults seek speech-language services because they desire to increase their English intelligibility for such reasons as job promotions, improved social interaction with native English speakers, and others. It is within the speech–language pathologist's purview to provide elective services to help EFL adults to increase their English intelligibility and thus enhance the quality of their lives in the United States.

Principles of Assessment

■ It is crucial that the clinician not view EFL clients generally as having a communication disorder; however, occasionally, an EFL client will have an actual communication disorder. Some experts estimate that in certain settings, approximately 25–30% of EFL clients who refer themselves for services have communication difficulties involving fluency, voice, and possible dyspraxia (Smit, 2004).

■ However, generally, EFL clients are intelligent, educated adults who choose to seek services to improve their English intelligibility. They do not have actual communication disorders. Rather, the impact of their first language or first-learned languages upon English is so great that their English intelligibility is substantially reduced. The first author has worked with adults from many countries who have shared that they perceived their limited English intelligibilty to be a barrier in vocational and social situations. These EFL clients, therefore, wished to enhance their communication in English on the job and in social situations.

■ When conducting an assessment, it is important for the clinician to understand exactly the types of English articulation errors clients will make based upon previously learned languages (see Chapter 9). Clinicians can refer to a variety of resources that describe the effects of other languages on English pronunciation (Brice, 2002; Goldstein, 2000; Goldstein & Iglesias, 2004; Roseberry-McKibbin, 2002).

■ Smit (2004, pp. 175–176) also recommends the following procedures in the assessment of an EFL client's intelligibility:

- Determine which important persons in the client's environment have difficulty understanding her English and first language (L1) skills (an employer, spouse, professor?).
- Make a high-quality recording of the client's conversational speech and transcribe the recording thoroughly. Determine the percentage of vowels correct and the percentage of consonants correct.
- Have one or two unfamiliar listeners listen to the sample, and from this determine the percent of intelligible words.
- List the client's speech-sound errors completely, using a phonemic inventory for both consonants and vowels.
- Determine the client's speaking rate.
- Assess word-level and sentence-level stress and prosody.
- Perform an oral peripheral examination.
- Carefully assess other factors that may be contributing to lack of intelligibility (e.g., very soft vocal volume, glottal fry, and others).

■ Clinicians can also use published tests to assess EFL clients. One such instrument is the *Proficiency in Oral English Communication: An Assessment of Accented Speech* (Sikorski, 1997).

Principles of Accent Training

■ Some clinicians do not use words such as *treatment* or *intervention* when referring to EFL clients because these terms imply that the client has a communication disorder. For the EFL client who has a communication difference based on first-language influence, the term *accent training* is preferable.

■ Many factors determine which parameters clinicians should target in training. Probably the most important deciding factor is selection of those parameters that contribute most to reduced intelligibility. For example, a client might have a very soft speaking volume that makes him difficult to understand. In intervention, the clinician would work on helping the client to increase his speaking volume. In another example, many EFL clients speak very quickly. Slowing down their rate of speech is often quite effective in making an immediate improvement in intelligibility.

■ Clinicians should also select consonants and vowels that the client rarely produces correctly in English and that contribute to reduced intelligibility. For example, the first author has worked with many Asian clients who do not produce /r/ correctly. Because /r/ is one of the most commonly used phonemes in English, it is an important target to work on in accent training.

■ Clinicians should use training activities and materials that are culturally sensitive and compatible with the client's interests. For example, many of the first author's clients have appreciated doing carryover activities involving reading and discussing information from the Internet about their countries of origin.

■ Many EFL clients benefit from increased exposure to English through more interactions with Americans as well as listening to American TV, radio, or both. However, this increased exposure to English is usually an adjunct to accent training; increased exposure to English alone is usually not as effective as a combination of accent training and increased English exposure.

■ It is usually ideal, in accent training, to use a multimodal approach involving visual cues (e.g., anatomical drawings), tactile cues, and auditory cues. Many clients benefit from the use of the VisiPitch (Kay Elemetrics) because they can see and hear precise feedback about their productions of various vowels and consonants. Most clients also appreciate receiving audiotapes of training targets so they can practice outside of training sessions.

SUMMARY

✓ Clinicians may encounter adults who have learned English as a foreign language (EFL). They seek speech-language services because they perceive that their accents reduce their English intelligibilty.

✓ Clinicians must conduct a thorough assessment that evaluates all parameters of intelligibility. These parameters include production of consonants and vowels, vocal volume and quality, fluency, and others. Most EFL adults have communication differences, not disorders.

✓ Some EFL adults elect to participate in accent training to improve their English intelligibility. These adults are often seeking to improve their English communication skills for vocational and social purposes. It is within the speech-language pathologist's purview to provide elective services to help EFL adults to increase their English intelligibility.

CHAPTER HIGHLIGHTS

◆ **THE TERM *ARTICULATION DISORDER*** generally refers to speech-motor-control problems, physical difficulty producing sounds. The term *phonological disorder* is usually used to describe an underlying difficulty with the phonological aspect of language knowledge displayed by a highly unintelligible child. Acknowledging that many children have a combination of motor and language knowledge difficulties, many professionals use the term *articulatory-phonological disorder.*

◆ **VARIOUS THEORIES OF PHONOLOGICAL** development have been proposed: structural, behavioral, biological, cognitive, prosodic, natural phonology, and generative phonology. These theories attempt to explain how children acquire phonological rules and the sounds of their speech communities. Most theories fall under the categories of linear and nonlinear phonology theories.

◆ **IN ORDER TO DIAGNOSE** articulatory-phonological delays in infants and children, many clinicians turn to developmental norms. Oller proposed five stages of normal infant articulatory-phonological development. Cross-sectional and longitudinal studies have yielded data about the speech sound acquisition of normally developing children. Some researchers have proposed time frames in which normally developing children use certain phonological processes for a time and then stop using those processes as they mature.

◆ **SOMETIMES CHILDREN DO NOT** develop articulatory-phonological skills normally. Such children are said to have an articulatory-phonological disorder. These disorders are generally viewed in one of two categories: *functional,* or *idiopathic* (no observable organic cause; the etiology is unknown), and *organic* (physical damage to the peripheral or central nervous system, the oral mechanism, or all of these).

◆ **SOME GENERAL FACTORS HAVE** been associated with articulatory-phonological disorders but have not been proven to be causal in nature. These factors include gender, intelligence, birth order and sibling status, socioeconomic status, language development and academic performance, and auditory discrimination skills.

◆ **ORGANICALLY BASED ARTICULATORY-PHONOLOGICAL DISORDERS** have been associated with oral structural variables such as ankyloglossia (tongue-tie), dental deviations such as malocclusions, poor oral-motor coordination skills, orofacial myofunctional disorders

CHAPTER HIGHLIGHTS

(tongue thrust), and hearing loss. Neuropathologies such as apraxia of speech and dysarthria directly cause articulatory-phonological disorders in children.

◆ **CLINICIANS ASSESS CHILDREN FOR** articulatory-phonological disorders using a general set of procedures. This includes, at a minimum, gathering a case history, conducting an orofacial examination, and conducting a hearing screening. If relevant, clinicians may also obtain information about other variables (e.g., hearing problems, dental abnormalities, mental retardation) that occur with the articulatory-phonological disorder.

◆ **WHEN CONDUCTING A FORMAL,** in-depth assessment, clinicians may use conversational speech samples, evoked speech samples, stimulability assessments, and standardized tests. The results are scored and analyzed, and then a statement of prognosis is made. Treatment goals are created.

◆ **TREATMENT OF ARTICULATORY-PHONOLOGICAL DISORDERS** can be artificially dichotomized into *motor approaches* and *cognitive-linguistic approaches*. Often a combination of the two approaches is used. Motor approaches are usually appropriate for a child with several discrete sounds in error (e.g., /s/, /r/, /θ/) who has physical difficulty producing those sounds correctly. Motor approaches, which focus generally on remediating motor difficulties and faulty perceptual abilities, include Van Riper's traditional approach, McCabe and Bradley's multiple phoneme approach, Baker and Ryan's Monterey Articulation Program, McDonald's sensory-motor approach, and Irwin and Weston's paired stimuli approach.

◆ **COGNITIVE-LINGUISTIC APPROACHES ARE GENERALLY** appropriate for highly unintelligible children who are assumed to have underlying phonological systems that differ from those of the adult speech community. Cognitive-linguistic approaches attempt to establish phonological rules in children's repertoires and treat underlying patterns or rules instead of discrete phonemes. Commonly known cognitive-linguistic approaches include the distinctive features approach, the minimal pair contrast approach, the phonological knowledge approach, and the phonological process approach (especially that of Hodson and Paden). Many children with phonological disorders profit from metaphon therapy and phonological awareness therapy.

CHAPTER HIGHLIGHTS

◆ **SOMETIMES ADULTS WHO SPEAK** English as a foreign language elect to receive accent training from speech–language pathologists to improve their English intelligibility. Usually these adults have communication differences, not disorders. Clinicians may provide elective services to these adults to help them improve their English intelligibilty for vocational, social, and personal purposes.

✎ **ADD YOUR OWN CHAPTER HIGHLIGHTS HERE:**

Study & Review Questions

Essay

1. Compare and contrast linear and nonlinear phonology theories.

2. Describe major categories of phonological processes in children. After 3 years of age, which phonological processes should children not be using?

3. What are the differences between dysarthria and developmental apraxia of speech in children? What are the ramifications of these differences for assessment and treatment?

4. Describe three specific components of a thorough assessment of a child with an Ar-Ph disorder.

5. Describe one assessment and one training concept or principle that clinicians should keep in mind when providing services for adults who refer themselves for accent training to increase their intelligibility.

Multiple Choice

6. You are working as a clinician in a private clinic. A father brings his son Johnny, age 4½ years old, for an evaluation. According to his father, Johnny is "hard to understand and sometimes the kids at preschool make fun of him." The pediatrician has told Johnny's father that Johnny will "outgrow this speech problem on his own," but the father wants to make sure that this advice is correct. Johnny will be starting kindergarten in 6 months, when he turns 5 years of age, and his father wants to be sure that Johnny speaks as intelligibly as possible so that he will not be teased in elementary school. When you evaluate Johnny, you find that he has θ/s, t/f, w/r, d/ð, and j/l substitutions. You decide to place him into therapy. You would begin therapy by addressing:

   A. θ/s substitution.
   B. t/f substitution.
   C. w/r substitution.
   D. d/ð substitution.
   E. j/l substitution.

7. In Oller's stages of infant phonological development, reduplicated babbling precedes:

   A. nonreduplicated or variegated babbling.
   B. expansion.
   C. cooing.
   D. phonation.
   E. reduplicated expansion.

8. A clinician evaluates the speech of a 5-year-old child with a phonological delay. The child is not intelligible to her kindergarten teacher or her peers, and is placed into therapy to improve her intelligibility. Assuming that this child uses the phonological process of consonant-cluster reduction, which of the following is the word you would most likely put on a word list used for treatment?

A. bus
B. stopped
C. horse

D. Lassie
E. shoes

9. The therapy technique of *phonetic placement* is used to teach or establish:

A. auditory discrimination.
B. stimulability.
C. production of a phoneme in isolation.

D. minimal pair contrasts.
E. phonological processes.

10. A speech–language pathologist's role in tongue thrust or oral myofunctional therapy may include:

A. none; SLPs do not work with those students.
B. working as a team member with a dentist, orthodontist, and physician.
C. evaluating and treating the effects of OMD on swallowing, rest postures, and speech.
D. A only
E. B and C

11. A child comes to you for an evaluation. According to her mother, Sharma has a history of middle-ear infections. Sharma's mother reports that Sharma is quite difficult to understand. For example, according to her mother, Sharma says things like gʌk/dʌk and koʊ/toʊ. This child is manifesting the phonological process of:

A. fronting.
B. stridency deletion.
C. backing.

D. glottal replacement.
E. progressive assimilation.

12. The articulation therapy approach that emphasizes the syllable as the basic unit of speech production and heavily utilizes the concept of phonetic environment is:

A. McDonald's sensory-motor approach.
B. Irwin and Weston's paired stimuli approach.
C. Baker and Ryan's Monterey Articulation Program.
D. Van Riper's traditional approach.
E. McCabe and Bradley's multiple phoneme approach.

13. A child is referred to you by his preschool teacher. This child, Damien, is 4 years 3 months old and has transferred from out of state. In his previous state, Damien was reportedly assessed by a speech–language pathologist who recommended that Damien receive intervention before kindergarten. According to the report from the previous clinician, Damien uses the phonological processes of gliding, consonant cluster reduction, stopping, reduplication, and final consonant deletion. Your assessment confirms the presence of these phonological processes. You would begin treatment by addressing:

A. final-consonant deletion.
B. gliding.
C. consonant-cluster reduction.

D. reduplication.
E. stopping.

14. Which one of the following is FALSE regarding dental deviations?

A. *Skeletal malocclusion* refers to deviations in the shape and dimensions of the mandible and maxilla.
B. *Dental malocclusion* refers to deviations in the positioning of individual teeth.
C. In *class I malocclusion,* the arches themselves are generally aligned properly; however, some individual teeth are misaligned.
D. In *class II malocclusion,* the maxilla is receded and the mandible is protruded.
E. *Overjet* occurs when a child has a Class II malocclusion and the upper teeth from the molars forward are positioned excessively anterior to the lower teeth.

15. Which of the following is/are TRUE with regard to treatment of articulatory-phonological disorders?

A. The *distinctive features approach* is used to find a child's underlying patterns (e.g., problems with the feature of nasality) and train one or several sounds in that pattern in hopes that generalization to other sounds in that pattern will occur.
B. *Hodson and Paden's cycles approach* involves treating children with phonological disorders in cycles in which the child is trained to a criterion of mastery for error patterns such as final-consonant deletion and fronting.
C. In *Elbert and Geirut's phonological knowledge approach,* the *least knowledge method* trains treatment targets that contain many new features that the child is missing.
D. A, B, C
E. A, C

Questions 16–18 *refer to the following scenario:*

A 5-year-old child, Crystal S., is brought to you for an evaluation of her speech. The family speaks only English in the home. According to Crystal's mother, Crystal "loves to talk but most people have trouble understanding her." As you play with Crystal informally, you estimate that she is approximately 50–60% intelligible. You conduct an oral peripheral evaluation, which reveals that Crystal does not have any anatomical or physiological anomalies that would explain why she is so unintelligible. You also conduct in-depth assessment in other areas to determine the nature of Crystal's unintelligibility and to determine therapy goals.

16. You discover through your assessment that there are some sounds that Crystal consistently misarticulates. For example, she usually makes a t/k substitution (e.g., *tea/key*). You want to know if Crystal can produce /k/ in isolation. You show her how to produce /k/ by giving her a model and tell her "watch me make the /k/ sound. Then you do it just like I did." When you are doing this, you are assessing Crystal's:

A. phonological knowledge.
B. receptive phonology skills.
C. overall intelligibilty.
D. stimulability.
E. diadochokinetic skills.

17. You find that Crystal uses a number of phonological processes. One of those processes is stopping. You know this when you hear Crystal make such substitutions as:

A. bae/bath
B. tu/shoe
C. ruz/rush
D. nake/snake
E. tuhree/three

18. You decide that for therapy, you would like to use the distinctive features approach to help Crystal become more intelligible. In this approach, you would:

A. use minimal pairs.
B. try to find Crystal's underlying patterns and train one or several sounds in those patterns in hopes that generalization to other sounds in that pattern would occur.
C. use auditory bombardment as a key component of each therapy session.
D. A, B
E. B, C

19. You are approached by Dr. Kim Lee, a 34-year-old university assistant professor from Korea. Dr. Lee has been in the United States for six years; she received her Ph.D. in chemistry in the United States. Dr. Lee now teaches undergraduate and graduate classes in chemistry at a local university. Dr. Lee reports that she usually gets good student evaluations; however, many students report that they have trouble understanding her speech. Dr. Lee states that "I feel frustrated because I know my accent is getting in the way of my teaching." Dr. Lee has no history of dyspraxia, voice problems, or other communication disorders in Korean or English. The best thing for you to do in this case is to:

A. give Dr. Lee standardized language and articulation tests in English because it is clear that Dr. Lee has a communication disorder that needs to be remediated, and these tests will spotlight Dr. Lee's weaknesses.
B. tell Dr. Lee that her accent makes her special, and that no accent training is necessary because Dr. Lee's accent is "a unique and beautiful part of who you are."
C. tell Dr. Lee that you will assess her English intelligibility using an accent assessment instrument as well as analysis of a conversational sample; if she would like to participate in elective accent training to become more intelligible, such training is available to her.
D. tell Dr. Lee to listen daily to more English TV and radio, and come back in 6 months if her student evaluations have not improved.
E. tell Dr. Lee that she has a communication disorder in both Korean and English, and that she will need intensive therapy to remediate this disorder.

20. A 3-year-old child is receiving therapy for remediation of several phonological processes. The child has difficulty acquiring the rules of the phonological system, and the clinician decides to help the child pay attention to the phonological structure of language as well as help the child develop awareness that sounds can be classified by characteristics such as place (front–back), duration (long–short), and others. To achieve this goal, the clinician will most likely use:

A. Hodson's cycles approach.
B. McDonald's approach.
C. metaphon therapy.
D. the distinctive feature approach.
E. Van Riper's traditional approach to therapy.

REFERENCES AND RECOMMENDED READINGS

American Speech-Language-Hearing Association. (1996). Orofacial myofunctional disorders. *Asha, 38*(2), 46–47.

Arlt, P. B., & Goodban, M. J. (1976). A comparative study of articulation acquisition as based on a study of 240 normals, age three to six. *Language, Speech, and Hearing Services in Schools, 7,* 173–180.

Baker, R. D., & Ryan, B. P. (1971). *Programmed conditioning for articulation.* Monterey, CA: Monterey Learning Systems.

Ball, M. J., & Kent, R. D. (1997). *The new phonologies: Developments in clinical linguistics.* San Diego, CA: Singular/ Del Mar Publishing.

Bankson, N. W., & Bernthal, J. E. (2004). Treatment approaches. In J. E. Bernthal & N. W. Bankson, *Articulation and phonological disorders* (5th ed., pp. 292–347). Boston: Allyn & Bacon.

Bauman-Waengler, J. (2004). *Articulatory and phonological impairments: A clinical focus* (2nd ed.). Boston: Allyn & Bacon.

Bernhardt, B., & Stemberger, J. P. (2000). *Workbook in nonlinear phonology for clinical application.* Austin, TX: PRO-ED.

Bernthal, J. E., & Bankson, N. W. (Eds.). (1994). *Child phonology: Characteristics, assessment, and intervention with special populations.* New York: Thieme Medical Publishers.

Bernthal, J., & Bankson, N. (2004). *Articulation and phonological disorders* (5th ed.). Boston: Allyn & Bacon.

Bleile, K. M. (2002). Evaluating articulation and phonological disorders when the clock is running. *American Journal of Speech–Language Pathology, 11,* 243–249.

Bleile, K. M. (2004). *Manual of articulation and phonological disorders: Infancy through adulthood* (2nd ed.) (Clinical Competence Series). San Diego, CA: Singular/DelMar Publishing Group.

Brice, A. E. (2002). *The Hispanic child: Speech, language, culture and education.* Boston: Allyn & Bacon.

Caruso, A. J. (1999). *Clinical management of motor speech disorders in children.* New York: Thieme Medical Publishers.

Cassar, M., & Treiman, R. (2004). Developmental variations in spelling: Comparing typical and poor spellers. In C. A. Stone, E. R. Silliman, B. J. Ehren, & K. Apel (Eds.), *Handbook of language and literacy: Development and disorders* (pp. 627–643). New York: The Guilford Press.

Chomsky, N., & Halle, M. (1968). *The sound pattern of English.* New York: Harper & Row.

Clarke-Klein, S., & Hodson, B. W. (1995). A phonologically based analysis of misspellings by third graders with disordered-phonology histories. *Journal of Speech and Hearing Research, 38,* 839–849.

Creaghead, N. A. (1989). Development of phonology, articulation, and speech perception. In N. A. Creaghead, P. W. Newman, & W. A. Secord, (Eds.), *Assessment and remediation of articulatory and phonological disorders* (pp. 35–68). Columbus, OH: Merrill Publishing Company.

Elbert, M., & Geirut, J. (1986). *Handbook of clinical phonology: Approaches to assessment and treatment.* San Diego, CA: College-Hill Press.

Ferguson, C. A. (1978). Learning to pronounce: The earliest stages of phonological development in the child. In F. D. Minifie & L. L. Lloyd (Eds.), *Communicative and cognitive abilities—Early behavioral assessment.* Baltimore: University Park Press.

Ferguson, C. A. (1986). Discovering sound units and constructing sound systems: It's child's play. In J. S. Perkell & D. H. Klatt (Eds.), *Invariance and variability of speech processes.* Hillsdale, NJ: Lawrence Erlbaum.

Fey, M. E., Catts, H. W., & Larrivee, L. S. (1995). Preparing preschoolers for the academic and social challenges of school. In M. E. Fey, J. Windsor, & S. F. Warren (Eds.), *Language intervention: Preschool through the elementary years* (Vol. 5, pp. 3–38). Baltimore: Paul H. Brookes.

Flynn, M. C., Dowell, R. C., & Clark, G. M. (1998). Aided speech recognition abilities of adults with a severe or severe-to-profound hearing loss. *Journal of Speech, Language, and Hearing Research, 41*(2), 285–299.

Forrest, K. (2002). Are oral-motor exercises useful in the treatment of phonological/articulatory disorders? *Seminars in Speech and Language, 23,* 15-25.

Goldstein, B. (2000). *Cultural and linguistic diversity resource guide for speech–language pathologists.* San Diego, CA: Singular/Thomson Learning.

Goldstein, B., & Iglesias, A. (2004). Language and dialectal variations. In J. E. Bernthal & N. W. Bankson, *Articulation and phonological disorders* (5th ed., pp. 348–374). Boston: Allyn & Bacon.

Goldsworthy, C. L. (2003). *Developmental reading disabilities: A language-based treatment approach* (2nd ed.). San Diego, CA: Singular/Del Mar Publishing Group.

Hall, P. K., Jordan, L. S., & Robin, D. A. (1993). Developmental apraxia of speech. Austin, TX: PRO-ED.

Haynes, W. O., & Pindzola, R. H. (2004). *Diagnosis and evaluation in speech pathology* (6th ed.). Boston: Allyn & Bacon.

Helfer, K. S. (1998). In C. M. Seymour & E. H. Nober (Eds.), *Introduction to communication disorders: A multicultural approach* (pp. 277–305). Newton, MA: Butterworth-Heinemann.

Hillis, A. E., & Bahr, D. C. (2001). Neurological and anatomical bases. In D. C. Bahr (Ed.), *Oral motor assessment and treatment: Ages and stages* (pp. 1–41). Boston: Allyn & Bacon.

Hodson, B. W., & Paden, E. P. (1991). *Targeting intelligible speech: A phonological approach to remediation* (2nd ed.). Austin, TX: PRO-ED.

Hodson, B. W., Scherz, J. A., & Strattman, K. H. (2002). Evaluating communicative abilities of a highly unintelligible preschooler. *American Journal of Speech–Language Pathology, 11,* 236-242.

Hoffman, P. R., & Norris, J. A. (2002). Phonological assessment as an integral part of language assessment. *American Journal of Speech–Language Pathology, 11,* 230–235.

Howell, J., & Dean, E. (1994). *Treating phonological disorders in children: Metaphon-theory to practice* (2nd ed.). London: Whurr.

Ingram, K., & Ingram, D. (2002). Commentary on "Evaluating articulation and phonological disorders when the clock is running." *American Journal of Speech–Language Pathology, 11,* 257–258.

Irwin, J. V., & Weston, A. J. (1975). The paired-stimuli monograph. *Acta Symbolica, 6,* 1–76.

Jakobson, R. (A. R. Keiler, Trans.). (1968). *Child language, aphasia, and phonological universals.* The Hague: Mouton.

Justice, L. M., & Schuele, C. M. (2004). Phonological awareness: Description, assessment, and intervention. In J. E. Bernthal & N. W. Bankson, *Articulation and phonological disorders* (5th ed., pp. 376–405). Boston: Allyn & Bacon.

Kamhi, A. G., & Pollock, K. E. (2005). *Phonological disorders in children: Clinical decision making in assessment and intervention.* Baltimore: Brookes Publishing Co.

Kellum, G. (1994). Overview of orofacial myology. In M. M. Ferketic & K. Gardner (Eds.), *Orofacial myology: Beyond tongue thrust.* Rockville Pike, MD: American Speech-Language-Hearing Association.

Kent, R. (2004). Normal aspects of articulation. In J. E. Bernthal & N. W. Bankson, *Articulation and phonological disorders* (5th ed., pp 1–62). Boston: Allyn & Bacon.

Klein, D., & Briggs, M. (1986). *Observation of communicative interaction,* (DHS Publication No. MCJ06351-01-0). Washington, DC: U.S. Government Printing Office.

Klein, E. S. (1996). *Clinical phonology: Assessment and treatment of articulation disorders in children and adults.* San Diego, CA: Singular Publishing Group.

Klein, H. B., & Moses, N. (1999). *Intervention planning for children with communication disorders: A guide for clinical practicum and professional practice* (2nd ed.). Needham Heights, MA: Allyn & Bacon.

Lewis, B. A., Freebairn, L. A., Hansen, A. J., Iyengar, S. K., & Taylor, H. G. (2004). School-age follow-up of children with childhood apraxia of speech. *Language, Speech, and Hearing Services in Schools, 35,* 122–140.

Locke, J. L. (1983). Phonological acquisition and change. New York: Academic Press.

Locke, J. L. (1990). Structure and stimulation in the ontogeny of spoken language. *Developmental Psychobiology, 23,* 621–643.

Lof, G. L. (2002). Two comments on this assessment series. *American Journal of Speech–Language Pathology, 11,* 255–256.

Lowe, R. J. (1994). *Phonology: Assessment and intervention applications in speech pathology.* Baltimore: Williams & Wilkins.

Lowe, R. J. (2002). *Workbook for the identification of phonological processes and distinctive features* (3rd ed.). Austin, TX: PRO-ED.

Lowe, R. J., & Weitz, J. M. (1994). Intervention. In R. J. Lowe (Ed.), *Phonology: Assessment and intervention applications in speech pathology* (pp. 175–206). Baltimore: Williams & Wilkins.

Macken, M. A., & Ferguson, C. A. (1983). Cognitive aspects of phonological development: Model, evidence and issues. In K. E. Nelson (Ed.), *Children's language* (Vol. 4). Hillsdale, NJ: Lawrence Erlbaum.

Marquardt, T. P., Sussman, H. M., Snow, T., & Jacks, A. (2002). The integrity of the syllable in developmental apraxia of speech. *Journal of Communication Disorders, 35,* 31–49.

McCabe, R., & Bradley, D. (1975). Systematic multiple phonemic approach to articulation therapy. *Acta Symbolica, 6,* 1–18.

McDonald, E. T. (1964). *Articulation testing and treatment: A sensory motor approach.* Pittsburgh, PA: Stanwix House.

Menn, L. (1983). Development of articulatory, phonetic, and phonological capabilities. In B. Butterworth (Ed.), *Language production* (Vol. 2). London: Academic Press.

Moller, K. T. (1994). Dental-occlusal and other oral conditions and speech. In J. E. Bernthal & N. W. Bankson (Eds.), *Child phonology: Characteristics, assessment, and intervention with special populations* (pp. 3–23). New York: Thieme Medical Publishers.

Mowrer, O. (1960). *Learning theory and symbolic processes.* New York: John Wiley.

Oller, D. K. (1980). The emergence of the sounds of speech in infancy. In G. Yeni-Komshian, J. Kavanagh, & C. A. Ferguson (Eds.), *Child phonology: Vol. 1, Production.* New York: Academic Press.

Olmsted, D. (1971). *Out of the mouth of babes.* The Hague: Mouton.

Owens, R.E. (2004). *Language disorders: A functional approach to assessment and intervention* (4th ed.). Boston: Allyn & Bacon.

Parker, F. (1994). Phonological theory. In R. J. Lowe (Ed.), *Phonology: Assessment and intervention applications in speech pathology* (pp. 17–34). Baltimore: Williams & Wilkins.

Peña-Brooks, A., & Hegde, M. N. (2000). *Articulatory and phonological disorders in children: A dual level text.* Austin, TX: PRO-ED.

Poole, E. (1934). Genetic development of articulation of consonant sounds in speech. *Elementary English Review, 11,* 159–161.

Prather, E. M., Hedrick, D. L., & Kern, C. (1975). Articulation development in children aged two to four years. *Journal of Speech and Hearing Disorders, 40,* 179–191.

Ray, J. (2002). Treating phonological disorders in a multilingual child: A case study. *American Journal of Speech–Language Pathology, 11,* 305–315.

Reed, V. A., & Baker, E. (2005). Normal language development: A review. In V. A. Reed, *An introduction to children with language disorders* (3rd ed., pp. 43–74). Boston: Allyn & Bacon.

Roseberry-McKibbin, C. (2002). *Multicultural students with special language needs: Practical strategies for assessment and intervention* (2nd ed.). Oceanside, CA: Academic Communication Associates.

Sander, E. (1972). When are speech sounds learned? *Journal of Speech and Hearing Disorders, 37,* 55–63.

Sikorski, L. D. (1997). *Proficiency in Oral English Communication: An Assessment of Accented Speech.* Santa Ana, CA: LDS & Associates, LLC

Smit, A. B. (2004). *Articulation and phonology resource guide for school-age children and adults.* Clifton Park, NY: Delmar/Thomson Learning.

Smith, N. V. (1973). *The acquisition of phonology: A case study.* Cambridge, England: Cambridge University Press.

Stampe, D. (1969). *The acquisition of phoneme representation.* Paper presented at the Fifth Regional Meeting of the Chicago Linguistic Society, Chicago, IL.

Stoel-Gammon, C., & Dunn, C. (1985). *Normal and disordered phonology in children.* Austin, TX: PRO-ED.

Swank, L. K., & Catts, H. W. (1994). *Phonological awareness and written word decoding. Language, Speech, and Hearing Services in Schools, 25,* 9–14.

Templin, M. (1957). *Certain language skills in children: Their development and interrelationships* (Institute of Child Welfare, Monograph 26). Minneapolis: University of Minnesota Press.

Troia, G. A. (2004). Phonological processing and its influence on literacy learning. In C. Stone, E. R. Silliman, B. J. Ehren, & K. Apel (Eds.), *Handbook of language and literacy: Development and disorders* (pp. 267–270). New York: The Guilford Press.

Tyler, A. A., Lewis, K. E., Haskill, A., & Tolbert, L. C. (2002). Efficacy and cross-domain effects of a morphosyntax and a phonology intervention. *Language, Speech, and Hearing Services in Schools, 33,* 52–66.

Tyler, A. A., & Tolbert, L. C. (2002). Speech-language assessment in the clinical setting. *American Journal of Speech-Language Pathology, 11,* 215–220.

Van Riper, C. (1978). *Speech correction: Principles and methods* (6th ed.). Englewood Cliffs, NJ: Prentice-Hall.

Vihman, M. M. (2004). Early phonological development. In J. E. Bernthal & N. W. Bankson (Eds.), *Articulation and phonological disorders* (4th ed., pp. 63–112). Boston: Allyn & Bacon.

Waterson, N. (1971). Child phonology: A prosodic view. *Journal of Linguistics, 7,* 179–211.

Waterson, N. (1981). A tentative developmental model of phonological representation. In T. Myers, J. Laver, & J. Anderson (Eds.), *The cognitive representation of speech.* Amsterdam: North-Holland.

Wellman, B. L., Case, I. M., Mengert, E. G., & Bradbury, D. E. (1931). *Speech sounds of young children* (University of Iowa Studies in Child Welfare). Iowa City: University of Iowa.

Williams, A. A. (2002). Epilogue: perspectives in the assessment of children's speech. *American Journal of Speech–Language Pathology, 11,* 259–263.

Yavas, M. (1998). *Phonology development and disorders.* San Diego, CA: Singular Publishing Group.

Study & Review
Answers

6. B. The /f/ sound is developed earlier than the /s/, /r/, /θ/, and /l/ sounds, thus beginning therapy by addressing /f/ would be the best approach.

7. A. In Oller's stages of infant phonological development, reduplicated babbling precedes nonreduplicated or variegated babbling.

8. B. *Stopped* is the only word in the list that contains a consonant cluster.

9. C. Phonetic placement is used when a client cannot imitate the modeled production of a phoneme such as /s/ or /r/. The clinician uses a combination of verbal instructions and physical guidance to show the client how target sounds are produced.

10. E. ASHA (1996) has stated that this therapy is appropriate for and within the purview of speech–language pathologists, who assess and treat the effects of OMD on swallowing, rest postures, and speech. Speech–language pathologists traditionally work on a team also composed of a dentist, orthodontist, and physician.

11. C. A child who says things like gʌk/dʌk and koʊ/toʊ is manifesting the phonological process of backing.

12. A. The articulation therapy approach that emphasizes the syllable as the basic unit of speech production and heavily utilizes the concept of phonetic environment is McDonald's sensory-motor approach.

13. D. Reduplication is the earliest of the listed phonological processes to be phased out. In normally developing children, reduplication is usually phased out by approximately 2 years 4 months of age.

14. D. The maxilla is receded and the mandible protruded in class III malocclusion. In class II malocclusion, the maxilla is protruded and the mandible receded.

15. E. In Hodson and Paden's cycles approach, children are *not* trained to a criterion of mastery for error patterns. Rather, the clinician introduces correct patterns, gives the child limited practice with production of those patterns, and moves on to other error patterns.

16. D. You are assessing Crystal's stimulability for the /k/ sound by evaluating whether or not she can imitate your model.

17. B. If Crystal says tu/shoe, she is demonstrating the phonological process of stopping.

18. D. If you use the distinctive feature approach, you would use minimal pairs and also try to find Crystal's underlying patterns and train one or several sounds in those patterns in hopes that generalization to other sounds in that pattern would occur.

19. C. Tell Dr. Lee that you will assess her English intelligibility using an accent assessment instrument as well as analysis of a conversational sample; if she would like to participate in elective accent training to become more intelligible, such training is available to her. It is highly unlikely that Dr. Lee has a communication disorder.

20. C. Metaphon therapy is designed to enhance children's metaphonological skills. The metaphon therapy approach is often used with preschool children who have moderate to severe phonological disorders. Metaphon therapy focuses on feature differences between sounds to help children develop an awareness that sounds can be classified by characteristics such as place (front–back), duration (long–short), and others.

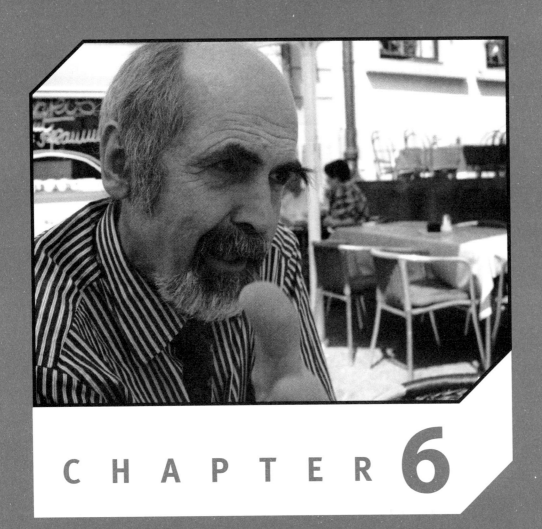

CHAPTER 6

FLUENCY AND

ITS DISORDERS

Disorders of fluency are speech disorders.

There are two main varieties of fluency disorders: stuttering and cluttering. Fluency may be impaired in such clinical conditions as aphasia, although a diagnosis of stuttering or cluttering may not be made in such cases. Fluency problems associated with aphasia are described in Chapter 8. In this chapter, research and clinical information on stuttering and cluttering are reviewed (Bloodstein, 1995; Conture, 2001; Culatta & Goldberg 1995; Curlee, 1999; Guitar, 1998; Myers & St. Louis, 1992; Onslow, Packman, & Harrison, 2001; Shapiro, 1999; Silverman, 2004; Van Riper, 1973, 1982).

FLUENCY AND STUTTERING: AN OVERVIEW

INTRODUCTION

Fluent speech is smooth, relatively easy, and flowing. Nonfluent or stuttered speech is effortful and defined according to various criteria. Various forms of dysfluencies make up the core behaviors of stuttering. Familial factors, gender, and ethnocultural variables affect the incidence and prevalence of stuttering. Stuttering onset can be more or less gradual but typically takes place in early childhood. Eventually, stuttering is associated with various types of abnormal motor behaviors (some describe them as *secondary behaviors* or *secondary stutterings*), muscular tension, breathing abnormalities, negative emotions, and avoidance behaviors. The loci of stuttering, or locations in the speech sequence where stutterings are typically observed, can often be predicted. Stuttering frequently varies when certain variables are manipulated, creating phenomena such as adaptation, consistency, and adjacency. Theories of stuttering have been built on environmental, genetic, and neurophysiological observations; none is universally accepted, although each line of investigation has contributed to a more comprehensive understanding of stuttering. Many treatment procedures are advocated for adults and children who stutter, but only a few are based on research evidence.

Definition and Description of Fluency

■ Fluency has not been studied as extensively as stuttering. For the most part, some rudimentary characteristics of fluency have been described. For example, fluent speech is:

- produced with relative ease (less effort and tension)
- flowing
- smooth
- continuous
- relatively rapid
- normally rhythmic
- free from an excessive amount or duration of dysfluencies

■ Characteristics of fluency contrast with those of stuttering. Stuttered speech is produced with greater than the normal amount of effort; it is halting, and thus does not flow. Perhaps for the same reason, it is discontinuous; it is not smooth, and it may be slow because of all the dysfluencies. The rhythm of stuttered speech may be abnormal because of the various kinds of dysfluencies (Bloodstein, 1995; Starkweather & Givens-Ackerman, 1997).

Definition and Description of Stuttering

General Principles

- It is generally agreed that stuttering is a *disorder of fluency*—it is the most researched of the fluency disorders—and historically, it has also been defined as a *disorder of rhythm*.
- Although it is agreed that stuttering is a disorder of fluency and rhythm, clinicians have further defined it in a variety of different ways. Much of this variation is due to theoretical orientation, not clinical approach. A few sample definitions illustrate the variety.

Definition in Terms of Non-Speech Behaviors

- Historically, some experts have defined stuttering in terms of variables that are not specific to speech characteristics. The following three definitions emphasize various personal and social consequences of dysfluent speech.
- First, stuttering is defined as an anticipatory, apprehensive, hypertonic, avoidance reaction. According to Johnson and Associates (1959), who offered this definition, stuttering is not the same as dysfluency. Stuttering begins when a child learns to avoid speech, speaking situations, and certain kinds of audiences. It consists of anticipating trouble in speaking situations, becoming apprehensive about the prospect of speaking, experiencing tension, and, finally, avoiding the speaking situation. According to this definition, a diagnosis of stuttering is not made on the basis of dysfluencies. Instead, it is based on the theory that avoidance is a result of parental disapproval or punishment of normal dysfluencies. The child seeks to avoid the parental disapproval of normal nonfluencies.
- Second, stuttering is defined as what a person does to avoid stuttering. This is an alternative definition offered by Johnson (1959), but it is consistent with the view that stuttering is essentially an attempt to avoid the negative consequences of normal nonfluencies.
- Third, stuttering is defined as a social role conflict. Sheehan (1970), who offered this definition, believed that the primary problem of stuttering is a social role conflict. The person who stutters cannot play certain social roles normally. For example, stuttering people typically speak with improved fluency when they talk to young children and pets and when they play theatrical roles. However, the same people may have difficulty talking to their bosses, ordering in restaurants, and speaking to strangers. To Sheehan, this indicated a problem in efficiently playing different social roles.

Definition in Terms of Unspecified Behaviors

- Some definitions do not specify any behaviors. They simply refer to stuttering in some molar or global terms. The central notion in these definitions is an expert judgment. In essence, an expert's judgment that stuttering has occurred is the definition of stuttering.
- For example, in one view, stuttering is defined as a *moment;* the moment of stuttering is what an expert observes in a time duration. This definition emphasizes a time duration during which something believed to be stuttering has occurred; it does not specify the behavior that is observed. Although it is widely used, this definition does not specify what stuttering is and thus does not help measure the behavior objectively.
- Another view defines stuttering as an *event:* stuttering is an event so recognized by an expert. This definition, also widely used, does not specify the behavior or action that constitutes stuttering. It is similar to the notion of a *stuttering moment* in that it is both nonspecific and not helpful in objective measurement.

Definition Limited to Certain Types of Dysfluencies

- There are many types of dysfluencies, and they play a major role in the varied definitions of stuttering and its diagnostic criteria. However, in some definitions, only certain types of dysfluencies are included. In other words, some forms of dysfluencies are of clinical significance, whereas others are considered a part of normal speech.
- Some classic definitions of stuttering have limited the term to part-word repetitions and speech-sound prolongations. All other forms of dysfluencies (e.g., word repetitions, interjections, pauses) are thought be normal kinds of nonfluencies.
- According to Van Riper, "stuttering occurs when the forward flow of speech is interrupted by a motorically disrupted sound, syllable, or word or by the speaker's reactions thereto" (1982, p. 15). This definition restricts stuttering to sound, syllable, or word repetitions and sound prolongations. An important aspect of the definition is its emphasis on speaker reactions.

Definition Based on Psychopathology (Neurosis)

- Psychoanalysts and psychologists believe that stuttering may be due to some kind of psychopathology or that it may be a neurotic reaction. Such psychological reactions as anxiety, frustration in self-expression, and apprehension about speaking situations or speaking certain kinds of words are all self-reported by many adults who stutter. These and other psychological reactions are the basis for definitions based on psychopathology or neurosis.
- Stuttering is a form of neurosis because it is based on some form of psychopathology. Freudian psychoanalysts believe that such psychological processes as fixation at an earlier stage of psychosexual development, frustration later in life, regression to the fixated stage of development, and subsequent symptom formation (conversion) explain stuttering.
- Psychologists who hold the view that stuttering is a form of neurosis need not believe in the Freudian fixation-regression-symptom formation model, however. Some may believe that stuttering is a form of learned neurotic reaction.

Definition Based on All Types of Dysfluencies

- Many experts tend to describe stuttering in terms of the frequency and duration of dysfluencies. Such experts tend to include all types of dysfluencies in their definitions or descriptions of stuttering. According to this view, all forms of dysfluencies disrupt fluency and create a fluency disorder if their frequencies or durations are excessive. The basis for this view is that

CONCEPTS TO CONSIDER

How is stuttering defined? Describe at least three definitions.

_____

_____

_____

_____

_____

listeners tend to classify as dysfluent or stuttered speech that contains only word repetitions or interjections at high frequencies (Bloodstein, 1995; Hegde & Hartman, 1979a, 1979b).

- Accordingly, stuttering is the production of dysfluencies of excessive frequency, excessive durations, or both. In this definition, stuttering includes all varieties of dysfluencies when they are excessive in frequency, duration, or both. In a later section of this chapter, different varieties of dysfluencies are described with examples. It is important to note that both excessive frequency and excessive duration of dysfluencies may be grounds for a diagnosis of stuttering.

Definition Based on Etiology

- Most definitions are descriptions of what constitutes stuttering. Very few include a hypothesized cause.
- One such definition says that stuttering is that class of fluency failure that is a result of classically conditioned negative emotion; only part-word repetitions and sound prolongations fall into this category; all other forms of dysfluencies are not stutterings but are operantly conditioned (Brutten & Shoemaker, 1967). In this definition, two types of etiology are hypothesized for two classes of dysfluencies. Part-word repetitions and speech-sound prolongations are said to fall into one category and all other forms into another. Repetitions and prolongations are hypothesized to be a result of negative emotion; their basis is negative emotion, which in turn is based on Pavlovian, or classical conditioning.
- All other forms of dysfluencies (including whole-word repetitions, interjections, pauses, etc.), according to this definition, are due to Skinnerian, or operant conditioning. Stuttering is diagnosed only on the basis of part-word repetitions and speech-sound prolongations that are due to classically conditioned negative emotion.
- Another definition incorporates the _cerebral dominance theory_. According to this theory, persons who stutter (as a group) are less likely than their fluent peers to have developed unilateral cerebral dominance; they are often ambidextrous. Thus, these people stutter because of their lack of unilateral cerebral dominance (Silverman, 2004). Today, there is little interest in this theory.

Forms of Dysfluencies

■ Regardless of definitional orientations, it is important to understand the different forms of dysfluencies, as they all interrupt fluency. The following are the major types of dysfluencies and their examples:

- *Repetitions.* Saying the same element of speech more than once.

  — *Part-word repetitions* (sound or syllable repetitions): Repetition of a part of a word or a sound or syllable (e.g., "S-S-S-Saturday" or "Sa-Sa-Sa-Saturday").
  — *Whole-word repetitions:* Repetition of an entire word more than once; word repeated may be of single or multiple syllables (e.g., "I-I-I am fine" or "could-could-could not do it").
  — *Phrase repetitions:* Repetition of more than one word (e.g., "I am–I am–I am fine" or "could not–could not–could not do it").

- *Sound prolongations.* Sounds produced for a duration longer than typical (e.g., "lllllike it" or "Mmmmommy").
- *Silent prolongations.* An articulatory posture held for a duration longer than average but with no vocalization (e.g., the articulatory position for producing the *p* sound in the word *pot* may be held too long; such postures are usually associated with increased muscular tension).
- *Interjections.* Extraneous elements introduced into the speech sequence. These may be one of the following:

  — sound or syllable interjections (e.g., the common *um* and the schwa interjections)
  — word interjections (e.g., interjections of *like, okay, well*)
  — phrase interjections (e.g., interjections of *you know, I mean*)

- *Pauses.* Silent intervals in the speech sequence at inappropriate junctures or of unusually long duration.
- *Broken words.* Silent intervals within words, also known as *intralexical pauses* (e.g., "Be [pause] fore you say it").
- *Incomplete sentences.* Often described as incomplete phrases, these are grammatically incomplete productions (e.g., "Last summer I was . . . last summer . . . we went to Paris this time").
- *Revisions.* Changes in wording that do not change the overall meaning of an utterance (e.g., "Let me have coffee, maybe tea").

Theoretical and Clinical Significance of Dysfluencies

■ As the different definitions of stuttering make evident, not all experts agree on how to evaluate various forms of dysfluencies. Some think that only certain forms of dysfluencies are stutterings; others think that all forms of dysfluencies, if they exceed certain quantitative limits of duration and frequency, are stutterings (or at least disorders of fluency even if not diagnosed as stuttering).

- There is evidence that forms of dysfluency that are traditionally not considered indicative of stuttering (e.g., whole-word repetitions or schwa interjections) may still evoke judgments of stuttering from listeners if the frequency exceeds certain limits (Hegde & Hartman, 1979a, 1979b).

- Generally, speech that contains 5% or more dysfluencies may be judged dysfluent or stuttered by most listeners. Bloodstein (1995), among others, has advocated that dysfluencies found in normally fluent speech, if they exceed certain limits, are grounds for diagnosing stuttering.

- Research also has shown that listeners may have different tolerance thresholds for different forms of dysfluencies. Part-word repetitions (e.g., "buh-buh-baby") and sound prolongations are judged abnormal at lower frequencies (as low as 2% of words spoken), whereas whole-word repetitions and schwa interjections must reach at least 5% to evoke judgments of dysfluent or stuttered speech.

- Thus, all forms of dysfluencies that exceed certain limits of frequency or duration may be judged abnormal, but some forms are judged abnormal at lower levels of frequency or duration.

Incidence and Prevalence of Stuttering

General Principles

- The *incidence* of a given disorder or disease is its rate of occurrence in a specified group of people. Incidence is studied by a longitudinal method. An incidence study starts with a healthy or normal group of subjects and repeatedly observes those individuals over a period of time, counting the number who begin to show a particular disease or disorder. Incidence is a predictive statement. Incidence studies are more expensive and time consuming than prevalence studies.
- *Prevalence* of a particular disorder or disease is determined by counting the number of individuals who currently have it. Thus, prevalence involves a head count. To establish the prevalence of a disorder, investigators use a cross-sectional method of study. A prevalence study starts with clinical records of individuals who already exhibit a disorder. The study's investigators collect information from various sources (e.g., clinics and hospitals) and add up the number of patients who are receiving clinical services or have received such services. Prevalence does not make a predictive statement; it simply gives the current number of people who exhibit a given disorder. Prevalence studies are less expensive and less time consuming than incidence studies. However, head counting often underestimates the prevalence of a disorder by missing those who have not received clinical services.
- Most available studies of stuttering are prevalence studies; most are rough estimates. There are only a few studies of the incidence of stuttering. However, incidence and prevalence can be derived from each other.

Incidence and Prevalence in the General Population

- A classic study of incidence was conducted in England and reported by Andrews and Harris in 1964. They studied more than 1,000 newborn babies and followed them for 15 years. This is the only longitudinal study of stuttering of such a long duration involving such a large number of subjects. This and other, less extensive, studies on the incidence and prevalence of stuttering have shown the following facts:

- The life time expectancy of stuttering is about 5%. This means that 5% of the population has a probability of ever stuttering, even if stuttering lasts only a few days, weeks, or months.
- The incidence of stuttering is about 1% in the general U.S. population. Somewhat higher incidence rates have been reported for European countries. Investigations have shown that the prevalence of stuttering is higher in African Americans than in other ethnic groups in the United States (Cooper & Cooper, 1998). Experts believe that in spite of variations, no society is completely free from stuttering.
- The risk of developing a stutter varies by age, but stuttering typically begins during early childhood. In the majority, stuttering begins between the ages of 3 and 6 years. The onset of stuttering is relatively rare after 12 years of age.
- Adult onset of stuttering is rare. In some cases, a reemergence may occur of early childhood stuttering, from which the individual had recovered. In most cases, adult onset of stuttering is associated with neurological damage or disease. For example, some adults begin to stutter after a stroke or as a result of Alzheimer's dementia.

Spontaneous Recovery

- *Spontaneous recovery from stuttering* refers to its disappearance without professional help. The term may be a misnomer, because such recovery may be associated with the use of certain techniques. For instance, a person who stutters may accidentally discover that a slower rate of speech reduces stuttering and adopt such a rate. That is not truly spontaneous recovery.
- That some children and adolescents recover from stuttering without professional help has been documented, but the percentage of such recovery has remained controversial. Some early studies have suggested a 60% or higher spontaneous recovery rate. A few recent studies also have reported high recovery rates.
- Others believe that a realistic spontaneous recovery rate is about 30–35%. Even then, the rate applies to groups of stuttering children, not to individual children. It is not possible to predict whether a given child will or will not recover spontaneously.

Prevalence and Gender Ratio

- It is well documented that stuttering is far more common in males than in females. The most frequently cited ratio is 3:1 (male:female) for children in earlier elementary grades.
- The ratio is larger in higher grades (perhaps 4:1). This may be because of a slightly higher spontaneous recovery of stuttering in girls or because of a greater number of new cases in boys.
- The documented gender ratio has given rise to hypotheses about possible genetic factors in the etiology of stuttering.

Familial Prevalence

- *Familial prevalence* is the frequency with which a given condition appears in successive generations of blood relatives.
- The familial prevalence of stuttering is higher than that in the general population. That is, if there is one stuttering person in a family, there are likely to be others among his or her blood relatives. It is estimated that the familial prevalence of stuttering is more than three times higher than that in the general population.
- Some evidence suggests that familial prevalence is higher in families that have a female who stutters than in families that have a male who stutters. Familial prevalence and gender ratio interact; sons of mothers who stutter run a greater risk of stuttering than sons of fathers who stutter.

- Daughters generally have a lower risk, but daughters of stuttering mothers have a higher risk than daughters of nonstuttering mothers or of stuttering fathers. Familial incidence may be explained on the basis of genetic or environmental factors; most experts tend to emphasize genetic factors.

Prevalence and Concordance Rates in Twins

- *Concordance* is the occurrence of the same clinical condition (or normal trait) in both members of a twin pair. If both members of a twin pair have the same condition, then they are *concordant* for that condition; if only one member of a twin pair has a particular condition, then the pair is *discordant* for that condition.
- A *concordance rate* for stuttering is based on the number of twin pairs studied and the number in whom stuttering is evident in both members. For instance, if in a hundred pairs of twins studied, stuttering is found in both members of 50 pairs, then the concordance rate would be 50%; the remaining 50% would be discordant (one twin member stutters; the other does not).
- Differential concordance rates in ordinary siblings, identical (monozygotic) twins, and fraternal (dizygotic) twins would suggest the importance of genetic variables in stuttering.
- The concordance rate of stuttering for identical twins is higher than that for fraternal twins; the rates reported vary across studies with a range of 30%–80% of identical twin pairs.
- The concordance rate for fraternal twins is higher than that for ordinary siblings; this suggests that at least a *portion* of the concordance rate for identical twins may be due to their common environment.
- Studies of identical twins who have been separated and brought up in different environments and of children who have been adopted by families with and without stuttering members might be more definitive; well-designed studies of this kind are nonexistent; a few observations have reported ambiguous or inconclusive results.
- Differential prevalence data suggest that both genetic factors (which predispose the individual to stutter) and environmental events (which may trigger the disorder) play a part in the etiology of stuttering.

CONCEPTS TO CONSIDER

List three facts about the incidence and prevalence of stuttering. What does current research state about the familial and gender prevalence of stuttering?

Prevalence in Other Selected Populations

- The prevalence of stuttering in several other specific populations has been studied. A somewhat *higher* prevalence of stuttering than that of the general population has been reported for:

    - people with developmental disabilities (especially children and adults with Down syndrome); some data suggest that many in this group may clutter (see "Cluttering" section later in chapter) or clutter and stutter.
    - people with neurological impairment (especially those who have brain injuries or epilepsy).

- A *lower* prevalence of stuttering has been reported for deaf and hard of hearing people; at one time, it was claimed that deaf people do not stutter. However, stuttering in deaf people with oral skills has been documented; the reported lower prevalence may be due to the limited oral language skills in many individuals who are deaf.

Prevalence and Ethnocultural Variables

- Some experts, Wendell Johnson among them, have claimed that stuttering is a culturally determined disorder. According to Johnson and Associates (1959), parents who are critical of their children's normal nonfluencies tend to encourage apprehension and avoidance reactions, which he called stuttering.
- Johnson has further stated that societies and cultures that place a heavy emphasis on verbal skills have a higher prevalence of stuttering; Native Americans, for example, do not stutter, according to him.
- Johnson's theory has been contradicted by data. Native Americans do stutter; as previously noted, stuttering is found in almost all societies and ethnocultural groups. The prevalence rates appear to be somewhat different in different ethnocultural groups, but those differences are hard to explain and may even be due to methodological variations across studies.

Onset and Development of Stuttering

- Stuttering begins as an increase in the frequency of dysfluencies. The increase may be sudden or gradual, but the dysfluency rate remains highly variable for some time, resulting in periods of normal or near-normal fluency alternating with periods of excessive dysfluency.

- In many cases, parents report nothing unusual about the time of onset. Excessive tension, facial grimaces, and breathing abnormalities may or may not be present at or soon after the onset.

- The frequency of dysfluencies may stabilize and become more consistent across situations and time, although some degree of variability is a basic characteristic of stuttering, even in adults with many years of stuttering history.

- Development of avoidance and negative emotions (described later) may occur as stuttering becomes more consistent across situations and on certain words.

Associated Motor Behaviors

■ Stuttering may be associated with various abnormal motor behaviors, including:

- excessive muscular effort
- various facial grimaces
- various hand and foot movements (e.g., wringing the hands, tapping the foot)
- rapid eye blinking
- knitting of the eyebrows
- lip pursing
- rapid opening and closing of the mouth
- tongue clicking

■ The number and severity of associated motor behaviors vary across individuals. Whereas some children who stutter show notable associated motor behaviors, others may show none or show several that are almost undetectable. Adults who stutter generally show at least a few associated motor behaviors; some show many and severe forms of such behaviors.

■ Associated motor behaviors may have been accidentally reinforced. For instance, just when a person who stutters experienced a release from stuttering, he or she may have jerked an arm. From then on, an arm jerk may be associated with stuttering. Such accidentally reinforced associated motor behaviors rarely help the stuttering persons speak fluently.

■ Associated motor behaviors are not crucial for a diagnosis of stuttering. Excessive frequency or duration of dysfluencies is sufficient to diagnose stuttering. However, the presence of severe forms of frequently exhibited motor behaviors associated with increased frequency or duration of dysfluencies virtually assures a diagnosis of stuttering.

Associated Breathing Abnormalities

■ In many people, stuttered speech is associated with certain breathing abnormalities. Although not crucial for a diagnosis of stuttering, it is important to consider the following kinds of associated breathing abnormalities:

- attempts to speak on inhalation
- holding breath before talking
- continued attempts to speak even when the air supply is exhausted
- interruption of inhalations by exhalations and vice versa
- speaking without first inhaling a sufficient amount of air
- rapid and jerky breathing during speech
- exhaling puffs of air during stuttered speech
- generally tensed breathing

■ The noted breathing abnormalities do not suggest an inherent respiratory disorder; they are a part of the stuttering symptom complex. Fluent speech in people who stutter is not characterized by severe forms of breathing abnormalities.

Negative Emotions and Avoidance Behaviors

■ When stuttering persists, negative emotions and avoidance of words and speaking situations tend to develop. Avoidance and negative emotions are not crucial to a diagnosis of stuttering, but they are important to consider in a comprehensive program of assessment and treatment.

■ Negative emotions associated with stuttering include anxiety and apprehension about stuttering, fear of certain speaking situations, possibly some hostility toward certain speakers, frustration in efforts to communicate, and, possibly, a sense of humiliation in certain difficult speaking situations.

■ Difficult speaking situations include speaking with strangers and formal audiences, speaking with people at counters where services or products are bought, speaking on the telephone, ordering in restaurants, speaking to authority figures, and self-introductions or introductions of other people; however, avoidance of listeners and speaking situations is typically client-specific.

■ Avoidance may occur of specific sounds and words on which stuttering is frequently experienced, resulting in circumlocution and use of nonspecific words. However, sounds and words avoided are typically client-specific. For example, one client might avoid words beginning with *b* because he stutters more when saying such words. Another client may avoid saying her boss's name because she stutters whenever she tries to say it.

■ People who stutter may anticipate or expect to have more or fewer problems in certain speaking situations. A majority of people who stutter can predict a certain amount of their stuttering; however, there is no one-to-one correspondence between the anticipation of and actual stuttering. Words not expected to be stuttered may be, and those that are expected to be stuttered may be spoken fluently.

The Loci of Stuttering

■ Certain classes of sounds, words in certain positions in a sentence, and certain kinds of words have a high probability of being stuttered. Based on such observations, it is possible to predict the loci of stuttering. The *loci of stuttering* refers to the locations in a speech sequence where stutterings are typically observed.

■ In the speech of *adults and school-age children* who stutter, stuttering is more likely to occur:

  • *with consonants than with vowels,* although some speakers stutter predominantly on vowels; this is explained partly on the basis of the greater complexity of consonantal productions than vowel productions;
  • *on the first sound or syllable of a word;* more than 90% of stutterings occur on the initial sound or syllable of a word; this suggests that stuttering is a phenomenon of either disturbed speech initiation or disturbed movement to the next element in the speech chain;
  • *on the first word in a phrase or sentence;* generally, the first few words are more likely to be stuttered than the last few words in a sentence; this again suggests that the initial components in a speech sequence are more difficult than subsequent components;
  • *on the first word in a grammatical clause;* this suggests that grammatical class initiation is

somewhat similar to sentence initiation;

- *on longer words;* this is explained on the basis that longer words may be generally more difficult to produce than shorter words;
- *with less frequently used words;* this may be because less frequently used words tend to be longer as well; and
- *on content words* (nouns, verbs, adjectives, and adverbs) more often than on function words (articles, conjunctions, prepositions, and pronouns); this tendency may partly be due to the word position; content words tend to initiate more sentences and phrases than do function words.

■ The loci of stuttering in *preschool children* are the same as those for adults and school-age children except for one factor: Preschool children's stuttering tends to occur on function words (especially pronouns, conjunctions, and prepositions). This contrasts with the adult and school-age stutterers, who tend to stutter more often on content words than on function words.

■ Preschool children's tendency to stutter more on function words than on content words is partly explained on the basis that preschool children tend to initiate their phrases and sentences with certain function words, especially pronouns and conjunctions. This suggests that it is the position of words in a sentence (especially the first position), rather than the grammatical class of words, that is important in affecting the loci of stuttering.

■ Preschool children also tend to exhibit many whole-word repetitions. Thus, an early characteristic of stuttering is an increase in whole-word repetitions (along with other forms of dysfluencies).

■ Generally, dysfluencies tend to occur at the same loci in the speech of stuttering and non-stuttering people. Dysfluencies in the speech of people who do not stutter also tend to occur on initial consonants, initial words, longer words, less frequently used words, and content words.

CONCEPTS TO CONSIDER

Summarize the results of the research on the loci of stuttering.

Stimulus Control in Stuttering

■ Most of the variations found in the frequency of stuttering are due to variations in stimuli. Such patterns of variation suggest a strong environmental control, called here *stimulus control*. Research has shown that stuttering varies systematically when certain variables are manipulated. A few important phenomena that suggest a strong stimulus control of stuttering include adaptation, consistency, adjacency, and audience size.

Adaptation

- The *adaptation effect* is systematic reduction in the frequency of stuttering when a short printed passage is repeatedly read aloud. Important characteristics of adaptation include the following:

    - The amount of reduction in stuttering is greatest during the first few oral readings of a passage; by about the fifth reading, most reduction will have occurred.
    - The magnitude of reduction is progressively less on subsequent readings of the same passage until the amount of reduction is negligible.
    - The greater the time interval between readings, the less the degree of adaptation.
    - There is no transfer of adaptation from one passage to another.
    - Adaptation is a temporary phenomenon; if the same passage is read after a few hours of rest, the amount of stuttering will have increased to the baseline level.
    - Silent reading of a passage does not produce greater adaption when the same passage is subsequently read orally.
    - Lipped or whispered reading may reduce stuttering to some extent, but repeated oral reading produces the most dramatic adaptation.
    - Less severe stuttering tends to adapt more than more severe stuttering.
    - Both children and adults, and those who stutter and those who do not, show adaptation.
    - There is a great deal of individual difference in the amount of adaptation exhibited; most people adapt to varying extents; some do not adapt at all; and some show an increase in stuttering upon repeated readings.

- Adaptation has been explained in various ways, including the following:

    - Adaptation is an experimental extinction of the stuttering response (Wischner, 1950).
    - Adaptation is due to a deconfirmation of the expectancy of stuttering, which results in reduced anxiety and reduced stuttering (Johnson, 1959).
    - Adaptation is due to a reactive inhibition; stuttering is reduced because it produces a reactive inhibition (fatigue), which suppresses further stuttering (Brutten & Shoemaker, 1967).
    - Adaptation is due to fear reduction; each instance of stuttering reduces fear of stuttering and hence further reduces stuttering (Sheehan, 1970).
    - Adaptation is due to the rehearsal effect; repeated reading of the same passage provides rehearsal of the material and hence a reduction in stuttering (Bloodstein, 1995).
    - There is no agreement on the explanation of adaptation. No theory is fully supported by data. The degree of adaptation is inconclusive evidence of the degree of improvement that will occur in therapy.

Consistency

- The *consistency effect* is the occurrence of stuttering on the same word or loci when a passage is read aloud repeatedly. In a sense, it is the opposite of the adaptation effect: While adaptation refers to a disappearance of stuttering on certain previously stuttered words, consistency refers to the occurrence of stuttering on the same words upon repeated reading.
- Aspects of the consistency effect include the following:

    - About 65% of stuttering in given individuals may be consistent; that is, stuttering tends to occur on the same words or loci in repeated readings.
    - Consistency remains when the subjects reread a passage after weeks of interval.

- The consistency effect is presumed to be an indicator of the strength of the stimuli that evoke stuttering. The consistency effect is a stimulus-response phenomenon.

Adjacency

- The *adjacency effect* is the occurrence of new stuttering on words that surround previously stuttered words. It is a striking phenomenon of stimulus control.
- This effect is studied by having a subject read a passage multiple times, blotting out or otherwise concealing the words on which stuttering occurs, and then having the subject read the passage again to note the occurrence of new stuttering.
- The results of such experiments have shown that:

    - In several subjects, words that were fluently read during earlier readings were eventually stuttered.
    - The newly stuttered words were often adjacent to those blotted out (previously stuttered words).
    - The adjacency effect is evident in adults and children who stutter.
    - The adjacency effect may be horizontal (new stuttering occurs on words to the right or left of the blotted-out word on which stuttering had occurred previously) or vertical (new stuttering occurs on words printed below or above the word previously stuttered).

- The adjacency effect is yet another powerful demonstration of stimulus control of stuttering. A stimulus associated with past stuttering may serve as a stimulus for new stuttering.

Audience Size

- The *audience size effect* refers to the observation that the frequency of stuttering increases with an increase in audience size.
- Yet another striking phenomenon of stimulus control, the audience size effect is characterized by:

    - a marked decrease in stuttering when there is no audience and the person is speaking to himself or herself (monologue);
    - a corresponding increase in the amount of stuttering with a systematic increase in the number of listeners;
    - a reduced amount of stuttering when a listener's hearing is visibly masked; and

FLUENCY AND ITS DISORDERS 293

- a greater amount of stuttering when listeners can hear the stutterer than when they can only see the stutterer.

■ The audience size effect is another demonstration of conditioning and stimulus control over stuttering. This phenomenon is sometimes explained on the basis of communicative pressure. The greater the number of listeners, the higher the communicative pressure.

People Who Stutter and Their Families

■ Various theories and viewpoints in the past held that certain "personality" variables might be the underlying cause of stuttering. This idea is especially inherent to psychoneurotic conceptions of stuttering, in which persons who stutter are thought to exhibit psychoneurotic tendencies.

■ Other conceptions, such as those of Johnson (1959), implied that parents of stutterers may hold unusually and unrealistically high standards of fluency.

■ Such parents are then likely to place undue pressure on their children or to misdiagnose stuttering based on normal nonfluency, as Johnson has hypothesized. Such views have led to an investigation of the personality of individuals who stutter and their families, especially their parents.

■ Personality variables such as anxiety, level of aspiration, obsessive–compulsive behaviors, oral and anal eroticism, passive dependency, hostility and aggression, self-concept, social adjustment, body image, and so forth, have been investigated over several decades. Various kinds of questionnaires and such projective tests as the Rorschach have been used.

■ This kind of research has shown that people who stutter:

- do not have a distinct personality that may be causally related to their stuttering;
- are not clinically maladjusted;
- are not clinically and chronically anxious (although many may have slightly elevated levels of anxiety in speaking situations which may be an effect, not a cause, of stuttering); and
- may have low self-esteem, possibly due to their stuttering.

■ Research on parents of people who stutter has shown that they:

- do not exhibit unique personality patterns that may be causally related to stuttering in their children;
- are not clinically maladjusted or neurotic;
- may exhibit a somewhat higher standard of behavior and be somewhat more critical of their children than are parents of children who do not stutter; however, the clinical significance of this finding is unclear and a general conclusion about its importance is unwarranted.

■ In essence, neither the personality of people who stutter nor that of their parents seems to provide strong clues to the etiology of stuttering. People who stutter and their parents are not a distinct and unique group of individuals who are neurotic or maladjusted. In most respects, they are like people who do not stutter and their parents.

CONCEPTS TO CONSIDER

Define the adaptation, consistency, and adjacency effects discussed in the literature on stuttering.

_____

_____

_____

_____

_____

Theories of Stuttering

Foundational Concepts

- There are environmental, genetic, and neurophysiological theories of stuttering. However, no theory explains all aspects of stuttering.
- Theories are likely to remain incomplete until the nature of causation is determined. Existing theories are at best hypotheses that require the support of additional research. Hence, none is universally accepted as an explanation of stuttering.
- The basic premise of genetic and neurophysiological theories of stuttering is that the person who stutters has a genetic basis for stuttering and that his or her neurophysiological speech system is deviant compared to that of nonstuttering individuals. Theories within this group differ in their emphasis on genetic and neurophysiological variables. Some place a greater emphasis on genetic variables, while others emphasize the neurophysiological organization involved in speech production.
- Other theories about stuttering include those that focus on the role of learning and conditioning as well as those that view stuttering as a form of psychoneurosis.

Genetic Hypothesis

- There is much speculation about the role genes play in the genesis of stuttering. A potential genetic basis of stuttering is suggested by the following observations:

    - Stuttering has a higher familial incidence.
    - There is a well-established gender ratio in the prevalence of stuttering.
    - Stuttering shows a higher concordance rate among identical twins.

- Although various kinds of data suggest a possible genetic basis, no gene or chromosomal abnormality responsible for stuttering has been identified. Also, no particular mechanism of inheritance of stuttering has been clearly established. Furthermore, in about half the number of cases, familial incidence may be negative.

- Evidence does not suggest a simple, Mendelian type of inheritance. Data do not support sex-linked, autosomal, or recessive inheritance patterns. Some investigators believe that patterns of familial prevalence suggest inheritance due to a single gene.
- Others believe that inheritance may be based on multiple genes (polygenic inheritance) that predispose an individual to stutter. Currently, no genetic transmission theory is universally accepted (Bloodstein, 1995).

Neurophysiological Hypotheses

- Several variations exist of the basic neurophysiological position that people who stutter have an abnormal neurophysiological or neuromotor organization.
- The *laryngeal dysfunction hypothesis* states that stuttering is due to aberrant laryngeal functions. The etiology of aberrant laryngeal function may be defective neuromotor control of the laryngeal mechanism, as no local laryngeal pathology has been documented in people who stutter.
- Evidence supporting the laryngeal dysfunction hypothesis includes the following:

  - *slightly delayed voice onset time* (VOT) in some people who stutter; VOT is measured by giving a visual or auditory signal to produce a simple vocal response (e.g., saying /ɑ/) and measuring the time between the offset of the stimulus and the onset of the vocal response; documented delay is in milliseconds and fades with repeated trials;
  - *increased tension in the laryngeal muscles* associated with stuttered speech, measured by such techniques as electromyography;
  - *aberrant muscle behavior* during stuttered speech (e.g., simultaneous activation of laryngeal abductors and adductors, which are normally active reciprocally); and
  - *excessive laryngeal muscle activity* during stuttered speech, also measured by such techniques as electromyography.

- Whether laryngeal abnormality, especially the delayed vocal reaction time, is due to potential respiratory problems is an unresolved issue. Vocal responses involve respiratory responses as well. Problems in respiratory control of the speech mechanism during stuttering could result in delayed vocal response.
- *Hypotheses on the brain and speech and language mechanisms and stuttering* suggest that the brain, which controls the speech mechanism, may not be working properly in speakers who stutter. Related hypotheses suggest that the auditory portion of the brain may not be functioning properly or that there may be an auditory feedback problem.
- Evidence suggesting potential brain dysfunction in people who stutter includes the following:

  - Some studies suggest that people who stutter may not have a *dominant hemisphere* to process language. This lack of dominance for language may cause inefficient or even confused neuromotor control of the speech mechanism, resulting in stuttering.
  - Some *electroencephalographic* studies suggest that the brain waves, especially the alpha waves, may be abnormal in some people who stutter. However, the evidence on abnormal brain waves is contradictory. While some studies report abnormal patterns of brain waves, others report essentially normal patterns.
  - Limited evidence suggests that in some people who stutter, *cerebral blood flow* may be reduced. Such a reduction has been noted in the frontal lobe involved in speech-motor control and the left temporal lobe.

- Some *cineradiographic* studies of face and oral structures suggest that even when speech is fluent, movements involved in speech are slower than normal in people who stutter; the brain may not be initiating and regulating speech activity in a smooth, efficient, and coordinated manner.

- Some studies on the *central auditory function* in people who stutter suggest potential involvement of the auditory portion of the brain, but the specific pathology is unclear. Studies on central auditory processing suggest that some people who stutter may have subtle central auditory problems. Such evidence has been reported with the ipsilateral competing message test, the acoustic reflex amplitude function, and the staggered spondaic word test. However, contradictory evidence suggests essentially normal central auditory function in most people who stutter.

- Unspecified *auditory feedback problems* are suggested by studies investigating delayed auditory feedback and auditory masking noise, both of which reduce most types of dysfluencies. Based on such outcomes, some experts have suggested a potential involvement of the auditory mechanism in the etiology of stuttering. Investigators have speculated that people who stutter may have a basic delay in processing auditory information, and thus delayed auditory feedback helps them achieve greater fluency. Masking noise was once hypothesized to prevent stuttering people from hearing their own stuttering or masking a defective auditory feedback mechanism. That hypothesis has been discredited by studies that show that stuttering is reduced under even mild masking that does not prevent auditory feedback. Some experts attribute increased fluency under altered auditory conditions to a decreased speech rate, which is dramatically evident in delayed auditory feedback.

Learning, Conditioning, and Related Hypotheses

- In contrast to neurophysiological theories, learning, conditioning, and a few other somewhat related theories emphasize the importance of environmental variables in the etiology of stuttering. These theories also have several variations, including those described below.

Stuttering as an Operant Behavior

- Some studies suggest that stuttering may be an operant behavior. An operant is a behavior that can be changed by changing its consequences. Thus, operant behaviors are learned.
- Some studies have shown that stuttering frequency may be decreased by corrective feedback (e.g., saying "No," or "Wrong," for every dysfluency), response-contingent electric shock or noise, time-out, or response cost. The evidence on the effect of shock on stuttering is somewhat controversial, whereas the evidence on the effects of time-out and response cost is more uniform and positive.
- Studies generally have shown that any stimulus can decrease stuttering. For example, the word "tree" presented response-contingently can reduce the frequency of stuttering. Such studies do suggest that stuttering may be an operant because to show that a behavior is an operant, one only needs to show that its frequency may be altered by certain consequences.

Stuttering as Speech Disruption Due to Classically Conditioned Negative Emotion

- Brutten and Shoemaker (1967) have proposed that stuttering consists of fluency disruption due to classically conditioned negative emotion.
- As noted earlier, this theory limits the term *stuttering* to part-word repetitions and sound prolongations that are based on negative emotion. The negative emotion may be classically conditioned to speaking situations, sounds, words, or audience factors. In this theory, all other

forms of dysfluencies (e.g., whole-word repetitions, interjections, pauses) are operant behaviors that can be changed by changing their consequences.
- Stutterings as defined in the theory are not operant behaviors and can be reduced only by counter-conditioning more positive emotional reactions that replace those negative emotions.

Stuttering as Avoidance Behavior

- This view, too, has several variations. An early and systematic theory of stuttering based on avoidance is that of Johnson (1959).
- His *diagnosogenic theory* states that when parents punish a child's normal nonfluencies, the child develops anticipatory, apprehensive, and hypertonic avoidance reactions that are indeed stutterings. Johnson asserted that dysfluencies are normal as they are found in almost all speakers; hence, stuttering could not be diagnosed based on a feature of normal dysfluency.
- It is only when a child begins to *avoid* the consequences of normal nonfluencies that the stuttering problem emerges. Johnson further asserted that stuttering is a cultural phenomenon created by parents who overly emphasize fluency.
- Consistent with that position, Johnson believed that among such cultures as those of Native Americans, who did not emphasize fluency, people did not stutter. However, it is now well known that Native Americans do stutter and that there is no conclusive evidence that parental punishment of normal nonfluency is the origin of avoidance behaviors (Bloodstein, 1995).

Stuttering as Approach Avoidance

- Sheehan's (1970) early version of stuttering theory emphasizes an approach-avoidance conflict. He believed that a stuttering person's hesitations and repetitions indicate a conflict between a desire to approach speaking situations and an equally strong desire to avoid them.
- Fluent speech is possible when the drive or desire to speak is stronger than the drive to avoid speech. When the drive to avoid speech is the stronger of the two, the person does not talk at all. However, when the two drive states are equal in strength, stuttering results.

Stuttering as a Reaction of Tension and Fragmentation

- Bloodstein (1995) has proposed that stuttering is essentially a response of tension and fragmentation in speech. Stuttering is not unlike normal nonfluency (dysfluency), though it is typically greater in quantity and more disruptive in quality. Such a response of tension and fragmentation may come about because of a child's belief that speech is a difficult task.
- Unlike Johnson, who proposed that the origin of stuttering (avoidance behavior) is parental disapproval of normal nonfluency, Bloodstein thinks that stuttering may have many origins, most of them related to various kinds of severe communicative pressure that leads to repeated communicative failures. This view is generally known as the *anticipatory struggle hypothesis*.

Stuttering Due to Demands Exceeding Capacities

- This view of stuttering implies an interaction between a child's inherent linguistic, cognitive, motoric, or emotional capacity for effective and fluent communication and environmental demands made on the child for realizing such communication.
- The theory essentially states that stuttering can result when a child faces demands for communication that he or she cannot meet because of limited capacities. This view, known as the *demands and capacities model,* is not unlike other approaches such as that of Bloodstein (1995), which states that continued and severe communicative pressure can result in chronic communicative failure.

CONCEPTS TO CONSIDER

Summarize the key points of the neurophysiological and the learning and conditioning hypotheses of stuttering.

_____

_____

_____

_____

_____

Stuttering as a Form of Psychoneurosis

- The hypothesis that stuttering may be a psychological disorder has a long history. A particular form of this hypothesis was proposed by Freudians, who considered stuttering a form of psychoneurosis.
- According to this hypothesis, stuttering is due to an underlying psychopathology, and stutterings themselves are merely symptoms of deep-seated psychological conflicts.
- These conflicts are generated and maintained by such psychological processes as infantile fixation, later frustration, regression to the fixated stage, and symptom formation. In this sense, stuttering is similar to other forms of neurosis, including anxiety, phobia, and hysterical (conversion) reaction. Such unconscious but socially unacceptable urges as oral or anal gratification may find socially acceptable forms of expression such as repetitions or prolongations. The main problems with the psychoanalytic explanation of stuttering are that it is unverifiable and that treatment based on it is generally ineffective.

SUMMARY

✓ Fluent speech is generally rhythmic, smooth, and produced with ease. Stuttered speech contains excessive amounts of dysfluencies, durations of dysfluencies, or both. Various definitions of stuttering exist.

✓ The incidence and prevalence of stuttering have been studied in relation to the general population, spontaneous recovery, prevalence and gender ratio, familial prevalence, and prevalence and concordance rates in twins and other selected populations.

✓ Stuttering onset may be gradual or sudden. It is usually characterized by abnormal associated motor behaviors, breathing abnormalities, negative emotions, and avoidance behaviors.

✓ Several phenomena such as adaptation, consistency, adjacency, and audience size suggest that various stimuli in the environment affect the frequency of stuttering (stimulus control).

✓ There are environmental, genetic, neurophysiological, and psychoanalytic theories of stuttering. No theory explains all aspects of stuttering, and hence none is universally accepted.

ASSESSMENT AND TREATMENT OF STUTTERING

INTRODUCTION

Assessment of stuttering includes standard procedures such as a hearing screening, a detailed case history obtained from the client or family members, measurement of stuttering, and obtaining information on related behaviors (e.g., associated motor behaviors and negative emotions). A detailed assessment of the stuttering includes evaluation of the frequency and types of dysfluencies, variability in stuttering, associated motor behaviors, avoidance behaviors, rate of speech, and negative emotional reactions. Methods of treatment of stuttering include psychological methods, the fluent stuttering method, the fluency shaping method, the fluency reinforcement method, masking and delayed auditory feedback techniques, and the direct stuttering reduction methods.

Assessment of Stuttering

■ Assessment includes procedures designed to evaluate stuttering and related behaviors. In addition to such standard procedures such as hearing screening and orofacial examination, the following are important considerations (Hegde, 2001a).

■ It is important to take a detailed case history by interviewing the client, family members, or both, to obtain information on:

- the onset of stuttering and any special circumstances associated with the onset;
- familial prevalence of stuttering;
- the earliest behaviors considered stuttering by the family members, other caretakers, or teachers who initially diagnosed the stuttering;
- the initial and subsequent course of the stuttering, including its variability and stability;
- prior clinical services and the names of the specialists who provided them;
- prior treatment procedures and their initial and subsequent effects;
- current education and occupation or future educational and occupational plans of the client;
- general health history; and
- language and speech development and educational performance in the schools, in the case of children who stutter.

■ Assessment of the frequency and types of dysfluencies or stutterings may be conducted by:

- recording an extended conversational speech sample with the clinician and with a member of the family (e.g., the child's mother or father engaged in conversation with the child); and
- recording an oral reading sample with reading material appropriate for the client's age, interest, reading skill level, and ethnocultural background.

- The clinician may make an assessment of variability in stuttering by:

  - having the client or a caretaker rate different speaking situations in which stuttering frequency varies;
  - obtaining verbal reports from family members regarding variability in stuttering across time and situations;
  - obtaining a tape-recorded sample of speech produced at home, school, or an occupational setting for the clinician's analysis of dysfluency rates;
  - comparing the frequency of dysfluencies produced in the clinic with that produced in naturalistic settings; and
  - repeating the clinic and the home measures if results of any two comparable dysfluency rates are discrepant.

- Assessment of associated motor behaviors may be carried out by:

  - taking note of the associated motor behaviors exhibited during assessment; and
  - describing those behaviors.

- The clinician may conduct an assessment of avoidance behaviors by:

  - having the client describe sounds, words, situations, and audiences typically avoided;
  - taking note of words and sounds avoided during the interview;
  - asking the client to make a list of sounds or words that are especially difficult and submit this list during the next clinical visit;
  - asking the client to make a hierarchy of most difficult (e.g., speaking to the boss) to least difficult (speaking to a close friend) speaking situations;
  - having family members describe a child's avoidance reactions; and
  - administering the *Behavior Assesment Battery* (Brutten & Vanryckeghem, 2001), which helps assess negative emotions and attitudes associated with speech, speaking situations, and avoidance behaviors of adults and children who stutter.

- Assessment of speech rate and articulatory rate may be carried out by:

  - counting the number of words or syllables spoken per minute in at least three 2-minute samples of continuous speech (speech rate); and
  - counting the number of syllables produced while discounting all stutterings and pauses that exceed 2 seconds (articulatory rate).

- Assessment of negative emotional reactions may be carried out by:

  - having the client describe his or her negative emotions about speech, particular speaking situations, specific audiences, and so forth;
  - administering the modified S-Scale by Andrews and Cutler (1974); administering Brutten's *Behavior Assessment Battery* (Brutten & Vanryckeghem, 2001), which helps assess negative attitudes and emotions associated with speech as well as avoidance behaviors of adults and children who stutter; and
  - asking family members or friends about negative emotions the client typically expresses.

- Diagnosis of stuttering may be made by using one of several diagnostic criteria:

  - a dysfluency rate that exceeds 5% of spoken words when all kinds of dysfluencies are

counted
- a certain frequency of part-word repetitions, speech sound prolongations, and broken words (at least 2% of the words spoken)
- excessive duration of dysfluencies (1 second or longer)
- other criteria the clinician adopts

Treatment of Stuttering

- There are several approaches to stuttering treatment, described in various sources (Bloodstein, 1995; Culatta & Goldberg, 1995; Curlee, 1999; Guitar, 1998; Hegde, 2001b; Onslow et al., 2001; Shapiro, 1999; Van Riper, 1982). Most of the treatment procedures can be classified and described as follows.

Psychological Methods of Treatment

- Psychological methods include Freudian psychoanalysis, non-Freudian psychotherapy, and counseling. Psychological methods are offered by psychiatrists, psychologists, and psychoanalysts. Various forms of counseling may be offered by qualified speech–language pathologists.
- These methods involve the assumption that stuttering is a psychological disorder and that underlying psychological conflicts, which may be conscious or unconscious, are the causes of stuttering. Treatment consists of attempts to resolve those conflicts.
- The somewhat varied methods include:

    - discussion of psychological problems associated with stuttering;
    - discussion of feelings, emotions, and attitudes associated with stuttering;
    - discussion and resolution of potential psychological conflicts, unconscious psychosexual conflicts, and various kinds of negative reactions; and
    - reeducation of the client about a more realistic and rational approach to the stuttering problem.

- There is no strong evidence that psychotherapy or counseling is effective in treating stuttering. Speech–language pathologists who offer counseling do so in conjunction with other methods designed to enhance fluency. In such cases, it is difficult to claim effectiveness for any one method used.

Fluent-Stuttering Method

- An established method of treating stuttering is Van Riper's fluent-stuttering approach, also called the *stutter-more-fluently* approach. Van Riper believed that modifying the severity and the visible abnormality of stuttering is the most realistic goal for many people who stutter. The goal of this approach is not normal fluency, but more fluent (less abnormal) stuttering. This method involves the following steps:
- *Teaching stuttering identification.* The client is taught to identify his or her stuttering and associated problems (e.g., feelings and attitudes) in both clinical and everyday situations.
- *Desensitizing the client to his or her stuttering.* The client is encouraged to be open and honest with his or her stuttering and voluntarily stutter in many speaking situations to get desensitized.
- *Modifying stuttering.* The client is taught to produce more fluent, easier, and less abnormal stuttering by the clinician, encouraging the client to:

  - face difficult speaking situations and use feared words without avoidance
  - use *cancellations* (pausing after a stuttered word and saying the word again with easy and more relaxed stuttering)
  - use *pull-outs,* or changing stuttering in mid-course (e.g., by slowing down and using soft articulatory contacts instead of blocking on sounds or words)
  - use *preparatory sets* (e.g., changing the manner of stuttering so that the client produces less abnormal stuttering)

- *Stabilizing the treatment gains.* The client is encouraged to use the techniques of stuttering modification (cancellations, pull-outs, and preparatory sets) in all speaking situations.
- *Counseling the client.* The client is encouraged to discuss the emotions and attitudes he or she associates with stuttering to gain a more realistic and accepting view of his or her difficulties.
- A limitation of the fluent-stuttering method is that it rarely establishes normal fluency, as only modified stuttering is its goal. Relapse of stuttering also may be a problem.

Fluency-Shaping Method

- The goal of fluency shaping (also called the *speak-more-fluently* approach) is to establish normal fluency (not fluent stuttering). Teaching the various skills of fluency (e.g., appropriate management of airflow to produce and sustain fluent speech, slower rate of speech, and gentle onset of phonation) is the main treatment task.
- In different treatment programs, one or more of such fluency skills may be emphasized or particular combinations of skills may be targeted. The treatment targets and procedures include the following:

  - Teach airflow management (i.e., inhalation of air and immediate slight exhalation before phonation; maintenance of an even airflow throughout an utterance).
  - Teach gentle, soft, relaxed, and easy onset of phonation, beginning after the initiation of exhalation.
  - Teach a reduced rate of speech through syllable prolongation, not by extending pause durations; typically, the vowel is prolonged; if preferred, delayed auditory feedback can be used to reduce the rate of speech.
  - Help the client achieve stutter-free speech, mostly by means of airflow management, gentle phonatory onset, and rate reduction through syllable prolongation.
  - Shape normal prosodic features (e.g., increased rate, normal vocal intensity, and normal intonation after stutter-free speech is stabilized).
  - Implement maintenance strategies (e.g., teaching self-monitoring skills and training family and friends to monitor and reinforce fluency in natural settings and over time).

- Use specific treatment procedures as follows:

  - Initially, teach specific skills individually and in the sequence of airflow management, gentle onset, and rate reduction to achieve stutter-free speech; then, shape normal prosodic features.
  - Start treatment starts with what the client can handle; words, phrases, or even short sentences can be the starting points to practice fluency skills. Move treatment gradually to controlled conversation and finally to more spontaneous conversation in natural settings.
  - Use such specific procedures as instruction, modeling, corrective feedback for mismanaged skills and dysfluencies, and positive reinforcement for correct responses.

- A limitation of the fluency-shaping method is that it generates slow, deliberate, and somewhat unnatural-sounding fluency. Clients tend not to maintain the slower rate needed to sustain that fluency, as such a rate is socially and personally unacceptable.

CONCEPTS TO CONSIDER

Compare and contrast the fluent-stuttering method and the fluency-shaping method. What are three key differences between the methods?

_____

_____

_____

_____

_____

Fluency Reinforcement Method

A simple method that works with many young children is to positively reinforce fluent speech in naturalistic conversational contexts. This method can be combined with such targets as reduced speech rate.

- In this method, the clinician:

    - arranges a pleasant and relaxed therapeutic setting;
    - evokes speech with the help of picture books, toys, and other play materials;
    - positively reinforces the child for fluent utterances with verbal praise, tokens, or both;
    - frequently models a slow, relaxed speaking rate that assures stutter-free speech; and
    - reshapes normal prosody if a slower rate is an added target.

- Clinical experience suggests that fluency reinforcement alone may be effective with young children, whereas with older children and adult clients, adding a slower speech rate as a target may increase the efficiency of the technique.

Masking and Delayed Auditory Feedback Techniques

- An approach popular for many years in the past involved altered auditory feedback of speech. As noted in a previous section, when a stuttering person hears his or her own speech with a fraction of a second's delay, most of the dysfluencies are reduced. Similarly, auditory masking noise improves fluency.
- Most experts now believe that both techniques may achieve their desirable effects by inducing syllable prolongation, especially the prolongation of vowels. Consequently, both techniques, especially the delayed auditory feedback (DAF), induce a slow speech with reduced prosodic features.

- In using the DAF technique, the clinician:

  - uses a DAF machine that allows for variable delays;
  - determines a client-specific duration of delay that assures stutter-free speech;
  - has the client practice stutter-free speech for varying lengths of time to eliminate stutterings; and
  - fades the delay in gradual steps to reshape normal prosody while maintaining fluency.

- The main advantage of DAF is its capacity to induce a slower rate of speech. Many clinicians, however, have found it unnecessary to use DAF to achieve that effect. Instruction and repeated modeling are often sufficient to induce a slow rate that assures stutter-free speech.
- In using the masking noise technique of DAF, the clinician:

  - determines a minimum level of auditory masking that induces stutter-free speech;
  - has the client practice stutter-free speech for variable lengths of time, depending on the client's progress; and
  - fades the masking noise to reshape normal prosody while maintaining fluency.

- The use of masking noise has decreased over the years, mainly because of the problems of maintaining fluent speech in natural settings. Even in therapy sessions, masking noise may eventually lose its effects because of adaptation to noise.

Direct Stuttering Reduction Methods

- Direct stuttering reduction methods seek to reduce stuttering directly, without teaching specific fluency skills or modifying stuttering into less abnormal forms. To reduce stuttering directly, behavioral methods of time-out or response cost may be used.
- *Time-out (pause-and-talk).* In this method, the person who stutters is taught to pause after each dysfluency and then resume talking. The specific procedures include the clinician:

  - saying "stop" or giving other signals (e.g., a light that comes on) as soon as a dysfluency is observed and making sure that the client completely ceases talking;
  - avoiding eye contact with the client for about 5 seconds;
  - reestablishing eye contact after the time-out duration and letting the client continue his or her speech; and
  - maintaining eye contact, smiling, and employing other social reinforcers for fluent speech.

- *Response cost.* In this method, for every instance of stuttering, the clinician takes away from the client a positive reinforcer while reinforcing fluency with the same reinforcer (being withdrawn). The specific procedure includes the following:

  - reinforcing the client for every fluently spoken word, phrase, or sentence with a token that is backed up with other kinds of reinforcers;
  - taking a token away in a matter-of-fact manner immediately following a stuttering or at the earliest sign of it; and
  - progressing from words and phrases to conversational speech.

- Both pause-and-talk and response cost can help establish more natural-sounding fluency. There is no need to teach such fluency skills as slow rate or airflow management. Of the two techniques, time-out is the better researched, although evidence on the effectiveness of response cost in treating young children, including preschoolers, is accumulating.

SUMMARY

✓ Assessment of stuttering includes standard assessment procedures and a detailed interview of the client, family, or both.

✓ Detailed assessment of the stuttering behavior includes assessment of frequency and types of dysfluencies, variability in stuttering, associated motor behaviors, avoidance behaviors, speech rate, and negative emotional reactions.

✓ Approaches to the treatment of stuttering include psychological methods, the fluent-stuttering method associated with Van Riper, and the fluency-shaping method.

✓ Other approaches to treatment include the fluency reinforcement method, masking and delayed auditory feedback techniques, and the direct stuttering reduction methods.

CLUTTERING

INTRODUCTION

Cluttering is a disorder of fluency that often coexists with stuttering. People described as clutterers often speak in a highly dysfluent, rapid, unclear, and disorganized manner that is jerky and monotonous. They do not manifest obvious concern about their speaking patterns. Little research exists on treatment of cluttering, although it has been found that decreasing the rate of speech and increasing the client's awareness of the problem are often effective.

Definition and Description of Cluttering

■ Compared to stuttering, less information is available on cluttering. The prevalence of cluttering in the United States is unknown, but in Germany it is reported to be 1.8% of 7- to 8-year-old children. Like stuttering, cluttering is more common in males than in females.

■ *Cluttering* is a disorder of fluency characterized by rapid but disordered articulation, possibly combined with a high rate of dysfluencies and disorganized thought and language. It tends to coexist with stuttering, but there is no strong tendency for stuttering to coexist with cluttering (Myers & St. Louis, 1992).

■ The characteristics of cluttering are as follows:

- impaired fluency with excessive amounts of dysfluencies
- rapid repetition of syllables, along with other forms of dysfluencies
- rapid but disordered articulation resulting in indistinct (unintelligible) speech
- clearer articulation and improved intelligibility at slower rate of speech
- omission and compression of sounds and syllables
- jerky or stumbling rhythm
- monotonous tone

- spoonerisms (unintentional interchanges of sounds in a sentence; e.g., *many thinkle peep so* instead of *many people think so*)
- reportedly, a lack of personal concern about or reduced awareness of one's speech problem
- lack of anxiety about or negative reactions to one's speech difficulty
- Disorganized thought processes, a controversial feature of cluttering

■ The causes of cluttering are unknown. Genetic transmission and subtle brain damage have been among suggested factors. No hypothesis or theory about its causation has received wide support. However, some experts think that it is a central language disorder (a disassociation between thought and language) for which there is very little empirical support.

CONCEPTS TO CONSIDER

Briefly define cluttering.

_____

_____

_____

_____

_____

Treatment of Cluttering

■ Little or no controlled treatment research exists on cluttering. Currently, most clinicians treat cluttering as they would stuttering.

■ Reducing the rate of speech usually improves clarity as well as fluency. If thought problems or language formulation problems are dominant, teaching the client to plan sentences and other forms of expression before actually producing them might be helpful.

■ Increasing the clutterer's awareness of his speech through the use of audiotapes or videotapes can be highly effective. Some people who clutter are surprised when confronted with recordings of their speech. Unfortunately, videotaped samples do not convince others who clutter that there is a problem with their rate of speech.

■ Maintenance of fluent and well-articulated speech is the major problem in treating persons who clutter. Systematic treatment research is needed to develop unique and more effective treatment procedures for cluttering.

SUMMARY

✓ Cluttering is a disorder of fluency characterized by rapid, imprecise, jerky, and disorganized speech.

✓ Little research exists about its treatment. Reducing the speaking rate and increasing self-awareness helps some people who clutter to sound more intelligible.

CHAPTER HIGHLIGHTS

◆ **FLUENT SPEECH IS FLOWING,** smooth, and relatively rapid and effortless. Stuttering and cluttering are two main forms of fluency disorders. Stuttering may be defined as: (a) all types of dysfluencies that exceed a measure such as 5% of words spoken, (b) production of part-word repetitions and speech-sound prolongations, (c) moments or events judged to be stutterings, (d) anticipatory, apprehensive, hypertonic, avoidance reaction.

◆ **DYSFLUENCIES INTERRUPT THE FLOW** of fluency; there are many forms including repetitions, prolongations, broken words, interjections, pauses, incomplete sentences, and revisions. When dysfluencies exceed 5% of words spoken, listeners tend to judge the speech as dysfluent or stuttered.

◆ **THE INCIDENCE OF STUTTERING** in the U.S. general population is about 1%. The lifetime expectancy of stuttering is about 5%. Stuttering is more prevalent in men than in women; there is a higher concordance rate for identical twins than for ordinary siblings. Neither those who stutter nor their parents constitute a unique group whose characteristics are causally related to stuttering.

◆ **IN EARLY CHILDHOOD, STUTTERING** begins as an initial increase in the amount of dysfluencies. Associated motor behaviors, breathing abnormalities, negative emotions, and avoidance behaviors tend to develop in due course and to varying extents across individuals.

◆ **STUTTERING OCCURS AT SUCH** predictable loci as initial sounds and words, consonants, longer and unfamiliar words, content words in older children and adults, function words in younger children.

◆ **STUTTERING IS UNDER STRONG** stimulus control, as evidenced by such phenomena as adaptation (progressive decrease in stuttering upon repeated oral reading of a passage), consistency (persistent stuttering on the same loci), adjacency (new stuttering on loci adjacent to old stuttering), and dependence on audience size (increased stuttering with increased number of listeners).

◆ **GENETIC EXPLANATIONS OF STUTTERING** include a single-gene hypothesis and a multiple-genes hypothesis, which presume that certain individuals may be predisposed to stutter. Neurophysiological hypotheses propose that stuttering people may have abnormal laryngeal control, abnormal cerebral language processing, or aberrant neuromotor control of the speech mechanism. Psychoanalytic hypotheses propose deep-seated psychopathology. Conditioning and learning hypotheses propose faulty learning and conditioning. None of the hypotheses is fully supported by experimental evidence.

◆ **ASSESSMENT OF STUTTERING INCLUDES** a detailed case history; measurement of types and frequency of dysfluencies in conversational speech and oral reading; evaluation of the variability of dysfluencies; assessment of negative emotions, avoidance reactions, and associated motor behaviors; measurement of speech and articulatory rates; and application of a chosen diagnostic criterion.

◆ **TREATMENT OF STUTTERING INCLUDES** a variety of procedures, including counseling and psychotherapy; the fluent-stuttering method (Van Riper's method aimed at reducing the abnormality of stuttering through cancellations, pull-outs, and preparatory sets); the fluency-shaping method (widely used procedures that include airflow management, gentle phonatory onset, rate reduction, and shaping normal prosody); fluency reinforcement and time-outs (teaching pausing after every instance of stuttering); response cost (losing a tangible reinforcer after every instance of stuttering); and delayed auditory feedback and use of masking noise.

◆ **CLUTTERING, ANOTHER DISORDER OF** fluency, includes rapid but disordered articulation, possibly combined with a high rate of dysfluencies and disorganized thought and language. Treatment of cluttering is similar to that of stuttering.

✎ **ADD YOUR OWN CHAPTER HIGHLIGHTS HERE:**

_____

_____

_____

_____

_____

Study & Review Questions

Essay

1. What do the terms *incidence* and *prevalence* mean? Describe.

2. Describe the various forms of dysfluencies (e.g., whole-word repetitions, interjections). Give examples of each.

3. Sometimes persons who stutter have associated motor behaviors and breathing abnormalities. List three associated motor behaviors and three breathing abnormalities that a stutterer might manifest.

4. Compare and contrast the stutter-more-fluently and the speak-more-fluently approaches to stuttering. How do they differ from one another?

5. Describe a direct stuttering reduction method. What is involved?

Multiple Choice

6. The position that stuttering indicates a social role conflict was taken by:

   A. Van Riper   D. Bloodstein
   B. Wischner   E. Brutten and Shoemaker
   C. Sheehan

7. Research on the prevalence of stuttering has shown that:

   A. familial incidence is higher than in the general population.
   B. sons of stuttering mothers run a greater risk than sons of stuttering fathers.
   C. blood relatives of a stuttering woman run a greater risk of stuttering themselves than those of a stuttering man.
   D. all of the above
   E. A, C

8. Stuttering in preschool children is more likely on:

   A. content words.   D. vowels.
   B. function words.   E. consonant clusters.
   C. final words in a sentence.

9. Facts about stuttering adaptation include:

CX

    A. The greatest reduction in stuttering occurs only on the seventh reading.

    B. There is transfer from one passage to the other.

    C. Most of the reduction in stuttering occurs by the fifth reading.

    (D.) A higher magnitude of adaptation occurs with an increased time interval between readings.

    E. Most people who stutter do not show the adaptation effect.

10. Brutten and Shoemaker proposed that:

X

D

    (A.) stuttering is limited to part-word repetitions and sound prolongations.

    B. stuttering is due to classically conditioned negative emotion.

    C. some dysfluencies are operantly conditioned.

    D. all of the above

    E. B, C

11. Bloodstein believes that stuttering may be caused by:

X

A

    A. any belief that speech is a difficult task, resulting in tension and speech fragmentation.

    B. parental diagnosis of stuttering in normally fluent children.

    (C.) demands exceeding a child's capacities for fluency.

    D. an approach-avoidance conflict.

    E. an emotionally traumatic experience in childhood.

12. The fluent-stuttering treatment:

    A. aims for reduced abnormality of stuttering.

    B. aims for normally fluent speech.

    C. was developed by Van Riper.

    D. all of the above

    (E.) A, C

13. Cancellations, pull-outs, and preparatory sets are taught in:

X

X

    A. the fluent-stuttering approach.

    (B.) the fluency-shaping approach.

    C. approach-avoidance reduction treatment.

    D. none of the above

    E. all of the above

14. Such skills as airflow management, gentle phonatory onset, and reduced rate of speech are targets in:

    A. the fluent-stuttering technique.

    (B.) the fluency-shaping technique.

    C. counseling to reduce psychological conflicts.

    D. all of the above

    E. B, C

15. A mother calls a clinician and shares concerns about her child's speech. According to the mother, her daughter, Rachel, is difficult to understand. The mother describes Rachel's speech as "sort of rushed, and she kind of stutters sometimes." When the clinician tests Rachel, he concludes that Rachel is a clutterer. Based upon this diagnosis, one would expect to see that Rachel:

A. is probably secretly very anxious about her speech and has a rapid rate of speech, but is intelligible.
B. is dysfluent but has clear articulation and no spoonerisms.
C. has excellent language skills and is not anxious about her speech, and is highly dysfluent with no articulation problems.
D. has a lack of anxiety or concern about her speech, uses spoonerisms, and has rapid, disordered articulation resulting in unintelligible speech.
E. has disorganized thought and language, little dysfluency, and poor intelligibility.

16. When the speech-language pathologist provides treatment for Rachel to help her become more intelligible, which techiques would probably be ideal for her?

A. Reducing Rachel's rate of speech, and increasing her awareness of her speech through audiotapes or videotapes
B. Reducing Rachel's rate of speech, but not increasing her awareness of her speech through audiotapes or videotapes because this could create self-consciousness, which could make the cluttering worse
C. Helping Rachel maintain a rapid rate of speech, but working on increasing her intelligibility through emphasizing the final consonants of words
D. Probing to see if Rachel has negative emotions (that her mother is unaware of) about her speech and spending most of therapy time helping Rachel deal with these emotions
E. Helping Rachel learn to use cancellations, pullouts, and easy onset of phonation

17. The theory that stuttering is caused by lack of a unilateral dominant hemisphere is the:

A. stuttering as psychoneurosis theory.
B. approach-avoidance theory.
C. diagnosogenic theory.
D. hemispheric domination theory.
E. cerebral dominance theory.

18. A researcher wants to study the occurrence of stuttering in a given city. She wants to know how many adults and children in Middletown city have officially been diagnosed as stutterers. The researcher does not necessarily want to give a predictive statement; rather, she just wants to know the number of individuals in Middletown who stutter. The researcher wants to study the _____ of stuttering.

A. incidence   D. population statistics
B. prevalence   E. none of the above
C. current sample

19. A 5-year-old child, Marcus, has been identified as needing treatment because he is a true stutterer. His parents share that he has been stuttering since he was 3 years old, and the stuttering has become worse. Now children tease him, and Marcus's parents are concerned that as he enters kindergarten, the teasing will become worse. The clinician decides to use the direct stuttering reduction method with Marcus. This method will involve which techniques?

A. delayed auditory feedback, response cost, and slowed speech
B. masking, response cost, and time-out
C. response cost, GILCU, and time-out
D. reduced rate of speech, airflow management, and GILCU
E. syllable prolongation, easy onset of phonation, and response cost

20. A 32-year-old man, Frank G., wants to go to law school. He is very bright, but has been working in minimum-wage jobs where he does not have to do much talking. Frank shares that he has passed the entrance examination to get into law school, but he is afraid to enroll in classes. He feels frustrated by his dilemma, and shares that he is experiencing a great deal of anxiety about his situation. The clinician decides to use the stutter-more-fluently approach. This would involve:

A. not discussing Frank's feelings and attitudes, but rather teaching and establishing skills such as airflow management, reduced rate, and easy onset of phonation.

B. encouraging Frank to discuss his feelings and attitudes about his stuttering, desensitizing Frank to his stuttering, and using procedures such as time out and response cost.

C. using DAF, masking, and procedures such as time-out and response cost.

D. using time-out, response cost, DAF, and allowing Frank to discuss his feelings and attitudes toward his stuttering.

E. allowing Frank to discuss his feelings and attitudes toward his situation, desensitizing Frank to his stuttering, and helping Frank to modify his stuttering through the use of such techniques as cancellations and pullouts.

REFERENCES AND RECOMMENDED READINGS

Andrews, G., & Cutler, J. (1974). Stuttering therapy: The relation between changes in symptom level and attitudes. *Journal of Speech and Hearing Disorders, 39,* 312–319.

Andrews, G., & Harris, M. (1964). The syndrome of stuttering. *Clinics in developmental medicine, 17.* London: Heinemann.

Bloodstein, O. (1995). *A handbook on stuttering* (5th ed.). San Diego, CA: Singular Publishing Group.

Bothe, A. K. (Ed.) (2004). *Evidence-based treatment of stuttering: Empirical bases and clinical applications.* Mahwah, NJ: Lawrence Erlbaum Associates.

Brutten, G. J., & Shoemaker, D. J. (1967). *The modification of stuttering.* Englewood Cliffs, NJ: Prentice-Hall.

Brutten, G. J., & Vanryckeghem, M. (2001). Behavior Assessment Battery: A research pathway.*Journal of Fluency Disorders, 26,* 349-352.

Conture, E. G. (2001). *Stuttering: Its nature, diagnosis, and treatment.* Boston: Allyn & Bacon.

Cooper, E. B., & Cooper, C. S. (1998). Multicultural considerations in the assessment and treatment of stuttering. In D. E. Battle (Ed.), *Communication disorders in multicultural populations* (2nd ed., pp. 247–274). Newton, MA: Butterworth-Heinemann.

Culatta, R., & Goldberg, S. A. (1995). *Stuttering therapy: An integrated approach to theory and practice.* Needham Heights, MA: Allyn and Bacon.

Curlee, R. F. (1999). *Stuttering and related disorders of fluency* (2nd ed.). New York: Thieme.

Curlee, R. F., & Siegel, G. M. (Eds.). (1997). *Nature and treatment of stuttering: New directions* (2nd ed.). Needham, MA: Allyn and Bacon.

Gregory, H. H., Campbell, J., Gregory, C. B., & Hill, D. G. (2003). *Stuttering therapy: Rationale and procedures.* Boston: Allyn & Bacon.

Guitar, B. (1998). *Stuttering: An integrated approach to its nature and treatment* (2nd ed.). Baltimore: Williams & Wilkins.

Hegde, M. N. (2001a). *Pocketguide to assessment in speech–language pathology* (2nd ed.). San Diego, CA: Singular Publishing Group.

Hegde, M. N. (2001b). *Pocketguide to treatment in speech–language pathology* (2nd ed.). San Diego, CA: Singular Publishing Group.

Hegde, M. N. (2004). *Treating stuttering in young children: An experimental evaluation of response cost.* Paper presented at the Special Interest Division 4 (Fluency Disorders) Leadership Conference, Portland, OR.

Hegde, M. N., & Hartman, D. (1979a). Factors affecting judgments of fluency: I. Interjections. *Journal of Fluency Disorders, 4,* 1–11.

Hegde, M. N., & Hartman, D. (1979b). Factors affecting judgments of fluency: II. Word repetitions. *Journal of Fluency Disorders, 4,* 13–22.

Johnson, W., & Associates. (1959). *The onset of stuttering.* Minneapolis: University of Minnesota Press.

Myers, F. L., & St. Louis, K. O. (1992). *Cluttering: A clinical perspective.* Kibworth, England: Far Communications.

Onslow, M., Packman, A., & Harrison, E. (2001). The *Lidcombe program of early stuttering intervention.* Austin, TX: PRO-ED.

Shapiro, D. A. (1999). *Stuttering intervention.* Austin, TX: PRO-ED.

Sheehan, J. G. (1970). *Stuttering: Research and therapy.* New York: Harper & Row.

Silverman, F. H. (2004). *Stuttering and other fluency disorders* (3rd ed.). Long Grove, IL: Waveland Press.

St. Louis, K. O. (1986). *The atypical stutterer.* New York: Academic Press.

Starkweather, W., & Givens-Ackerman, J. (1997). *Stuttering.* Austin, TX: PRO-ED.

Van Riper, C. (1973). *The treatment of stuttering.* Englewood Cliffs, NJ: Prentice-Hall.

Van Riper, C. (1982). *The nature of stuttering.* Englewood Cliffs, NJ: Prentice-Hall.

Wall, M. J., & Myers, F. L. (1995). *Clinical management of childhood stuttering* (2nd ed.). Austin, TX: PRO-ED.

Wischner, G. J. (1950). Stuttering behavior and learning: A preliminary theoretical formulation. *Journal of Speech and Hearing Disorders, 15,* 324–335.

Yairi, E., & Ambrose, N. G. (2004). *Early childhood stuttering.* Austin, TX: PRO-ED.

Study & Review
Answers

6. C. The position that stuttering indicates a social role conflict was taken by Sheehan.

7. D. Research on the prevalence of stuttering has shown all of the above—that familial incidence is higher than in the general population, that sons of stuttering mothers run a greater risk than sons of stuttering fathers, and that blood relatives of a stuttering woman run a greater risk than those of a stuttering man.

8. B. Stuttering in preschool children is more likely on function words.

9. C. One fact about stuttering adaptation is that most of the reduction in stuttering occurs by the fifth reading.

10. D. Brutten and Shoemaker proposed all of the above—that stuttering is limited to part-word repetitions and sound prolongations, that stuttering is due to classically conditioned negative emotion, and that some dysfluencies are operantly conditioned.

11. A. Bloodstein suggests that stuttering may be caused by any belief that speech is a difficult task, resulting in tension and speech fragmentation.

12. E. The fluent-stuttering treatment aims for reduced abnormality of stuttering and was developed by Van Riper.

13. A. Cancellations, pull-outs, and preparatory sets are taught in the fluent-stuttering approach.

14. B. Such skills as airflow management, gentle phonatory onset, and reduced rate of speech are targets in the fluency-shaping technique.

15. D. Because Rachel is a clutterer, one would expect to see a lack of anxiety or concern about her speech, use of spoonerisms, and rapid, disordered articulation resulting in unintelligible speech.

16. A. Reducing Rachel's rate of speech, and increasing her awareness of her speech through audiotapes or videotapes is the best method of helping her become more intelligible.

17. E. The theory that stuttering is caused by lack of a unilateral dominant hemisphere is the cerebral dominance theory.

18. B. When one wants a headcount or to establish the number of individuals who currently have a particular disorder, one is determining the prevalence of the disorder.

19. C. The direct stuttering reduction method uses response cost, GILCU, and time-out procedures.

20. E. The stutter-more-fluently approach of Van Riper would involve allowing Frank to discuss his feelings and attitudes toward his situation, desensitizing Frank to his stuttering, and helping Frank to modify his stuttering through the use of such techniques as cancellations and pull-outs.

CHAPTER **7**

VOICE AND

ITS DISORDERS

The area of voice and its disorders is becoming a topic of greater interest to communicative disorders professionals and members of the public alike. Society is increasingly recognizing the value of a clear, professional-sounding, and pleasing voice for optimal communication. Communicative disorders professionals, due to more sophisticated instrumentation, are learning more about how to treat voice disorders and help patients achieve maximally competent voice production. In this chapter, we discuss normal aspects of voice, evaluation of voice disorders, disorders of resonation, disorders of phonation, and aspects of treatment.

VOCAL ANATOMY AND PHYSIOLOGY

INTRODUCTION

Optimal voice production is based upon intact anatomy and physiology of the larynx and surrounding structures. The human voice undergoes certain changes throughout the life span; between birth and death, everyone experiences vocal changes. In this section, the topics of laryngeal anatomy and physiology and voice changes through the life span are discussed. (*Note:* Chapter 1 contains more detailed information about laryngeal anatomy and physiology and the neurological mechanisms that control vocalization. These concepts are briefly reviewed in this chapter.)

The Larynx

Basic Principles

- The larynx is a biological valve located at the top of the trachea. It helps close the entry into the trachea so food, liquids, and other particles do not enter the lungs. The larynx connects superiorly to the oral cavity and vocal tract and inferiorly to the lungs and trachea.

- The larynx builds air pressure below it to assist in the performance of biological functions such as getting rid of body wastes, coughing, doing heavy lifting, and child bearing.
- The larynx houses the vocal folds, which vibrate to produce voice. The vocal folds *adduct* (move toward the midline) or *abduct* (move away from the midline). The opening between the vocal folds is called the *glottis.*
- The vocal folds have a layered structure that is composed of the epithelium, the thyroarytenoid (TA) muscle, and the lamina propria (see Chapter 1). According to the *cover-body theory of phonation,* the epithelium, the superficial layer of the lamina propria, and much of the intermediate layer of the lamina propria vibrate as a "cover" on a relatively stationary "body." This body is composed of the remainder of the intermediate layer, the deep layer, and the TA muscle (Hirano, 1977, as cited in Malmgren & Glaze, 2004).
- The *ventricular* or *false* vocal folds lie above the "true" vocal folds described above. They do not usually vibrate during normal phonation and are used only during activities such as lifting and coughing.
- The *aryepiglottic folds* lie above the ventricular folds. They separate the pharynx and the laryngeal vestibule and help preserve the airway.
- *Cranial nerve VII* innervates the posterior belly of the digastric muscle of the vocal folds. The primary cranial nerve involved in laryngeal innervation is *Cranial nerve X* (vagus nerve). The primary branches of the vagus nerve that innervate the larynx are the superior laryngeal nerve (SLN) and the recurrent laryngeal nerve (RLN).
- The *superior laryngeal nerve* has internal and external branches. The internal branch provides all sensory information to the larynx, and the external branch supplies motor innervation solely to the cricothyroid muscle.
- The *recurrent laryngeal nerve* supplies all motor innervation to the interarytenoid, posterior cricoarytenoid, thyroarytenoid, and lateral cricoarytenoid muscles. It supplies all sensory information below the vocal folds. If there is a lesion of the recurrent laryngeal nerve, the patient may experience (among other problems) difficulty adducting the vocal folds (Boone, McFarlane, & von Berg, 2005).
- In terms of vascular supply of the larynx, the three primary "feeding" arteries are the superior laryngeal, cricothyroid, and inferior laryngeal arteries. The superior laryngeal and cricothyroid arteries are usually branches of the superior thyroid artery, which is part of the external carotid artery (Lyon & Barkmeier-Kraemer, 2004).

Key Structures and Cartilages

Hyoid Bone

- The larynx is suspended from the hyoid bone. Many extrinsic laryngeal muscles are attached to the hyoid bone. Figure 7.1 illustrates the hyoid bone in relation to other key laryngeal structures.

Epiglottis

- This leaf-shaped cartilage is attached to the hyoid bone.
- The epiglottis protects the trachea by closing down inferiorly and posteriorly over the laryngeal area, directing liquids and food into the esophagus during swallowing.

Thyroid Cartilage

- The largest of all the laryngeal cartilages, the thyroid cartilage is sometimes called the *Adam's*

Figure 7.1. A front and back view of key laryngeal structures. *Note.* From *Introduction to Communicative Disorders*, 3rd ed. (p. 233), by M. N. Hegde, 2001, Austin, TX: PRO-ED. Copyright 2001 by PRO-ED, Inc. Reprinted with permission.

apple. It is particularly prominent in men. The thyroid cartilage shields other laryngeal structures from damage.

- The thyroid cartilage is composed of two lamina, or plates of cartilage, that are joined at midline and form an angle. Figure 7.2 shows the thyroid cartilage and its relation to the vocal folds.

Cricoid Cartilage

- This is the second-largest laryngeal cartilage and is sometimes called the uppermost tracheal ring (however, it is quite different from the other tracheal rings).
- The cricoid cartilage completely surrounds the trachea. It is linked with the paired arytenoid cartilages and the thyroid cartilage.

Arytenoid Cartilages

- The arytenoid cartilages are positioned on the supraposterior surface of the cricoid cartilage on either side of the midline.
- The arytenoid cartilages are shaped like pyramids. The *vocal processes* are the most anterior angle of the base of the arytenoids; the true vocal folds attach at the vocal processes.

Corniculate Cartilages

- The corniculate cartilages sit on the apex of the arytenoids and are small and cone-shaped.
- They play a minor role in vocalization.

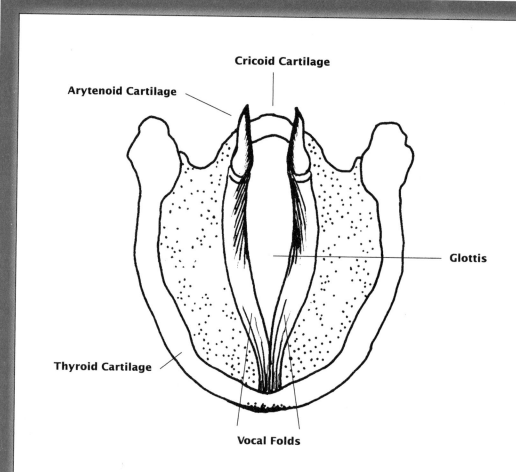

Figure 7.2. The thyroid cartilage and surrounding structures. *Note.* From *Introduction to Communicative Disorders,* 2nd ed. (p. 233), by M. N. Hegde, 2001, Austin, TX: PRO-ED. Copyright 2001 by PRO-ED, Inc. Reprinted with permission.

Cuneiform Cartilages

- The cuneiform cartilages are tiny, cone-shaped cartilage pieces under the mucous membrane that covers the aryepiglottic folds.
- They play a very minor role in the phonatory functions of the larynx.

Intrinsic Laryngeal Muscles

- These pairs of muscles have both of their attachments to structures within the larynx (see Figure 7.3). With one exception, all are adductors. The intrinsic laryngeal muscles are primarily responsible for controlling vocalization.
- The sets of intrinsic laryngeal muscles are:

    - thyroarytenoids
    - cricothyroids
    - posterior cricoarytenoids (the only abductors)
    - lateral cricoarytenoids

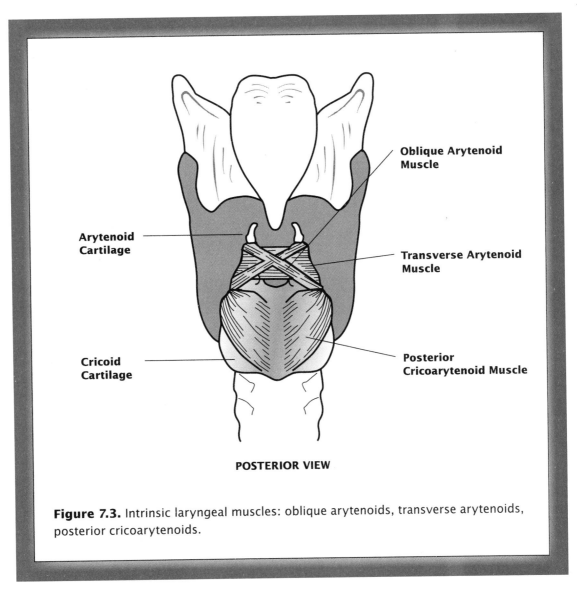

Figure 7.3. Intrinsic laryngeal muscles: oblique arytenoids, transverse arytenoids, posterior cricoarytenoids.

- transverse arytenoids
- oblique arytenoids

Extrinsic Laryngeal Muscles

- These muscles have one attachment to a structure outside the larynx and one attachment to a structure within the larynx. All extrinsic laryngeal muscles are attached to the hyoid bone.
- These muscles elevate or lower the position of the larynx in the neck. They give the larynx fixed support.
- The *infrahyoid* laryngeal muscles lie below the hyoid bone; their primary function is to depress the larynx. They are sometimes called the *depressors*. They have a strong impact upon vocal pitch. The infrahyoid muscles are listed below (one can remember them by the acronym TOSS):

  - thyrohyoids
  - omohyoids

- sternothyroids
- sternohyoids

- *The suprahyoid* laryngeal muscles lie above the hyoid bone; their primary function is to elevate the larynx. They are sometimes called *elevators*. The suprahyoid muscles are:

  - digastrics
  - geniohyoids
  - mylohyoids
  - stylohyoids
  - genioglossus
  - hyoglossus

CONCEPTS TO CONSIDER

List and briefly describe two key laryngeal cartilages, two sets of intrinsic laryngeal muscles, and two sets of extrinsic laryngeal muscles.

_____

_____

_____

_____

_____

Voice Changes Through the Life Span

Infancy Through Adolescence

Mean Fundamental Frequency (MFF)

- There is a gradual and discernible decline in MFF from birth on. As people grow older, their voices become lower in pitch with some gender differences in old age.
- Most studies suggest that boys' and girls' voices are similar before adolescence. During adolescence, changes in pitch become noticeable.
- The MFF of 7- and 8-year-old children ranges from 281 to 297 Hz. The MFF of 10- and 11-year-old children ranges from 238 to 270 Hz.
- Nineteen-year-old females have an MFF of 217 Hz; nineteen-year-old males have an MFF of 117 Hz.

Maximum Phonation Time (MPT)

- This refers to a client's ability to sustain "ah." Usually, the client is asked to breathe deeply and "say ah for as long as you can."
- Three- and 4-year-old children have an MPT ranging from 7.50 to 8.95 seconds. Five- to 12-year-old children have an MPT ranging from 14.97 to 17.74 seconds.

Changes Resulting from Puberty

- Girls' voices may lower by 3–4 semitones.
- Boys' voices may lower by as much as an octave. Boys may show pitch breaks, huskiness, and hoarseness as their pitch lowers due to laryngeal growth.

Adulthood

- Men have an MFF of 100–150 Hz. The typical fundamental frequency for men is approximately 125 Hz. Women have an MFF of 180–250 Hz, and the average fundamental frequency for women is approximately 225 Hz (Boone et al., 2005).
- Adults aged 18–39 have an MPT ranging from 20.90 to 24.60 seconds.

The Geriatric Voice

- Females 70–94 years old have an MFF of 201 Hz; males 70–89 years old have an MFF that ranges from 132 to 146 Hz.
- Adults aged 66–93 years have an MPT ranging from 14.20 to 18.10 seconds.
- It is difficult to make generalizations about the geriatric voice because an older person's vocal quality and overall health are significantly related to whether or not the person has a disease (e.g., Parkinson's disease) or is disease-free. However, several generalizations can be made (Boone et al., 2005).
- A person's fundamental frequency appears to lower with each successive decade of life through 50 years of age. A female's voice continues to lower in fundamental frequency as long as she lives, whereas a male's fundamental frequency begins to get slightly higher in the sixties and in every decade after that.
- Some older people speak more slowly and with decreased loudness. The decreased loudness may be related to increases in breathiness (Linville, 2002).

SUMMARY

✓ The larynx is used as a biological valve for helping humans perform certain functions. It also houses the vocal folds, which vibrate to produce voicing.

✓ Key structures in the laryngeal area include the hyoid bone, epiglottis, thyroid cartilage, cricoid cartilage, arytenoid cartilages, corniculate cartilages, and cuneiform cartilages. There are two groups of laryngeal muscles: the intrinsic and the extrinsic laryngeal muscles.

✓ There are three sets of vocal folds: the aryepiglottic folds, the ventricular or false vocal folds, and the true vocal folds, which vibrate to produce voice.

✓ Cranial nerve X, with its superior and recurrent laryngeal nerve branches, which innervate the larynx, is the key cranial nerve in laryngeal function.

✓ The voice changes throughout the life span. Mean fundamental frequency declines from birth on, with more dramatic changes for the male in adolescence. Older males and females differ in fundamental frequency changes. Maximum phonation time grows greater between childhood and adulthood. It usually decreases as people age.

VOCAL PITCH, VOLUME, AND QUALITY

INTRODUCTION

Pitch, volume, and quality are important characteristics of the voice. People's personality, intelligence, and competence are often judged by these parameters. Voice disorders tend to affect vocal pitch, volume, and quality. Experienced clinicians listen for disturbances in these aspects of voice when evaluating clients with voice disorders.

Pitch

■ The perceptual correlate of frequency, pitch is largely based on the frequency with which the vocal folds vibrate. This rate is often described as the *fundamental frequency*. Fundamental frequency is generally considered an individual's habitual or typical pitch.

■ Pitch is determined by mass, tension, and elasticity of the vocal folds. Higher pitch results when the vocal folds are thinner, more tense, or both; lower pitch results when the folds are thicker, more relaxed, or both.

■ *Frequency perturbation*, or *jitter*, refers to variations in vocal frequency that are often heard in dysphonic patients. Jitter can be measured instrumentally as a patient sustains a vowel. Patients with voice problems such as tremor or hoarseness might show a large amount of jitter. People with no laryngeal pathology are able to sustain a vowel with less than 1% jitter (Case, 2002).

Volume

■ The perceptual correlate of intensity, volume, or loudness, is determined by the intensity of the sound signal; the more intense the sound signal, the greater its perceived loudness.

■ The sound is a disturbance in air particles; it takes the form of waves that move forward and backward in a medium such as air or water. The extent of such movements is amplitude. The greater the *amplitude*, the louder the voice.

■ *Amplitude perturbation*, or *shimmer*, refers to the cycle-to-cycle variation of vocal intensity. It can be measured instrumentally as a patient sustains a vowel. A speaker with no laryngeal pathology should have a very small amount of variation of intensity with each vibratory cycle. Some experts (e.g., Case, 2002) believe that more than 1 dB of variation across cycles makes a patient sound dysphonic. Patients who have difficulties with regularity of vocal fold vibration (e.g., roughness) might show large amounts of shimmer.

■ Measures of shimmer and jitter are becoming more common because they can be useful in early detection of vocal pathology. Laryngologists may ask speech–language pathologists to obtain these measures because they can help to detect vocal pathology even when the laryngologist sees no obvious tissue or lesion change (Haynes & Pindzola, 2004).

Quality

Definition

Voice quality is the perceptual correlate of complexity. It refers to the physical complexity of the laryngeal tone, which is modified by the resonating cavities (Aronson, 1990). The determination of voice quality is frequently subjective.

Types of Vocal Quality

Hoarseness

- The voice shows a combination of breathiness and harshness, which results from irregular vocal fold vibrations. In such cases, the fundamental frequency of the speaker varies randomly due to aperiodic vibration.
- Hoarse voices often sound breathy, low-pitched, and husky. There may also be pitch breaks and excessive throat clearing.

Harshness

- The voice is described as rough, unpleasant, and "gravelly" sounding. It is associated with excessive muscular tension and effort. The vocal folds are adducted too tightly, and the air is then released too abruptly.

Strain-Strangle

- Phonation is effortful, and the patient sounds as if she is "squeezing" the voice at the glottal level. Initiating and sustaining phonation are both difficult.
- Talking fatigues patients, and they experience much tension when they speak.

Breathiness

- The breathy voice results from the vocal folds being slightly open, or not firmly approximated, during phonation. Air escapes through the glottis and adds noise to the sound produced by the vocal folds (see Figure 7.4).
- Breathiness may be due to *organic* (physical) or *nonorganic* (nonphysical, or *functional*) causes. Patients often complain that they feel like they are running out of air.
- Breathy voices are often soft, with little variation in loudness. Patients frequently show restricted vocal range.

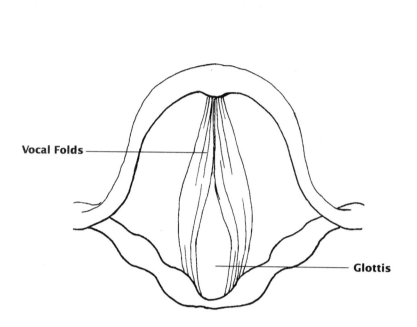

Figure 7.4. Partially open vocal folds, allowing air to escape through the open glottis and create a breathy voice. *Note.* From *Introduction to Communicative Disorders,* 3rd ed. (p. 236), by M. N. Hegde, 2001, Austin, TX: PRO-ED. Copyright 2001 by PRO-ED, Inc. Reprinted with permission.

Glottal Fry

- Also called *vocal fry,* glottal fry is heard when the vocal folds vibrate very slowly. The resultant sound occurs in slow but discrete bursts and is of extremely low pitch. The voice sounds "crackly."
- Vocal fry may be the vibratory cycle we use near the bottom of our normal pitch range. Typically, it is produced near the end of a long phrase or sentence when air flow rate and subglottal air pressure are both low and lung volume is less.
- For some patients, use of vocal fry may help modify vocal quality problems such as stridency. Other patients work to eliminate vocal fry by slightly increasing subglottal air pressure and slightly elevating their pitch level (Boone et al., 2005).

Diplophonia

- This means "double voice." It occurs when one can simultaneously perceive two distinct pitches during phonation.

- Diplophonia usually occurs when the vocal folds vibrate at different frequencies due to differing degrees of mass or tension. A client with a unilateral polyp, for example, might sound diplophonic.

Stridency

- A patient with a strident voice sounds shrill, unpleasant, somewhat high pitched, and "tinny."
- Physiologically, stridency is often caused by hypertonicity or tension of the pharyngeal constrictors and elevation of the larynx. Tense patients may sound strident.

SUMMARY

✓ Pitch (the perceptual correlate of frequency) and volume (the perceptual correlate of intensity) are important vocal parameters that clinicians must evaluate in all voice patients. Measures of jitter and shimmer can be helpful in evaluating the dysphonic patient.

✓ Vocal quality, the perceptual correlate of complexity, is often affected by pathological changes of the laryngeal mechanism. Patients can manifest such vocal qualities as hoarseness, harshness, strain-strangle, breathiness, glottal fry, diplophonia, and stridency.

✓ Experienced clinicians evaluate patients' pitch, volume, and quality in making a determination of whether a voice disorder exists.

EVALUATION OF VOICE DISORDERS

INTRODUCTION

A thorough voice evaluation is critical to creating an individualized, successful treatment program. When conducting evaluations, clinicians must remember to carry out a thorough oral peripheral examination, a hearing screening, and collect a speech–language sample. Gathering a complete case history is important. A team-oriented approach to evaluation is always necessary; the team may consist of specialists from medicine, education, and professional voice pedagogy. Clinicians, depending upon their settings and the availability of technology, use both instrumental and perceptual tools to evaluate patients' voices.

Case History: Purposes and Goals

The clinician needs to:

- Obtain information about variables such as onset, duration, causes, and variability of the voice problem. Ask for the perceptions of the patient as well as significant others about these variables.

- Obtain information about any associated symptoms or problems such as slurring of speech, difficulty swallowing, excessive coughing, and others.

- Identify factors (e.g., health, environment, family history) that might be contributing to the problem.

■ Gather information regarding previous therapy, medical intervention, or other attempts to deal with the voice problem.

■ Obtain patient and significant others' descriptions of daily vocal use and possible abuse or misuse patterns.

■ For culturally and linguistically diverse clients, obtain their specific perceptions of what constitutes a "normal-sounding" voice in their particular culture (DeJarnette & Holland, 1998).

A Team-Oriented Approach

■ A multidisciplinary, team-oriented approach is critical to a thorough evaluation. Before beginning therapy, it is always necessary to obtain a medical evaluation of the vocal mechanism; this is performed by an otolaryngologist. In some cases, it may also be necessary to refer the patient to a neurologist before treatment is initiated.

■ The team always includes the speech–language pathologist, but teams may be oriented differently, as follows, for example (Andrews, 1999; Rubin, Sataloff, & Korovin, 2003):

- A *medical team* would consist of a general practitioner, neurologist, otolaryngologist, radiologist, orthodontist, social worker, psychiatrist or psychologist, pulmonary specialist, and gastroenterologist.
- An *educationally oriented team* would consist of a classroom teacher, school nurse, school psychologist, and counselor.
- A *team oriented toward professional voice users* could consist of voice scientists, psychologists, and vocal pedagogy teachers such as singing and vocal coaches.

Instrumental Evaluation

■ All forms of instrumental evaluation are used to view the vocal folds. Instrumentation is increasingly being used to provide an objective, data-based description of the dysphonic patient's vocal characteristics (Kent & Ball, 2000). A description of each type of evaluation follows.

Indirect Laryngoscopy (Mirror Laryngoscopy)

- The specialist uses a bright light source and a small, round, 21–25 mm mirror, angled on a long, slender handle, to lift the velum and press gently against the patient's posterior pharyngeal wall area.
- The specialist maneuvers the mirror to view the laryngeal structures during phonation (usually the patient's production of "eeeee") and during quiet respiration. Figure 7.5 shows a patient undergoing indirect laryngoscopy.

Direct Laryngoscopy

- This procedure is performed by a surgeon when the patient is under general anesthesia in outpatient surgery. The laryngoscope is introduced through the mouth into the pharynx and positioned above the vocal folds.

Figure 7.5. Indirect laryngoscopy. *Note.* From *Clinical Management of Voice Disorders,* 4th ed. (p. 48), by J. L. Case, 2002, Austin, TX: PRO-ED. Copyright 2002 by PRO-ED, Inc. Reprinted with permission.

- The patient cannot phonate, thus vocal function cannot be determined. However, the surgeon can obtain a direct microscopic view of the larynx.
- Direct laryngoscopy is valuable when a biopsy is required due to the suspicion of laryngeal cancer.

Flexible Fiber-Optic Laryngoscopy

- This procedure utilizes a thin, flexible tube containing a lens and fiberoptic light bundles.
- The specialist inserts the tube through the patient's nasal passage, passes it over the velum, and maneuvers it into position above the larynx. The fibers transmit the laryngeal image to the specialist's eyepiece.
- The patient is able to speak and sing. The specialist can obtain an excellent, prolonged view of the vocal mechanism and photograph rapid vocal fold movement.

Endoscopy

- There are two kinds of endoscopes: *flexible* and *rigid*. The rigid endoscope is introduced orally; the flexible endoscope is introduced nasally, using a 3.6 mm tube (see Figure 7.6).
- There is a light at the tip of the scope; this light is fiber optic and comes from an external light source.
- The structures are illuminated by the light and viewed by the specialist at the other end of the endoscope through a window lens.
- The endoscope can be attached to a videocamera (*videoendoscopy*). A stroboscopic (*flashing*) light source can also be used.
- With the flexible endoscope, the specialist can view the velopharyngeal mechanism, including velopharyngeal valving. The endoscope (also called a nasopharyngoscope) can be lowered further to view the laryngeal mechanism (see Figure 7.7).
- Because the patient can perform a variety of phonatory tasks, endoscopy may be used to study laryngeal anatomy and physiology in detail, including the mucosal wave.

Figure 7.6. Flexible fiber-optic endoscopy. *Note.* From *Clinical Management of Voice Disorders*, 4th ed. (p. 50), by J. L. Case, 2002, Austin, TX: PRO-ED. Copyright 2002 by PRO-ED, Inc. Reprinted with permission.

Figure 7.7. Model showing placement of nasopharyngolaryngoscope. *Note.* From *Clinical Management of Voice Disorders,* 4th ed. (p. 50), by J. L. Case, 2002, Austin, TX: PRO-ED. Copyright 2002 by PRO-ED, Inc. Reprinted with permission.

Spectrograph

- The sound or speech spectrograph is extremely useful for quantitative analysis of speech. Kay Elemetrics Corporation has a Digital Sona-Graph 5500, which is a DC-16 kHz Spectrum Analyzer. It produces waveform displays of amplitude and frequency, spectrograms, and other analysis displays in real time.
- The Sona-Graph's memory can store up to two megabytes of sampled data; this translates to approximately 50 seconds of speech sampled at 20 kHz. These same analyses can also be made on the Computer Speech Laboratory (CSL; also made by Kay Elemetrics).
- Clinicians can use the above-described instruments to obtain baseline measurements prior to therapy or surgery. Post-therapy or -surgery measurements may be obtained and compared to the baseline measurements of a patient's voice to quantitatively document vocal improvement or decline (Case, 2002).

Videostroboscopy

- Videostroboscopy can be helpful in differentiating between functional and organic voice problems. It can also be used to detect laryngeal neoplasms (tumors) (Bless & Poburka, 2002).
- The specialist can perform videostroboscopy by using a flexible fiber-optic laryngoscope, a rigid endoscope, or both.
- The strobe light is a pulsing light that permits the optical illusion of slow-motion viewing of the vocal folds during a variety of tasks. The observer perceives the rapidly presented images as a complete picture of cycle-to-cycle vibration (vibratory pattern of phonation).
- The specialist places a microphone on the patient's neck along the thyroid cartilage to record the voice signal. Then he introduces the scope, switches on the stroboscopic light, and asks the

patient to phonate.
- The resulting image on the monitor screen is projected through optic devices such as a camera lens, an endoscope, and pixels on the monitor screen.
- The stroboscopic image yields information about the periodicity or regularity of vocal fold vibrations, vocal fold amplitude (horizontal excursion), glottal closure, presence and adequacy of the mucosal wave, and the possible presence of lesions or neoplasms.

Electroglottography (EGG)

- This noninvasive procedure yields an indirect measure of vocal fold closure patterns.
- Surface electrodes are placed on both sides of the thyroid cartilage, and a high-frequency electric current is passed between the electrodes while the patient phonates. The laryngeal and neck tissue conducts the current.
- A glottal wave form results, and the specialist is able to observe vocal fold vibration. EGG can also detect breathy and abrupt glottal onset of phonation.
- Researchers and practitioners disagree about the efficacy of EGG as a diagnostic technique; many variables can impact its accuracy. It is currently recommended as a cross-validation tool with other measures of vocal fold functioning.

Electromyography (EMG)

- This invasive procedure directly measures laryngeal function to study the pattern of electrical activity of the vocal folds and to view muscle activity patterns.
- The specialist inserts needle electrodes into the patient's peripheral laryngeal muscles; the resulting electrical signals are judged as either normal or indicative of pathology.
- When the specialist interprets the electrical signals, she is looking for: (a) reduced or increased speed of muscle activation, (b) extraneous bursts of muscle activity, or (c) onset or termination of muscle activity.
- EMG is useful when attempting to determine vocal fold pathology, especially that caused by neurological and neuromuscular diseases. It is also useful in verifying excessive muscle activity prior to the injection of BOTOX (botulinus toxin; described later) for patients with spasmodic dysphonia.

Aerodynamic Measurements

- Aerodynamic measurements refer to the airflows, air volumes, and average air pressures produced as part of the peripheral mechanics of the respiratory, laryngeal, and supralaryngeal airways.
- Specialists use aerodynamic measurements to evaluate dysphonia, monitor voice changes and treatment progress, and differentiate between laryngeal and respiratory problems.
- Many specialists want to assess patients' lung volume because breath support for optimal voice may be lacking. Specific measures can be made of the following parameters:

  - *tidal volume* (amount of air inhaled and exhaled during a normal breathing cycle)
  - *vital capacity* (the volume of air that the patient can exhale after a maximal inhalation)
  - *total lung capacity* (total volume of air in the lungs)

- Various instruments may be used to obtain aerodynamic measurements. Some of the most common include *wet spirometers, dry spirometers, manometric devices,* and *plethysmographs.* (For further description of these forms of instrumentation, see Boone et al., 2005; Case, 2002; Kent & Ball, 2000.)

Describe two types of instrumental evaluation that might be appropriate for a patient with laryngeal lesions that might be indicative of laryngeal cancer.

_____

_____

_____

_____

_____

Pitch Measurements

- Many instruments can be used to measure pitch. One of the most popular is the *Visi-Pitch* (see Figure 7.8).

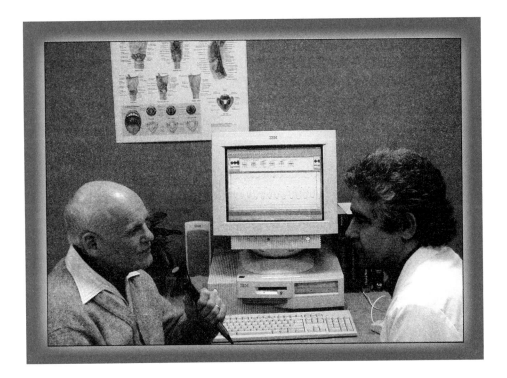

Figure 7.8. Visi-Pitch Voice Analyzer. *Note.* From *Clinical Management of Voice Disorders*, 4th ed. (p. 50), by J. L. Case, 2002, Austin, TX: PRO-ED. Copyright 2002 by PRO-ED, Inc. Reprinted with permission.

- To use it, the patient speaks into a microphone, and the Visi-Pitch displays his or her frequencies visually on a computer monitor. The Visi-Pitch can indicate the patient's frequency range, optimal pitch, and habitual pitch. It can also give a printout of these factors.
- The Visi-Pitch enjoys widespread use among clinicians because it is noninvasive and affordable, and it gives instant visual feedback to both clinician and patient. Printouts give documented, quantitative measurements of a patient's pitch characteristics.

Perceptual Evaluation

Basic Principles

- In perceptual voice evaluation, the clinician makes subjective judgments of many vocal parameters, including the patient's pitch, volume, vocal quality, resonance, respiration, and ability to sustain phonation.
- Many rating scales are available for making these judgments; Table 7.1 is an example of a scale that the clinician can use for making subjective judgments.

Pitch Assessment

- To assess pitch, clinicians make subjective judgments about the following:

    - the patient's habitual pitch, or typical conversational pitch;
    - whether the client is using optimal pitch (judged to be the most appropriate, comfortable pitch for that individual);
    - whether the pitch is appropriate to the client's gender and age, rather than too high or too low; and
    - whether the patient is *monopitched,* with lack of appropriate inflections as judged by members of his or her culture.

Loudness Assessment

- To assess loudness, clinicians make subjective judgments about the following:

    - parameters such as harshness, hoarseness, breathiness, and vocal tension;
    - whether the client's loudness is appropriate to daily situations; and
    - whether the client's voice is too soft or too loud due to possible physical factors (e.g., asthma, a hearing loss).

Resonance Assessment

- To assess resonance, clinicians subjectively judge the presence of:

    - *hyponasality* (when nasal resonance is absent on nasal sounds); and
    - *hypernasality* (when too much nasal resonance is present on non-nasal sounds).

Table 7.1 SUMMARY OF VOICE ASSESSMENT DATA USING A RATING SCALE

UNIVERSITY SPEECH AND HEARING CENTER

Client _____ Age _____ Sex _____

Clinician _____ Date/time _____

	Normal	Mild	Moderate	Severe	Profound

1. **Voice quality** — Breathy/Harsh/Hoarse — 1 2 3 (4) 5

The voice was judged hoarse on 90% of the utterances produced in conversational speech.

2. **Pitch** — Too high/Too low — 1 2 3 (4) 5

The client's pitch was judged too high on 80% of the utterances produced in conversational speech.

3. **Loudness** — Too loud/Too soft — 1 2 (3) 4 5

The client's voice was judged too loud during most of the assessment time.

4. **Nasal resonance** — Hypernasal/Hyponasal — 1 2 (3) 4 5

The client's voice was judged hypernasal on 45% of the utterances produced in conversational speech.

5. **Oral resonance** — Reduced oral resonance — 1 (2) 3 4 5

The client spoke with limited mouth opening; on most utterances, the oral resonance was reduced.

6. **Muscle tension** — Hypertense/Hypotense — 1 2 (3) 4 5

The client's muscles of the face, neck, and chest were judged hypertense during conversational speech.

7. **Abusive vocal behaviors** — 1 2 3 (4) 5

Client has a history of vocally abusive behaviors including loud and excessive talking, loud cheering at games, and screaming and yelling while playing with friends.

Comments and Recommendations: The client speaks with excessive muscular tension and effort; voice is excessively hoarse most of the time; there is a history of frequent and severe abusive vocal behaviors. Voice therapy is recommended to reduce the frequency and severity of such behaviors.

Note. The comments are for illustration only; a given client may not exhibit all the problems described. From *Introduction to Communicative Disorders,* 3rd ed. (p. 265) by M. N. Hegde, 2001, Austin, TX: PRO-ED. Copyright 2001 by PRO-ED, Inc. Reprinted with permission.

Respiration Assessment

- To assess respiration, many clinicians look for the following types of breathing:

  - *Clavicular breathing.* When the patient inhales, the shoulders elevate. Often there is strain and tension. Clavicular breathing is inefficient.
  - *Diaphragmatic-abdominal breathing.* This appropriate, efficient breathing utilizes the abdominal region and the lower thoracic cavity. There is little to no chest or shoulder movement. Diaphragmatic-abdominal breathing is ideal for professional voice users, including singers, teachers, and public speakers.
  - *Thoracic breathing.* The patient who uses thoracic breathing exhibits characteristics of both clavicular and diaphragmatic-abdominal breathing. There is no observable abdominal or upper thoracic expansion upon inspiration.

Phonation Assessment

- To assess a patient's ability to sustain phonation, clinicians use simple measures such as the following:

  - *Maximum phonation time (MPT).* As mentioned earlier, MPT is a measurement of the patient's ability to sustain phonation (e.g., "ah") during one exhalation. The clinician generally gives the patient three trials and compares the patient's MPT (in seconds) with norms. MPT enables the clinician to observe adequacy of respiration, glottal efficiency, and the possible presence of vocal pathology such as nodules.
  - *S/z ratio.* This procedure is used to help determine whether there is laryngeal pathology present. The patient is asked to produce two long /s/ phonemes, then two long /z/ phonemes. The clinician divides the longest /s/ by the longest /z/. An s/z ratio of more than 1.4 is indicative of possible laryngeal pathology.
  - For example, a patient may sustain /s/ for 15 seconds and /z/ for 9 seconds. This would yield an s/z ratio of 15/9, or 1.6, indicating possible laryngeal pathology.

SUMMARY

✓ A comprehensive, multidisciplinary team assessment of the voice patient is necessary as a foundation for appropriate treatment. A key component of assessment is a thorough case history.

✓ Instrumentation procedures that various specialists can use to assess a patient's voice include indirect or mirror laryngoscopy, direct laryngoscopy, flexible fiber-optic laryngoscopy, endoscopy (flexible or rigid), spectrogram, videostroboscopy, electroglottography, and electromyography. Instruments may also be used to obtain aerodynamic and pitch measurements.

✓ In a perceptual evaluation (which can occur alone or accompany instrumental evaluation), clinicians often use rating scales and informal tasks to assess pitch, loudness, vocal quality, resonance, respiration, and the ability to sustain phonation.

✓ Ideally, each patient is evaluated through a combination of measures that permit both qualitative and quantitative baseline measures and documentation of progress in voice therapy.

DISORDERS OF RESONANCE AND THEIR TREATMENT

INTRODUCTION

Resonance is the modification of sound by the structures through which the sound passes. The resonating structures that lie below and above the larynx (e.g., the oral and nasal cavities) modify the laryngeal tone. Voice disorders of resonance include an absence of a desired resonance, inadequate resonance, or inappropriate resonance. Appropriate resonance or lack thereof is based in part on cultural and linguistic norms. Among some cultural and linguistic groups (e.g., Americans living in the United States), there is little tolerance for hypernasality in conversational speech. Some Asians (speakers of Chinese, for example) may have slightly more hypernasality than Americans perceive as normal or desirable. Clinicians must always take patients' cultural and linguistic backgrounds into account when judging resonance.

Hypernasality

- Hypernasality is the most common resonance disorder presented by patients who come for services. A person who exhibits hypernasality, or excessive nasality, sounds like he or she is speaking through the nose.

- Hypernasality results when the velopharyngeal mechanism does not close the opening to the nasal passage during the production of non-nasal sounds. The air and sound escape through the nose, adding unnecessary nasal resonance to non-nasal speech sounds.

- Hypernasality can occur due to functional or organic factors. In the case of functional hypernasality, there is no physical reason for the hypernasality; the patient has made a habit of "talking through the nose." Functional nasality is often found in the speech of deaf people; they have adequate velopharyngeal mechanisms but are unable to monitor the sound of their own voices.

- Patients who are hypernasal due to organic factors have a physical problem that may need to be corrected surgically. *Cleft palate* is a major cause of hypernasality. Patients with inadequate cleft repairs are often severely hypernasal.

- *Velopharyngeal inadequacy* or *insufficiency (VPI)*, another cause of hypernasality, means that the velopharyngeal mechanism is inadequate to achieve closure; as a result, the nasal cavities are not sealed off appropriately from the oral cavity. According to Pannbacker (2004), the etiology of VPI is heterogeneous and may be neurological, structural, or learned. Major causes of VPI are (Nicolosi, Harryman, & Kresheck, 2004):

  - *Decreased muscle mass of the velum* (not enough velar tissue) to achieve closure.
  - *Adenoidectomy or tonsillectomy.* This occurs especially when a child's velo-pharyngeal mechanism initially did not have sufficient muscle mass. The adenoids and tonsils are masses that can help compensate for an otherwise inadequate velopharyngeal mechanism. When these masses are surgically removed, the basic velopharyngeal inadequacy may become apparent.
  - *Paresis (weakness) or paralysis of the velum,* which reduces its mobility so it is unable to assist in achieving adequate closure. Velar paresis and paralysis frequently occur secondarily to cerebral palsy, stroke, head injury, debilitative diseases such as Parkinson's disease, and other conditions of neuropathology.

- Assessment of hypernasality can include subjective, perceptual judgments as well as use of instrumentation such as the Nasometer (described later).

Hyponasality

- Hyponasality, or *denasality,* is a lack of appropriate nasal resonance on nasal sounds /m, n, ng/. Patients often substitute oral sounds for nasal sounds (e.g., "*b*aby" instead of "*m*aybe"). Frequent substitutions are b/m, d/n, and g/ng (Haynes & Pindzola, 2004).

- Hyponasality can be temporary, due to conditions such as colds and allergies. It can also occur due to obstructions in the nasal cavity (e.g., nasal polyps or papilloma), enlarged adenoids or tonsils, or a deviated septum. Hyponasal patients may be mouth breathers.

- Enlargement of the tonsils and adenoids is common in young children and can result in marked hyponasality. Hypertrophy of the tonsils and adenoids can block both the oropharyngeal and nasal pathways; in severe cases, sleep apnea can result. Assessment of the degree of obstruction may be performed using lateral X-ray studies of the nasopharyngeal area (Dworkin, Marunick, & Krouse, 2004).

- Assessment of hyponasality can include subjective, perceptual judgments as well as use of instrumentation such as the Nasometer (described later).

Assimilative Nasality

- Assimilative nasality occurs when the sound from a nasal consonant carries over to adjacent vowels. For example, in the word *ba__na__na*, the /ə/ and /æ/ sounds appear hypernasal because they are next to the nasal sound /n/.

- In assimilative nasality, the velar openings begin too soon and last too long, thus nasalizing vowels that occur next to nasal phonemes.

- Assimilative nasality can be functionally or organically based; assessment and treatment depend on etiology.

Cul-de-Sac Resonance

- *Cul-de-sac* (bottom of the sack) *resonance* is produced by backward retraction of the tongue; the tongue is carried too far posteriorly in the oral cavity.

- The oral cavity is partially closed at the back and open in the front. Because the tongue blocks some of the sound waves generated by the larynx from reaching the oral cavity, the perceptual result is distorted voice and resonance. The person's voice can sound muffled or hollow.

- Deaf people and those with neurological disorders often have difficulty making proper tongue adjustments, resulting in cul-de-sac resonance. People with no organic deviations also may acquire the habit of carrying the tongue too far back in the oral cavity while speaking. In addition, children with hypertrophied tonsils and adenoids may demonstrate cul-de-sac resonance.

CONCEPTS TO CONSIDER

Describe the differences between hypernasality and hyponasality. What are some causes of each?

_____

_____

_____

_____

_____

Treatment Principles

Medical Intervention

- It is always imperative, as a first step, to determine whether the disorders of resonance are due to functional or organic factors. Organically based resonance problems must be treated medically before therapy can be successful (Case, 2002).
- Medical treatment can take the form of surgery, prostheses, or both. For example, a child with a cleft palate may undergo surgery to repair the cleft and then be fitted with a prosthesis. (A more detailed description of medical intervention is presented in the section on craniofacial anomalies in Chapter 13.)

Treatment of Hypernasality

- Biofeedback can be effective in treating hypernasality. Electronic instruments instantaneously display the amount of oral and nasal resonance as the patient talks. Such visual displays give the patient immediate feedback.
- The *Nasometer,* an instrument created by Kay Elemetrics, allows the patient to receive visual feedback through a computer display. Feedback includes the target level of *nasalance* (oral–nasal ratio) and the amount of nasalance the patient is producing. The patient's productions can be shaped so they increasingly reflect an oral–nasal resonance balance that is within normal limits.
- Specific treatment techniques for hypernasality include:

  - employing *visual aids* such as a piece of tissue or a mirror, which can be put under a patient's nose so he or she can see appropriate vs. inappropriate nasal airflow during phonation;
  - *ear training,* or helping patients learn to monitor their own productions (instruments such

as the Nasometer and even a tape recorder [video or audio] are helpful);

- *increasing the patient's mouth opening* so that oral resonance is enhanced;
- *increasing the patient's loudness,* which can be accompanied by respiration training;
- *improving the patient's articulation,* which often results in the voice being perceived as less hypernasal; exaggerating consonants can contribute to a perception of less hypernasality;
- *changing the patient's speaking rate;* the clinician must first assess whether increasing or decreasing the rate decreases hypernasality; and
- *decreasing pitch,* which can contribute to greater oral resonance, especially if the patient's habitual pitch is too high.

Treatment of Hyponasality

- As with hypernasality, hyponasality can often be effectively treated through feedback such as that provided by the Nasometer and video or audio recordings.
- Specific techniques that can decrease hyponasality involve increasing the patient's awareness of the nasal cavity as a resonator. These techniques include:

  - *Focusing,* or directing of the tone into the facial "mask," which is the area above the maxillary sinuses and around the nasal bridge. The clinician demonstrates and then has the patient say words with nasal sounds (e.g., *moon, me*) in an exaggerated way. This produces vibrations in the mask. The patient is asked to feel the vibrations, focusing his or her attention in the mask area. Appropriate resonance is then shaped from that point of reference.
  - *Nasal-glide stimulation.* The clinician selects words with many glides and nasals (e.g., *lawnmower, many, manners, lemon*). The patient practices saying these words in various combinations. The combination of glides and nasals helps direct resonance more appropriately into the nasal cavity and gives the patient auditory and kinesthetic feedback about proper utilization of the nasal cavity.
  - *Visual aids.* A piece of tissue or a mirror may be put under the patient's nose so he or she can see appropriate vs. inappropriate nasal airflow during phonation.

SUMMARY

✓ Resonance is an important component of voice and must be evaluated as part of a thorough voice assessment. Difficulties with resonance include hypernasality, hyponasality, assimilative nasality, and cul-de-sac resonance.

✓ Treatment may include medical intervention if necessary; the patient with medical-physical needs will not progress until those needs are dealt with.

✓ When the clinician has ascertained that physical factors have been accounted for and treated appropriately, then he or she can use appropriate treatment techniques to help patients achieve optimal resonance patterns.

DISORDERS OF PHONATION AND THEIR TREATMENT

INTRODUCTION

Many disorders of phonation are associated with physical factors. Some patients have cancer of the larynx; others have progressive diseases of the central nervous system. Some patients present with pathological changes in the vocal folds due to vocally abusive habits, with consequent perceptual sequelae such as hoarseness, breathiness, harshness, and low pitch. In this section, we describe some of the major physical factors associated with voice disorders of phonation. Basic treatment principles are also discussed.

Carcinoma and Laryngectomy

Basic Principles

■ The larynx is one of the most common sites of cancer, accounting for approximately 1–2% of all cancers and 20% of all head and neck cancers (American Cancer Society, 2003). Laryngeal cancer is found more frequently in men than in women and is considered a multifactorial disease.

■ Alcohol, tobacco, exposure to environmental toxins (e.g., irradiation, asbestos), gastroesophageal reflux, and a combination of these cofactors all can contribute to laryngeal cancer.

■ Early warning signs of laryngeal cancer include hoarseness, difficulty swallowing, and pain in the laryngeal area. Successful treatment of laryngeal cancer is highly dependent upon early detection and intervention.

Medical Treatment

▪ Medical treatment depends on the site, type, and extent of the cancer (Casper & Colton, 1998). Tumors can be *supraglottic* (above the vocal folds), *glottic* (at the level of the vocal folds), or *subglottic* (below the vocal folds). *Metastasis* (spread of the cancer to other regions) and *node involvement* are also major considerations.

▪ Doctors classify and treat laryngeal cancer based upon three primary categories: *T* (primary site of tumor), *N* (involvement of the lymph nodes), and *M* (metastasis). Thus, the patient's medical chart will probably feature a TNM designation to describe the site(s) and extent of the cancer.

▪ There are three basic types of medical treatment for laryngeal cancer: surgery, chemotherapy, and radiation.

▪ A *laryngectomy*, or surgery to remove the larnyx, can consist of a *total laryngectomy* (in which the entire larynx is removed) or a *hemilaryngectomy* (in which only the diseased part of the larynx is removed). Patients with advanced laryngeal cancer involving lymph nodes and metastasis may undergo total laryngectomy with *radical neck dissection,* in which the lymphatic system in the neck is removed. The person who has had his larynx removed is known as a *laryngectomee.*

▪ *Chemotherapy* may be used alone or in conjunction with other measures to increase the survival of patients with advanced cancer when the original tumor is large and metastasis is a risk. Side effects of chemotherapy include weight and hair loss, nausea, and weakness.

▪ *Radiation therapy,* used alone or combined with surgery, may be used for some patients. Doctors often use radiation therapy, before surgery is attempted, to try to eliminate the cancer. Some patients prefer radiation therapy to laryngectomy if given a choice. Side effects of radiation can include skin burns, risk of cavities, edema, swallowing problems, diminished taste, sore throat, and *xerostomia* (dry mouth due to trauma to the salivary glands).

General Issues in Rehabilitation of the Laryngectomee

▪ A team approach is critical in rehabilitation. Laryngectomees and their families need support from the surgeon, speech–language pathologist, social worker, nurse, vocational counselor, nutritionist, and maybe a counselor or psychologist to deal with accompanying emotional issues (Shipley & Roseberry-McKibbin, 2006).

- It is critical for the speech–language pathologist to acknowledge that the patient and family will most probably need both pre- and postoperative counseling to deal with the substantial emotional issues and life changes that accompany a laryngectomy. The first few days after the surgery often constitute the emotional "low point" for patients (Haynes & Pindzola, 2004).
- Experienced, rehabilitated laryngectomees can be substantially helpful in providing information and support both pre- and postsurgically. Some cities have established support groups for laryngectomees and their families.
- Consultation and support, both written and verbal, are needed pre- as well as postsurgery. Patients and families who do not receive presurgical support tend to suffer more depression and isolation than those who receive information and support prior to surgery. Clinicians must remember that spouses and significant others need support just as the patient does.

Types of Alaryngeal Speech

- Because the vocal folds are gone, after a laryngectomy normal voicing is not possible and breathing is different. To allow the patient to breathe, the surgeon creates a *stoma* or opening in the lower part of the neck and connects it with the trachea. The patient now breathes through that opening.
- Figure 7.9 illustrates the anatomy and physiology of the head and neck before and after a total laryngectomy. Because of the altered anatomy and physiology, a new source of sound is needed for voicing.
- Laryngectomees produce vocalizations in three ways: *external devices, esophageal speech,* and *surgical modifications or implanted devices* in the laryngeal area.
- A widely used external device is the artificial larynx, a mechanical, hand-held device that generates sound. Many types of artificial larynxes exist on the market. The patient presses the *artificial larynx* against the neck, and turns on the unit with the thumb. The sound generated by the vibrator is transferred to the mouth, and the patient then articulates in a slightly exaggerated manner to increase intelligibility.
- The esophagus is also a source of sound. Patients can be taught *esophageal speech,* in which they literally speak on burps or belches. There are two methods of esophageal speech:

    - In the injection method, the patient impounds the air in the mouth as in saying /t/ or /p/. The impounded air is pushed back into the esophagus and then expelled, producing vibrations of the soft tissues of the esophagus—particularly the *cricopharyngeus* muscle. The patient shapes the resulting belch into speech.
    - In the *inhalation method,* the patient is taught to inhale rapidly while keeping the esophagus open and relaxed. The inhaled air passes through the esophagus and sets its tissues into vibratory motion. The resulting sound is shaped into speech.

- *Surgical modifications and implanted devices* can also serve as sound sources. In the popular *Blom-Singer tracheoesophageal puncture* (TEP), the tracheoesophageal wall, which separates the trachea and the esophagus, is punctured. A shunt or tunnel is opened to connect the two structures. To keep the tunnel open, the Blom-Singer prosthetic device (see Figure 7.10) is inserted. The device, which is a small 1.8–3.6 cm plastic or silicone tube, is designed to prevent the passage of fluid and food into the trachea. There are two major types of devices: one that the patient herself can insert and manipulate, and an indwelling device that can only be inserted and removed by the physician (Boone et al., 2005).
- To speak, the patient exhales and occludes the stoma with a finger; the pulmonary air enters through the anterior opening of the tube, passing from the trachea to the esophagus. This sets the esophagus into vibration, resulting in sound production. The patient modifies the sound into speech.

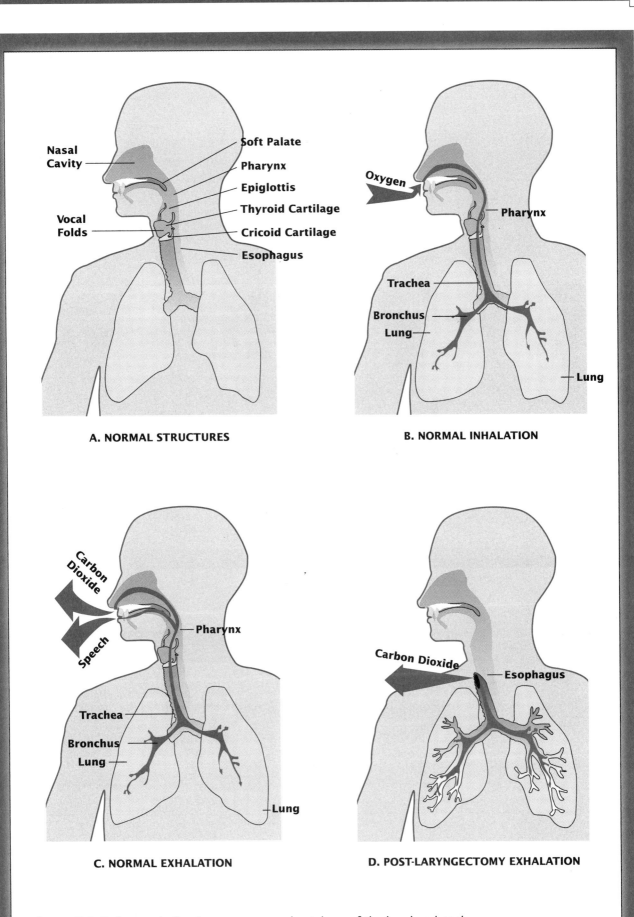

A. NORMAL STRUCTURES

Nasal Cavity
Soft Palate
Pharynx
Epiglottis
Vocal Folds
Thyroid Cartilage
Cricoid Cartilage
Esophagus

B. NORMAL INHALATION

Oxygen
Pharynx
Trachea
Bronchus
Lung
Lung

C. NORMAL EXHALATION

Carbon Dioxide
Speech
Pharynx
Trachea
Bronchus
Lung
Lung

D. POST-LARYNGECTOMY EXHALATION

Carbon Dioxide
Esophagus

Figure 7.9. Before and after laryngectomy: physiology of the head and neck.

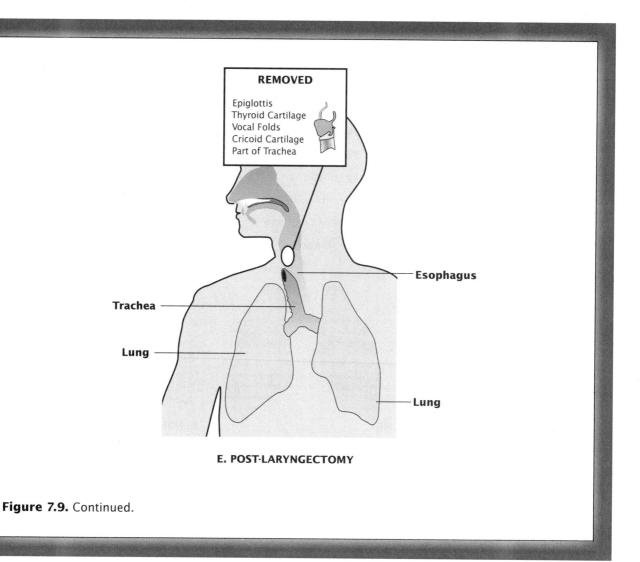

E. POST-LARYNGECTOMY

Figure 7.9. Continued.

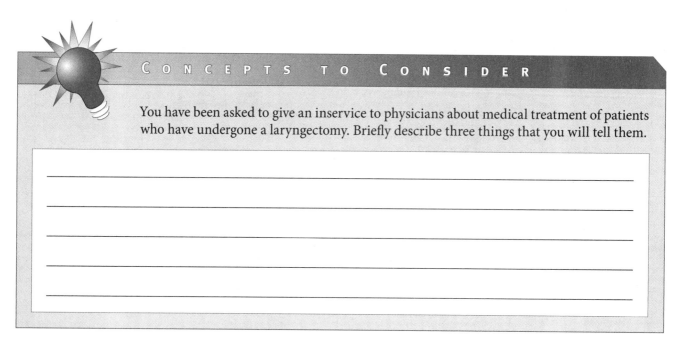

CONCEPTS TO CONSIDER

You have been asked to give an inservice to physicians about medical treatment of patients who have undergone a laryngectomy. Briefly describe three things that you will tell them.

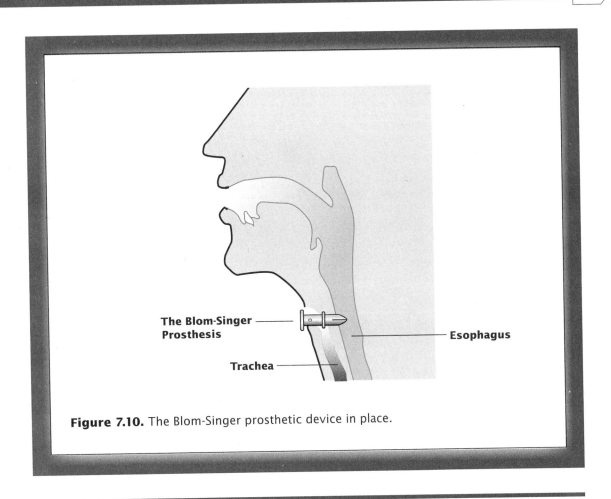

The Blom-Singer Prosthesis

Esophagus

Trachea

Figure 7.10. The Blom-Singer prosthetic device in place.

Physically and Neurologically Based Disorders of Phonation

Granuloma

- A *granuloma* is a localized, inflammatory, vascular lesion, that is usually composed of granular tissue in a firm, rounded sac. Granulomas frequently develop on the vocal processes of the arytenoid cartilages in the posterior laryngeal area. They can be unilateral or bilateral. An example is shown in Figure 7.11.
- Granulomas may be caused by vocal abuse, intubation during surgery, injury to the larynx, and gastroesophageal reflux. Granulomas are most often associated with contact ulcers.
- Patients with granulomas often sound breathy and hoarse; they feel the need to frequently clear their throat. The degree of dysphonia depends on the granuloma size and how much it interferes with glottal efficiency.
- Granulomas are treated by surgery, voice therapy, or both.

Hemangioma

- *Hemangiomas* are similar to granulomas, but are soft, pliable, and filled with blood. They occur in the posterior glottal area.
- Hemangiomas are usually caused by intubation or hyperacidity due to gastroesophageal reflux. They can also be congenital.
- Usually hemangiomas are surgically excised. Follow-up voice therapy is often necessary to improve vocal quality.

Figure 7.11. Contact ulcer with granuloma. *Note.* From *Clinical Management of Voice Disorders*, 4th ed. (p. 162), by J. L. Case, 2002, Austin, TX: PRO-ED. Copyright 2002 by PRO-ED, Inc. Reprinted with permission.

Leukoplakia

- *Leukoplakia* are benign growths of thick, whitish patches on the surface membrane of the mucosa. These growths may extend into the subepithelial space.
- Leukoplakia occur due to tissue irritation, especially that caused by smoking, alcohol, or vocal abuse. They may appear on the anterior third of the vocal folds and under the tongue.
- Though benign, leukoplakia are considered precancerous and must be monitored to ensure that they do not develop into squamous cell carcinoma.
- Patients with leukoplakia may sound hoarse, low-pitched, breathy, and soft in volume. Diplophonia may also be present. Treatment usually involves a combination of surgery, voice therapy, and eliminating exposure to tissue irritants.

Hyperkeratosis

- *Hyperkeratosis* refers to a rough, pinkish lesion that can appear in the oral cavity, larynx, or pharynx. Hyperkeratosis of the vocal folds may involve the epithelial cover of the folds as well as the superficial layer of the lamina propria. These lesions are often benign but may be precursors to malignancy.
- Hyperkeratotic growths occur due to tissue irritation and may arise in response to such causes as smoking, gastroesophageal reflux, and vocal abuse.
- The voice symptoms presented by patients range from mild to severe hoarseness or harshness,

reduced loudness, and low pitch. Treatment involves eliminating the tissue irritants, possible ablative surgery, and voice therapy.

Laryngomalacia

- A congenital condition also known as *congenital laryngeal stridor, laryngomalacia* involves soft, "floppy" laryngeal cartilages, particularly the epiglottis.
- The epiglottis is very soft and pliable due to abnormal development. When the child breathes, the epiglottis resists the airstream, causing *stridor,* or rough, breathy noise upon inhalation.
- Because this condition usually resolves spontaneously by the time the child is 2 or 3 years old, no treatment is normally required after the initial diagnosis. However, in severe cases, the child may have substantial breathing problems, which will require treatment.

Papilloma

- Papillomas are sometimes called *juvenile papillomas* because they tend to occur primarily in children (although they can occur in adults as well). When children reach puberty, papillomas often cease to be a problem.
- Papillomas are wart-like growths caused by the human papilloma virus. They are pink, white, or both and may be found anywhere in the airway (including but not limited to the larynx) (see Figure 7.12).
- Hoarseness, breathiness, and low pitch are the most frequent perceptual symptoms of papilloma. Airway obstruction is a major and potentially life-threatening concern.

Figure 7.12. Laryngeal papillomas. *Note.* From *Clinical Management of Voice Disorders,* 4th ed. (p. 335), by J. L. Case, 2002, Austin, TX: PRO-ED. Copyright 2002 by PRO-ED, Inc. Reprinted with permission.

- At present, most patients with papilloma are treated through multiple surgeries; some patients have had 30–100 surgeries for papilloma removal.
- Repeated surgeries strip the mucosa and create vocal fold scar tissue, which impacts vocal quality. After surgery children often sound even more hoarse and low-pitched than before. Laryngeal webbing (discussed later) can also occur. However, doctors are most concerned about airway preservation; thus, sequelae like hoarseness and laryngeal webbing are not considered high-priority problems.
- Treatments include *cup forceps surgery* (diminishing in popularity), *Interferon* medication, and CO_2 *laser surgery* (widely used). Carefully performed, CO_2 laser surgery helps preserve mucosa and surrounding tissue while ablating the papillomas. Interferon can be effective but has potentially serious side effects, including induced autoimmune diseases.
- In 1998, Rosen, Woodson, Thompson, Hengesteg, and Bradlow shared preliminary results of a trial using indole-3-carbinol to treat recurrent respiratory papillomatosis. This FDA-approved nutritional supplement is highly concentrated in broccoli, cabbage, cauliflower, and brussels sprouts. Eighteen months after treatment with indole-3-carbinol, one third of the subjects in this study had not responded to the treatment, one third of the subjects had reduced growth of the papillomas, and one third of the subjects had complete cessation of the papilloma growth.
- Voice therapy can be helpful after surgical treatment. Therapy can involve relaxation exercises, teaching the patient to use amplification devices, and helping the patient decrease supraglottic hyperfunction. Therapy does not prevent recurrences of the papilloma, but it can help patients make the best use of their weakened and scarred vocal mechanism.

Laryngeal Trauma

- Seen more frequently in children than in adults, *laryngeal trauma* refers to many kinds of injury to the larynx. Causes of laryngeal trauma include burns (thermal or chemical), motor vehicle accidents, sports-related accidents, attempted strangulations, and gunshot wounds. Young children may suffer trauma by swallowing sharp objects.
- Patients who suffer laryngeal trauma generally undergo surgery designed to reconstruct the vocal mechanism. The success of surgery depends on several factors, including the health of the overall vocal tissue prior to surgery. Patients who smoke or have gastroesophageal reflux disease (GERD), for example, must cease smoking or have treatment for the GERD before surgery occurs so that the vocal tissue will be as optimal as possible. If vocal tissue is compromised before surgery, more scarring from surgery can occur (Thibeault & Gray, 2004).
- Most patients undergo voice therapy after surgery. The postsurgical necessity of voice therapy varies from patient to patient, depending on the degree of dysphonia displayed. Voice therapy success depends largely on the proficiency of the remaining or surgically reconstructed laryngeal mechanism.

Laryngeal Web

- A *laryngeal web* is a membrane that grows across the anterior portion of the glottis.
- There are two basic types of laryngeal webs: *congenital,* or present at birth; and *acquired,* due to trauma to the inner edges of the vocal folds. The vocal folds may be traumatized by forceful or prolonged intubation, surgery, severe laryngeal infections, or accidental injury.
- Treatment for infants with congenital webs involves immediate surgery followed by tracheostomy.
- Treatment for webbing in adults involves surgery to remove the web. After surgery, the surgeon places a *laryngeal keel* (a fingernail-sized, rudder-shaped device) between the vocal folds to prevent them from growing back together. The patient generally undergoes 6–8 weeks of

voice rest while the keel is in place. After the keel is removed, voice therapy may be required to assist in return of normal phonation.

Paradoxical Vocal Fold Motion (PVFM)

- In PVFM, also called *laryngeal dyskinesia* and *episodic paroxysmal laryngospasm (EPL)*, there is an inappropriate closure or adduction of the true vocal folds during inhalation, exhalation, or both (see Figure 7.13) (Gallivan & Adrianopoulos, 2004).
- Patients with PVFM often appear asthmatic (Davenport & Sapeinza, 2004). Sometimes they undergo tracheotomy to relieve their symptoms. Some patients display stridor and dysphonia; others display only stridor.
- PVFM has been attributed to both psychological and physiological causes. Some experts view it as a conversion disorder in patients with psychological problems. Others believe it may be due to pharmacological, neurological, and other variables.
- For example, some persons with PVFM have upper airway sensitivity to laryngeal irritants. Irritants in the airway are likely to contribute to PVFM in children. These irritants include sinus drainage/postnasal drip, laryngopharyngeal reflex, and exposure to irritating smoke, fumes, gas, dust, mist, or vapors (Sandage & Zelazny, 2004).
- Identification of PVFM has increased a great deal in recent years, and has been documented in both males and females of all ages. Most clients with PVFM fall between 10 and 40 years of age, but the condition has been identified in children as young as 4 months old (Sandage & Zelazny, 2004).

Figure 7.13. Paradoxical vocal fold movement (larynx shown during inhalation). *Note.* From *Clinical Management of Voice Disorders,* 4th ed. (p. 247), by J. L. Case, 2002, Austin, TX: PRO-ED. Copyright 2002 by PRO-ED, Inc. Reprinted with permission.

- Treatment may include a combination of psychological, medical, and behavioral approaches. Some patients respond well to voice therapy involving endoscopy and direct feedback, in which they learn the nature of the disorder as well as how to relax the entire vocal mechanism. Children and adolescents may respond well to visual biofeedback techniques and relaxation exercises.

Gastroesophageal Reflux Disease (GERD)

- GERD, mentioned earlier, occurs when gastric contents spontaneously empty into the esophagus when the person has not vomited or belched. Patients may experience heartburn, acid indigestion, sore throat, and hoarseness. Consequent pathological vocal fold changes may also occur, such as *contact ulcers* (bilateral ulcerations on the medial surfaces of the vocal processes of the arytenoid cartilages).
- Manometric evaluation (a form of aerodynamic evaluation) for patients with GERD can be very effective. When a team of professionals is planning for antireflux surgery, esophageal manometric evaluation is critical (Collins & Samlan, 2004).
- Treatment options include antacids, propping up the head at night, use of prescription medications, not exercising directly after eating, and changes in dietary habits. Some patients may need to decrease the amount of coffee they drink, because coffee drinking has been associated with GERD.
- Medical personnel should usually be involved in treatment of patients with GERD. Treatment plans for these patients usually include behavioral, medical, and surgical therapies as well as voice therapy.

Paralysis and Ankylosis

- Because the vocal folds are composed primarily of muscle, they can be paralyzed when their nerve supply is cut off. Muscles that are not stimulated by the nerves do not move, resulting in paralysis.
- Vocal folds can become paralyzed due to the following:

  - accidental injury of the recurrent laryngeal nerve during certain *surgical procedures* (e.g., a thyroidectomy, in which a cancerous thyroid gland is surgically removed);
  - progressive, debilitative *neurological diseases,* such as amyotrophic lateral sclerosis;
  - *malignant diseases,* causing tumors outside the larynx to impact vocal fold mobility;
  - *intubation trauma,* causing compression of the recurrent laryngeal nerve, dislocation of the arytenoids, and other difficulties;
  - *laryngeal trauma* that is so severe it is irreparable (e.g., gunshot wound);
  - *stroke;* and
  - *vagus nerve deficits.*

- Even in patients who can achieve a near-normal-sounding voice despite vocal fold paralysis, coughing is not vigorous because of the difficulty in achieving the necessary amount of subglottal pressure for the vocal folds to close firmly. Some patients demonstrate dysphagia, breathiness, and reduced pitch and volume.
- In *unilateral paralysis,* only one vocal fold is paralyzed and assumes a static position. In some cases, the normal fold may move toward the paralyzed fold to make contact; the voice in such cases may sound almost normal. In other cases, the paralyzed fold may be so far away from midline that the healthy fold cannot make contact to achieve closure. This causes aphonia.
- *Bilateral paralysis,* or paralysis of both vocal folds, may lead to a wide-open glottis, causing aphonia. When the vocal folds are paralyzed in an abducted position, aspiration can occur. If

the vocal folds are paralyzed in an adducted position, the patient struggles for breath but the voice is not significantly dysphonic (Case, 2002).

- In *ankylosis,* or stiffening of the joint(s), the movement of the arytenoids is restricted because of a bone-joint disease such as arthritis. Cancer can also cause ankylosis. The vocal folds are attached to the arytenoids; when the arytenoids are stiff, the vocal folds do not close fully.

- A number of treatment techniques are available for patients with vocal fold paralysis. In cases of unilateral paralysis, doctors create a bulge in the paralyzed fold so that the healthy fold meets it more readily. Substances used to create the bulge include *Teflon, collagen, Gelfoam,* and *autologous fat* (the patient's own fat).

- One popular technique used to achieve vocal fold medialization is *thyroplasty I.* The surgeon creates a small window in the thyroid cartilage, medializes the vocal fold, and places a small Silastic implant to keep the paralyzed fold medialized.

- In *nerve-muscle pedicle reinnervation,* the surgeon takes a pedicle of a neck strap muscle with innervation and sutures it either into the adductors for medialization purposes or into the posterior cricoarytenoids in order to promote abduction (Case, 2002).

- Depending on the type of paralysis, the following treatment techniques have been used to help patients achieve firmer vocal fold closure:

  - elevation in pitch
  - increased loudness
  - increased breath support, as well as breathing more often between phrases
  - pushing approach, in which the patient activates the glottal effort closure reflex by pushing against an object to increase vocal fold medialization
  - hard glottal attacks
  - head turning or positioning, in which the patient changes head position to see which position creates the best voice

Spasmodic Dysphonia

- Spasmodic dysphonia (SMD) is a focal laryngeal dystonia. Although it has traditionally been considered psychologically based, most experts today believe that SMD has neurogenic causes with possible emotional side effects. Currently, SMD is thought to involve brain stem dysfunction (Woodson & Murry, 2004). The onset of SMD usually occurs in adults; the average age of onset is 38 years. There are two types.

- *Abductor spasmodic dysphonia* is created by intermittent, involuntary, fleeting vocal fold abduction when the patient tries to phonate. Loudness is reduced, and the patient is occasionally aphonic, with breathy or whispered speech. Treatment options include BOTOX (Botulinus toxin) injections, speech therapy involving relaxation techniques and continuous voicing, and pharmacological intervention.

- *Adductor spasmodic dysphonia,* the most common type, is characterized by overpressure due to prolonged overadduction or tight closure of the vocal folds. The voice may sound choked and strangled. Popular current treatment techniques include:

  - *CO_2 laser surgery.* The paralyzed fold is thinned with a CO2 laser beam. This creates a 2-mm-wide groove, whose healing and scarring action pulls the vocal fold away from the midline, widening the glottis. Repeated surgeries may be necessary.
  - *Recurrent laryngeal nerve (RLN) resection.* Here, the RLN is cut in order to paralyze the vocal fold on that side. This reduces vocal fold hyperadduction. RLN resection has met with mixed success. RLN is currently considered to be a viable option for patients with severe SMD who do not wish to have repeated, frequent BOTOX injections (Woodson &

Murry, 2004).

- *BOTOX injections.* BOTOX, a neurotoxin injected directly by needle into the vocal folds, creates a flaccid paralysis, and hyperadduction ceases. Injections are usually repeated every 3–6 months. BOTOX is currently the treatment of choice among many specialists.
- *Voice therapy.* Voice therapy can include inhalation phonation, increased pitch, relaxation, head turning, counseling, the yawn-sigh approach, and soft, breathy phonation onset using /h/. (*Note:* Pushing techniques are counterproductive for patients who have RLN; recurrence of spasticity can occur.)

Neurological Diseases

Multiple Sclerosis (MS)

- Patients with MS experience progressive and diffuse demylination of white matter, with corresponding preservation of axons at the brainstem, cerebellum, and spinal cord.
- Patients may have impaired prosody, pitch, and loudness control, harshness, breathiness, hypernasality, articulation breakdown, and nasal air escape.
- Pharmacological intervention may include ACTH (adrenocorticotrophic hormone) to reduce acute symptoms. Corticosteroids such as Prednisone may also be used.

Myasthenia Gravis

- This neuromuscular autoimmune disease produces fatigue and muscle weakness. There is a decreased amount of acetylcholine at the myoneuronal junction.
- Patients often sound hypernasal, breathy, hoarse, and soft in volume. Dysphagia and distorted articulation may also be present.
- Myasthenia gravis is often treated with corticosteroids, which improve strength and endurance of the bulbar musculature.

Amyotrophic Lateral Sclerosis (ALS)

- ALS, or *Lou Gehrig's disease,* is a progressive, fatal disease involving degeneration of the upper and lower motor neuron systems.
- Patients with ALS often sound breathy, low pitched, and monotoned. There is poor respiratory control.
- Patients with ALS do not respond well to medications, but Riluzole has been shown to slow muscle deterioration in some patients.
- Because ALS is progressive, many clinicians focus treatment efforts on augmentative/alternative forms of communication that can be used even in the later stages of the disease.

Parkinson's Disease

- Parkinson's is caused by a lack of dopamine (a neurotransmitter) in the substantia nigra of the basal ganglia. It can be idiopathic (occurring in isolation or primary form) or secondary to other conditions such as dementia.
- Patients with Parkinson's disease often sound breathy, low pitched, and monotoned.
- Treatment includes *L-dopa* (levodopa) to increase dopamine in the substantia nigra; voice treatment may also be indicated. The currently popular *Lee Silverman Voice Treatment* program emphasizes stimulating patients to increase respiratory and phonatory efforts and to sustain those efforts over time (Brin, Velickovic, Ramig, & Fox, 2004).

Treatment Techniques for Patients with Neurological Diseases

- Because patients with neurological diseases tend to manifest dysarthria, with some exceptions, treatment techniques often follow principles based upon therapy for dysarthria.
- Although patients will differ and have individual needs, many of them will benefit from the following therapy strategies designed to improve the efficiency of the overall system and increase general intelligibility:
  - improve articulation through exaggerating consonants and slowing rate of speech;
  - improve resonance through increasing mouth opening, decreasing posterior tongue tension, and improving velopharyngeal closure;
  - improve prosody to decrease monopitch;
  - improve respiration through relaxation, increasing efficiency of breathing (e.g., teaching diaphragmatic-abdominal breathing), and teaching the patient to breathe as often as necessary; and
  - improve vocal fold approximation through activities already mentioned (see "Paralysis and Ankylosis").

CONCEPTS TO CONSIDER

Describe two neurologically based disorders of phonation. What types of treatment might be appropriate for those disorders?

_____

_____

_____

_____

_____

Abuse-Based Disorders of Phonation

Vocally Abusive Practices

- Many disorders of voice occur due to vocally abusive behaviors. The sophisticated vocal mechanism works well when used properly, but it is extremely sensitive to abuse, which often causes a variety of voice problems. These problems are sometimes described as resulting from *phonotrauma,* or trauma or injury to the vocal folds (Lyon & Barkmeier-Kraemer, 2004).
- *Abusive behaviors* that can damage the vocal mechanism include: excessive shouting; screaming; cheering; excessive talking; coughing; hard glottal attacks; throat clearing; strained and explosive vocalizations; excessive laughing and crying; speaking with inappropriate pitch, loudness, or both; and speaking in noisy environments.
- Adults in occupations such as teaching or coaching may be more vulnerable to vocal abuse

than adults in vocations that do not require a great deal of speaking (especially at a loud volume) (Roy, Merrill, Thibeault, Gray, & Smith, 2004).

- The majority of vocally abusive behaviors are associated with excessive muscular effort, tension, and consequent irritation of the vocal folds. Excessive effort and tension can cause physical damage to the vocal folds (phonotrauma) and create physical pathologies. Patients who abuse their voices often demonstrate increased laryngeal airway resistance (Davenport & Sapienza, 2004). The voice problems that result from vocally abusive behaviors are due to such physical damage to and pathological states of the larynx.

- Therapy, medication, surgery, or a combination of those treatments are generally used to correct voice disorders resulting from pathological changes to the vocal folds due to abuse. However, if patients continue the abusive practices and do not change their vocal habits, pathological changes to the vocal folds with consequent voice problems are likely to recur.

Vocal Nodules

- Vocal nodules are small nodes that develop on the vocal folds and protrude from surrounding cells (see Figure 7.14). In the beginning, the nodules are reddish or pinkish. As they develop over time, they appear white or grayish because they become fibrous.

- Vocal nodules can be unilateral; however, they are typically bilateral and sit opposite each other on the two folds. Nodules typically appear at the junction of the anterior and middle-third portion of the folds.

- Nodules are well defined in the beginning stages but become more diffuse later because of inflammation of the surrounding tissue. Nodules develop over time as the result of prolonged

Figure 7.14. Vocal folds with nodules. *Note.* From *Clinical Management of Voice Disorders,* 4th ed. (p. 123), by J. L. Case, 2002, Austin, TX: PRO-ED. Copyright 2002 by PRO-ED, Inc. Reprinted with permission.

vocally abusive behaviors.

- Vocal nodules increase the mass of the vocal folds. Consequently, the folds vibrate at a slower rate, resulting in lower pitch. The nodules also make smooth vocal fold approximation impossible, contributing to breathiness and hoarseness of voice.

- Vocal nodules are seen most frequently in children who scream and yell on playgrounds and in adults whose career or leisure activities involve vocally abusive practices (e.g., yelling at sports events). Singers are especially susceptible to vocal nodules.

- Vocal rest usually clears up the nodules, but prolonged abuse of the vocal folds will result in larger and more persistent nodules. Unless the patient changes his or her abusive behaviors, the nodules will rarely disappear.

- Persistent nodules are frequently treated in two ways: voice therapy (described later) or surgery. Surgery involves tissue excision, or removal of the nodules through microdissection or laser.

- Recently, some doctors have been using cold steel lasers or microspot CO_2 (heat) lasers, whose beam is so small that heat cannot penetrate the surrounding tissues. The goal of laser and microdissection is to remove the nodules while disturbing as little of the mucosa and surrounding tissue as possible.

Polyps

- Polyps, like nodules, are masses that grow and bulge out from surrounding tissue. Polyps are softer than nodules and may be filled with fluid or have vascular tissue. Polyps tend to be unilateral as opposed to the typically bilateral nodules. Figure 7.15 shows a vocal polyp.

Figure 7.15. Vocal polyp. *Note.* From *Clinical Management of Voice Disorders,* 4th ed. (p. 336), by J. L. Case, 2002, Austin, TX: PRO-ED. Copyright 2002 by PRO-ED, Inc. Reprinted with permission.

- *Sessile polyps* have a broad base on the vocal fold; *pedunculated polyps* are attached to the vocal folds by a stalk.
- It is believed that traumatic use of the vocal folds results in submucosal hemorrhage (bleeding within the folds), which leads to the formation of tumorlike polyps. Polyps can grow over time or can be created after just one instance of severe vocal abuse (e.g., screaming if attacked).
- Polyps are more frequently seen in adults than in children, who are more susceptible to developing vocal nodules. Patients with polyps usually sound breathy and hoarse. They may also have *diplophonia* ("double voice," in which two different pitches are heard simultaneously) because the healthy fold vibrates at a different rate than the fold with the polyp.
- Polyps may disappear with voice rest and changes in vocal habits, or they may persist and become worse with time and no treatment. Techniques for treating patients with vocal polyps are described later.

Contact Ulcers

- Contact ulcers are sores or craterlike areas of ulcerated, granulated tissue that develop (usually bilaterally) along the posterior third of the glottal margin.
- The causes of contact ulcers include:

    - *The slamming together of the arytenoid cartilages* that occurs during low-pitched phonation accompanied by hard glottal attack and sometimes by increased loudness. Frequently, contact ulcers are seen in hard-driving patients who speak forcefully and talk excessively.
    - *Gastroesophageal reflux* (discussed earlier), in which stomach acid is forced into the esophagus. The acid pools in and irritates the area between the arytenoid cartilages; this can occur especially at night when one is sleeping.
    - *Intubation* for surgery, especially if intubation is prolonged or the tube is too large for the patient's larynx. Seventy percent of children who are intubated have a lacerated glottal area; this can cause permanent scarring and dysphonia.

- Patients with contact ulcers may complain of vocal fatigue and pain in the laryngeal area. They frequently sound hoarse and often clear their throats.
- Depending on the etiology, contact ulcers may require medical treatment (e.g., medication for gastroesophageal reflux). Surgery is not recommended; because the area is already ulcerated and highly irritated, healing is usually poor. Voice therapy techniques (described later) are geared toward taking the extra effort out of phonation.

Vocal Fold Thickening

- Prolonged use of vocally abusive behaviors such as throat clearing, screaming, and others can cause the vocal folds to thicken slowly and gradually. The vocal folds usually thicken along the anterior two thirds of the glottal margin.
- Vocal fold thickening results in a breathy voice with lowered pitch. Vocal fold thickening is often a precursor to nodules or polyps. When these appear, the voice becomes increasingly hoarse. Vocal fold thickening can be reduced through elimination of the vocally abusive behaviors.

Traumatic Laryngitis

- *Traumatic laryngitis* differs from *infectious,* or *organic,* laryngitis, which occurs due to infections, colds, or allergies (of bacterial or viral origin). Traumatic laryngitis is created when the patient engages in vocally abusive behaviors such as continual yelling.

- Vocally abusive behaviors irritate the vocal folds, which get swollen. Consequently, the voice is hoarse and may be low pitched with pitch breaks.
- Voice therapy usually consists of vocal rest and strategies for changing the vocally abusive behaviors.

Treatment for Abuse-Based Voice Disorders

Basic Principles

- As described above, abuse-based voice disorders are the result of a chain of causes and effects:

    vocally abusive behaviors, which cause

    laryngeal tissue changes, which in turn cause

    voice disorders, which then may cause

    personal, social, emotional, and occupational problems that cause additional stress and more vocal strain

- The clinician's goal, in voice therapy, is to help the patient achieve the best-sounding voice possible. This can involve either *restoration* of the previous healthy voice, or *compensation,* by which the patient produces the best voice possible given damage already done to the laryngeal mechanism.
- As mentioned, treatment for abuse-based voice disorders usually involves *voice therapy, medication, surgery,* or a combination thereof.
- Patients with voice disorders due to vocal abuse and consequent pathological changes in the vocal mechanism must reduce or eliminate vocal abuses and learn to regularly use healthy vocal habits. Laryngeal lesions and resulting voice problems will recur unless patients permanently alter their ways of speaking.
- Clinicians can facilitate medical evaluations, awareness of vocally abusive habits, and the learning of new, healthy habits that will ensure optimal vocal health and voice production.
- Clinicians can also help clients, especially adults, to ascertain whether environmental modifications within their workplaces (e.g., using a microphone for voice amplification in a noisy classroom) can help decrease the need for using vocally abusive behaviors such as shouting (Roy et al., 2004).

Fundamental Steps in Therapy

- Most adults and children who undergo voice therapy benefit from the foundational treatment steps listed below.
- Make a thorough evaluation of the voice disorder.
- Always ensure a medical evaluation is completed before starting voice therapy.
- Maintain a cooperative working relationship with a laryngologist; be knowledgeable about laryngeal surgical procedures and medications and their effects on and interactions with voice treatment methods.
- Ensure periodic medical examinations are completed during the course of voice therapy.
- Combine, in most cases, techniques designed to reduce vocally abusive behaviors with those that facilitate efficient and normal voice production.
- Individualize the facilitating techniques to each patient.
- Help patients understand the nature of the disorder, what habits are maintaining the disorder,

and the harmful results of the vocally abusive behaviors.

- Give adults readings, illustrations of vocal anatomy and physiology, and explanations.
- Children may enjoy computer games that motivate them to change their vocally abusive behaviors to improve their voices (Hooper, 2004). For example, Kay Elemetrics (2004) has voice games contained in software packages.
- Design a program to help patients reduce abusive behaviors and establish vocally appropriate behaviors.
- Help all patients understand what their specific treatment goals are.
- Work closely with the patient's significant others (e.g., parents, siblings, spouses) to help reduce vocally abusive behaviors and to reinforce healthy vocal behaviors.
- Establish baselines of vocally abusive behaviors and the frequency of abnormal voice productions in and outside the clinic.
- Ask patients (or parents of young children) to measure their vocally abusive behaviors for a few days and graph their frequency on a daily basis to establish the baselines of vocally abusive behaviors in natural settings.
- Encourage patients to monitor their voice production both inside and outside the clinic setting.
- Consistently use audio recordings for feedback, ear training, and development of patients' ability to self-monitor; video recordings are even better.
- Use visual monitoring and feedback such as that provided by the Visi-Pitch.
- Support patients, especially adults, in identifying and making needed lifestyle changes such as avoiding smoke (including secondhand smoke) and alcohol, taking appropriate allergy medications, and drinking enough water.
- Phonotraumatic behaviors such as chronic throat clearing and coughing can be virtually eliminated with hydration therapy. The patient should adjust his water intake as needed. When he feels a need to cough or clear his throat, he can take a sip of water first; this often eliminates the need for coughing or throat clearing (Gallivan & Adrianopoulos, 2004).

Specific Treatment Techniques

- Not every client needs every technique. Clinicians can select individually appropriate techniques that are designed to reduce vocally abusive habits and replace them with positive, nonabusive practices that will promote optimal vocal health. See the following list for examples.
  - Use the *open mouth approach.* Teach the patient to speak with a wider mouth opening; this helps increase volume and improve the oral–nasal resonance balance. Use a mirror if necessary.
  - Help the patient speak with *appropriate pitch and volume.*
  - Teach the patient to *reduce the frequency of coughing* and throat clearing.
  - Teach the patient to *relax the body* and the oral–laryngeal area when speaking; reduce tension.
  - Use the *chant-talk method,* in which words are spoken in a connected manner, with soft glottal attack, even stress, prolongation of sounds, and the absence of stress for individual words.
  - Use *digital manipulation* of the larynx, which will lower pitch and decrease laryngeal tension. Here, the clinician gently places her thumb and fingers on either side of the patient's thyroid cartilage and gently pushes downward while the patient phonates. The clinician can then fade the model, and the patient can perform the manipulation.
  - Use *respiration training* to teach thoracic and diaphragmatic–abdominal breathing to increase breath support for vocalization.
  - *Encourage voice rest,* which can range from no vocalizations at all for a time period to specific, planned periods of the day when the client does not vocalize. Clients who have

to rest their voices often need positive reinforcement for implementing voice rest because curtailing voice use can substantially impact their lifestyles (van der Merwe, 2004).

- Teach *gentle voice onset,* in which the client initiates phonation using an /h/ or /h/ + vowel (e.g., "ha" or "hi"). Voice initiation is gentle, relaxed, and whispered.
- Teach the *yawn-sigh method* to relax the oral–laryngeal mechanism and increase the mouth opening. The client inhales on a wide yawn, which is followed by an expiratory sigh and phonation.
- For clients with pharyngeal focus, or voices coming from too deep in the throat, teach *appropriate focus* in the facial mask (referred to earlier).

CONCEPTS TO CONSIDER

A 43-year-old high school football coach comes to you for an evaluation. He states that he has been hoarse for approximately 10 months. A subsequent medical evaluation reveals the presence of well-developed vocal nodules. Describe some treatment techniques you will use with this patient.

_____

_____

_____

_____

_____

Disorders of Loudness and Pitch

Basic Principles

- Frequently, the problems of loudness and pitch are components of other voice disorders. For example, the breathy and hoarse voice is typically low pitched. Laryngeal pathologies may prevent a loud enough voice.
- However, several disorders of loudness and pitch occur independently of other problems. When treating patients with these disorders of loudness and pitch, clinicians must rule out physical problems such as hearing loss, asthma, and others.

Disorders of Loudness

Key Facts

- Vocal loudness varies among individuals and is determined by variables such as culture and gender of the patient as well as health issues.

- Few people seek professional help for loud speech unless it is part of a larger problem such as vocal nodules or polyps, which in turn create a voice problem.
- The typical patient who seeks treatment speaks too softly. Patients may speak too softly, as judged by mainstream listeners, for a variety of reasons: hearing loss, cultural mores, clinical depression, psychological trauma, or sheer habit.

Treatment

- Most patients with inadequate loudness and no contraindicating health problems can be easily trained. The clinician can help them maintain enough air pressure while speaking and can systematically reinforce progressively louder speech.
- Auditory and visual feedback such as that provided by a tape recorder, the Visi-Pitch, or a computer program can be very helpful.

Disorders of Pitch

Key Facts

- The typical pitch disorder consists of either too high or too low a pitch considering the age and sex of the speaker. Due to mainstream cultural expectations, an unusually high pitch in a man or an unusually low pitch in a woman might be considered abnormal or undesirable.
- Most clients with pitch disorders are men who speak with too high a pitch and wish to speak with a lower, more appropriate pitch. A high pitch in a man can be due to psychological factors, physical factors, or both.
- In *mutational falsetto,* or *puberphonia,* a young man speaks with a high pitch although the larynx has grown normally and puberty is completed. This can occur due to psychosocial factors (e.g., embarrassment about the newly developing low voice), endocrine disorders, or neurologic diseases.
- For patients with puberphonia, it is optimal for treatment to be initiated in the teens or early twenties. Some atrophy of the vocal muscles may occur if the mutational falsetto persists untreated.
- Pitch disorders due to *hormonal changes* may impact some patients, especially women. Menstruation, menopause, use of oral contraceptives, and virilization (increased masculinity) of the female voice have all been associated with pitch changes.
- Pitch changes before and during menstruation are not usually a major problem. However, such changes are troublesome to professional singers. Lowered levels of estrogen and progesterone before menses can cause vocal fold thickening, with consequent hoarseness and lowered pitch.
- Drugs containing male hormones are sometimes used to treat cancer. For example, uterine cancer is often treated with testosterone. Such drugs can thicken the vocal folds and decrease vocal pitch; those changes may be irreversible.

Treatment

- In patients with a pitch that is too high, especially young men with puberphonia, the larynx is often elevated, with accompanying tension of the laryngeal musculature.
- Because of this tension, relaxation, yawn-sigh, the open-mouth approach, and digital manipulation are often successful in lowering pitch. The use of nonspeech vocalizations such as coughing and glottal fry can also be helpful.
- Speech-range masking can be an effective treatment technique for individuals (especially

men) who wish to lower their vocal pitch. The clinician asks the patient to begin oral reading and records the patient's reading. Near the tenth word, masking is introduced. Utilizing the *Lombard effect* (where the patient's voice becomes louder in the presence of background noise) with the introduction of masking noise, the voice usually spontaneously becomes louder and lower. The patient can then listen back to his lower voice and be encouraged that he is able to produce this type of voice (Boone et al., 2005).

- Visual and auditory feedback such as that provided by tape recordings and instruments such as the Visi-Pitch are quite helpful to patients with pitch problems.
- Some patients may need psychological counseling in conjunction with voice therapy. This is dependent upon the needs and background of the individual.
- Clients from linguistically and culturally diverse backgrounds should be asked to describe their perception of a voice with normal pitch; the clinician should then conduct the therapy accordingly (DeJarnette & Holland, 1998).

Psychogenic Voice Disorders

Basic Principles

- *Psychogenic,* or "functional," voice disorders occur when the voice is abnormal in the presence of normal laryngeal structures. A laryngoscopic examination reveals essentially normal vocal structures; however, during attempted phonation, the vocal folds may remain fully or partially abducted.
- In *hysterical,* or *conversion aphonia,* there is usually no evidence of a structural pathology. There is no known physiological or neurological basis for the patient's voice loss. The loss can be sudden or gradual.
- Patients with conversion aphonia often experience voice loss after an emotionally traumatic event such as a violent crime. The voice loss may represent an unconscious attempt to avoid dealing with the traumatic event. The voice problem is thus viewed as a conversion reaction, or translation of the emotional trauma into another set of symptoms.
- Aphonia in the absence of any organic cause has been treated with either counseling/psychotherapy or behavior therapy.
- For counseling/psychotherapy, clinicians often refer the patient to a professional psychologist, psychiatrist, or marriage and family counselor. During therapy sessions, clients are encouraged to speak freely about themselves and their problems. With the support of a sympathetic listener, clients are expected to resolve their psychological conflicts and return to normal phonation.
- Clinicians who employ *behavior therapy* treat conversion aphonia by modifying the client's behaviors. Specific therapy techniques can include:

  - masking, or the Lombard effect, mentioned earlier, (when the patient receives masking noise and is asked to vocalize, he or she may do it reflexively; the clinician should tape-record this)
  - progressive relaxation techniques and reduction in muscle tension
  - encouraging coughing, grunting, throat clearing, laughing, humming, and other non-speech vocalizations
  - prolonging a cough into a normal vowel
  - inhalation phonation
  - the yawn-sigh approach
  - production of vowels, monosyllabic words, and polysyllabic words

- progression to simple phrases, oral reading
- engaging in simple conversation alone with the clinician
- engaging in conversations with an increased variety of interlocutors in an increased variety of settings
- generalization to daily communication activities

- For many patients with conversion aphonia, the prognosis for return to normal voice is quite good. Clinicians must, after gathering an extensive case history and viewing the overall situation, make accurate decisions about the most effective course of treatment for conversion aphonia patients.

Gender Issues and the Voice

Basic Principles

- Sometimes clinicians encounter clients who are experiencing gender reassignment. Some clients go from female to male, but more typically clients go from male to female. In these types of cases, the term *transsexual* has been used; however, today, the term *transgender* is most commonly used (Boone et al., 2005; Case, 2002).
- The Henry Benjamin International Gender Dysphoria Association (HBIGDA, 2003) has introduced guidelines for service delivery to and care of persons who are undergoing gender identity changes. These guidelines recognize that these clients can be supported by receiving assistance in changing their voice, speech patterns, and overall communication style. (See References and Recommended Reading for how to contact HBIGDA for more information.)
- For most transgender clients, the primary voice concern is achieving appropriate pitch. Vocal pitch factors that need to be modified include intonational variability, fundamental frequency, lower and upper limits of the frequency range, and others (Gelfer & Schofield, 2000).

Treatment

- The female-to-male transgender client can often achieve lowered vocal pitch through hormonal therapy. Testosterone thickens the vocal folds, thus helping produce a lower pitch. Testosterone also increases muscle definition and increases facial and bodily hair.
- Male-to-female clients generally take estrogen, which successfully produces some physical changes such as the softening of overall muscle definition. However, estrogen does not impact the vocal folds; the vocal folds remain the same as they always were, and the client's pitch remains masculine sounding.
- Some male-to-female clients undergo vocal surgery to achieve a higher-pitched voice. For example, thyroplasty and longitudinal incision of the vocal folds can help the male-to-female client talk with a higher-pitched voice. Even with surgery, however, experts still recommend that these clients undergo voice therapy (Boone et al., 2005).
- Voice therapy for male-to-female clients includes several components (Andrews, 1999; Case, 2002; Gelfer, 1999; Hooper, 2000). One is teaching the client to use a greater number of rising pitch inflections at the ends of utterances. Another technique to help the client sound more feminine is to teach the client to use greater articulatory precision, use a softer voice, and use more modals (*can, may, will, shall, must*) (Case, 2002). The clinician can also help the client learn to adopt more feminine body language, including gestures and facial expressions.
- Transgender clients often need psychological support and counseling as well as voice therapy. Clinicians must recognize that the issues experienced by transgender clients are quite com-

plex and affect every area of the clients' lives—social, professional, personal, and others (Sue & Sue, 2003).

SUMMARY

✓ Patients often seek evaluation and treatment for voice disorders that have been caused by physical changes to the larynx. One major physical change, for some patients, involves laryngeal cancer.

✓ Patients who have surgery for total removal of the larynx need specific rehabilitation to learn alaryngeal speech. Other patients present voice disorders that result from physical changes caused by abusive vocal habits, neurological problems, or irritation by environmental agents.

✓ Disorders of loudness and pitch can be caused by organic or functional factors. Treatment will depend upon the etiology of the problem, as well as the patient's cultural perception of what constitutes a normal voice.

✓ Patients who have psychogenic voice disorders have frequently undergone emotional trauma with consequent loss of voice. For many of these patients, behavioral therapy, counseling/psychotherapy, or a combination is quite successful in voice restoration. Clinicians sometimes see transgender patients who are going from female to male; more typically, these clients are going from male to female. For the latter group, surgery combined with voice therapy to help the client sound more feminine appears to be an optimal situation.

◆ **HAVING A NORMAL, OPTIMAL-SOUNDING** voice depends on the health and intactness of the larynx and its structures. Key structures include the major laryngeal cartilages: thyroid cartilage, cricoid cartilage, arytenoid cartilages, and the corniculate and cuneiform cartilages. Cranial nerve X, the vagus nerve, is the nerve primarily responsible for innervation of the larynx.

◆ **KEY LARYNGEAL MUSCLES INCLUDE** the intrinsic laryngeal muscles: thyroarytenoids, cricothyroids, posterior cricoarytenoids, lateral cricoarytenoids, and interarytenoids. The extrinsic laryngeal muscles include: (a) the infrahyoids or laryngeal depressors—thyrohyoids, omohyoids, sternothyroids, and sternohyoids—and (b) the suprahyoids or laryngeal elevators—digastrics, geniohyoids, mylohyoids, stylohyoids, genioglossus, and hyoglossus.

◆ **EACH INDIVIDUAL'S VOICE UNDERGOES** changes during his or her life span. These changes involve mean fundamental frequency and maximum phonation time.

◆ **VOCAL PITCH (FREQUENCY) AND** volume (intensity) are important parameters of the voice. Vocal quality is greatly impacted by patients' daily vocal habits.

◆ **EVALUATION OF VOICE DISORDERS** should be comprehensive and based on a multidisciplinary team approach. A medical evaluation should be conducted before any therapy is initiated.

◆ **OPTIMALLY, A VOICE EVALUATION** should include: (a) gathering a thorough case history, (b) conducting additional assessments such as an oral peripheral examination and hearing screening, (c) performing instrumental analysis, and (d) conducting perceptual analysis of vocal characteristics.

◆ **DISORDERS OF RESONANCE INCLUDE** hypernasality, hyponasality, assimilative nasality, and cul-de-sac resonance. For the patient with resonance problems, it is critical to rule out organic causes such as velopharyngeal inadequacy. Therapy will not succeed unless the physical basis for the resonance problem is resolved.

◆ **DISORDERS OF VOICE ARE** often associated with physical factors involving pathological changes of the laryngeal mechanism. These factors include carcinoma, physical changes due to vocal abuse, neurological problems, and vocal fold irritation created by environmental agents. Treatment often involves medication, surgery, therapy, or a combination of these approaches.

◆ **DISORDERS OF LOUDNESS AND** pitch are associated with functional causes, organic causes, or both. Common problems associated with pitch and loudness include mutational falsetto, hormonal changes, and hearing loss.

◆ **PSYCHOGENIC VOICE DISORDERS OCCUR** when the voice is abnormal in the presence of normal laryngeal structures. Hysterical or conversion aphonia is often attributed to an underlying emotional etiology. Patients with psychogenic voice disorders can often be successfully treated with a variety of behavioral strategies. However, some patients may require psychotherapy or counseling. Transgender patients who are going from male-to-female status or female-to-male status have unique needs that must be sensitively and thoroughly addressed.

✎ **ADD YOUR OWN CHAPTER HIGHLIGHTS HERE:**

Study & Review Questions

Essay

1. List and briefly describe the key structures and cartilages of the larynx.

2. When a client is undergoing a voice evaluation, the clinician will probably use both instrumental and perceptual tools. Describe five types of instrumental evaluation tools and techniques that can be used to evaluate a client's voice.

3. Compare and contrast the terms *hypernasality* and *hyponasality*. What do these terms mean? What are the possible causes of each one? What treatment techniques can be used with clients who present with these disorders of resonance?

4. Describe types of alaryngeal speech that can be used by a patient who has undergone a laryngectomy.

5. What are some of the physical results of vocal abuse? (e.g., vocal nodules) Describe these results and list four treatment techniques that can be used with clients who present with phonotrauma based on vocally abusive practices.

Multiple Choice

6. The infrahyoid laryngeal muscles lie below the hyoid bone; they are sometimes called *depressors*. These muscles are the:

   A. digastrics, omohyoids, thyrohyoids, and hyoglossus.
   B. hylohyoids, genioglossus, digastrics, and sternothyroids.
   C. thyrohyoids, omohyoids, sternothyroids, and sternohyoids.
   D. digastrics, geniohyoids, thyrohyoids, stylohyoids, genioglossus, and sternothyroids.
   E. sternothyroids, hylohyoids, digastrics, and omohyoids.

7. The suprahyoid laryngeal muscles lie above the hyoid bone; they are sometimes called *elevators*. The suprahyoid muscles are the:

   A. digastrics, geniohyoids, thyrohyoids, stylohyoids, genioglossus, and sternothyroids.
   B. thyrohyoids, digastrics, stylohyoids, and hyoglossus.
   C. geniohyoids, hylohyoids, stylohyoids, genioglossus.
   D. hylohyoids, digastrics, hyoglossus, and sternothyroids.
   E. digastrics, geniohyoids, hylohyoids, stylohyoids, genioglossus, and hyoglossus.

8. Sometimes specialists assess the lung volume of voice patients because breath support is inadequate. Specialists can measure _____, or the total volume of air in the lungs; other measurements can include _____, or the amount of air inhaled and exhaled during a normal breathing cycle, and _____, or the volume of air that the patient can exhale after a maximal exhalation.

   A. total lung capacity, tidal volume, vital capacity
   B. vital capacity, tidal capacity, total lung volume
   C. vital capacity, total lung capacity, tidal volume
   D. tidal volume, total lung capacity, vital volume
   E. vital capacity, total lung volume, tidal volume

9. You have been asked to counsel with Doug Y., a 45-year-old man who has smoked and drunk alcohol since he was a teenager. He now has laryngeal cancer, and before surgery, the surgeon asks you to talk with Doug about esophageal speech. You explain to Doug that there are two basic types of esophageal speech. In one method, the patient is taught to keep the esophagus open and relaxed while inhaling rapidly. In the other method, the patient impounds the air in the oral cavity, pushes it back into the esophagus, and vibrates the cricopharyngeus muscle. The second method is called the:

   A. inhalation method.
   B. injection method.
   C. inhalatory injection method.
   D. laryngeal airway resistance method.
   E. injection resistance method.

10. The cranial nerve primarily responsible for innervating the larynx is:

   A. nerve V
   B. nerve X
   C. nerve XI
   D. nerve VI
   E. nerve IV

11. A 67-year-old man comes to you for a voice evaluation. He was referred by his primary care doctor. He states that his voice has been getting "weaker" for the last 5–6 months. Upon oral peripheral examination, you find that he has fasciculations (tremors) of the tongue and some general facial weakness. The first thing you would do is:

   A. refer him to a psychologist for an evaluation.
   B. take detailed notes and tell him to come back in 6 months.
   C. begin voice therapy, focusing on strengthening exercises.
   D. refer him to a pulmonary specialist.
   E. refer him to a neurologist for an evaluation.

12. You are asked to see an 8-year-old boy, Jason, for potential therapy because he is very hoarse. Jason has been hoarse for approximately 8 months. He is an active, happy third grader who loves sports and is engaged in various types of sports year-round (soccer, baseball, etc.). Reportedly, Jason frequently screams at games. At the school, there is one 15-minute recess in the morning and a 30-minute recess after lunch. You observe Jason on the playground at recess several times over a period of 2 weeks, and see that he loves to run, play, and yell loudly with his friends. Jason's parents have given you a letter from the ENT that definitively states that Jason has vocal nodules. After an evaluation, the first thing you would do is:

   A. prescribe 2–3 weeks of almost total voice rest, telling Jason and his parents that he can speak only when he absolutely has to—no yelling at recess or when he plays sports.
   B. monitor Jason's vocal status by seeing him once every 2 months for the next year to observe whether or not his hoarseness gets better or worse.
   C. focus on identification and reduction of vocally abuse behavior such as yelling and screaming, using computer games to help motivate Jason to use better vocal habits.

    D. send Jason to a counselor to probe into any possible emotional/psychological factors that are contributing to his vocally abusive behavior.

    E. give Jason and his parents reading materials that discuss vocal abuse, and tell the parents that if the hoarseness does not resolve in 1–2 months, you will probably see Jason for voice therapy.

13. Vivian B., a 72-year-old woman, has just had surgery for laryngeal cancer. The clinician is trying to support Vivian in many ways, including asking several laryngectomy patients from a local support group to come and talk with Vivian about her options for speech. The support group members strongly recommend the Blom-Singer prosthetic device. They explain that the Blom-Singer prosthetic device is used by laryngectomees to:

    A. clean the surgically created fistula.

    B. shunt air from the esophagus to the trachea so that the salpingopharyngeus muscle will vibrate during inhalation.

    C. assist in the development of competent esophageal speech.

    D. prevent particles of food from entering the trachea.

    E. shunt the air from the trachea to the esophagus so that the patient can speak on pulmonary air entering the esophagus.

14. Patients who might be treated with CO_2 laser surgery, recurrent laryngeal nerve resection, BOTOX, voice therapy, or a combination would probably have:

    A. contact ulcers.
                              D. spasmodic dysphonia.

    B. paradoxical vocal fold motion.
             E. Myasthenia gravis.

    C. hemangioma.

15. A client comes to a clinician seeking voice therapy. Sam M. is a 25-year-old male transgender client who has undergone several procedures to become more feminine. He tells you that he is taking estrogen also. Sam shares that he needs help to speak in a more feminine way, but he does not know how to go about this. He is also dealing with emotional issues surrounding his gender reassignment. In this case, the clinician should ideally:

    A. tell Sam that various surgical procedures such as thyroplasty are available and that having surgical procedures will be sufficient to help him change his voice to sound more feminine.

    B. advise Sam that surgical procedures are unnecessary, but that voice therapy will help him to sound more feminine by teaching new communication patterns such as higher pitch and more feminine intonation patterns.

    C. advise Sam that a combination of voice therapy and counseling will be the best way for him to sound more feminine and also receive emotional support as he deals with gender reassignment issues.

    D. share with Sam that frequently it is ideal to have a combination of surgery and voice therapy to teach such feminine communication patterns as increased pitch, increased upward inflection at the ends of utterances, and female body language.

    E. advise Sam that a combination of counseling, surgery, and voice therapy to teach more feminine pitch levels and communication patterns would best serve his needs.

16. The cover-body theory of phonation states that:

    A. the epithelium, the superficial layer of the lamina propria, and much of the intermediate layer of the lamina propria vibrate as a "cover" on a relatively stationary "body," which is made up of the remainder of the intermediate layer, the deep layer, and the TA muscle.

    B. the epithelium, the deep layer of the lamina propria, and much of the superficial layer of the lamina propria vibrate as a "cover" on a relatively stationary "body," which is made up of the remainder of the superficial layer, the deep layer, and the TA muscle.

C. the superficial layer of the lamina propria and much of the intermediate layer of the lamina propria vibrate as a "cover" on a relatively stationary "body," which is made up of the remainder of the intermediate layer, the deep layer, and the TA muscle.

D. the epithelium and much of the intermediate layer of the lamina propria vibrate as a "cover" on a relatively stationary "body," which is made up of the remainder of the intermediate layer and the TA muscle.

E. the epithelium, the superficial layer of the lamina propria and much of the intermediate layer of the lamina propria vibrate as a "cover" on a relatively stationary "body," which is made up of the remainder of the intermediate layer and the deep layer.

Questions 17–20 *refer to the following scenario.*

As a clinician in a medically based private practice, you receive a referral of 22-year-old Juanita L., a college cheerleader. Juanita has been a cheerleader since her freshman year at Freeport College; she is now a senior. Juanita works part time as a telemarketer, and according to her boyfriend she "is glued to her cell phone." Juanita also sings in the college chorus. She has been hoarse for several years and tells you during the case history that "I've ignored the way I sound—it's just me. I haven't felt like I've needed to change anything." However, Juanita shares that lately, she has been feeling a lot of pain and the hoarseness is substantially worse. She says that "sometimes when I talk, it's almost like there's a 'double voice.'" Juanita tells you that she is worried because she will graduate from college in three months, and will be looking for a job. She is worried that employers will not want to hire someone who "sounds like a frog." You immediately refer Juanita to an otolaryngologist for a thorough examination of her vocal folds. You then proceed to do your own instrumental and perceptual evaluation. You come up with a number of findings, including the fact that Juanita has increased laryngeal airway resistance, a maximum phonation time of 6 seconds, and dysphonia. You think that Juanita is a probable candidate for phonosurgery, but will wait for the otolaryngologist's diagnosis and recommendations.

17. When you assess Juanita, you indeed find the presence of "double voice." The perception of two distinct simultaneous pitches during phonation is:

A. glottal fry.
B. diplophonia.
C. strain-strangle.
D. cul-de-sac resonance.
E. harshness.

18. You need to view Juanita's vocal folds. You know that the otolaryngologist will do this also, but you are fortunate to have instrumentation available to you. You decide to use a procedure that uses a pulsing light to permit the optical illusion of slow-motion viewing of the vocal folds. This is called:

A. electroglottography.
B. stroboscopy.
C. electromyography.
D. videofluoroscopy.
E. nasoendoscopy.

19. Measures of jitter and shimmer are becoming more common in use with voice patients because they can be useful in early detection of vocal pathology. Although you suspect that the otolaryngologist will find obvious vocal pathology given Juanita's history of prolonged hoarseness, you still want to obtain measures of jitter and shimmer because these can serve as an excellent baseline—especially if Juanita has phonosurgery. When you take these measures, you might expect to see:

A.   a small amount of shimmer and a large amount of jitter.
B.   a large amount of jitter with only a small-moderate amount of shimmer.
C.   large amounts of both jitter and shimmer, with more than 1 dB of variation across vibratory cycles when jitter is measured.
D.   large amounts of both jitter and shimmer, with more than 1 dB of variation across vibratory cycles when shimmer is measured.
E.   large amounts of both jitter and shimmer, with Juanita being able to sustain a vowel with approximately 15% shimmer.

20. You receive a phone call and a report from the otolaryngologist that Juanita will indeed need phonosurgery for the presence of bilateral vocal fold polyps (the right polyp is larger than the left). The otolaryngologist wants you to obtain quantitative measurements of Juanita's voice before phonosurgery; he wants to use these baseline measures as a comparison with measures taken after phonosurgery to evaluate whether or not the phonosurgery was successful. To obtain these quantitative measurements, you will probably use:

A.   esophageal manometry.
B.   indirect laryngoscopy.
C.   a sound spectrograph.
D.   a plethysmograph.
E.   a Nasometer.

REFERENCES AND RECOMMENDED READINGS

American Cancer Society, The National Cancer Information Center. (2003). 1825B Kramer Lane, Ste 200, Austin, TX 78758.

Andrews, M. L. (1999). *Manual of voice treatment: Pediatrics through geriatrics* (2nd ed.) New York: Thomson Delmar Learning.

Andrews, M. L. (2001). *Voice treatment for children and adolescents.* New York: Thomson Delmar Learning.

Aronson, A. (1990). *Clinical voice disorders: An interdisciplinary approach* (3rd ed.). New York: Thieme.

Baken, R. J., & Orlikoff, R. F. (2000). *Clinical measurement of speech and voice.* New York: Thomson Delmar Learning.

Bless, D. M., & Poburka, B. (2002). *Video laryngeal stroboscopy.* New York: Thomson Delmar Learning.

Boone, D. R., McFarlane, S. C., & von Berg, S. (2005). *The voice and voice therapy* (7th ed.). Boston: Allyn & Bacon.

Brin, M. F., Velickovic, M., Ramig, L. O., & Fox, C. (2004). Dysphonia due to Parkinson's disease: Pharmacological, surgical, and behavioral management perspectives. In C. M. Sapienza & J. Casper (Eds.), *Vocal rehabilitation for medical speech–language pathology* (pp. 209–270). Austin, TX: PRO-ED.

Case, J. L. (2002). *Clinical management of voice disorders* (4th ed.). Austin, TX: PRO-ED.

Casper, J. K., & Colton, R. H. (1998). *Clinical manual for laryngectomy and head/neck cancer rehabilitation.* New York: Thomson Delmar Learning.

Collins, S., & Samlan, R. (2004). Gastroesophageal reflux/extraesophageal reflux disease: Medical, behavioral, and pharmacological perspectives. In C. M. Sapienza & J. Casper (Eds.), *Vocal rehabilitation for medical speech–language pathology* (pp. 293–330). Austin, TX: PRO-ED.

Davenport, P., & Sapienza, C. (2004). Pulmonary function and breathing for speech. In C. M. Sapienza & J. Casper (Eds.), *Vocal rehabilitation for medical speech–language pathology* (pp. 331–364). Austin, TX: PRO-ED.

Deem, J. F., & Miller, L. (2000). *Manual of voice therapy* (2nd ed.). Austin, TX: PRO-ED.

DeJarnette, G., & Holland, R. W. (1998). Voice and voice disorders. In D. E. Battle (Ed.), *Communication disorders in multicultural populations* (2nd ed., pp. 275–308). Newton, MA: Butterworth-Heinemann.

Dworkin, J. D., Marunick, M. T., & Krouse, J. H. (2004). Velopharyngeal dsyfunction: Speech characteristics, variable etiologies, evaluation techniques, and differential treatments. *Language, Speech, and Hearing Services in Schools, 35,* 333–352.

Gallivan, G., & Adrianopoulos, M. (2004). Dysphonia due to paradoxical vocal fold movement/episodic paroxysmal laryngospasm: Medical and pharmacological perspectives. In C. M. Sapienza & J. Casper (Eds.), *Vocal rehabilitation for medical speech-language pathology* (pp. 165–208). Austin, TX: PRO-ED.

Gelfer, M. P. (1999). Voice treatment for the male-to-female transgendered client. *American Journal of Speech–Language Pathology, 8,* 201–208.

Gelfer, M. P., & Schofield, K. J. (2000). Comparison of acoustic and perceptual measures of voice in male-to-female transsexuals perceived as female versus those perceived as male. *Journal of Voice, 14,* 22–23.

Haynes, W. O., & Pindzola, R. H. (2004). *Diagnosis and evaluation in speech pathology* (6th ed.). Boston: Allyn & Bacon.

Henry Benjamin International Gender Dysphoria Association (HBIGDA) (2003). 1-612-625-1500. Address: 1300 South Second Street, Suite 180, Minneapolis, MN 55454.

Hirano, M. (1977). Structure and vibratory behavior of the vocal folds. In M. Sawashima & F. S. Cooper (Eds.), *Dynamic aspects of speech production* (pp. 13–30). Tokyo: University of Tokyo Press.

Hooper, C. R. (2000). Voice treatment for the male-to-female transsexual. In J. C. Stemple (Ed.), *Voice therapy clinical studies* (2nd ed.). San Diego, CA: Singular Publishing.

Hooper, C. R. (2004). Treatment of voice disorders in children. *Language, Speech, and Hearing Services in Schools, 35,* 320–326.

Kay Elemetrics. (2004). Computerized Speech Lab, Model 4500 [computer software]. Lincoln Park, NJ: Author.

Kent, R. D., & Ball, M. J. (2000). Voice quality measurement. San Diego, CA: Singular Publishing Group.

Linville, S. E. (2002). Source characteristics of aged voice assessed from long-term average spectra. *Journal of Voice, 16,* 472–479.

Lyon, M., & Barkmeier-Kraemer, J. (2004). Vascular supply of the larynx. In C. M. Sapienza & J. Casper (Eds.), *Vocal rehabilitation for medical speech–language pathology* (pp. 69–108). Austin, TX: PRO-ED.

Malmgren, L. T., & Glaze, L. (2004). Intervention for vocal fold atrophy, vocal fold bowing, and immobility. In C. M. Sapienza & J. Casper (Eds.), *Vocal rehabilitation for medical speech–language pathology* (pp. 109–144). Austin, TX: PRO-ED.

Nicolosi, L., Harryman, E., & Kresheck, J. (2004). *Terminology of communication disorders: Speech-language-hearing* (5th ed.). Baltimore: Lippincott Williams & Wilkins.

Pannbacker, M. (2004). Velopharyngeal incompetence: The need for speech standards. *American Journal of Speech-Language Pathology, 13,* 195–201.

Prater, R. J., & Swift, R. W. (1984). *Manual of voice therapy.* Boston: Little, Brown.

Ramig, L. O., Bonitati, C. M., Lemke, J. H., & Horii, Y. (1994). Voice treatment for patients with Parkinson's disease: Development of an approach and preliminary efficacy data. *Journal of Medical Speech–Language Pathology, 2,* 191–209.

Rammage, L., Morrisson, M., & Nichol, H. (2001). *Management of the voice and its disorders.* New York: Thomson Delmar Learning.

Rosen, C. A., Woodson, G. E., Thompson, J. W., Hengesteg, A. P., & Bradlow, H. L. (1998). Preliminary results of the use of indole-3-carginol for recurrent respiratory papillomatosis. *Current Opinion in Otolaryngology and Head and Neck Surgery, 118,* 810–815.

Roy, N., Merrill, R. M., Thibeault, S., Gray, S. D., & Smith, E. M. (2004). Voice disorders in teachers and the general population: Effects on work performance, attendance, and future career choices. *Journal of Speech, Language, and Hearing Research, 47,* 542–551.

Rubin, J. S., Sataloff, R. T., & Korovin, G. S. (2003). *Diagnosis and treatment of voice disorders* (2nd ed.). New York: Thomson Delmar Learning.

Sandage, M. J., & Zelazny, S. K. (2004). Paradoxical vocal fold motion in children and adolescents. *Language, Speech, and Hearing Services in Schools, 35*, 353–362.

Sapienza, C. M., & Casper, J. (Eds.). (2004). *Vocal rehabilitation for medical speech–language pathology.* Austin, TX: PRO-ED,

Shipley, K. G., & Roseberry-McKibbin, C. (2006). *Interviewing and counseling in communicative disorders: Principles and procedures* (3rd ed.). Austin, TX: PRO-ED.

Stemple, J. C. (2000). *Voice therapy, clinical case studies.* New York: Thomson Delmar Learning.

Stemple, J. C., Glaze, L. E., & Klaben, B. G. (2000). *Clinical voice pathology, theory, and management.* New York: Thomson Delmar Learning.

Sue, D. W., & Sue, D. (2003). *Counseling the culturally diverse: Theory and practice* (4th ed.). New York: John Wiley & Sons.

Thibeault, S. L., & Gray, G. (2004). Response of the vocal mechanism to trauma. In C. M. Sapienza & J. Casper (Eds.), Vocal rehabilitation for medical speech–language pathology (pp. 11–28). Austin, TX: PRO-ED.

van der Merwe, A. (2004). The voice use reduction program. *American Journal of Speech-Language Pathology, 13*, 208–218.

Woodnorth, G. H. (2004). Assessing and managing medically fragile children: Tracheostomy and ventilatory support. *Language, Speech, and Hearing Services in Schools, 35*, 363–372.

Woodson, G. E., & Murry, T. (2004). Spasmodic dysphonia: Medical, pharmacological, and behavioral perspectives. In C. M. Sapienza & J. Casper (Eds.), *Vocal rehabilitation for medical speech–language pathology* (pp. 145–164). Austin, TX: PRO-ED.

Study & Review
Answers

6. C. The infrahyoid laryngeal muscles that lie below the hyoid bone (sometimes called *depressors*) are the: thyrohyoids, omohyoids, sternothyroids, and sternohyoids (TOSS).

7. E. The suprahyoid muscles or elevators are the: digastrics, geniohyoids, hylohyoids, stylohyoids, genioglossus, and hyoglossus.

8. A. Sometimes specialists assess the lung volume of voice patients because breath support is inadequate. Specialists can measure total lung capacity, or the total volume of air in the lungs; other measurements can include tidal volume, or the amount of air inhaled and exhaled during a normal breathing cycle, and vital capacity, or the volume of air that the patient can exhale after a maximal exhalation.

9. B. In the injection method, the patient impounds the air in the oral cavity, pushes it back into the esophagus, and vibrates the cricopharyngeus muscle.

10. B. Cranial nerve X, the vagus nerve, is primarily responsible for laryngeal innervation.

11. E. The first thing a clinician must do with a patient who exhibits potential signs of a neurological problem is refer the patient to a neurologist.

12. C. Voice rest for an 8-year-old boy is somewhat unrealistic. There is no indication that he needs a counselor. He is old enough to identify and reduce vocally abusive behaviors.

13. E. The Blom-Singer device is used to shunt air from the trachea to the esophagus so that the patient can speak on that air.

14. D. The above-listed treatment techniques are commonly used with patients who have spasmodic dysphonia.

15. E. It would be best for the clinician to advise Sam that a combination of counseling, surgery, and voice therapy to teach more feminine pitch levels and communication patterns would best serve his needs.

16. A. The cover-body theory of phonation states that the epithelium, the superficial layer of the lamina propria, and much of the intermediate layer of the lamina propria vibrate as a "cover" on a relatively stationary "body," which is made up of the remainder of the intermediate layer, the deep layer, and the TA muscle.

17. B. The term diplophonia refers to the perception of a "double voice."

18. B. Stroboscopy is the only procedure that uses a pulsing "strobe" light for perceived slow-motion viewing of the vocal folds.

19. D. Measurements of jitter, or frequency perturbation, indicate that in a normal speaker with no vocal pathology, jitter should be less than 1% as the speaker sustains a vowel. Measurements of shimmer, or amplitude perturbation, evaluate the cycle-to-cycle variation of vocal intensity. Some experts believe that more than 1 dB of variation across cycles causes a patient to sound dysphonic.

20. C. The sound or speech spectrograph is very useful for quantitative analysis of speech, and is often used to obtain baseline measurements of a patient's vocal characteristics prior to phonosurgery. Postsurgery measures can be obtained and compared to the baseline measurements of Juanita's voice to quantitatively document vocal improvement or decline.

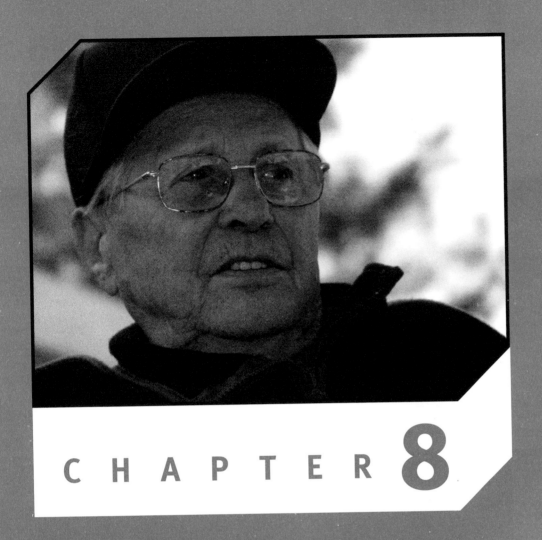

CHAPTER 8

NEUROLOGICALLY BASED

COMMUNICATIVE

DISORDERS

AND DYSPHAGIA

Neuropathologies or brain trauma cause

several disorders of communication. In this chapter, we provide an overview of the nature, assessment, and treatment of such communicative disorders, which include aphasia, apraxia of speech, dysarthrias, dementia, right hemisphere syndrome, traumatic brain injury, and swallowing disorders (dysphagia).

Strokes often cause aphasia, a neurologically based language disorder. There are different types of aphasia, depending upon the area(s) of the brain in which the stroke(s) occurred. Apraxia is a neurogenic speech disorder characterized by sensorimotor problems in volitional production of speech. Dysarthrias (all types) are a group of motor speech disorders that result from impaired muscular control of the speech mechanism due to nervous system pathology. Dementia is an acquired neurological syndrome that is usually accompanied by progressive deterioration in intellectual functioning. Right hemisphere syndrome describes a group of characteristics—mostly related to perceptual and attentional deficits—demonstrated by patients with neurological insult to the right hemisphere. Traumatic brain injury refers to injury to the brain due to external force or physical trauma. Finally, dysphagia refers to swallowing disorders, which are not necessarily related to communication disorders.

To understand communication disorders described in this chapter, an adequate knowledge of neuroanatomy and the basic neuroscience is essential. See Chapter 1 and consult other sources (Bhatnagar, 2002; Webster, 1999).

APHASIA

INTRODUCTION

Aphasia, a neurologically based language disorder, is caused by various types of neuropathologies (most commonly stroke). Aphasia can be classified as fluent, nonfluent, and subcortical. Aphasia may or may not be accompanied by alexia, agraphia, or agnosia. Assessment of patients with aphasia may involve standardized tests and functional assessment tools. Treatment of aphasia is concerned with verbal expression, auditory comprehension, reading, writing, and nonverbal modes of communication.

Foundational Concepts

- *Aphasia* is a neurologically based language disorder, contrasted with such neurologically based speech disorders as apraxia and dysarthria.

- Aphasia is caused by various kinds of neuropathologies. The third leading cause of death in the United States, cerebrovascular accidents (CVA), popularly known as strokes, are the most common causes of aphasia.

- About 750,000 new cases of stroke are reported each year. Incidence of strokes increases with advancing age; two thirds of strokes are associated with age 65 and older.

- Although men are more prone to CVAs, because of their longevity more women experience them.

- More than 50% of those who survive a stroke have aphasia.

- Strokes cause permanent disability in more than 300,000 people.

- African American men and women have higher incidence of strokes than white men and women.

- South Asians have a high prevalence of strokes.

- Native Americans tend to have more hemorrhagic strokes than whites.

- Hispanics and African Americans tend to have strokes at an earlier age than whites.

- Whites are more prone to ischemic strokes than Hispanics; African Americans, Hispanics, and Asians are more prone to hemorrhagic strokes than whites.

- Strokes may be ischemic or hemorrhagic. *Ischemic* strokes are caused by a blocked or interrupted blood supply to the brain. Blockage or interruption may be caused by two kinds of arterial diseases: thrombosis or embolism.

- A *thrombus* is a collection of blood material that blocks the flow of blood. An *embolus* is a traveling mass of arterial debris or a clump of tissue from a tumor that gets lodged in a smaller artery and thus blocks the flow of blood.

- *Hemorrhagic strokes* are caused by bleeding in the brain due to ruptured blood vessels. Ruptures may be *intracerebral* (within the brain) or *extracerebral* (within the meninges, resulting in subarchnoid, subdural, and epidural varieties).

- Other causes of aphasia include brain trauma, intracranial tumors, and infections. Tumors may be *primary intracranial* (grown within the brain) or *secondary*, or *metastatic* (grown elsewhere but migrated and attached to brain tissue and still growing). Infections may be bacterial or viral.

Definition and Classification of Aphasia

- There are numerous definitions of aphasia. Some are nontypological and others are typological. *Nontypological definitions* suggest a single disorder. Other definitions are based on cognitive functions. *Typological definitions* classify aphasia into types (Hegde, 2005).

- A general definition of aphasia is that it is a loss or impairment of language caused by a recent brain injury (Benson & Ardila, 1996). Comprehension and expression of language, along with reading and writing, may be impaired.

- Darley's (1982) definition of aphasia as "an impairment, as a result of brain damage, of the capacity for interpretation and formulation of language symbols" (p. 42) illustrates a nontypological definition. The definition suggests a unitary language disorder due to recent brain injury.

- There are several typological definitions. For example, Goodglass, Kaplan, and Barresi (2001a) define aphasia as the "disturbance of any or all of the skills, associations and habits of spoken or written language, produced by injury to certain brain areas that are specialized for these functions" (p. 5). The terms *any disturbance* and *all disturbance* can refer to different types of aphasia. Most contemporary experts classify aphasia into fluent aphasias, nonfluent aphasias, and subcortical aphasias.

- Cognitive definitions base their description on impaired cognition. For example, Davis (2000) defines aphasia as "a selective impairment of the cognitive system specialized for comprehending and formulating language, leaving other cognitive capacities intact" (p. 17).

- Communication disorders that are progressive and are due to such neurological diseases as Alzheimer's disease and Parkinson's disease are *not* aphasia. Also, confused or abnormal language associated with psychiatric disorders (e.g., schizophrenia) is not aphasia.

Nonfluent Aphasias

- Varieties of nonfluent aphasias are characterized by limited, agrammatic, effortful, halting, and slow speech with impaired prosody.

Broca's Aphasia

- This nonfluent variety of aphasia is caused by damage to Broca's area (Brodmann's areas 44 and 45) in the posterior inferior frontal gyrus of the left hemisphere. Broca's area is supplied by the upper division of the middle cerebral artery. Damage to Broca's area is not essential to produce this type of aphasia, because symptoms characteristics of Broca's aphasia may be observed in patients who have *intact* Broca's area.

- Broca's aphasia is characterized by:

    - nonfluent, effortful, slow, halting, and uneven speech
    - limited word output, short phrases and sentences
    - misarticulated or distorted sounds
    - agrammatic or telegraphic speech (often limited to nouns and verbs, with omission of articles, conjunctions, and prepositions)
    - impaired repetition of words and sentences, especially the grammatic elements of a sentence
    - impaired naming, especially confrontation naming
    - rarely normal, but better auditory comprehension of spoken language than production
    - difficulty in understanding syntactic structures
    - poor oral reading and poor comprehension of material read
    - writing problems (slow and laborious writing that is full of spelling errors and letter omissions, possibly because patients are forced to use their nonpreferred left hand due to paralysis of the right hand)
    - monotonous speech

- Although not a characteristic of aphasia, patients with Broca's aphasia may exhibit apraxia of speech and dysarthria. In essence, patients who have Broca's aphasia also may have one or more, independent, speech disorders.
- Patients with Broca's aphasia may have right-sided paralysis or weakness (paresis).
- Some patients with Broca's aphasia may be depressed or react emotionally when confronted with difficult assessment tasks.

Transcortical Motor Aphasia (TMA)

- This nonfluent variety of aphasia is caused by lesions in the anterior superior frontal lobe, often below or above Broca's area, which is not affected. The areas supplied by the anterior cerebral artery and the anterior branch of the middle cerebral artery are affected in TMA.
- Transcortical motor aphasia is characterized by:

    - initial speechlessness
    - echolalia and perseveration
    - absent or reduced spontaneous speech
    - nonfluent, paraphasic, agrammatic, and telegraphic speech
    - *intact repetition skill,* a distinguishing characteristic
    - awareness of grammaticality (patients may correct a grammatically incorrect model)
    - refusal to repeat nonsense syllables
    - unfinished sentences
    - limited word fluency
    - simple and imprecise syntactic structures
    - attempts to initiate speech with the help of such motor activities as clapping, vigorous head nodding, and hand waving
    - generally good comprehension of simple conversation; possibly impaired for complex speech
    - slow and difficult reading aloud
    - seriously disturbed writing

- Patients with TMA tend to exhibit such motor disorders as rigidity of upper extremity, absence or poverty of movement (akinesia), lowness of movement (bradykinesia), buccofacial apraxia, and weakness of the legs.
- Apathy, withdrawal, and little interest in communication may be additional behavioral characteristic of some patients with TMA.

Mixed Transcortical Aphasia (MTA)

- This somewhat rare variety of nonfluent aphasia is caused by lesions in the watershed area or the arterial border zone (between the areas supplied by the middle cerebral arteries and the anterior and posterior arteries, described in Chapter 1).
- MTA is characterized by:

  - limited spontaneous speech
  - automatic, unintentional, and involuntary nature of communication
  - severe echolalia (parrotlike repetition of what is heard)
  - repetition of an examiner's statement
  - severely impaired fluency
  - severely impaired auditory comprehension for even simple conversation
  - marked naming difficulty and neologism; impaired confrontation naming
  - mostly unimpaired automatic speech (e.g., recitation of months in a year or a number series) if somehow initiated and not interrupted
  - severely impaired reading, reading comprehension, and writing

- Varied neurologic symptoms are seen across patients; these may include bilateral uppermotor neuron paralysis (spastic paralysis that affects the volitional muscles), weakness of all limbs (quadriparesis), and visual field defects.

Global Aphasia

- This is the most severe form of nonfluent aphasia. It is caused by extensive lesions affecting all language areas (the perisylvian region). Widespread destruction of the fronto-temporo-parietal regions is common. The more common sites of damage are supplied by the middle cerebral artery.
- Global aphasia is characterized by:

  - profoundly impaired language skills and no significant profile of differential skills
  - greatly reduced fluency
  - expressions limited to a few words, exclamations, and serial utterances
  - impaired repetition
  - impaired naming
  - auditory comprehension limited to single words at best
  - perseveration (repetition of short utterances)
  - impaired reading and writing

- Verbal and nonverbal apraxia, although technically not a part of aphasia, may be present in patients with global aphasia.
- Strong neurological symptoms, including right-side paresis or paralysis, right-sided sensory loss, and neglect of the left side of the body, may be observed in many patients.

Fluent Aphasias

- Varieties of fluent aphasias are characterized by relatively intact fluency but generally less meaningful, or even meaningless, speech.

- The speech is generally flowing, abundant, easily initiated, and well articulated with good prosody and phrase length.

Wernicke's Aphasia

- This common variety of fluent aphasia is caused by lesions in Wernicke's area (the posterior portion of the superior temporal gyrus in the left hemisphere). Wernicke's area is supplied by the posterior branch of the left middle cerebral artery.
- Wernicke's aphasia is characterized by:

    - incessant, effortlessly produced, flowing speech with normal, or even abnormal, fluency (*logorrhea,* or *press of speech*) with normal phrase length
    - rapid rate of speech with normal prosodic features and good articulation
    - intact grammatical structures
    - severe word-finding problems
    - paraphasic speech containing semantic and literal paraphasias, extra syllables in words, and creation of meaningless words (neologisms)
    - circumlocution (talking around words that cannot be recalled)
    - empty speech (substitution of such general words as *this, that, stuff,* and *thing*)
    - poor auditory comprehension, especially for sentences and names of common objects; much worse comprehension of speech when there is background noise, movements, and background conversation
    - impaired conversational turn taking
    - impaired repetition skill
    - reading comprehension problems, including difficulty recognizing sounds associated with written words, meanings of printed words
    - writing problems, including excessive but meaningless writing, frequent misspellings, and neologistic writing
    - generally poor communication in spite of fluent speech

- Patients with Wernicke's aphasia may sound confused. Because of lack of insight into their language problems, the patients are less frustrated with their failed attempts at communication. The patients also may be paranoid, homicidal, suicidal, and depressed; therefore, they may be confused with psychiatric patients.
- Patients with Wernicke's aphasia are generally free from obvious neurological symptoms; paresis and paralysis are uncommon.

Transcortical Sensory Aphasia (TSA)

- This variety of fluent aphasia is caused by lesions in the temporo-parietal region, especially in the posterior portion of the middle temporal gyrus. This region is supplied by the posterior branches of the left middle cerebral artery.

- TSA is characterized by:

    - fluent speech with normal phrase length, good prosody, normal articulation, and apparently appropriate grammar and syntax
    - paraphasic and empty speech
    - severe naming problems and pauses due to those problems
    - good repetition skills but poor comprehension of repeated words
    - echolalia of grammatically incorrect forms, nonsense syllables, and words from foreign languages (unlike patients with TMA)
    - impaired auditory comprehension of spoken language
    - difficulty in pointing, obeying commands, or answering simple yes/no questions
    - normal automatic speech (e.g., counting)
    - tendency to complete poems and sentences started by the clinician
    - good reading (aloud) but poor comprehension of material read
    - generally better oral reading skills than other language skills
    - writing problems that parallel those in expressive speech

- A hemiparesis associated with the onset of TSA may disappear, leaving the patient with no obvious neurologic impairment. Neglect of one side of the body may be common.
- Patients with TSA sound similar to those with Wernicke's aphasia; however, *repetition is intact in patients with TSA, whereas it is impaired in patients with Wernicke's aphasia.*

Conduction Aphasia

- This rare variety of fluent aphasia is caused by lesions in the region between Broca's area and Wernicke's area, especially in the supramarginal gyrus and the arcuate fasciculus. Lesion sites of conduction aphasia are controversial, as is this aphasia type.
- Conduction aphasia is characterized by:

    - disproportionate impairment in repetition (a distinguishing characteristic); especially impaired repetition of longer words, function words, and longer phrases and sentences
    - variable speech fluency across patients; generally less fluent than patients with Wernicke's aphasia
    - paraphasic speech
    - marked word-finding problems, especially for content words
    - empty speech because of omitted content words
    - efforts to correct errors in speech, though not always successful
    - good syntax, prosody, and articulation
    - severe to mild naming problems
    - near-normal auditory comprehension, especially for routine conversational speech
    - being better at pointing to a named stimulus than at confrontation naming
    - highly variable reading problems; better comprehension of silently read material
    - writing problems in most cases
    - buccofacial apraxia (difficulty in performing buccofacial movements when requested) in most patients

- Symptoms of conduction aphasia are similar to those of Wernicke's aphasia. A main difference is that unlike patients with Wernicke's aphasia, those with conduction aphasia have good to normal auditory comprehension.
- While some patients may have no neurological symptoms, others may have paresis of the right

side of the face, limb, or oral apraxia and right sensory impairment; patients may recover from most of these impairments.

Anomic Aphasia

- This variety of fluent aphasia is controversial and may be caused by lesions in different regions, including the angular gyrus, the second temporal gyrus, and the juncture of the temporo-parietal lobes.
- Anomic aphasia is a syndrome, whereas *anomia* is a naming difficulty (a symptom) common to most forms of aphasia.
- Anomic aphasia is characterized by:

  - a most debilitating and pervasive word-finding difficulty, which is the distinguishing feature; however, pointing to named objects is unimpaired
  - generally fluent speech
  - normal syntax except for pauses (possibly due to word-finding problems)
  - use of vague and nonspecific words, resulting in empty speech
  - verbal paraphasia (word substitutions)
  - circumlocution (beating around the bush because of lack of access to precise words)
  - good auditory comprehension of spoken language
  - intact repetition
  - unimpaired articulation
  - normal oral reading skills and good reading comprehension
  - normal writing skills

- The distinguishing feature of anomic aphasia is that, generally, most language functions, except for naming, are relatively unimpaired.
- A residual symptom of most patients who recover from any type of aphasia is a naming difficulty.

Subcortical Aphasia

- Aphasia is typically produced by cortical damage; however, aphasia due to subcortical injury has been reported in recent years.
- Extensive subcortical damage, with possible involvement of left cortical areas, may underlie this type of aphasia. Lesions in areas surrounding the basal ganglia and the thalamus have been linked to subcortical aphasia.
- Subcortical aphasia caused by lesions in the basal ganglia and surrounding structures in the left hemisphere is characterized by:

  - fluent speech, which may include pauses and hesitations
  - intact repetition skills
  - normal auditory comprehension for routine conversation; may be defective for complex material
  - articulation problems (similar to those in Broca's aphasia)
  - prosodic problems
  - word-finding problems
  - semantic paraphasia in some cases
  - relatively preserved writing skills
  - limb apraxia if the lesions extend posteriorly to deep white matter in the parietal area

- Subcortical aphasia caused by lesions or hemorrhages in the left thalamus is characterized by:

  - hemiplegia, hemisensory loss, right-visual field problems, and, in some cases, coma
  - initial mutism, which may improve to paraphasic speech
  - severe naming problems
  - good auditory comprehension of simple material and poor comprehension of complex material
  - good repetition skills
  - impaired reading and writing skills

CONCEPTS TO CONSIDER

Describe the major characteristics of fluent and nonfluent aphasias. Describe common as well as unique symptoms.

_____

_____

_____

_____

_____

Aphasia in Bilingual Populations

- Aphasia in bilinguals constitutes an interesting clinical entity that needs more research (Paradis, 1998).

- In the United States, about 150,000 bilingual individuals have aphasia in any given year; about 45,000 new cases of bilingual aphasia are reported every year.

- In bilingual speakers, as in unilingual speakers, language is represnted in the left hemisphere (contrary to some suggestion of right dominance).

- Systematic research on aphasia in both the languages of bilingual speakers is limited.

- Patterns of recovery from aphasia in bilingual individuals vary. Some may recover both the languages, some only one language, and some only the dominant language. Some patients may recover one language first and the other after months. Some patients may lose the recovered language as they begin to recover the other language.

- Some patients may mix languages or automatically translate their utterances or those they hear into one of their languages.

■ Clinicians should analyze individual patterns, not just known patterns, in persons who are bilingual and have aphasia.

Aphasia in Left-Handed Individuals

■ Aphasia in left-handed individuals is another interesting clinical entity, but research information is slow to accumulate because of its limited incidence (Basso & Rusconi, 1998).

■ Of the 4% of the general population that is left-handed, half have language representation in the left hemishpere, and the other half in the right. In essence, only 2% of the population has a right dominance for language.

■ Incidence of aphasia due to left hemisphere damage in left-handed individuals is the same as that in right-handed persons who suffer a left-hemisphere damage.

■ Incidence of aphasia caused by a right-hemisphere damage in left-handed persons is higher than the incidence of the same kind of aphasia in right-handed individuals.

■ The symptom complex and recovery patterns of aphasia in left-handed individuals (with either left or right damage) seem to be comparable to those found in typical patients (right-handed, left-language dominant).

Assessment of Aphasia

Foundational Concepts

- Assessment of aphasia involves an evaluation of speech and language skills along with reading and writing skills.
- Related cognitive functions also may be assessed, depending on the clinician's theoretical view and treatment goals. Both standardized and client-specific procedures may be used.

Standardized Aphasia Tests

- Aphasia screening tests include the *Aphasia Language Performance Scales* (ALPS) (Keenan & Brassell, 1975); *Sklar Aphasia Scale* (SAS) (Sklar, 1983); *Aphasia Screening Test* (Whurr, 1996); *Bedside Evaluation and Screening Test–Second Edition* (BEST–2) (West, Sands, & Ross-Swain, 1998); *Aphasia Screening Test* (Reitan, 1991); and *Quick Assessment for Aphasia* (Tanner & Culbertson, 1999).
- Screening tests should not replace diagnostic tests and extended client-specific observations. The following are among the more frequently used diagnostic tests:

  - The *Boston Diagnostic Aphasia Examination–Third Edition* (BDAE) (Kaplan & Barresi, 2001). Helpful in evaluating articulation, fluency, word-finding, repetition, serial speech, grammar, paraphasias, auditory comprehension, oral reading, reading comprehension, writing, and musical skills (e.g., singing), this test tries to classify aphasia into types.
  - The *Western Aphasia Battery* (WAB) (Kertesz, 1982). This test evaluates speech content, fluency, auditory comprehension, repetition, naming, reading, writing, calculation,

drawing, nonverbal thinking, and block design, this test also tries to classify aphasia into types.

- The *Minnesota Test for Differential Diagnosis of Aphasia* (MTDDA) (Schuell, 1972). MTDDA evaluates five areas of performance: auditory disturbances, visual and reading disturbances, speech and language disturbances, visuomotor and writing disturbances, and numerical and arithmetic disturbances.

- The *Neurosensory Center Comprehensive Examination for Aphasia* (NCCEA) (Spreen & Benton, 1977). This test evaluates such language functions as comprehension, production, reading, writing, word fluency, digit and sentence repetition, visual object naming, sentence construction, and articulation. The test also evaluates visual and tactile functions.

- *Multilingual Aphasia Examination* (Benton & Hamsher, 1978). This test is similar to the NCCEA in its contents. It evaluates such language functions as naming, repetition, fluency, auditory comprehension, spelling, and writing. It comes in English, French, German, Italian, and Spanish versions.

- *Bilingual Aphasia Test* (BAT) (Paradis, 1987). A comprehensive test that helps evaluate skills in forty languages with parallel forms. A patient's phonologic, morphologic, syntactic, lexical, and semantic skills in a primary and a secondary language may be assessed.

- The *Porch Index of Communicative Ability* (PICA) (Porch, 1981). A limited measure of language, the Porch evaluates auditory comprehension, reading, oral expressive language, pantomime, visual matching, writing, and copying. However, the test requires intensive training to administer and score.

- *Aphasia Diagnostic Profile* (Helm-Estabrooks, 1992). This test helps assess overall severity of aphasia along with such specific skills as comprehension, word retrieval, repetition, and alternative communication. The test helps classify aphasia.

Functional Assessment Tools

- Some assessment tools target functional communication. These are useful in evaluating daily communication in everyday settings. Functional assessment tools may be less biased than standardized tests in evaluating clients from linguistically and culturally diverse backgrounds. Changes in functional communication during treatment may be measured.

- Most tools require clinicians to make extensive and systematic observation of their clients and rate them on variables being measured. Commonly used functional communication tools include the following:

  - *Functional Communication Profile* (Sarno, 1969). This test evaluates 45 behaviors in five categories: movement, speaking, understanding, reading, and "other." A 9-point rating scale is used to evaluate the performance.

  - *Communicative Abilities in Daily Living–Second Edition* (Holland, Frattali, & Fromm, 1998). This test emphasizes daily communication in everyday situations. Such skills as reading, writing, estimation of time, use of verbal and nonverbal contexts in communication, role playing, social conventions, nonverbal symbolic communication, humor, absurdity, and metaphor are rated.

  - *Communicative Effectiveness Index* (Lomas, Pickard, Bester, Elbard, Finlayson, & Zoghaib, 1989). This test helps assess four domains of functional communication skills, including social needs, life skills, basic needs, and health threats. Such specific skills as giving yes/no answers, expressing physical pain or discomfort, and starting a conversation are rated.

  - *Communication Profile: A Functional Skills Survey* (Payne, 1994). An advantage of this test is that its sample included patients from African American, Native American/Alaska Native, Asian American/Pacific Islander, and Asian American ethnic groups. Therefore, this test is especially useful in evaluating patients from those ethnocultural backgrounds. The test uses a 5-point scale to rate the importance of selected skills in daily living.

- *Functional Assessment of Communication Skills for Adults* (ASHA FACS) (Frattali, Thompson, Holland, Wohl, & Ferketic, 1995). This test was developed for the American Speech-Language-Hearing Association. It helps rate social communication; communication of basic needs; reading, writing, and number concepts; and daily planning. Clinicians or others familiar with the patient may make the observations and complete the rating form.
- *Amsterdam Nijmegan Everyday Language Test* (ANELT) (Blomert, Kean, Koster, & Schokker, 1994). This test has two parallel forms, each containing ten items to assess pragmatic language skills related to familiar daily living activities.
- *Revised Edinburgh Functional Communication Profile* (Wirz, Skinner, & Dean, 1990). This test evaluates such pragmatic communication skills as greeting, acknowledging, responding, requesting, and initiating conversation.

- In addition to diagnostic aphasia tests, clinicians may use independent tests of specific skills such as auditory comprehension and reading.
- Various tests of auditory comprehension include the *Token Test* (DeRenzi & Vignolo, 1962); the *Auditory Comprehension Test for Sentences* (Shewan, 1979); *Functional Auditory Comprehension Task* (LaPointe & Horner, 1978); and the *Discourse Comprehension Test* (Brookshire & Nichols, 1993).
- Tests of reading skills include the *Reading Comprehension Battery for Aphasia–Second Edition* (LaPointe & Horner, 1998); the *Nelson Reading Skills Test* (Hanna, Schell, & Schreiner, 1977); and the *Gates-MacGinitie Reading Test* (Gates, 1978).

CONCEPTS TO CONSIDER

Briefly describe two standardized tests and two functional assessment tools that can be used with patients who have aphasia.

_____

_____

_____

_____

_____

An Outline of Aphasia Assessment

- Aphasia assessment includes such standard procedures as a detailed case history, orofacial examination, and hearing screening. Beyond these basic procedures, the clinician must assess specific speech and language skills that affect a diagnosis of aphasia (Brookshire, 2003; Chapey, 2001; Davis, 2000; Hegde, 2001a, 2005; Helm-Estabrooks & Albert, 2004). The following lists describe the skills to be assessed.

Assessment of Repetition Skills

- repetition of single words (single-syllable words with visible voiced consonants—e.g., *bed*—and blends and multisyllable words)
- repetition of object names, verbs, numbers, letters, and function words
- repetition of sentences (short and commonly used sentences—e.g., "Sit down"—first and progressively longer sentences next)
- Repetition of a few short but infrequently used sentences

Assessment of Naming Skills

- responsive naming (naming with contextual cues—e.g., the clinician asks, "What do you use to write?" or "What color is snow?")
- confrontation naming (e.g., the clinician asks "What is this?" while showing a picture)
- word fluency (recalling names that belong to a specific category—e.g., the clinician asks the client to "name all the animals you can think of")

Assessment of Auditory Comprehension of Spoken Language

- hearing evaluation
- visual evaluation
- comprehension of natural commands given without gestures (e.g., "Move your chair a little closer" or "Close your eyes")
- comprehension of multistep commands (e.g., "Pick up the pencil and the comb and place them in the box")

Assessment of Comprehension of Single Words

- comprehension of single items ("red" or "cat") and semantic groups of items ("colors" or "animals")
- comprehension of words that vary in number of syllables, emotionality, frequency of usage, semantic class, and phonemic similarity

Assessment of Comprehension of Sentences and Paragraphs

- comprehension of a brief and simple story that is told
- comprehension of more complex stories

Assessment of Reading Skills

- comprehension of silently or orally read material (e.g., matching single printed words to pictures, matching printed words with spoken words, crossing out words that do not belong in a list)
- completion of printed sentences (e.g., reads the printed incomplete sentence "We wear hats on our..." and completes it with the verbal response "head")

Assessment of Writing Skills

- graphomotor skills (letter formation)
- general writing skills
- automatic writing

- propositional writing
- confrontation writing (e.g., the clinician says, "Write the names of these pictures")
- writing to dictation
- narrative writing (e.g., the clinician says, "Write a story about this picture")
- premorbid writing samples for comparison

Assessment of Gestures and Pantomime

- expression through gestures and pantomime
- comprehension of gestures and pantomime

Assessment of Automated Speech and Singing

- recitation of the alphabet, days of the week, months of the year, and numbers
- recitation of prayers, poems, and nursery rhymes
- singing
- humming a tune

Treatment of Aphasia

Foundational Concepts

- Most current research shows that aphasia treatment is effective. Many treatment approaches are available (Basso, 2003; Brookshire, 2003; Chapey, 2001; Davis, 2000; Hegde, 2001b, 2005; Helm-Estabrooks & Albert, 2004; LaPointe, 1997; Robey, 1998; Rosenbek, LaPointe, & Wertz, 1989).
- Treatment must take into account the client's cultural and linguistic background. For example, in many minority groups, family and extended family members may be extremely helpful in assisting with home carryover of treatment targets (Wallace, 1998).
- Prognosis for treatment is better in the case of patients:

  - who are younger and healthier
  - who are better educated and in verbally demanding occupations
  - whose lesions are smaller
  - who have no other medical or behavioral disorders
  - who have good hearing acuity
  - who have normal or adequately corrected vision
  - who have better motor skills
  - who have better preserved language skills
  - whose aphasia is less severe
  - whose treatment is initiated soon after onset
  - who receive effective treatment techniques in an accurate manner for a long enough duration
  - whose family members are involved in treatment
  - who maintain their health during the course of treatment

Treatment of Auditory Comprehension

- Lesions within the posterior superior temporal lobe (PST) suggest a better prognosis than those outside the PST.
- Comprehension is generally better for frequently used words, nouns, picturable words, shorter sentences, syntactically simpler sentences, active sentences, personally relevant sentences, slower speech, words that are stressed, speech in quiet surroundings, redundant messages, repeated phrases, speech preceded by alerting stimuli (e.g., "Ready?" "Listen!"). Louder speech and video presentation of stimuli are ineffective.
- Auditory comprehension treatment is sequenced as follows:

  - *comprehension of single words:* understanding nouns and verbs (e.g., the clinician asks the patient to point to named body parts and objects, to specific named actions pictured)
  - *comprehension of spoken sentences:* question comprehension, following spoken directions, and sentence verification (e.g., the clinician asks yes/no questions and open-ended questions; following simple and more complex directions, and verifying the meaning of sentences by matching a sentence to a picture that represents it)
  - *discourse comprehension:* understanding narratives and questions (e.g., retelling a story the clinician narrates and responding to such personally relevant questions as "Do you like to watch football games?")

Treatment of Verbal Expression: Naming

- Naming skills are the most frequently targeted expressive verbal skills. These skills are subsequently expanded into longer and grammatically more correct and communicatively more functional utterances.
- In treating naming, it is important to select words that are client specific (e.g., names of family members, activities the client engages in) and words that are functional (that enhance communication in a variety of settings).
- Naming treatment techniques include a variety of special cues that help evoke the target responses which are promptly reinforced:

  - modeling of responses
  - incomplete sentences (e.g., the clinician says, "You write with a _____")
  - phonetic cues (e.g., the clinician says, "The word starts with a *p*")
  - syllabic cues (e.g., the clinician says, "The word starts with *spoo_____*")
  - silent phonetic cues (e.g., the clinician exhibits a silent articulatory posture for /p/ for *pen*)
  - personalized verbal cues (e.g., instead of prompting "it starts with an *m* for the word *mechanic,*" the clinician may say " he works on your Toyota"—a cue that is specific to the experience of the patient) (Freed, Celery, & Marshall, 2004)
  - functional descriptions of objects (e.g., the clinician says, "It is something you roll or kick")
  - descriptions and demonstrations of actions (e.g., the clinician says, "You use this to write like this" followed by writing)
  - patient's description as stimulus for naming (e.g., the clinician says, "Tell me what you do with this and then say its name")

- patient's demonstration of function as stimulus for naming (e.g., the clinician says, "Show me how to use this and tell me its name")
- paired objects or pictures with their printed name as stimuli for naming (e.g., the clinician shows a book and the printed word *book* and asks "What is this?")
- patient's spelling as stimulus for naming (e.g., the clinician says, "Spell this word first and then say it")
- patient's spelling and writing as stimuli for naming (e.g., the clinician says, "Spell this word, write the word, and then say it")
- associated sounds as stimulus (e.g., the clinician says, "It makes an arf-arf sound")
- rhyme as stimulus (e.g., the clinician says, "What is this? It rhymes with _____")
- synonyms (e.g., "dwelling" to evoke "house"); antonyms (e.g., "woman" to evoke "man"); associated words (e.g., "plate" to evoke "cup"); generic words (e.g., "man" to evoke "husband"); superordinates (e.g., "flower" to evoke "rose")

Treatment of Verbal Expression: Expanded Utterances

- *Expansion of verbal expression* involves systematically increasing the length and complexity of target responses. Names taught may be expanded into phrases and sentences that are functional and effective in naturalistic communication. The clinician initially uses modeling and subsequently fades it.
- Action-filled pictures and stories may be used to teach narratives and discourse. Sequenced pictures also will help evoke narratives with temporal sequences.
- Eventually, conversational speech involving topics of relevance and interest to the client is targeted for treatment. Description of daily activities (e.g., cooking) and special events (e.g., planning a vacation) may be used to promote conversational speech.

Treatment of Reading Skills

- Target reading skills are selected based on an assessment of premorbid reading skills and the current need for reading.
- Functional reading skills may be sequenced as follows:

    - survival reading skills (e.g., reading letters, menus, bank statements, and maps)
    - reading newspapers, books, and letters
    - reading and comprehension of printed words
    - reading and comprehension of phrases and sentences
    - reading and comprehension of paragraphs and extended material

Treatment of Writing Skills

- Target writing skills also are selected based on an assessment of premorbid reading skills and the current need for writing.
- Functional writing skills may be sequenced as follows:

    - initially writing functional words (e.g., one's own name, names of family members)
    - writing functional lists (e.g., a grocery list)
    - writing short notes, reminders, addresses, and so forth
    - filling out forms
    - writing letters

- Depending on current writing skills, treatment procedures include the following:

    - pointing to the correct printed letter the clinician names
    - pointing to printed words and phrases
    - saying the sound of a printed letter shown
    - saying a printed word shown
    - tracing printed letters
    - copying printed words and phrases
    - spelling words correctly
    - writing to dictation
    - spontaneous writing of phrases and sentences
    - spontaneous extended writing (e.g., making a grocery list, writing a note to a spouse, writing a letter to a friend)

CONCEPTS TO CONSIDER

List one treatment technique that can be used with patients with aphasia in each of the following areas: auditory comprehension, naming, reading, and writing.

_____

_____

_____

_____

_____

Alexia, Agraphia, and Agnosia

- *Alexia* is loss of previously acquired reading skills due to recent brain damage. *Dyslexia*, on the other hand, is a difficulty in learning to read; this difficulty is often genetically based and is manifested beginning in childhood. Some patients with aphasia manifest alexia (Benson & Ardila, 1996; Brookshire, 2003; Hegde, 2005; Helm-Estabrooks & Albert, 2004).

- *Agraphia* is the loss or impairment of normally acquired writing skills due to lesions in the foot of the second frontal gyrus, sometimes referred to as *Exner's writing area*. Various kinds of writing problems are evident in most patients with aphasia (Hegde, 1998).

- *Agnosia* is impaired understanding of the meaning of certain stimuli even though there is no peripheral sensory impairment. Patients can see, feel, and hear stimuli but cannot understand their meaning. Impairment often is limited to one sensory modality; the meaning of stimuli may be grasped in another modality. There are several forms of agnosia (Benson & Ardila, 1996).

Auditory Agnosia

- *Auditory agnosia* is caused by bilateral damage to the auditory association area and is characterized by:

    - impaired understanding of the meaning of auditory stimuli
    - normal peripheral hearing
    - difficulty in matching objects with their sound
    - normal visual recognition of objects

Auditory Verbal Agnosia

- *Auditory verbal agnosia* (pure word deafness) is caused by bilateral temporal lobe lesions that isolate Wernicke's area; it is characterized by:

    - impaired understanding of spoken words
    - normal peripheral hearing
    - normal recognition of nonverbal sounds
    - normal recognition of printed words
    - normal or near-normal verbal expression and reading

Visual Agnosia

- *Visual agnosia* is a rare disorder caused by bilateral occipital lobe damage or posterior parietal lobe damage; it is characterized by:

    - impaired visual recognition of objects, which may be intermittent
    - normal auditory or tactile recognition of objects

Tactile Agnosia

- *Tactile agnosia* is caused by lesions in the parietal lobe and is characterized by:

    - impaired tactile recognition of objects when visual feedback is blocked (as with a blindfold)
    - impaired naming of objects clients can feel in their hands
    - impaired description of objects clients can feel in their hands

SUMMARY

✓ Aphasia, a neurologically based language disorder, is most frequently caused by stroke. Aphasia may be categorized as fluent, nonfluent, or subcortical in nature. Clinicians must take into account individual issues such as the presence of bilingualism or left-handedness when assessing patients with aphasia.

✓ Assessment of patients with aphasia may include use of standardized aphasia tests. Clinicians may also use functional assessment tools, which target the patient's daily communication skills in everyday settings.

✓ Treatment of patients with aphasia generally involves the following skill areas: auditory comprehension, verbal expression (naming), verbal expression (expanded utterances), reading, and writing.

✓ Aphasia may be accompanied by alexia, agraphia, or agnosia. Types of agnosia include auditory, auditory verbal, visual, and tactile agnosia.

APRAXIA OF SPEECH

INTRODUCTION

Apraxia of speech (AOS) is a neurogenic speech disorder. Patients with AOS have sensorimotor problems in positioning and sequentially moving muscles for volitional speech production. AOS is caused by damage or injury to speech-motor programming areas (e.g., Broca's area) in the dominant hemisphere. Patients with AOS have a number of communication deficits, especially those caused by groping and struggling to speak. Assessment and treatment for patients with AOS involve detailed procedures related to evaluating and improving articulatory accuracy, speech rate, and self-monitoring (Caruso & Strand, 1999; Dabul, 1979; Duffy, 2005; Freed, 2000; Halpern, 2000; Hegde, 2001a; Vogel & Cannito, 2001; Yorkston, Beukelman, Strand, & Bell, 1999).

Definition and Distinctions

■ *Apraxia of speech* is a neurogenic speech disorder characterized by sensorimotor problems in positioning and sequentially moving muscles for the volitional production of speech.

■ AOS is primarily an articulatory-phonologic disorder, although its etiology and characteristics are different from those of similar disorders in children. Adult patients with AOS will have acquired articulation normally. Their current articulatory problems are due to recent neuropathology.

■ However, adults with AOS have unimpaired reflex and automatic acts. The difficulty they have is mostly in executing the voluntary movements involved in speech. AOS may be associated with prosodic problems (Duffy, 2005).

■ AOS is not caused by muscle weakness or neuromuscular slowness. It is thought that a disorder of motor programming for speech causes it. More frequently, AOS and aphasia may coexist, and less frequently, dysarthria of unilateral upper motor neuron type may coexist with AOS.

■ Pure apraxia is rare. Technically, and in its pure form, AOS should not affect language skills, as it is a speech-motor programming problem. However, language skills are affected if there is a coexisting aphasia. Coexistence of apraxia and aphasia (esecially of the Broca's type) is common.

■ *Apraxia* is a basic disorder of volitional movement in the absence of muscle weakness, paralysis, or fatigue. As such, AOS is a special case of apraxia.

■ *Nonverbal oral apraxia* is a disorder of nonverbal movement involving the oral muscles. AOS is frequently associated with nonverbal oral apraxia.

Neuropathology of AOS

■ AOS is caused by injury or damage to speech-motor programming areas in the dominant hemisphere; such areas as Broca's and supplementary motor areas often are involved.

■ Specific types of pathology include vascular lesions that cause strokes; specifically affected are the speech programming structures and pathways. In a majority of cases, the cause is a single left hemisphere stroke; in a few, the cause is multiple strokes.

■ Frontal lesions may be associated with parietal lesions as well; temporal lobe lesions are observed occasionally but only in combination with lesions elsewhere.

■ AOS may also be caused by such degenerative neural diseases as Alzheimer's disease, multiple sclerosis (MS), and primary progressive aphasia.

■ AOS can also be caused by left hemisphere trauma, surgical trauma, tumors in the left hemisphere, and seizure disorders.

General Symptoms of AOS

■ General symptoms of AOS include impaired oral sensation in some patients. When dysarthria is a coexisting condition, facial and lingual weakness may also be present. Some patients may also have limb apraxia.

■ An independent nonverbal oral apraxia (NVOA) is present in many patients. In some cases, there also may be right hemiparesis and sensory deficits.

Communication Deficits in AOS

■ Patients may have an independent problem of auditory processing deficits.

■ Most patients have a general awareness of their speech problems.

■ Patients' initiation of speech may be slow or delayed.

■ Patients may use a compensatory strategy of reduced rate.

■ Speech programming and production errors are the dominant symptoms of apraxia:

- problems in volitional or spontaneous sequencing of movements required for speech with relatively unaffected automatic speech;
- high variability of speech errors; changing patterns of errors on repeated attempts; normal production of difficult words on occasion;
- speech sound substitutions (more common), distortions, and omissions of speech sounds; voicing errors may be frequent, especially the substitution of a voiceless phoneme for a

voiced (e.g., *pet* for *bet*);

- more pronounced difficulty with consonants than vowels; more severe problems with affricates and fricatives and consonant clusters; more frequent errors on infrequently occurring sounds;
- anticipatory substitutions (a phoneme that occurs later in the word may replace the one that occurs earlier; e.g., "lelo" for "yellow");
- postpositioning errors (a phoneme that occurs earlier replaces the one that occurs later; e.g., "dred" for "dress");
- metathetic errors (switched position of phonemes in words; e.g., "tefalone" for "telephone");
- insertion of schwa into consonant clusters or between syllables;
- increased frequency of errors on longer words;
- trial-and-error groping and struggling associated with speech attempts;
- greater difficulty with word-initial sounds in some cases;
- easier automatic productions than volitional/purposive productions; and
- attempts at self-correction, often unsuccessful.

■ Patients with apraxia of speech frequently have prosodic problems, which include:

- a slower rate of speech, difficulty in increasing or changing the rate when requested
- silent pauses between words
- impaired intonation because of increased duration of consonants and vowels, even stress on syllables, even loudness or restricted range of loudness, and limited pitch range
- fluency problems including silent pauses, especially at the beginning of speech initiation, and repetitions because of false starts and attempts at self-correction.

Assessment of AOS

■ A detailed case history, careful examination of the medical records, interview of the client and his or her family members, and detailed observation of speech production are necessary to make a diagnosis of AOS in adults.

■ Procedures designed to diagnose aphasia (problems with language production and comprehension, reading, and writing) should be used when the patient shows signs of a coexisting aphasia, often Broca's aphasia (Duffy, 2005; Freed, 2000; Hegde, 2001a).

■ Assessment of speech to diagnose AOS involves the following procedures:

- tape-recording the patient's speech samples and transcribing the responses phonetically; taking note of struggle and groping, self-correction, repetition and other forms of dysfluencies, errors of articulation, delayed reaction, facial grimacing, and other behaviors that suggest apraxia;
- evoking imitative production of a speech sound;
- evoking repetitive production of syllables (e.g., asking the patient to say "pʌ-pʌ-pʌ," "tʌ-tʌ-tʌ," and "kʌ-kʌ-kʌ" as long and as evenly as possible);
- evoking the repetitive production of multiple syllables (e.g., asking the patient to say "pʌ-tʌ-kʌ" as long and as evenly as possible);
- evoking the imitative production of progressively longer words when modeling is provided (e.g., asking the patient to imitate such words as *several, tornado, artillery, linoleum, snowman, television, catastrophe, unequivocally, parliamentarian, statistical analysis,*

Encyclopedia Britannica);
- evoking repeated, imitative production of words and phrases (e.g., asking the patient to say such words as *artillery, impossibility,* and *disenfranchised* five times);
- evoking the imitative production of sentences;
- evoking counting responses (e.g., asking the patient to count from 1 to 20);
- evoking picture descriptions;
- assessment of oral reading;
- administration of a complete *diadochokinetic test* to assess oral, nonverbal movement (e.g., various tongue, lip, and jaw movements), oral apraxia, or a coexisting dysarthria in case of significant muscle weakness or paralysis;
- assessment of limb movements to evaluate limb apraxia by asking the patient to perform certain actions (e.g., demonstration of how an accordion works, how one salutes or waves good-bye); and
- administration of a standardized test of apraxia (e.g., the *Apraxia Battery for Adults* (Dabul, 1979) or the *Comprehensive Apraxia Test* (DeSimoni, 1989).

CONCEPTS TO CONSIDER

Describe the neuropathology of apraxia of speech. What are two important components of an assessment for this disorder?

_____

_____

_____

_____

_____

Treatment of AOS

- Treatment should be carefully sequenced to move from more automatic speech to less automatic speech and eventually to spontaneous speech.

- Treatment on simpler productions should precede that on more complex productions (e.g., visible sounds before nonvisible sounds, singletons before clusters).

- Treatment targets include articulatory accuracy, slower rate, systematic practice, gradual increase in the rate, and normal prosody.

- Treatment should be primarily concerned with speech movements as opposed to nonspeech movements.

- Treatment should include practice with a variety of sounds and sound combinations.

- Treatment procedures should include instructions, demonstration, modeling, shaping, phonetic placement, frequent cueing, use of rhythm, and immediate positive or corrective feedback.

- Cueing techniques may include tactile cues for placement of articulators, simultaneous production by the clinician and the client, clinician's modeling (immediately followed by client's imitation), delayed imitation (waiting for a few seconds before imitating the clinician's model), and so forth.

- Any special cues and modeling should be faded to promote more spontaneous productions.

- Contrastive stress tasks, phonetic contrasts, carrier phrases, and singing may all be useful.

- Pushing on the abdomen to achieve vocal fold closure and phonation or use of an artificial larynx may be helpful for a speechless client.

- Emphasis on total communication (combined use of verbal expressions, gestures, writing, augmentative devices) may be desirable.

- Teaching accurate sound productions in conversational speech should be an important goal.

- Increasing the speech rate to the near-normal also should be an important goal.

- Teaching self-monitoring skills is important for maintenance.

- Techniques of treating articulation and phonological disorders are generally useful.

- In the case of severe apraxia, family members and health care workers should be asked to speak slowly, use shorter sentences, reduce background noise, talk only when the client is focused, and use total communication. In the case of most severe apraxia, augmentative communication techniques may be necessary.

SUMMARY

✓ AOS is a neurogenic speech disorder characterized by sensorimotor problems in positioning and sequentially moving muscles for production of speech. AOS is caused by damage to speech-motor programming areas in the dominant hemisphere.

✓ Communication deficits to be assessed and treated in patients with AOS include highly variable speech errors, significant articulatory problems, increased frequency of errors on long words, prosodic problems, and groping and struggling behaviors.

✓ Assessment of patients with AOS may include detailed, individualized procedures as well as the administration of standardized tests. Treatment should be carefully sequenced to move from automatic, simple productions to less automatic, more spontaneous productions.

THE DYSARTHRIAS

The dysarthrias are a group of neurologically based speech-motor disorders. These disorders result from impaired muscular control of the speech mechanism, involving peripheral or central nervous system pathology. There are seven types of dysarthria: ataxic, flaccid, hyperkinetic, hypokinetic, mixed, spastic, and unilateral upper-motor neuron dysarthria. Patients with dysarthria typically manifest problems in respiration, phonation, articulation, prosody, and resonance. Assessment and treatment of patients with dysarthria involve addressing those problems (Caruso & Strand, 1999; Dabul, 1979; Duffy, 2005; Freed, 2000; Halpern, 2000; Hegde, 2001a; Vogel & Cannito, 2001; Yorkston et al., 1999).

Definition of the Dysarthrias

- Dysarthrias are neurologically based speech disorders contrasted with such similarly based language disorders as aphasia. Dysarthria also is contrasted with apraxia of speech, a neurogenic speech disorder of motor planning of speech movements with no muscular weakness or paralysis.

- There are different types of dysarthria but all share certain characteristics. Dysarthrias are a group of speech-motor disorders resulting from impaired muscular control of the speech mechanism, involving peripheral or central nervous system pathology.

- The oral communication problems that accompany dysarthria include respiratory, articulatory, phonatory, resonatory, and prosodic disturbances that are caused by weakness, incoordination, or paralysis of speech musculature. Dysarthrias are classified into ataxic, flaccid, hyperkinetic, hypokinetic, mixed, spastic, and unilateral upper motor neuron types (Duffy, 2005; Freed, 2000).

Neuropathology of the Dysarthrias

- Some of the common etiological factors include degenerative neurological diseases such as Parkinson's disease, Wilson's disease, progressive supranuclear palsy, dystonia, Huntington's disease, amyotrophic lateral sclerosis (ALS), multiple sclerosis, and myasthenia gravis.

- Dysarthria can also be caused by nonprogressive neurological conditions, including stroke, infections, traumatic brain injury, and surgical trauma, as well as congenital conditions, including cerebral palsy, Moebius syndrome, encephalitis, toxic effects from alcohol or drugs, and so forth.

- Common sites of lesion include lower motor neuron, unilateral or bilateral upper motor neuron, cerebellum, and the basal ganglia (extrapyramidal system) (Davis & Strand, 2004).

- Pathophysiology and neuromuscular problems include muscle weakness, spasticity, incoordination, and rigidity. There is usually a variety of movement disorders, including reduced or variable range and speed of movement, involuntary movements, reduced strength of movement, unsteady or inaccurate movement, and abnormal tone (increased, decreased, or variable).

Communicative Disorders Associated with Dysarthria

- *Respiratory problems* include forced inspirations or expirations that interrupt speech, audible or breathy inspiration, and grunting at the end of expiration.

- *Phonatory disorders* include:

  - pitch disorders characterized by abnormal pitch, pitch breaks, abrupt variations in pitch, monopitch, diplophonia, shaky or tremulous voice;
  - loudness disorders characterized by too soft or too loud speech, monoloudness, sudden and excessive variation in loudness, progressive decrease in loudness throughout an utterance, or alternating changes in loudness; and
  - vocal-quality problems characterized by a harsh, rough, gravelly voice, a hoarse voice (especially the "wet" variety), a continuously or intermittently breathy voice, a strained or strangled voice, effortful phonation, or a sudden and uncontrolled cessation of voice.

- *Articulation disorders* include imprecise production of consonants, prolongation and repetition of phonemes, irregular breakdowns in articulation, distortion of vowels, and weak production of pressure consonants.

- *Prosodic disorders* include a variety of rate problems, including slower, excessively faster, or variable rate of speech, shorter phrase lengths, and linguistic stress problems such as reduced, even, or excessive stress. There may also be prolongation of intervals between words or syllables, inappropriate pauses in speech, and short rushes of speech.

- *Resonance disorders* include hypernasality, hyponasality, and nasal emission.

- *Other characteristics* include slow, fast, or irregular diadochokinetic rate and palilalia (compulsive repetition of one's own utterances with increasing rate and decreasing loudness), as well as decreased intelligibility of speech.

Classification of the Dysarthrias

Ataxic Dysarthria

- *Ataxic dysarthria* results from damage to the cerebellar system. It is characterized predominantly by articulatory and prosodic problems.
- Neuropathology that results in ataxic dysarthria includes bilateral or generalized cerebellar lesions, degenerative ataxia (e.g., Friedreich's ataxia and olivopontocerebellar atrophy), cerebellar vascular lesions, tumors, traumatic brain injury, toxic conditions (e.g., alcohol abuse and drug toxicity), and inflammatory conditions (e.g., meningitis and encephalitis).
- The major characteristics of ataxic dysarthria include:

  - *gait disturbances:* instability of the trunk and head, tremors and rocking motions; rotated or tilted head posture; hypotonia
  - *movement disorders:* over- or undershooting of targets; uncoordinated, jerky, inaccurate, slow, imprecise, and halting movements

- *articulation disorders:* imprecise production of consonants; irregular articulatory break-downs and distortion of vowels
- *prosodic disorders:* excessive and even stress; prolonged phonemes and intervals between words or syllables; slow rate of speech
- *phonatory disorders:* monopitch, monoloudness, and harshness
- *speech quality:* impression of drunken speech

Flaccid Dysarthria

- *Flaccid dysarthria* results from damage to the motor units of cranial or spinal nerves that supply speech muscles (lower motor neuron involvement).
- Neuropathology that results in flaccid dysarthria includes such diseases as myasthenia gravis and botulism, vascular diseases and brain stem strokes, infections (e.g., polio and infections secondary to AIDS), demyelinating diseases (e.g., Guillain-Barré syndrome), degenerative diseases (e.g., motor neuron diseases, progressive bulbar palsy, and amyotrophic lateral sclerosis), and surgical trauma during brain, laryngeal, facial, or chest surgery.
- Specific cranial nerves that may be involved in flaccid dysarthria include the trigeminal (V), facial (VII), glossopharyngeal (IX), vagus (X), and hypoglossal (XII) nerves.
- The major characteristics of flaccid dysarthria include:

  - various muscular disorders (e.g., weakness, hypotonia, atrophy, and diminished reflexes)
  - isolated twitches of resting muscles (fasciculations) and contractions of individual muscles (fibrillations)
  - rapid and progressive weakness with the use of a muscle and recovery with rest
  - respiratory weakness in combination with cranial nerve weakness
  - phonatory disorders, including breathy voice, audible inspiration, and short phrases
  - resonance disorders, including hypernasality; imprecise consonants, nasal emission, and short phrases
  - phonatory-prosodic disorders, including harsh voice, monopitch, and monoloudness
  - articulation disorders, which are more pronounced with lesions of cranial nerves V, VII, and XII

Hyperkinetic Dysarthria

- *Hyperkinetic dysarthria* results from damage to the basal ganglia (extrapyramidal system). Dysarthria is associated with involuntary movement and variable muscle tone. Prosodic disturbances are dominant.
- Varied causes of hyperkinetic dysarthria include degenerative, vascular, traumatic, infectious, neoplastic, and metabolic factors. Such degenerative diseases as Huntington's disease also may be associated with this type of dysarthria. Causes are unknown in a majority of cases. The muscles of the face, jaw, tongue, palate, larynx, and respiration may be involved.
- The major characteristics of hyperkinetic dysarthria include the following:

  - movement disorders (because of damage to the basal ganglia control circuit); abnormal and involuntary movements of the orofacial muscles
  - myoclonus (involuntary jerks of body parts), tics of the face and shoulders, tremor, chorea; abrupt and severe contractions of the extremities; writhing, involuntary movements, often in hands (athetosis); spasms (sudden and involuntary contractions of a muscle or group of muscles)

- dystonia, which results from contractions of antagonistic muscles resulting in abnormal postures; spasmodic torticollis (intermittent dystonia and spasms of the neck muscles) blepharospasm (forceful and involuntary closure of the eyes due to spasm of the orbicularis oculi muscle)
- communicative disorders, specific symptoms depending on the dominant neurological condition (e.g., chorea, dystonia, athetosis, spasmodic torticollis)
- phonatory disorders, including voice tremor, intermittently strained voice, voice stoppage, vocal noise, and harsh voice
- resonance disorders, predominantly intermittent hypernasality
- prosodic disorders, including slower rate, excess loudness variations, prolonged interword intervals, and equal stress
- respiratory problems, including audible inspiration and forced and sudden inspiration or expiration
- inconsistent articulation problems, including imprecise consonant productions and distortion of vowels

Hypokinetic Dysarthria

- *Hypokinetic dysarthria* results from damage to the basal ganglia (extrapyramidal system). It results from a variety of causes including such degenerative diseases as progressive supranuclear palsy, Parkinson's (much more commonly), Alzheimer's, and Pick's diseases.
- Hypokinetic dysarthria can also occur due to vascular disorders that cause multiple or bilateral strokes, repeated head trauma (such as that sustained by boxers), inflammation, tumor, antipsychotic or neuroleptic drug toxicity, and normal-pressure hydrocephalus. Parkinson's disease produces the most typical form, although dysarthria occurs only in about half the patients with that disease.
- Hypokinetic dysarthria is characterized by:

  - tremors in the resting facial, mouth, and limb muscles that diminish when moved voluntarily;
  - mask-like face with infrequent blinking and no smiling;
  - micrographic writing (small print);
  - walking disorders (slow to begin, then short, rapid, shuffling steps);
  - postural disturbances (involuntary flexion of the head, trunk, and arm; difficulty changing positions);
  - decreased swallowing (accumulation of saliva in the mouth and drooling);
  - phonatory disorders, including monopitch, low pitch, monoloudness, and harsh and continuously breathy voice;
  - prosodic disorders, including reduced stress, inappropriate silent intervals, short rushes of speech, variable and increased rate in segments, and short phrases;
  - articulation disorders, including imprecise consonants, repeated phonemes, resonance disorders, and mild hypernasality (in about 25% of cases); and
  - respiratory problems, including reduced vital capacity, irregular breathing, and faster rate of respiration.

Mixed Dysarthrias

- *Mixed dysarthrias* are a combination of two or more pure dysarthrias. All combinations of pure dysarthrias are possible, although a combination of two types is more common than a combination of three or more. The two most common mixed forms are flaccid-spastic dysarthria and ataxic-spastic dysarthria.

- Mixed dysarthrias are characterized by:

  - symptoms characteristic of two or more individual types of dysarthria that are mixed in a given patient; and
  - the range of most to least severe symptoms of mixed flaccid-spastic dysarthria, associated with amyotrophic lateral sclerosis, includes imprecise production of consonants, hypernasality, harsh voice, slow rate, monopitch, short phrases, distorted vowels, low pitch, monoloudness, excess and equal stress or reduced stress, prolonged intervals, prolonged phonemes, a strained and strangled quality, breathiness, audible inspiration, inappropriate silences, and nasal emission.

Spastic Dysarthria

- *Spastic dysarthria* results from bilateral damage to the upper motor neurons (direct and indirect motor pathways). Lesions in multiple areas, including the cortical areas, basal ganglia, internal capsule, pons, and medulla are common.
- Spastic dysarthria is characterized by:

  - spasticity and weakness, especially bilateral facial weakness, though jaw strength may be normal and lower face weakness may be less severe;
  - movement disorders, including reduced range and slowness, loss of fine and skilled movement, and increased muscle tone;
  - hyperactive gag reflex;
  - hyperadduction of vocal folds and inadequate closure of the velopharyngeal port;
  - prosodic disorders, including excess and equal stress, slow rate, monopitch, monoloudness, reduced stress, and short phrases;
  - articulation disorders, including an imprecise production of consonants and distorted vowels;
  - phonatory disorders, including continuous breathy voice, harshness, low pitch, pitch breaks, strained-strangled voice quality, short phrases, and slow rate; and
  - resonance disorders with a predominant hypernasality.

Unilateral Upper Motor Neuron Dysarthria

- *Unilateral upper motor neuron (UUMN) dysarthria* results from damage to the upper motor neurons that supply cranial and spinal nerves involved in speech production.
- Dysarthria due to vascular disorders that produce left-hemisphere lesions may coexist with aphasia or apraxia, and disarthria due to right-hemisphere lesions may coexist with right hemisphere syndrome.
- UUMN dysarthria is characterized by:

  - unilateral lower face weakness, unilateral tongue weakness, unilateral palatal weakness, and hemiplegia/hemiparesis;
  - articulation disorders, including imprecise production of consonants and irregular articulatory breakdowns;
  - phonatory disorders, including harsh voice, reduced loudness, and strained harshness;
  - prosodic disorders, including slow rate, increased rate in segments, excess and equal stress, monopitch, monoloudness, low pitch, and short phrases;

- resonance disorders, predominantly hypernasality; and
- dysphagia, aphasia, apraxia, and right hemisphere syndrome.

CONCEPTS TO CONSIDER

How is dysarthria classified? What are the major symptoms of the different types of dysarthria?

_____

_____

_____

_____

_____

Assessment of the Dysarthrias

■ Assessment of the dysarthrias involves multiple procedures because of the wide range of symptoms that must be evaluated (Caruso & Strand, 1999; Duffy, 2005; Freed, 2000; Hegde, 1998, 2001a; Vogel & Cannito, 2001; Yorkston et al., 1999). The following procedures are appropriate in assessment.

- *Record an extended conversational speech sample* and a reading sample.
- *Use a variety of speech tasks,* including imitation of syllables, words, phrases, and sentences; production of modeled syllables, words, phrases, and sentences; and sustained phonation (vowel prolongation).
- *Assess the diadochokinetic rate* or alternating motion rates (AMRs) and sequential motion rates (SMRs).
- *Assess the speech production mechanism* during nonspeech activities through the following activities:
  — observing facial symmetry, tone, tension, droopiness, expressiveness, and so forth;
  — observing the movements of the facial structures as the patient puffs the cheeks, retracts and rounds the lips, bites the lower lip, and so forth;
  — observing the patient's emotional expressions;
  — taking note of the patient's jaw movements and deviation during movement and observing the tongue movements;
  — observing the velopharyngeal mechanism and its movements;
  — assessing nasal airflow by holding a mirror at the nares as the patient prolongs the vowel /ɪ/; and
  — assessing laryngeal functions by asking the patient to cough to take note of weak cough associated with weak adduction of the cords, inadequate breath support, or both.

- *Assess respiratory problems* by observing the patient's posture and breathing habits during quiet and speech, taking note of rapid, shallow, or effortful breathing, signs of shortness of breath and irregularity of inhalation and exhalation, and so forth.
- *Assess phonatory disorders* through the following activities:
  — having the patient say "ah" after taking a deep breath and sustain it as steadily and for as long as the air supply lasts;
  — taking note of the patient's pitch, pitch breaks, diplophonia, abrupt variations in pitch, and lack of normal pitch variations;
  — taking note of voice tremors, assessing the presence of diplophonia, and judging vocal loudness, its appropriateness, variations, decay, and alternating changes; and
  — judging the quality of voice, including hoarseness, harshness, and breathiness, taking note of strained or effortful voice production or sudden cessation of voice.

- *Assess articulation disorders* by evaluating consonant productions, duration of speech sounds, phoneme repetitions, irregular breakdowns in articulation, the precision of vowel productions, phoneme distortions, and the adequacy of pressure consonantal productions.
- *Assess prosodic disorders* by evaluating the rate of speech, phrase lengths in selected portions of speech, stress patterns in speech, pauses in speech, and the presence of short rushes of speech.
- *Assess resonance disorders* by making clinical judgments about hypo- and hypernasality and nasal emission.
- *Assess speech intelligibility* by making clinical judgments on the percentage of words or phrases understood and by using a rating scale if warranted.
- *Use such standardized tests* as the *Assessment of Intelligibility of Dysarthric Speakers* (Yorkston & Beukelman, 1981) and *Frenchay Dysarthria Assessment* (Enderby, 1983).

Treatment of the Dysarthrias

Goals and Procedures

- Treatment of dysarthria includes a wide range of techniques partly because the communication disorders themselves have a wide range. Techniques to modify respiratory, phonatory, articulatory, and resonatory problems are all necessary (Caruso & Strand, 1999; Duffy, 2005; Freed, 2000; Hegde, 1998, 2001a; Vogel & Cannito, 2001; Yorkston et al., 1999).
- *Treatment goals* include modification of respiratory, phonatory, articulatory, resonatory, and prosodic problems and increasing the efficiency, effectiveness, and naturalness of communication.
- Treatment goals also include increasing physiological support for speech and teaching self-correction, self-evaluation, and self-monitoring skills. Teaching compensatory behaviors for lost or reduced functions is important, and teaching the use of alternative or augmentative communication systems may be necessary.
- *Treatment procedures* include intensive, systematic, and extensive drill, instruction, demonstration, modeling (followed by imitation), shaping, prompting, fading, differential reinforcement, and other proven behavioral management procedures. When necessary, phonetic placement and its variations can be taught. Instrumental feedback or biofeedback may be used when needed.

Specific Treatment Targets

- In treating patients with dysarthria, the clinician needs to target specific skills:
- *Modification of respiration* by:

  - training, with the help of a manometer or air pressure transducer, consistent production of subglottal air pressure;
  - training maximum vowel prolongation;
  - shaping production of longer phrases and sentences;
  - teaching controlled exhalation;
  - teaching the client to push, pull, or bear down during speech or nonspeech tasks;
  - using a manual push on the client's abdomen;
  - modifying postures that promote respiratory support, including using neck and trunk braces if helpful; and
  - teaching the client to inhale more deeply and exhale slowly and with greater force during speech.

- *Modification of phonation* by using biofeedback to shape desirable vocal intensity, and training the client in the use of portable amplification systems if the voice is too soft. Phonation modification may also include training aphonia clients in the use of an artificial larynx and teaching the client to initiate phonation at the beginning of an exhalation.
- *Modification of resonance* disorders by providing feedback on nasal airflow and hypernasality by using a mirror, nasal flow transducer, or nasendoscope; training the client to open the mouth wider to increase oral resonance and vocal intensity; and using a nasal obturator or nose clip.
- *Modification of articulation* by:

  - training the client to assume the best posture for good articulation;
  - using a bite block to improve jaw control and strength;
  - using such methods as simplifying the target, instruction, demonstration, modeling, shaping, and immediate feedback in teaching correct articulation;
  - using phonetic placement, slower rate, and minimal contrast pairs;
  - providing instructions and demonstrations and teaching self-monitoring skills; and
  - teaching compensatory articulatory movements (e.g., use of tongue blade to make sounds normally made with tongue tip).

- *Modification of speech rate* by using delayed auditory feedback (DAF), a pacing board, an alphabet board, a metronome, hand or finger tapping, and by reducing excessive pause durations in speech.
- *Modification of prosody* by reducing the speech rate and teaching appropriate intonation.
- *Modification of pitch* with the help of instruction, modeling, differential feedback, or with the help of such instruments as Visi-Pitch.
- *Modification of vocal intensity* through behavioral methods of modeling, shaping, and differential reinforcement of greater inhalation, increased laryngeal adduction, and wider mouth opening.

SUMMARY

✓ The dysarthrias are a group of speech-motor disorders resulting from impaired muscular control of the speech mechanism, involving peripheral or central nervous system pathology.

✓ Dysarthrias are classified into ataxic, flaccid, hyperkinetic, hypokinetic, mixed, spastic, and unilateral upper-motor neuron types.

✓ The oral communication problems that accompany dysarthria include respiratory, articulatory, phonatory, resonatory, and prosodic disturbances that are caused by weakness, incoordination, or paralysis of speech musculature.

✓ These problems are assessed and treated in most patients with dysarthria. Treatment may involve the use of augmentative devices for patients with severe dysarthria.

DEMENTIA

INTRODUCTION

Dementia is a major health problem primarily found in people 65 years of age and older. It is an acquired neurological syndrome associated with persistent or progressive deterioration in intellectual functions (cognition, visuospatial skills), language, memory, emotion, and behavior. Dementia is commonly classified as cortical, subcortical, or mixed in nature. Assessment of dementia includes informal procedures and standardized tests. In treating dementia, the clinician helps clients manage their daily routines and families cope with the dementia (Bayles & Kaszniak, 1987; Cummings & Benson, 1992; Lubinski, 1995; Payne, 1997; Ripich, 1995; Shadden & Toner, 1997).

Definition and Classification of Dementia

■ Dementia, a major health care problem, may be as high as 25% in people 65 years and older. After the age of 65, the prevalence of dementia doubles every five years.

■ In most cases, dementia is an acquired neurological syndrome associated with persistent or progressive deterioration in intellectual functions (cognition, visuospatial skills), language, memory, emotion, and personality.

■ Most clinicians require that impairment be evident in at least three of those functions. The American Psychiatric Association's (2000) definition of dementia requires that memory impairment be evident to diagnose dementia.

■ Dementia can be related to *Wernicke-Korsakoff syndrome,* which is caused by prolonged alcohol abuse. Characteristics of Wernicke-Korsakoff syndrome include impaired learning, reduced memory, difficulty with visual-spatial integration, and difficulty processing abstract information (Wallace, 1998).

■ Dementia is typically progressive, but there are exceptions. It is reversible in about 20% of cases. Reversible dementia is a temporary intellectual impairment due to such factors as metabolic disturbances, nutritional deficiencies, chronic renal failure, persistent anemia, drug toxicity, and lung and heart diseases.

■ Classification of dementia is controversial. In one classification, dementia is classified as cortical, subcortical, and mixed (Cummings & Benson, 1992). Others simply describe the various forms of dementia. In some sources, dementia is classfied as *reversible* and *progressive* (American Psychiatric Association, 2000). Although information on various forms of dementia is accumulating at a fast rate, much of what we know about progressive dementia is based on studies of Alzheimer's disease. We will summarize the basic information on some major forms of dementia.

Dementia of the Alzheimer Type (DAT)

- Dementia associated with Alzheimer's disease is a form of cortical dementia. In this form of dementia, intellectual and language deterioration precedes motor deficits. In forms classified as subcortical, motor deficits precede intellectual deterioration.

- Approximately 50% of irreversible dementia is due to Alzheimer's disease.

- In a majority of the cases of DAT, onset takes place when people are in their 70s and 80s. More women than men are affected. DAT is associated with a family history of Down syndrome and also with a history of brain injury.

- Genetic inheritance accounts for some cases of DAT; the prevalence is 50% among the first-degree relatives. Genetic mutations in mitochondria and disturbed immune functions may also be etiological factors. Possible abnormalities in chromosomes 21, 17, 19, 12, 10, and 3 have been identified.

- Neuropathology of DAT involves the following:

  - *Neurofibrillary tangles.* Neurofibrils are filamentous structures in the nerve cells, dendrites, and axons; these structures are thickened, twisted, and tangled; they form unusual loops and triangles.
  - *Neuritic plaques.* Also known as *senile plaques,* neuritic plaques are minute areas of cortical and subcortical tissue degeneration. The cerebral cortex and hyppocampus (concerned with memory) are especially vulnerable to plaques. The result is destroyed cortical and subcortical synaptic connections.
  - *Neuronal loss.* Nerve cells are destroyed by fluid-filled cavities containing granular debris. The loss of neurons results in a shrunken brain; the shrinkage is most obvious in the cerebral hemispheres, especially in temporal and parietal lobes.
  - *Neurochemical changes.* Depletion of neurochemicals that help transmit messages across brain structures is a hallmark of dementia. Such neurochemicals as acetylcholine, somatostatin, vasopressin, and corticotropin are severely depleted in patients with Alzheimer's disease.

- Symptoms of early-stage DAT include:

  - subtle memory problems (especially for remote events)
  - somewhat pronounced difficulty in new learning and visuospatial problems (e.g., copying three-dimensional figures)
  - poor reasoning and judgment in social situations
  - behavior changes, including self-neglect and avoidance of routine tasks (e.g., cooking, asking a partner to keep the score while playing tennis)
  - other potential symptoms include depression, slight disorientation in new surroundings, and subtle language changes that are not evident to the family members

- Symptoms of later-stage DAT include:

  - intensified early-stage symptoms
  - severe problems in recalling remote and recent events
  - intensified visuospatial problems
  - widespread intellectual deterioration
  - hyperactivity, restlessness, agitation, meaningless handling of objects
  - problems in arithmetic calculations
  - profound disorientation to place, time, and person; wandering
  - problems in self-care (e.g., difficulty dressing, bathing)
  - difficulty in managing daily routines
  - lack of affect, tact, and judgment
  - loss of initiative, indifference
  - paranoid delusions and hallucinations
  - aggressive or disruptive behaviors
  - inappropriate humor and laughter
  - seizures, myoclonic jerks (sudden muscular contractions), incontinence, and physical deterioration in the very late stage

- Language problems associated with DAT include:

  - naming problems, verbal and literal paraphasias, and circumlocution
  - problems in comprehending abstract meanings
  - impaired picture description
  - difficulty in generating a list of words that begin with a specific letter
  - echolalia (repeating what others say), palilalia (repeating one's own utterances), and logoclonia (repeating the final syllable of words)
  - empty speech, jargon, and hyperfluency
  - incoherent, slurred, and rapid speech
  - pragmatic language problems, including inattention to social conventions (e.g., greetings), difficulty initiating conversation, and difficulty maintaining topics of conversation
  - reading and writing problems
  - in the final stages, no meaningful speech, mutism, and complete disorientation to time, place, people, and self

Frontotemporal Dementia (Including Pick's Disease)

- Frontotemporal dementia (FTD) is a group of heterogenous diseases that includes Pick's disease (PiD).

- FTD constitutes 12% of dementia cases diagnosed in people under 65; the typical onset of PiD takes place between age 40 and 60.

- FTD is often underdiagnosed and sometimes confused with DAT.

- Neuropathology of frontotemporal dementia include:

  - degeneration of nerve cells in the left and right frontal lobe, temporal lobe, or both the lobes in the two hemispheres
  - in the classic Pick's disease, atrophy may be focal, involving the anterior frontal and tem-

poral lobes, the orbital frontal lobe, and the medial temporal lobe
- Presence of Pick bodies (dense intracellular formation in the neuronal cytiplasm) and the presence of Pick cells (ballooned and inflated neurons) in the cortical layers
- Absence of Pick bodies and Pick cells in some variants of FTD, but the presence of atrophied, gliosed, and swollen brain cells

■ Symptoms of frontotemporal dementia include:

- notable behavioral changes as initial symptoms in patients with marked right-sided atrophy and notable language changes in those with marked left atrophy
- behavior disorders, including uninhibited and inappropriate social behaviors; compulsive behaviors, excessive eating (and weight gain); and delusions; these are more pronouned in patients with right-sided atrophy
- emotional disturbances, including depression, withdrawal, irritability, mood fluctuations, occasional euphoria, excessive jocularity, and exaggerated self-esteem
- impaired judgment and reasoning and lack of insight

■ Language problems associated with frontotemporal dementia include:

- dominant language problems with somewhat better preserved memory and orientation (contrasted with patients who have DAT)
- anomia (word-finding problems), more pronounced with temporal lobe atrophy
- progressive loss of vocabulary and consequent paraphasia and circumlocution
- difficulty defining common words and problems in reciting category-specific words (e.g., animals)
- limited spontaneous speech, echolalia, and nonfluent speech
- impaired comprehension of speech and printed material

Dementia Associated with Parkinson's Disease

■ Only about 35–55% of patients with Parkinson's disease (PD) have dementia.

■ PD is more common in males than in females, and onset is typically between 50 and 56 years of age.

■ Some experts classify dementia associated with Parkinson's disease as *subcortical* (motor symptoms precede intellectual deterioration).

■ The term *Parkinson's disease* refers to a single disease entity; the term *parkinsonism* refers to a group of neurological disorders that include hypokinesia, tremor, and muscular rigidity.

■ Both genetic factors and such environmental factors as pesticide and herbicide exposure are hypothesized causal factors.

■ Neuropathology of Parkinson's disease includes:

- brainstem degeneration
- presence of abnormal structures called Lewy bodies, small pathologic spots typically found in the substantia negra (a structure at the top of the brainstem)
- frontal-lobe atrophy resulting in widened sulci

- reduced inhibitory dopamine due to loss of cells in the substantia nigra
- neurofibriallary tangles and plaques of the kind found in Alzhemier's disease

■ Neurologic symptoms of Parkinson's disease include:

- slow voluntary movements (bradykinesia)
- tremors in resting muscles, starting in hand or foot, and spreading; tremors exacerbate during stress
- muscle rigidity (increased tone and resistance to movement)
- a mask-like face
- reduced eye blinking, festinating gait, disturbed posture, frequent falls, and freezing during movement
- swallowing disorders
- sleep disturbances

■ Speech, language, and related problems associated with Parkinson's disease (Brin, Velickovic, Ramig, & Fox, 2004):

- reduced speech volume
- voice problems that include monopitch and monoloudness
- long and frequent pauses in speech
- slow, fast, or festinating speech rate
- dysarthric speech
- serious memory problems, problems in abstract reasoning and problem solving
- impaired visuospatial perception
- impaired word-list generation
- severe naming and language comprehension problems in later stages of the disease
- apathy, confusion, hallucination, and delerium
- micrographia (writing in extremely small letters)

Dementia Associated with Huntington's Disease

■ Some classify dementia associated with Huntington's disease as *subcortical*.

■ Huntington's disease affects about 40–70 persons in a million; the typical age of onset is 35–40 years; it affects males and females equally.

■ Genetic etiology is supported; mutation on the short arm of chromosome 4 has been documented; half the offspring of a patient may have the disease.

■ A malformed protein called *huntingtin* kills the brain cells that control movement.

■ Neuropathology of Huntington's disease includes:

- a loss of neurons in the basal ganglia; significant loss of neurons in the caudate nucleus, putamen, and substantia nigra
- atrophy may be found in the prefrontal and parietal lobes as well
- reduced levels of inhibitory neurotransmitters, expecially GABA (gamma-amino butyric acid) and acetylcholine

■ Symptoms of Huntington's disease include:

- chorea (irregular, spasmodic, involuntary movement of the neck, head, and face)
- increasingly uncontrollable tic-like movement disorders
- gait disturbances, and progressively reduced voluntary movements
- slow movement in the advanced stages of the disease, leading to little or no voluntary movement
- behavioral disorders that include excessive complaining, nagging, eccentricity, irritability, emotional outbursts, a false sense of superiority, depression or euphoria, schizophrenic-like behaviors (delusion and hallucination), and suicide attempts

■ Speech, language, and cognitive-linguistic problems associated with the later stages of Huntington's disease include:

- deterioration in intellectual functions
- impaired word-list generation
- naming problems
- dysarthria
- incontinence, sleep disturbances, sleep reversal, and dysphagia
- muteness in the final stages

Infectious Dementia

■ Several infectious diseases lead to dementia. Dementia due to human immunodeficiency virus (HIV) infection or Jakob-Creutzfeldt disease is well known.

■ Dementia due to HIV infection is subcortical and is known as *AIDS dementia complex* or *human immunodeficiency virus encephalopathy;* it has the following features:

- opportunistic brain infections in people infected with the AIDS virus (e.g., cryptococcal meningitis) can lead to dementia
- HIV infection itself can cause dementia
- dementia is of slow onset, but the deterioration is rapid in the final stages
- neurologic symptoms include disturbed gait, tremor, headache, seizures, ataxia, rigidity, motor weakness, facial nerve paralysis, and incontinence
- dementia symptoms include forgetfulness, poor concentration, slow or impaired thinking, apathy and loss of interest in work, depression, mania, confusion, hallucinations, delusions, and memory loss
- language problems less prominent until mutism that settles in the final stage

■ Dementia due to Jakob-Creutzfeldt disease is another form of infectious dementia. Although no virus has been microscopically found, it is thought to be caused by an unconventional infectious agent called a *prion* (the word stands for *proteinacious infectious particle,* a form of abnormal protein found in the brains of people with the disease); the features of this disease include:

- neuropatholgy of Jakob-Creutzfeldt disease is a widespread spongiform state in the brain; neuron loss may be found in cortical areas, the basal ganglia, the thalamas, the brainstem, and the spinal cord

- physical symptoms include fatigue and sleep disturbances
- neurological symptoms include cerebellar ataxia, tremor, rigidity, chorea, athetosis, and visual problems
- symptoms of dementia include memory problems and reasoning impairments
- psychiatric symptoms include depression, anxiety, euphoria, hallucinations, and delusions
- the final stage is characterized by stupor, mutism, seizures, and pneumonia that often lead to death

Other Forms of Dementia

There are many other forms of dementia that space does not allow us to describe (Bayles & Kaszniak, 1987; Cummings & Benson, 1992; Lubinski, 1995; Payne, 1997; Ripich, 1995; Shadden & Toner, 1997). Notable among them:

- Vascular dementia. Vascular diseases may cause bilateral cortical, subcortical, or mixed damage resulting in dementia. More common in men than in women, and more common in African Americans than in whites, vascular dementia is associated with chronic hypertension. A distinguishing feature of vascular dementia is its sudden onset.

- Dementia associated with multiple cerebrovascular accidents, infarctions within the deep structures of the brain, and atrophy of subcortical white matter caused by repeated infarcts is also associated with a long-standing hypertension.

- Dementia associated with traumatic brain injury. Repeated brain injuries, especially those that cause prolonged periods of unconciousness, are a cause of dementia. Cortical, subcortical, and mixed types of damage may be associated with this type of dementia.

CONCEPTS TO CONSIDER

How is dementia classified? What is the major neuropathology of dementia?

Assessment of Dementia

■ A thorough case history, clinical examination, neurological assessment, including brain imaging and laboratory tests, communication assessment, and assessment of intellectual functions are a part of the diagnostic activities (Bayles & Kaszniak, 1987; Cummings & Benson, 1992; Hegde, 2001a, 2005; Lubinski, 1995; Payne, 1997; Ripich, 1995; Shadden & Toner, 1997). A definitive diagnosis of dementia is possible only after an autopsy, however.

■ Neither pointing to stimuli nor automatic speech tasks is useful in diagnosing mild forms of dementia. They are best diagnosed on the basis of verbal description, storytelling of both immediate and delayed variety, and word fluency (saying words that belong to a class, such as forms of transportation).

■ In assessing dementia, the following skills or domains are typically sampled:

  ▪ awareness and orientation to surroundings
  ▪ mood and affect, to assess depression or lack of emotional responses
  ▪ speech and language
  ▪ memory and other cognitive functions
  ▪ abnormal thinking (e.g., hallucinations or delusions)
  ▪ visuospatial skills

■ Various tests of aphasia may be helpful in assessing communication problems associated with dementia. There are only a few standardized tests of dementia. The *Arizona Battery for Communication Disorders of Dementia* (Bayles & Tomoeda, 1991) has been especially designed to assess dementia associated with Alzheimer's disease. It screens speech discrimination, visual perception and literacy, visual fields, visual agnosia, mental status, linguistic expression, linguistic comprehension, and visual–spatial construction.

■ The *Blessed Dementia Scale* (Hachinsky, Illiff, Zilhka, & Associates, 1975) helps evaluate changes in performance in eight everyday activities (e.g., inability to perform household tasks or to find way indoors) and changes in fourteen habits (e.g., changes in eating and dressing habits). Parents, caregivers, and medical records are the sources of information. Scores are specified for no impairment (below 4), mild impairment (4–9), and moderate to severe impairment (10 and higher).

■ The *Global Deterioration Scale* (Reisberg, Ferris, DeLeon, & Crook, 1982) also helps evaluate levels of functioning ranging from *no cognitive decline* to *very severe decline*. Information is gathered from a variety of sources.

■ Tests of language comprehension (e.g., the *Peabody Picture Vocabulary Test*) are useful in assessing receptive language skills of patients with dementia.

■ Intellectual skills may be assessed by administering selected tests of memory and general intelligence.

■ In addition to standardized dementia tests, the clinician may use such client-specific tasks as picture description to help assess various intellectual and language skills, including temporal sequencing, logical connections, grammaticality of sentences, topic maintenance, and so forth.

Clinical Management of Dementia

- ◼ The main clinical concerns are to help the client manage his or her daily routine and help the family cope with the progressively deteriorating dementia, for which there is no cure. In the early and intermediate stages, communication, memory, and behavioral management are targeted.

- ◼ Management of daily activities may include teaching the following strategies to the client (Brookshire, 1997):

  - ▪ establishing a simple routine
  - ▪ using various reminders: alarms, written instructions, staff reminders, self-monitoring devices, signs as reminders of activities and their times, and so forth
  - ▪ writing down a list of things to do every morning
  - ▪ always keeping phone numbers and possessions in a specific place
  - ▪ writing a checklist of things to do before leaving the house
  - ▪ always carrying a card with the names, addresses, and phone numbers of caregivers
  - ▪ always wearing a bracelet that contains identifying information and names, addresses, and phone numbers of caregivers
  - ▪ writing down important information when memory begins to fail

- ◼ Family members and caregivers need counseling and support. The family members should be (a) educated about dementia, (b) urged to monitor their emotional reactions, including depression, (c) offered counseling and other support services, and (d) offered respite care of patients. In addition, the family members may be counseled to manage the patient better by teaching them to (Shekim, 1997):

  - ▪ approach the patient slowly, touch the patient gently, establish eye contact, and speak clearly and slowly;
  - ▪ use gestures, smiling, posture, and other cues;
  - ▪ talk about simple and concrete events and talk in simple, short sentences;
  - ▪ point out the topic, person, or thing before speaking about it;
  - ▪ ask yes or no questions;
  - ▪ restate important information;
  - ▪ structure the client's room and the living environment to establish a routine;
  - ▪ always say good-bye or give other departing signals;
  - ▪ reduce emotional outbursts by analyzing the conditions under which they occur and eliminating those conditions; and
  - ▪ minimize demands made on the client.

SUMMARY

✓ Dementia, an acquired neurological syndrome associated with progressive deterioration in many functions (especially cognition), is usually found in people over 65 years of age.

✓ Dementia takes various forms; some are reversible, but most are progressive. A common type of cortical dementia is dementia of the Alzheimer's type. Frontotemporal dementia, which includes Pick's disease, is also a form of cortical dementia. Two major forms of subcortical dementia are those associated with Parkinson's disease and Huntington's disease. Various forms of infections cause dementia. The most prominent of this variety is the AIDS dementia complex and dementia associated with Creutzfeldt-Jakob disease.

✓ Assessment of patients with dementia includes administration of informal tasks and standardized tests. Treatment of patients with dementia is concerened with helping them manage their daily routines as effectively as possible and helping families cope with the dementia.

RIGHT HEMISPHERE SYNDROME

INTRODUCTION

The left and the right hemispheres specialize in somewhat different functions, although the brain works as an integrated whole. The corpus callosum, a thick bundle of fibers, connects the two hemispheres. Nonetheless, there are subtle structural differences between the two hemispheres. The left hemishpere is slightly larger in diameter. The lateral sulcus in the left hemisphere is slightly longer than that in the right hemisphere. The left planum temporale (a part of the superior surface of the superior temporal gyrus) is also larger than the right (Nolte, 2002). The symptoms of *right hemisphere damage* (RHD), also referred to as *right hemisphere syndrome,* vary depending upon the site of lesion. Typically, however, symptoms include attentional and perceptual, affective, symptoms; communicative deficits are found in 50% of the cases. Assessment of patients with RHD is mostly client specific, although a few standardized tests are available. Treatment often addresses such problems as impaired attention, impulsive behavior, pragmatic impairments, and visual neglect.

Foundational Concepts

■ While the left hemisphere specializes in most aspects of language, the right hemisphere either specializes in or, to some extent, controls:

- understanding holistic-gestalt stimuli, visual perception, geometric and spatial information
- facial recognition, drawing, and copying
- arousal, attention, and orientation
- emotional experience and expression
- perception of musical harmony
- certain prosodic features of communication, understanding ambiguous meanings, expressing and understanding the emotional tone of speech, understanding discourse, and pragmatic language skills (e.g., socially appropriate communication, turn taking, topic maintenance)

■ Right hemisphere functions are more diffusely organized than the left hemisphere functions.

■ The left and the right hemispheres are susceptible to the same kinds of neuropathology, including cerebrovascular accidents, tumors, head trauma, and various neurological diseases.

■ *Right hemisphere syndrome* varies in symptom complex. Posterior lesions do not produce motor problems, whereas frontal lobe injuries do. Patients with frontal lobe injuries are hospitalized longer than those with posterior lesions.

Symptoms of Right Hemisphere Syndrome

■ Symptoms of RHD include perceptual and attentional deficits, affective deficits, and communicative deficits. However, pure linguistic deficits are not typical of RHD. Attentional and perceptual deficits are dominant (Hegde, 2001a, 2005; Myers, 1999; Tompkins, 1995).

Attentional and Perceptual Deficits

- *Left neglect:* This is reduced awareness of the left side of the body and generally reduced awareness of stimuli in the left visual field. It consists of paying attention only to the right side of stimuli (e.g., copying only the right side of the face of a clock). Other characteristics of left neglect include failure to allow for a right margin in writing, reading only the right side of a printed page, bumping into things or people on the left side, and using only right-side pockets.
- *Denial of illness (anosagnosia):* The patient may deny the existence of the paralyzed arm or leg and be indifferent to admitted deficits or problems.
- *Confabulation regarding disability:* This refers to exaggerated claims regarding a disabled body part (e.g., a man with a paralyzed hand may claim to be painting with that hand).
- *Facial recognition deficits:* These deficits are characterized by failure to recognize a familiar face until the person begins to speak, difficulty remembering faces shown through pictures, and difficulty distinguishing faces of older and younger or male or female people.
- *Constructional impairment:* This impairment includes difficulty in reproducing block designs, drawing or copying geometric shapes, and reproducing two-dimensional stick figures.
- *Attentional deficits:* The patient may experience reduced awareness and arousal, difficulty sustaining attention, and difficulty in paying selective attention.
- *Disorientation:* Types of disorientation include topographic disorientation (confusion about space), geographic disorientation (not knowing where one is), and reduplicative paramnesia (e.g., a patient's belief that he has two left legs or two wives).
- *Visuoperceptual deficits:* These deficits involve difficulty recognizing line drawings; drawings that are distorted in size, dimension, or orientation; and drawings that are superimposed on another.

C O N C E P T S   T O   C O N S I D E R

You have been asked to give a workshop to physicians about recognizing right hemisphere syndrome in patients. List four things you will tell them.

_____

_____

_____

_____

_____

Affective Deficits

- Affective deficits found in people with right hemisphere syndrome include difficulty in:

  - understanding emotions other people express
  - describing emotions expressed on printed faces in storybooks
  - recognizing emotions expressed in isolated verbal productions
  - understanding emotional tone of voice
  - expressing emotions (not necessarily *experiencing* emotions)

Communicative Deficits

- As noted, only about half the number of patients with RHD have communicative deficits. These deficits are not so much related to syntactic and morphologic aspects of language as to an overall communicative effectiveness in social situations:

  - *Prosodic deficits.* These include monotone, impaired stress patterns, reduced speech rate, lack of affect, and difficulty understanding prosodic meanings of other people's speech.
  - *Impaired discourse and narrative skills.* These involve confusion between significant and irrelevant or trivial pieces of information in a picture description or conversational speech, making premature inferences during discourse, and unelaborated narratives.
  - *Confabulation and excessive speech.* These are characterized by excessive inference, too much attention to minor details, and saying too much, which borders on confabulation.
  - *Difficulty understanding implied, alternate, or abstract meanings.* This difficulty includes failure to grasp the overall meaning of situations or stories; difficulty understanding the central message of conversation; difficulty in describing the underlying theme of a picture or a story; literal interpretation of proverbs and sayings; and problems in appreciating humor, sarcasm, and irony.
  - *Pragmatic deficits.* These are characterized by problems in conversational turn taking, topic maintenance, and maintaining eye contact as well as rambling, excessive speech with little communicative value, and impulsive speech.
  - *Other communicative deficits.* These include naming problems, especially of collective nouns (e.g., problem in saying "flowers," but no problem in naming a particular type of flower); difficulty comprehending complex verbal material; and impaired oral reading of sentences.

Assessment of Right Hemisphere Syndrome

- Assessment of right hemisphere syndrome can be client specific, standardized, or both. For standardized testing, published assessment tools are available, which include the following:

  - The *Mini Inventory of Right Brain Injury* (Pimental & Kingsbury, 1989) helps evaluate such skills as visual scanning, integrity of gnosis (finger identification, tactile perception, two-point discrimination), integrity of body image, reading and writing, drawing, and affective and abstract language.
  - The *Right Hemisphere Language Battery,* 2nd edition (Bryan, 1995) helps assess comprehension of spoken and printed metaphors, inferred meanings, appreciation of humor, and discourse.

- The *Rehabilitation Institute of Chicago Clinical Management of Right Hemisphere Dysfunction* (Halper, Cherney, & Burns, 1996) helps assess typical skills impaired in RHD. In addition, the protocol includes an interview schedule and observation of a patient's interaction with others. Also helps assess nonverbal communication skills.
- The *Test of Visual Neglect* (Albert, 1973) helps assess neglect by asking the patient to cross out short lines randomly printed on a page.
- *Bells Test* (Gauthier, Dehaut, & Joanette, 1989) presents tasks in which the patient is asked to circle only the bells printed on a page that also contains other objects.
- The *Behavioral Inattention Test* (Wilson, Cockburn, & Halligan, 1987) contains both paper-and-pencil tests and techniques to assess neglect in such functional tasks as reading maps, menus, and newspapers and using a telephone.

■ Client-specific measures include language samples, narratives, discourse, and analysis of these observations; the clinician may assess visual–perceptual deficits by asking the client to draw simple pictures (e.g., the face of a clock, a human face).

Treatment of Right Hemisphere Syndrome

■ Treatment of patients with RHD is relatively new, and not much treatment research has been published. However, the treatment targets and strategies described below are generally considered appropriate (Brookshire, 2003; Hegde, 2001a, 2005; Myers, 1999; Tompkins, 1995).

- *Denial and indifference.* The clinician provides immediate feedback on errors to increase awareness. Videotaped sessions to give visual feedback on errors are helpful.
- *Impaired attention.* This involves drawing attention to treatment stimuli, giving specific directions to follow, repeating such directions throughout treatment, reinforcing attention during discourse training, and stopping the patient whenever he or she wanders away from topic of discourse.
- *Impulsive behavior.* Treatment includes nonverbal signals to wait a few seconds before giving an impulsive response (e.g., a hand gesture or a tone that signals the patient to wait). *Also helpful* are such verbal stimuli as "Wait for a few seconds and then tell me."
- *Pragmatic impairments.* Helpful techniques include videotaped conversations that show appropriate and inappropriate pragmatic behaviors to draw the patient's attention to such behaviors. The clinician may also give frequent reminders to maintain eye contact, continue talking on the same topic, and so forth.
- *Impaired reasoning.* The clinician can use activities that require reasoning (e.g., planning a vacation) and prompt and reinforce correct and logically sequenced descriptions.
- *Impaired inference.* Helpful treatment techniques include use of pictures that depict situations that require inference and reinforcement for correct inferences.
- *Impaired comprehension of metaphors and idioms.* Treatment involves practice in the correct interpretations of metaphors and idioms by asking the client to select printed statements or make comments that give literal, metaphoric, and implied meanings.
- *Visual neglect.* Treatment techniques include a thick and colorful line drawn on the left margins of printed pages to force attention to the text on the left side; teaching the patient to keep a finger on the left side of the page; pointing to the beginning of each line; frequent verbal prompts to pay attention to the neglected side of the body; and, generally, providing plenty of positive reinforcement for attending to objects on the left side and to left side of the body.

SUMMARY

✓ The left hemisphere specializes in most aspects of language. The right hemisphere specializes in processing holistic-gestalt stimuli, visual and spatial information, facial recognition, drawing, and copying.

✓ Patients with injury to the right hemisphere manifest various problems. These often include attentional and perceptual deficits, affective deficits, and communicative deficits with reasonably intact grammar.

✓ Client-specific and standardized methods may be used to assess patients with RHD. Treatment is targeted at impaired attention and behavior, pragmatic problems, impaired reasoning and inference, and visual neglect.

TRAUMATIC BRAIN INJURY

INTRODUCTION

Traumatic brain injury (TBI), also known as cranicerebral trauma, is injury to the brain sustained by physical trauma or external force. TBI is a frequently encountered medical emergency. Brain injuries can be penetrating or nonpenetrating. Assessment includes client-specific and standardized measures and is dependent upon the patient's level of postaccident consciousness. The two most common approaches to treatment of patients with TBI include the cognitive rehabilitation approach and the behavioral communication treatment approach (Adamovich, 1997; Bigler, 1990; Cooper & Golfinos, 2000; Hartley, 1995; Hegde, 2001a, 2005; Murdoch & Theorodos, 2001).

Definition and Incidence of TBI

■ *Traumatic brain injury* is injury to the brain sustained by physical trauma or external force. TBI does not include brain damage due to strokes, tumors, and progressive temporary neuropatholgies.

■ Estimates of the incidence of TBI vary within a range of about 150–200 cases to 367 cases per 100,000 persons in the United States.

■ The prevalence rate is the highest for the age group 15–19 years (400–700 per 100,000 individuals, depending on the studies). For the age group 75 and older, the prevalence is higher than it is for the general population (about 300 per 100,000 persons).

■ More males than females are affected. For every female with a TBI, there are three to five males with TBI.

■ TBI is a significant problem for people living in high-density urban areas, many of whom are from linguistically and culturally diverse backgrounds. There is limited and suggestive evidence that TBI is more common among African Americans and Hispanic Americans than the rest of the population (Wallace, 1998).

■ About 500,000 people are hospitalized with TBI annually, and 900,000 may sustain permanent disability (Cooper & Golfinos, 2000; Payne, 1997).

Common Causes of TBI

■ Automobile accidents, including pedestrian injuries, account for up to 50% of TBI; motor cycle riders have a higher risk of TBI than car drivers.

■ Falls are the second most common cause of TBI. Children and the elderly are especially vulnerable.

■ Interpersonal violence (including child and spousal abuse) accounts for up to 40% of TBI reported from urban areas.

■ Other causes include alcohol and drug abuse, serious and preexisting learning disorders, psychiatric disturbances, and prior history of TBI.

Types and Consequences of TBI

■ *Penetrating* and *nonpenetrating injuries* are two classifications of TBI; they produce different neuroanatomic and behavioral consequences. Also known as *open-head injuries,* penetrating brain injuries involve a fractured or perforated skull, torn or lacerated meninges, and an injury that extends to brain tissue. High-velocity missiles (e.g., bullets) and low-velocity impacts (e.g., blows to the head) are the most frequent causes of penetrating brain injuries.

■ Also known as *closed-head injuries,* nonpenetrating brain injuries involve no open wound in the head, a damaged brain within the skull, and no penetration of a foreign substance into the brain. Even when the skull is fractured, the injury is classified as nonpenetrating if the meninges are intact. Nonpenetrating injuries may be of acceleration-deceleration type or nonacceleration type:

   ▪ *Acceleration-deceleration injuries* are more serious than nonacceleration injuries. In acceleration-deceleration, a head is set into motion by physical forces; when the head begins to move, the brain inside is still static. Soon, the brain begins to move. When the head stops moving, the brain keeps moving inside the skull and thus strikes the skull on the opposite side of the initial impact. The moving brain is lacerated or torn because of the bony projections on the base of the skull. The acceleration-deceleration movement of the head in an automobile accident is an example.
   ▪ *Nonacceleration injuries* occur when a restrained head is hit by a moving object. A collapsing car crushing the head of a mechanic working under it is an example. A great deal of force may crush the head and kill a person; in most cases, however, nonacceleration injuries may fracture the skull, but they produce much less serious consequences for the brain and the behavior of the person.
   ▪ The brain injury at the point of impact (e.g., a blow to the head) is called the *coup injury;* the injury at the opposite side of the impact because the moving brain struck the skill is called the *contrecoup* injury.

■ Consequences of TBI include immediate or subsequent death in some cases, loss of consciousness, coma, destruction of brain tissue, diffuse axonal injury, diffuse vascular injury, brainstem injury, focal lesions, infection, penetration of foreign objects, reduced cerebral blood flow, increased blood pressure, swelling of the brain tissue, hydrocephalus, and various types of hematomas (accumulation of blood in an area of the brain).

- Other consequences of TBI may include increased intracranial pressure; ischemic brain damage (damage due to lack of blood); seizures; and long-term physical, language, and cognitive deficits.

- Additional consequences of TBI include altered consciousness (stupor, coma); confusion and disorientation; posttraumatic amnesia; dysphagia; behavior changes, including hallucinations, delusions and confabulations; poor emotional control; social withdrawal; irritability; childishness; and unreasonable behaviors.

- Communication disorders associated with TBI include an initial mutism that may last varying periods of time, confused language, dysarthria, naming difficulties, perseveration of verbal responses, reduced word fluency, difficulty initiating conversation, lack of turn taking in conversation, problems in topic initiation and maintenance, lack of narrative cohesion, impaired prosody, imprecise language, difficulty with abstract language, reading and writing problems, auditory comprehension deficits, and generally disturbed social interaction.

General Assessment of Patients with TBI

- In the assessment of patients with TBI, it is critical to gather a comprehensive case history, observe the client, interview family members and health-care workers, and review medical records to understand the nature and extent of TBI.

- Initial assessment depends on the medical condition of the client and may be brief. The client regaining consciousness may be inconsistent, disorganized, disoriented, restless, distracted, and irritated. The initial assessment may be done at the bedside. Major assessment tools used in the initial and subsequent stages of recovery include those described below.

    - The *Glasgow Coma Scale* (Teasdale & Jennett, 1976) helps make an initial assessment of eye opening, motor responses (e.g., flexing the body in response to pain), and verbal responses.
    - The *Brief Test of Head Injury* (Helm-Estabrooks & Hotz, 1991) is a brief screening test to evaluate adults with severe head injury. It helps assess orientation, following commands, and other relevant behviors of patients with head injury.
    - The *Comprehensive Level of Consciousness Scale* (Stanczak & Associates, 1984) also helps assess initial status by rating posture, resting eye position, spontaneous eye opening, ocular movements, pupillary reflexes, motor functioning, responsiveness, and communicative effort.
    - The *Galveston Orientation and Amnesia Test* (Levin, O'Donnell, & Grossman, 1979) helps assess amnesia, orientation, and memory.
    - The *Disability Rating Scale* (Rappoport, Hall, Hopkins & Associates, 1982) helps assess changes in patients with head injury; it helps assess eye opening, verbal responses, motor responses, feeding, toileting, and so forth.
    - The *Rancho Los Amigos Scale of Cognitive Levels* (Hagen & Malkamus, 1979) helps assess cognition and behavior at the levels of no response, generalized response, localized response, confused-agitated, confused-appropriate, automatic-appropriate, and purposeful-appropriate.

- Assessment of memory impairments includes assessment of posttraumatic amnesia (loss of memory for events following the trauma) and pretraumatic amnesia (loss of memory for events preceding the trauma). The clinician may use client-specific questions surrounding the trauma.

Assessment of Communicative Deficits Associated with TBI

■ Pure linguistic problems may not be severe or significant in patients with TBI. Articulatory or phonological disorders may be noted only if the patient sustained injury to the cerebellum, brain stem, or peripheral nerves. The patient's verbal expressions may be grammatically correct.

■ Assessment procedures may include selected tests of aphasia and client-specific procedures that the clinician develops (Brookshire, 2003; Hegde, 2001a, 2005). Initial and persistent communicative problems that must be assessed include the following:

- *dysarthria:* spastic dysarthria or mixed dysarthria in some patients with TBI are noted; these disorders may be assessed with standard dysarthria assessment tools described in a previous section
- *confused language:* if evident initially, may be assessed with standard interviews and bedside examinations
- *auditory comprehension problems:* possibly more pronounced for complex or abstract material; both clinical examinations and selected standardized assessment tools may be helpful in assessing auditory comprehension deficits
- *confrontation naming problems:* standard naming tests described in the section on aphasia and client-specific procedures the clinician devises (showing objects from the client's environment and asking him or her to name them) will be helpful in assessing these problems
- *perseveration of verbal responses:* repetitive verbal responses that may be observed and recorded during interview and conversations with the patient
- *pragmatic language problems:* difficulty in initiating conversation, turn taking, selecting appropriate topics for conversation, maintaining topic and cohesion, rambling, and understanding the meaning of facial expressions and gestures are best assessed during interview and conversation with the patient
- *reading and writing difficulties:* either specific reading and writing tests or such client-specific tasks as having the client read familiar print and write to dictation or copying printed material will help assess these difficulties

Treatment of Patients with TBI

■ Of the variety of treatment approaches advocated for patients with TBI, cognitive rehabilitation and direct communication training are the two most important (Hegde, 2001b, 2005).

■ *Cognitive rehabilitation* is preferred by some clinicians. In cognitive rehabilitation, clinicians train such components as attention, visual processing, and memory, which may not result in improved communication. Attempts to improve memory, reasoning skills, and other cognitive functions may be better integrated with communication training.

■ *Communication treatment* for patients with TBI often involves direct behavioral procedures. Systematic reinforcement of attending behaviors, appropriate discourse, topic maintenance, self-correction, and so forth, will result in their increase and a concomitant decrease in many inappropriate behaviors.

CONCEPTS TO CONSIDER

Discuss two approaches to rehabilitation of patients with TBI.

_____

_____

_____

_____

_____

- Communication treatment goals should be functional, with the initial focus on effectiveness of communication, not grammatical correctness. Family members should be involved in treatment. Other treatment goals are described below; the clinician can be involved in:

  - *increasing the patient's orientation and attention to place, person, and time* by asking questions about the patient's whereabouts; using written signs to help the patient remember the day of the week or the name of the hospital;
  - *increasing the patient's memory for daily routines* through written signs that remind the patient of routines and lists of daily activities;
  - *increasing the patient's memory for the names of significant people* by asking the patient to name pictures of family members;
  - *decreasing the variability in activities and schedules* by initially creating a simple, structured routine with few activities for the patient;
  - *increasing the patient's attention to communication partners and topics* to promote better comprehension by giving such signals as "Listen carefully, now," "I want to say something to you," and "Are you listening?";
  - *improving communicative attention* by introducing new topics and warning about topic changes in conversation;
  - *teaching the client to ask questions* when something said is not clear to him by modeling such questions and statements as "What do you mean?" "I do not understand that," "Tell me more about that," and so forth;
  - *withholding attention from irrelevant, inappropriate, or tangential responses* to reduce their frequency;
  - *teaching narrative skills in graded steps* by initially telling a brief and simple story, asking the patient to retell it, and eventually having the client retell more complex stories;
  - *integrating such pragmatic skills as topic maintenance and topic initiation into narrative skills teaching* by such prompts as "Say more" and "Give details";
  - *integrating work- or school-related words, phrases, and narratives into communication training* at all levels by selecting client-specific work or school-related vocabulary and expressions for treatment;

- *using tangible reinforcers* when necessary because some patients with TBI may not respond to verbal reinforcers in the early stages of recovery;
- *teaching self-monitoring skills* by including them at all levels of training;
- *teaching compensatory strategies* to handle residual deficits (e.g., writing down instructions and important information, requesting information, requesting people to speak slowly or repeat, requesting others to write down messages, establishing simple and invariable routines, reducing environmental distractions, and self-cueing);
- *training family members and others* to recognize, prompt, model, and reinforce appropriate communication and general behavior;
- *promoting community reentry* by preparing the patient for reentry to school or work; educating family members, teachers, and supervisors about the patient's strengths and weaknesses; teaching family members, teachers, colleagues, and supervisors to change their style of communication if needed; and modifying teacher or supervisor demands if necessary.

SUMMARY

✓ TBI, or injury to the brain sustained by physical trauma or external force, can involve penetrating or nonpenetrating injuries.

✓ Patients with TBI should undergo general assessment as well as assessment of communicative deficits such as possible dysarthria, pragmatic language and auditory comprehension problems, and written-language deficits.

✓ The two primary treatment approaches for patients with TBI include the cognitive rehabilitation and communication treatment approaches. These two approaches may be integrated to help the patient reenter the community to the greatest extent possible.

SWALLOWING DISORDERS

INTRODUCTION

Swallowing disorders (dysphagia) involve impaired execution of the oral, pharyngeal, and esophageal phases of a normal swallow. Dysphagia may be caused by strokes, TBI, and other factors. Assessment of dysphagia involves screening communication skills and evaluating the patient's swallowing skills. Treatment of dysphagia may be direct, indirect, medical, or a combination of these (Groher, 1997; Hegde, 2001a, 2001b; Logemann, 1998; Perlman & Schulze-Delrieu, 1997). Swallowing disorders, also known as *dysphagia or deglutition disorders,* are technically not disorders of communication. However, except for esophageal swallowing disorders, which are handled medically, speech–language pathologists are the recognized experts in the assessment and management of swallowing disorders.

Nature and Etiology of Swallowing Disorders

- *Dysphagia* involves impaired execution of the oral, pharyngeal, and esophageal stages of swallow. The patient may have problems in chewing the food, preparing it for swallow, initiating the swallow, propelling the bolus through the pharynx, and passing the food through the esophagus. There are many causes of swallowing disorders:

- strokes, especially brain stem and anterior cortical strokes, resulting in poor motor control of structures involved in swallowing
- oral and pharyngeal tumors and various neurologic diseases (e.g., Parkinson's disease, amyotrophic lateral sclerosis, multiple sclerosis, myasthenia gravis, muscular dystrophy, and dystonia)
- surgical or radiation treatment of oral, pharyngeal, and laryngeal cancer; any form of brain, head, neck, or gastrointestinal surgery
- traumatic brain injury; cervical spine disease
- poliomyelitis (polio), chronic and obstructive pulmonary disease, and cerebral palsy
- genetic factors (e.g., *dysautonomia,* an inherited disorder associated with autonomic imbalance, sensory deficits, and motor incoordination)
- side effects of certain prescription drugs (e.g., antispasticity, antipsychotic, and neuroleptic drugs)

Typical and Disordered Swallow

- There are various phases of dysphagia involving mastication as well as the oral preparatory, oral, pharyngeal, and esophageal phases and their disorders. The following are descriptions of these phases:

    - *Mastication and its disorders.* Mastication is chewing solid or semisolid food before initiating swallow. Disorders of mastication include problems in chewing food because of reduced range of lateral and vertical tongue movement, reduced range of lateral mandibular movement, reduced buccal tension, and poor alignment of the mandible and maxilla.
    - *Oral preparatory phase and its disorders.* Masticated food is prepared for swallow in the oral preparatory phase by making a *bolus* (a rounded mass of food that is ready to be swallowed). Disorders of the oral preparatory phase include difficulty in forming and holding the bolus, abnormal holding of the bolus, slippage of food into anterior and lateral sulcus, aspiration before swallow due mostly to weak lip closure, reduced tongue movement, and inadequate tongue and buccal tension.
    - *Oral phase and its disorders.* This phase begins with the posterior tongue action that moves the bolus posteriorly; the phase ends as the bolus passes through the anterior faucial arches when the swallowing reflex is initiated. Disorders of the oral phase include:

        — such problems in tongue movements as anterior instead of posterior movement and weak movement
        — food residue in various places (e.g., anterior and lateral sulcus and the floor of the mouth)
        — premature swallow and aspiration before swallow, caused by apraxia of swallow
        — tongue thrust
        — reduced labial, buccal, and tongue tension and strength
        — reduced range of tongue movement and elevation

    - *Pharyngeal phase and its disorders.* This phase consists of reflex actions of the swallow. Reflexes are triggered by the contact the food makes with the anterior faucial pillars. The pharyngeal phase involves velopharyngeal closure, laryngeal closure by an elevated larynx to seal the airway, reflexive relaxation of the cricopharyngeal muscle for the bolus to enter, and reflexive contractions of the pharyngeal contractors to move the bolus down and eventually into the esophagus. Disorders of the pharyngeal phase include:

— difficulties in propelling the bolus through the pharynx and into the P-E (pharyngo-esophageal sphincter) segment
— delayed or absent swallowing reflex
— nasal and airway penetration of food
— food coating on the pharyngeal walls
— food residue in *valleculae* (space between the base of the tongue and the epiglottis), on top of airway, in pyriform sinuses, and throughout the pharynx
— aspiration before and after swallow
— delayed pharyngeal transmit time
— reduced *pharyngeal peristalsis,* or the constricting and relaxing movements of the pharynx
— pharyngeal paralysis
— reduced movement of the base of the tongue
— reduced laryngeal movement
— inadequate closure of the airway
— cricopharyngeal dysfunctions

- *Esophageal phase and its disorders.* This swallowing phase is not under voluntary control. It begins when the food arrives at the orifice of the esophagus; food is propelled through the esophagus by peristaltic action and gravity and into the stomach. Bolus entry into the esophagus results in restored breathing and a depressed larynx and soft palate. Disorders of this phase include the following problems, which are generally caused by a weak crico-pharyngeus:

— difficulties in passing the bolus through the cricopharyngeus muscle and past the 7th cervical vertebra
— backflow of food from esophagus to pharynx
— reduced esophageal contractions due to surgery, neurologic damage, or radiation therapy
— formation of diverticulum (a pouch that collects food)
— development of tracheo esophageal fistula (a hole); and
— esophageal obstruction (e.g., by a tumor)

CONCEPTS TO CONSIDER

Describe the stages of a normal swallow.

_____

_____

_____

_____

_____

Assessment of Swallowing Disorders

■ Such standard procedures as taking a detailed case history, reviewing medical records, and interviewing the patient, family, and health-care workers are a part of the total assessment. In addition, the clinician may implement the following specific procedures (Hegde, 2001a):

- *Screen speech, voice, language, and writing skills* using the clinical interview. Errors of articulation, voice quality, pitch and loudness characteristics, and the presence of hyponasality and hypernasality may be noted.
- *Screen concrete and abstract language comprehension* by giving a few simple verbal commands and by asking the patient to give the meaning of common proverbs and phrases. Deviations in the use of language, if any, may be noted.
- *Conduct a laryngeal examination* with indirect laryngoscopy or endoscopic examination to inspect the base of the tongue, vallecula, epiglottis, pyriform sinuses, vocal folds, and ventricular folds and their functioning.
- *Administer test swallows*, taking into consideration the patient's medical condition and the type of swallowing disorder. Collect the necessary materials (a laryngeal mirror, a tongue blade, a cup, a spoon, a straw, a syringe, and various foods of different consistencies).
- *Correctly position the patient for test swallows*. For example, in the case of tongue weakness and bolus manipulation problems, the patient should tilt the head downward as food is placed in the mouth and tilt the head backward when the swallow is initiated. In the case of hemilaryngectomy, delayed triggering of swallowing reflex, and inadequate laryngeal closure, the patient should tilt the head downward to hold the food in the valleculae until the reflex is triggered.
- *Appropriately place the food in the mouth*. For example, place food in the more normal side of the mouth, or use a straw or a syringe to place liquids posteriorly.
- *Use different kinds of foods in evaluating test swallows*. For example, use liquid foods or foods of thin consistency when the patient has limited oral control and foods of thicker consistency when the patient's swallowing reflex is delayed.
- *Give appropriate instructions* for head position and swallowing.
- *Manually examine the swallowing movements* by placing the index finger just below the chin, the middle finger on the hyoid, and the third and fourth fingers at the top and bottom of the thyroid to take note of the submandibular, hyoid, and laryngeal movements during swallowing or aspiration.
- *Conduct a videofluorographic assessment* (modified barium swallow) of oropharyngeal swallow involving lateral and anterior-posterior (A-P) plane examinations.
- *Conduct a manometric assessment* with the help of an esophageal manometer, which measures pressure in the upper and lower esophagus.
- *Conduct an electromyographic assessment* by attaching electrodes on structures of interest (e.g., oral, laryngeal, or pharyngeal muscles).
- *Conduct an endoscopic assessment* to examine the movement of the bolus until it triggers the pharyngeal swallow and of any food residue after swallow.
- *Conduct ultrasound examination* to measure oral tongue movement and hyoid movement.

Treatment of Swallowing Disorders

■ Clinicians who treat patients with swallowing disorders should always take into account the patient's cultural background. Patients may have food preferences or religious beliefs that affect the type of food and the timing of feeding that occur as part of treatment (Wallace, 1998).

■ Direct, indirect, and medical procedures are used to treat swallowing disorders. Speech–language pathologists are involved in both direct and indirect treatment (Groher, 1997; Hegde, 2001b; Logemann, 1998; Perlman & Schulze-Delrieu, 1997).

Direct Treatment of Swallowing Disorders

• In direct treatment, food or liquid is placed in the patient's mouth to shape appropriate swallowing. Direct treatment is designed to reduce problems that are evident in the different stages of swallow, as follows:

  ▪ *Treatment of disorders of mastication* involves teaching the patient to better handle food in the mouth. The clinician may use such procedures as:

    — teaching the patient to press the tongue against the hard palate;
    — teaching the patient to keep the food on the more mobile side of the tongue or on the stronger side of the mouth;
    — applying a gentle pressure with one hand on the damaged cheek to increase cheek tension; and
    — teaching the patient to keep the head tilted to the stronger side to maintain food on that side.

  ▪ *Treatment of disorders of the preparatory phase of the swallow* involves such procedures as teaching the patient to tilt the head forward to keep the food in the front of the mouth until ready to swallow, tilting the head back to promote the swallow, holding the bolus in the anterior or middle portion of the mouth, and so forth.

  ▪ *Treatment of disorders of the oral phase of the swallow* involves:

    — teaching the patient to place the tongue on the alveolar ridge and initiate a swallow with an upward and backward motion to prevent tongue thrust swallow
    — teaching the patient to compensate by placing food at the back of the tongue and then initiating a swallow
    — teaching the patient to compensate for tongue elevation problems by placing food posteriorly in the patient's oral cavity, placing a straw almost at the level of the faucial arches to help the patient swallow liquid, and then tilting the patient's head back and letting gravity push the food from the oral cavity into the pharynx

  ▪ *Treatment of disorders of the pharyngeal stage of the swallow* can be carried out by:

    — teaching the patient to tilt the head forward while swallowing, to compensate for delayed or absent swallowing reflex;
    — teaching the patient to switch between liquid and semisolid swallows so that the liquid swallows help clear the pharynx to compensate for reduced peristalsis;
    — teaching the patient to tilt the head toward the stronger side if the patient has a unilateral paralysis in lingual function and the pharynx; and
    — teaching the patient to tilt the head forward while swallowing or placing pressure on the thyroid cartilage on the damaged side to improve laryngeal closure.

Indirect Treatment of Swallowing Disorders

- Indirect treatment of swallowing disorders does not involve food. Instead, various exercises designed to improve muscle strength are prescribed and practiced.
- *Oral-motor control exercises* are numerous, and each is designed to reduce a particular problem. For example, various exercises are designed to:

  - increase the range of tongue movements (e.g., raising the tongue, holding the tongue as high as possible, alternating raising and lowering the tongue);
  - increase buccal tension (e.g., stretching the lips as tightly as possible and saying "ee," rounding the lips tightly and saying "oh," and rapidly alternating between "ee" and "oh");
  - increase the range of lateral movements of the jaw (e.g., wide opening and sideways movement of the jaw) and of tongue resistance (e.g., pushing the tongue against a tongue depressor); and
  - strengthen lip closure (e.g., stretching the lips to stimulate the production of /i/; puckering the lips tightly; tightly closing the lips).

- Some exercises are designed to *stimulate the swallow reflex* by:

  - touching the base of the anterior faucial arch with a laryngeal mirror dipped in ice water for about 10 seconds (*thermal stimulation*);
  - asking the patient to swallow after the stimulation without food;
  - practicing liquid swallow after stimulation; and
  - progressively increasing the consistency of food introduced after stimulation.

- Some exercises are designed to *improve adduction of tissues at the top of the airway* by lifting and pushing exercises to improve laryngeal adduction to protect the airway during swallowing (e.g., holding his or her breath, the patient pushes down on the chair or pulls up on it; subsequently, the patient may lift or push with simultaneous voicing).

Medical Treatment of Swallowing Disorders

- Surgeons are mostly involved in the medical treatment of swallowing disorders as most of the medical procedures are surgical. These procedures are described briefly below:

  - *Cricopharyngeal myotomy.* In this surgical procedure, the cricopharyngeal muscle is split from top to bottom to create a permanently open sphincter for swallowing. Fibers of the inferior constrictor above and the esophageal musculature below also may be slit. Eating may be resumed within about a week. This procedure is recommended for patients with Parkinson's disease, amyotrophic lateral sclerosis, and oculopharyngeal dystrophy, whose main problem is cricopharyngeal dysfunction.
  - *Esophagostomy.* This is designed for patients who cannot tolerate oral feeding. The procedure involves inserting a feeding tube into the esophagus and stomach through a hole (stoma) that has been surgically created through cervical esophagus.
  - *Gastrostomy.* Also designed for patients who cannot tolerate oral feeding, this procedure involves insertion of a feeding tube into the stomach through an opening in the abdomen; blended table food is directly transported to the stomach.
  - *Nasogastric feeding.* This is another surgical method for dysphagic patients who cannot tolerate oral feeding. A tube, inserted through the nose, pharynx, and esophagus into the stomach, feeds the patient.

- *Pharyngostomy.* In this variation of nonoral, surgical feeding methods, a tube is inserted into the esophagus and stomach through a hole that has been surgically created through the pharynx.
- *Teflon injection into the vocal folds.* This is a surgical implant method designed to improve airway closure during swallowing. Teflon is injected to a normal or reconstructed vocal cord or any remaining tissue on top of the airway to increase the muscle mass that will help close the airway.

SUMMARY

✓ Dysphagia, which involves impaired execution of the oral, pharyngeal, and esophageal phases of a swallow, can be caused by many factors, including strokes and TBI.

✓ Phases of swallowing include the oral preparatory phase, oral phase, pharyngeal phase, and esophageal phase. A thorough assessment involves evaluation of all these phases.

✓ Treatment for dysphagia should take cultural factors into account. It can be direct, indirect, medical, or a combination of these. In direct treatment, food and liquid are placed in the patient's mouth to shape appropriate swallowing. In indirect treatment, food is not involved; exercises to improve muscle strength are practiced. Medical treatment may involve various surgical procedures.

◆ **APHASIA IS A NEUROGENIC** language disorder caused by a stroke. Strokes have many causes, including thrombosis and embolism. Aphasia is often classified into nonfluent, fluent, and subcortical varieties.

◆ **VARIETIES OF NONFLUENT APHASIA** include Broca's aphasia, transcortical motor aphasia, mixed transcortical aphasia, and global aphasia. Varieties of fluent aphasia include Wernicke's aphasia, transcortical sensory aphasia, conduction aphasia, and anomic aphasia. Nonfluent aphasias are generally caused by lesions in the anterior brain structures, and fluent aphasias are caused by lesions in the posterior structures; subcortical aphasia is caused by lesions in the basal ganglia and surrounding structures and the thalamus.

◆ **RELATIVELY INTACT AUDITORY COMPREHENSION** and agrammatic, anomic, telegraphic, dysfluent, effortful, and sparse speech characterize nonfluent aphasia. Impaired auditory comprehension and relatively fluent, jargon-filled, and grammatically correct but semantically impaired speech characterize fluent aphasia. Treatment of aphasia targets both auditory comprehension and verbal expression; functional communication is a realistic goal for many severely involved clients.

◆ **ALEXIA IS A READING** disorder due to cortical damage. Agraphia is a writing disorder due to cortical damage. Agnosia is a sensory disorder in which the meaning of sensory input in one modality is not perceived (even though peripheral sensory organs are normal), while the same input in another modality may be normally perceived.

◆ **APRAXIA IS A MOTOR-PLANNING** disorder due to cerebral damage. Apraxia of speech is a speech-motor planning disorder due to cerebral damage; it is characterized by articulation errors and difficulty in executing volitional movements needed for speech, with relatively intact automatic movements.

◆ **DYSARTHRIA IS A SPEECH-MOTOR** disorder due to impaired muscular control of the speech mechanism, involving peripheral or central nervous system pathology and affecting respiratory, articulatory, phonatory, resonatory, and prosodic aspects of speech.

◆ **DEMENTIA IS AN ACQUIRED** neurological syndrome associated with persistent or progressive deterioration in intellectual functions (cognition, visuospatial skills), language, memory,

CHAPTER HIGHLIGHTS

emotion, and personality. It is often seen in the elderly and is typically progressive but, in some cases, is reversible.

◆ **RIGHT HEMISPHERE SYNDROME IS** a symptom complex including perceptual, attentional, affective, and communicative deficits associated with injury to the right cerebral hemisphere.

◆ **TRAUMATIC BRAIN INJURY (TBI)** is injury to the brain sustained by physical trauma or external force. Penetrating injury involves a fractured or perforated skull, torn or lacerated meninges, and an injury that extends to brain tissue. Nonpenetrating brain injury involves no open wound in the head, a damaged brain within the skull, and no penetration of a foreign substance into the brain; the skull may be fractured, but the injury is nonpenetrating when the meninges are intact.

◆ **DYSPHAGIA IS A SWALLOWING** disorder involving impaired execution of the oral, pharyngeal, and esophageal stages of swallow. Patients with dysphagia may receive direct treatment, indirect treatment, medical treatment, or a combination.

✎ **ADD YOUR OWN CHAPTER HIGHLIGHTS HERE:**

Study & Review Questions

Essay

1. Compare and contrast aphasia and dementia. What are some general characteristics of both conditions? How would a clinician differentiate between the two, especially in an elderly patient?

2. Describe the differences between fluent aphasias and nonfluent aphasias.

3. List and briefly describe the types of dysarthria. What are the causes of each one?

4. Describe right hemisphere syndrome. How is this condition different than aphasia caused by left hemisphere damage?

5. What types of treatment are available for patients with swallowing disorders? Describe these types of treatment and when a clinician might use one or more of them.

Multiple Choice

6. A clinician in a hospital setting is asked to evaluate a 64-year-old patient who appears to have dementia. The referring physician wishes to have a specific diagnosis, and the clinician is asked to gather detailed case history information as well as to conduct a thorough assessment of the patient. In gathering the case history from the patient's adult daughter, the clinician finds out that the patient began drinking alcohol as a 15-year-old and has been a heavy drinker since that time. A detailed evaluation shows that the patient presents with memory problems, difficulty processing abstract information, and visual–spatial deficits. This patient most likely has:

   A. dementia of the Alzheimer's type.
   B. Parkinson's disease.
   C. Wernicke-Korsakoff Syndrome.
   D. aphasia.
   E. ataxic dysarthria.

7. Conduction aphasia is caused by lesions:

   A. between the areas supplied by the middle cerebral arteries and the anterior and posterior arteries.
   B. in the region between Broca's area and Wernicke's area, especially in the supramarginal gyrus and the arcuate fasciculus.
   C. in Brodmann's areas 44 and 45 in the posterior-inferior gyrus of the left hemisphere.
   D. in the angular gyrus, the second temporal gyrus, and the juncture of the temporo-parietal lobe.
   E. in the basal ganglia and the thalamus.

8. Among the following standardized tests of aphasia, the one that samples speech and language skills to only a limited extent is:

    A. the Neurosensory Center Comprehensive Examination for Aphasia.
    B. the Porch Index of Communicative Ability.
    C. the Boston Diagnostic Aphasia Examination.
    D. the Western Aphasia Battery.
    E. the Functional Living Assessment.

Questions 9–11 *refer to the following scenario:*

A hospital-based clinician receives a referral of a woman, Fran K., who is 76 years old. An active grandmother of six grandchildren, Fran enjoys walking, swimming, driving her grandchildren to various activities (e.g., soccer practice), and participating in her local church where she sings in the choir and attends weekly Bible study. When Fran comes for the initial interview, she tells the clinician that she has had to stop her daily walks with her dog because when she walks, she is slow to begin, then takes short, rapid, shuffling steps. She shares that her writing has become smaller, and that her friends and family say that she is "expressionless" these days. The clinician notices decreased intelligibility also.

9. Fran probably has:

    A. right hemisphere syndrome.
    B. unilateral upper motor neuron dysarthria.
    C. Broca's aphasia.
    D. Alzheimer's dementia.
    E. Parkinson's disease.

10. Based on your diagnosis, you would expect Fran's speech and language to be characterized by:

    A. fluency problems, including silent pauses as well as repetitions because of false starts and attempts at self-correction.
    B. quality and rate that are "drunken" and slow, with excessive and even stress.
    C. incoherent, slurred, and rapid speech accompanied by metathetic errors.
    D. monopitch, a harsh and breathy voice, short rushes of speech, imprecise consonants, and respiratory problems.
    E. problems in volitional or spontaneous sequencing of movements required for speech with relatively unaffected automatic speech.

11. Other symptoms the clinician might expect Fran to manifest would include:

    A. chorea, emotional outbursts, schizophrenic-like behaviors, and dysarthria.
    B. hallucinations, masklike face, confabulation.
    C. mask-like face, slow voluntary movements, tremors in resting muscles, and disturbed posture.
    D. circumlocutions, repetitive verbal responses, festinating speech.
    E. substitutions and distortions of speech sounds, high variability of errors, occasional normal production of difficult words.

12. Functional communication tests seek to assess:

    A. communication in natural or everyday situations.
    B. grammatically correct communication.

C. comprehension of both daily and academic vocabulary necessary for effective functioning in the "real world."

D. syntactially correct communication.

E. communication in formal settings (e.g., speaking in front of a group).

13. Apraxia of speech is often associated with:

A. lesions in Broca's area.

B. lesions in Wernicke's area.

C. lesions in subcortical structures.

D. lesions in the occipital area.

E. lesions in the cerebellum.

14. Dysarthria is:

A. a speech disorder in the absence of muscle weakness or paralysis.

B. a speech disorder never associated with aphasia.

C. a single disorder with a unitary etiology.

D. a speech disorder associated with muscle weakness or paralysis.

E. a speech disorder characterized by groping, effortful speech.

15. Of the following, the one associated with dysarthria is:

A. even and consistent breakdowns in articulation

B. impaired syntactic structures

C. forced inspirations and expirations that interrupt speech

D. an invariably slower rate of speech

E. an increased rate of speech under pressure

16. A clinician in a skilled nursing facility (SNF) receives a note that a new 80-year-old patient, Dick C., has been transferred to her facility. The note states that Dick was assessed by the clinician in the previous SNF, but there is no diagnosis in the papers that have been sent from the previous clinician. However, the previous clinician reported that Dick manifested the following symptoms: general awareness of his speech problems, significant articulation problems; problems with volitional speech with relatively intact automatic speech; more difficulty with consonants than vowels; intonation and fluency problems; and trial-and-error groping and struggling associated with speech attempts. Therapy was recommended. Dick C. most likely has:

A. hyperkinetic dysarthria.

B. unilateral upper motor neuron dysarthria.

C. right hemisphere syndrome.

D. apraxia of speech.

E. dementia of the Alzheimer's type (DAT).

17. Lucien N., a 22-year-old male, is hospitalized after sustaining traumatic brain injury from a motor vehicle accident. There is no injury to the cerebellum, brain stem, or peripheral nerves. When assessing Lucien, the clinician might expect to find:

A. dysarthria, confused language (e.g., confabulation), auditory comprehension problems, confrontation naming problems, perseveration of verbal responses, pragmatic language problems, and reading and writing difficulties.

B. dysarthria, confused language (e.g., confabulation), auditory comprehension problems, no confrontation naming problems, and agrammatic or telegraphic speech.

C. confrontation naming problems, perseveration of verbal responses, pragmatic language problems, intact reading and writing skills, and echolalia.

D. severely impaired fluency, severe echolalia, and agrammatic and telegraphic speech, intact auditory comprehension skills.

E. good syntax, prosody, and articulation; no naming problems; intact auditory comprehension skills; confabulation and circumlocution when speaking.

18. A hospital-based clinician receives a referral of Mary G., a 71-year-old woman. Her family is concerned about her; Mary's 35-year-old son says: "Mom just isn't herself anymore; we don't know what's wrong or what to do. We don't know if she had a stroke or what's going on." After talking with Mary in the initial interview, the clinician realizes that he will have to assess Mary in depth to evaluate whether she has aphasia or DAT (dementia of the Alzheimer's type). If Mary has DAT, which of the following symptoms will she show?

A. normal syntax except for word-finding problems; good auditory comprehension of spoken language; slurred and rapid speech; disorientation to time and place; visuospatial problems; difficulty with self-care and daily routines; intact repetition skills

B. visuospatial problems; widespread intellectual deterioration; intact picture description ability; slow but coherent speech; reading and writing problems; disorientation to time and place

C. severe problems in recalling remote and recent events; relatively intact syntactic skills; appropriate humor and laughter; disorientation to time and place; intact ability to initiate interactions

D. severely impaired fluency; severe echolalia; agrammatic and telegraphic speech; intact auditory comprehension skills; no difficulty with self-care or managing daily routines

E. poor judgment; impaired reasoning; disorientation in new places; widespread intellectual deterioration; empty speech; jargon; incoherent, slurred, and rapid speech; problems in comprehending abstract messages

19. A 54-year-old pastor, Rev. Johnson, has a stroke and takes a leave of absence from his job while he recovers. After a 3–4 month period, he tells his doctor that he feels well enough to go back to work. When Rev. Johnson begins his job again, he goes back to his usual duties: preaching sermons on Sunday mornings, teaching Bible study, visiting church members who are sick. Rev. Johnson says that he is "100% back"; however, his parishioners and family notice some subtle problems. For example, he tends to bump into people who walk on his left; when he writes, he does not use the left side of the page. He does not recognize parishioners whom he has known for 30 or more years until they begin to speak. When people tell jokes, Rev. Johnson does not laugh or appear to understand the jokes as he used to. He does not detect sarcasm in other people's speech. Rev. Johnson probably has:

A. dementia.
B. Wernicke-Korsakoff syndrome.
C. right hemisphere syndrome.
D. apraxia of speech.
E. Parkinson's disease.

20. A clinician is asked to give a workshop to graduate students about evaluation of patients with swallowing disorders. She discusses evaluation in depth. Which one of the following facts in the clinician's workshop would be *inaccurate*?

A. An ultrasound examination can measure oral tongue movement and hyoid movement.
B. A manometric assessment can assess the preparatory phase of the swallow using posterior and lateral plane examinations.
C. An electromyographic assessment can be conducted by attaching electrodes on structures of interest (e.g., oral, laryngeal, or pharyngeal muscles).

D. A laryngeal examination can be conducted with indirect laryngoscopy or endoscopic examination to inspect the base of the tongue, vallecula, epiglottis, pyriform sinuses, vocal folds, and ventricular folds.

E. A videofluorographic assessment (modified barium swallow) can be conducted to evaluate oropharyngeal swallow involving lateral and anterior-posterior (A-P) examinations.

REFERENCES AND RECOMMENDED READINGS

Adamovich, B. L. (1997). Traumatic brain injury. In L. L. LaPointe (Ed.), *Aphasia and related neurogenic language disorders* (2nd ed., pp. 226–237). New York: Thieme Medical Publishers.

Albert, M. L. (1973). A simple test of visual neglect. *Neurology, 23,* 658–664.

American Psychiatric Association (2000). *Diagnostic and statistical manual of mental disorders (DSM IV): Fourth edition, text revision.* Washington, DC: Author.

Bear, M. F., Connors, B. W., & Paradiso, M. A. (2001). *Neuroscience: Exploring the brain* (2nd ed.). Baltimore: Lippincott Williams & Wilkins.

Basso, A. (2003). *Aphasia and its therapy.* New York: Oxford University Press.

Basso, A., & Rusconi, M. L. (1998). Aphasia in left-handers. In P. Coppens, Y. Lebrun, & A. Basso (Eds.), *Aphasia in atypical populations* (pp. 1–34). Malhwa, NJ: Lawrence Erlbaum Associates.

Bayles, K. A., & Kaszniak, A. W. (1987). *Communication and cognition in normal aging and dementia.* Austin, TX: PRO-ED.

Bayles, K. A., & Tomoeda, C. (1991). *Arizona Battery for Communication Disorders of Dementia* (research edition). Tucson, AZ: Canyonlands Publishing.

Benson, D. F., & Ardila, A. (1996). *Aphasia: A clinical perspective.* New York: Oxford University Press.

Benton, A. L., & Hamsher, K. (1978). *Multilingual Aphasia Examination* (rev. ed.). Iowa City: University of Iowa Press.

Beukelman, D. R., & Yorkston, K. M. (1991). *Communication disorders following traumatic injury: Management of cognitive, language, and motor impairments.* Austin, TX: PRO-ED.

Bhatnagar, S. C. (2002). *Neuroscience for the study of communicative disorders* (2nd ed.). Baltimore: Williams & Wilkins.

Bigler, E. D. (Ed.). (1990). *Traumatic brain injury.* Austin, TX: PRO-ED.

Blomert, L., Kean, M. L., Koster, C., & Schokker, J. (1994). Amsterdam-Nijmegen Everyday Language Test: Construction, reliability, and validity. *Aphasiology, 8*(4), 381–407.

Boyle, M. (2004). Semantic feature analysis treatment for anomia in two fluent aphasia syndromes. *American Journal of Speech–Language Pathology, 13,* 236–249.

Brin, M. F., Velickovic, M., Ramig, L. O., & Fox, C. (2004). Dysphonia due to Parkinson's disease. In C. M. Sapeinza and J. Casper (Eds.), *Vocal rehabilitation for medical speech–language pathology* (pp. 209–270). Austin, TX: PRO-ED.

Brookshire, R. (2003). *An introduction to neurogenic communication disorders* (6th ed.). St. Louis, MO: Mosby-Year Book.

Brookshire, R., & Nichols, L. E. (1993). *The Discourse Comprehension Test.* Minneapolis, MN: BRK Publishers.

Brown, J. I., Bennet, J. M., & Hanna, G. (1981). *The Nelson-Denny Reading Test.* Chicago: Riverside.

Bryan, K. L. (1995). *The Right Hemisphere Language Battery* (2nd ed.). Leicester, England: Far Communications.

Caruso, A. J., & Strand, E. A. (1999). *Clinical management of motor speech disorders in children.* New York: Thieme.

Chapey, R. (Ed.). (2001). *Language intervention strategies in aphasia and related neurogenic communication disorders* (4th ed.). Philadelphia: Lippincott Williams & Wilkins.

Cooper, P. R., & Golfinos, J. G. (Eds.) (2000). *Head injury* (4th ed.). New York: McGraw-Hill.

Cummings, J. L., & Benson, D. F. (1992). *Dementia: A clinical approach* (2nd ed.). Boston: Butterworth-Heinemann.

Dabul, B. (1979). *Apraxia Battery for Adults.* Tigard, OR: C. C. Publications.

Darley, F. L. (1982). *Aphasia.* Philadelphia: W. B. Saunders.

Davis, G. A. (2000). *Aphasiology.* Boston: Allyn & Bacon.

Davis, P., & Strand, E. (2004). Neurophysiology of vocal rehabilitation. In C. M. Sapienza & J. Casper (Eds.), *Vocal rehabilitation for medical speech–language pathology* (pp. 29–68). Austin, TX: PRO-ED.

DeRenzi, E., & Vignolo, L. A. (1962). The token test: A sensitive test to detect receptive disturbances in aphasics. *Brain, 85,* 665–678.

DeSimoni, F. G. (1989). *Comprehensive Apraxia Test* (CAT). Dalton, PA: Praxis House.

Duffy, J. R. (2005). *Motor speech disorders (2nd ed.).* St. Louis, MO: Mosby.

Enderby, P. (1983). *Frenchay Dysarthria Assessment.* San Diego, CA: College-Hill Press.

Frattali, C. M., Thompson, C. K., Holland, A. L., Wohl, C. B., & Ferketic, M. M. (1995). *Functional assessment of communication skills for adults* (ASHA FACS). Rockville, MD: American Speech-Language-Hearing Association.

Freed, D. (2000). *Motor speech disorders: Diagnosis and treatment.* Albany, NY: Thomson Learning.

Freed, D., Celery, K., & Marshall, R. C. (2004). Effectiveness of personalized and phonological cueing on long-term naming performance by aphasic subjects: A clinical investigation. *Aphasiology, 18*(8), 743–757.

Gates, W. H. (1978). *Gates-MacGinitie Reading Test.* Chicago: Riverside.

Gauthier, L., Dehaut, F., & Joanette, Y. (1989). The Bells test: A quantitative and qualitative test for visual neglect. *International Journal of Clinical Neuropsychology, 11,* 49–54.

Gillis, R. J. (1996). *Traumatic brain injury: Rehabilitation for speech–language pathologists.* Boston: Butterworth-Heinemann.

Goodglass, H., Kaplan, E., & Barresi, B. (2001a). *The assessment of aphasia and related disorders* (3rd ed.). Philadelphia: Lippincott Williams & Wilkins.

Goodglass, H., Kaplan, E., & Barresi, B. (2001b). *The Boston Diagnostic Aphasia Examination* (3rd ed.). Philadelphia: Lippincott Williams & Wilkins.

Groher, M. E. (1997). *Dysphagia: Diagnosis and management* (3rd ed.). Boston: Butterworth-Heinemann.

Hachinsky, V. F., Illiff, L. D., Zilhka, E., & Associates (1975). Cerebral blood flow in dementia. *Archives of Neurology, 32,* 632–637.

Hagen, C., & Malkamus, D. (1979). *Interaction strategies for language disorders secondary to head trauma.* Paper presented at the annual convention of the American Speech-Language-Hearing Association, Atlanta, GA.

Halper, A., Cherney, L. R., & Burns, M. S. (1996). *Clinical management of right hemisphere dysfunction* (2nd ed.). Gaithersburg, MD: Aspen.

Halpern, H. (2000). *Language and motor speech disorders in adults* (2nd ed.). Austin, TX: PRO-ED.

Hanna, G., Schell, L. M., & Schreiner, R. (1977). *The Nelson Reading Skills Test.* Chicago: Riverside.

Hartley, L. L. (1995). *Cognitive-communicative abilities following brain injury: A functional approach.* San Diego, CA: Singular Publishing Group.

Hegde, M. N. (1998). A coursebook on aphasia and other neurogenic language disorders (2nd ed.). San Diego, CA: Singular Publishing Group.

Hegde, M. N. (2001a). *Hegde's pocketguide to assessment in speech–language pathology* (2nd ed.). Albany, NY: Thomson Learning.

Hegde, M. N. (2001b). *Hegde's pocketguide to treatment in speech–language pathology* (2nd ed.). Albany, NY: Thomson Learning.

Hegde, M. N. (2005). *A coursebook on aphasia and other neurogenic language disorders* (3rd ed.). Albany, NY: Thomson Learning.

Helm-Estabrooks, N. (1992). *Aphasia Diagnostic Profiles.* Austin, TX: PRO-ED.

Helm-Estabrooks, N., & Albert, M. L. (2004). *Manual of aphasia and aphasia therapy* (2nd ed.). Austin, TX: PRO-ED.

Helm-Estabrooks, N., & Hotz, G. (1991). *A brief test of head injury.* Chicago: Riverside.

Holland, A. L., Frattali, C. M., & Fromm, D. (1998). *Communicative abilities in daily living* (2nd ed.). Austin, TX: PRO-ED.

Kaplan, E., & Barresi, B. (2001). Boston Diagnostic Aphasia Examination (3rd.). Austin, TX: PRO-ED.

Keenan, J. S., & Brassell, E. G. (1975). *Aphasia Language Performance Scales.* Murphreesboro, TN: Pinnacle Press.

Kertesz, A. (1982). *Western Aphasia Battery.* New York: Gruene & Stratton.

LaPointe, L. L. (Ed.). (1997). *Aphasia and related neurogenic language disorders* (2nd ed.). New York: Thieme Medical Publishers.

LaPointe, L. L., & Horner, J. (1978). The functional auditory comprehension task (FACT): Protocol and test format. *FLASHA Journal,* 27–33.

LaPointe, L. L., & Horner, J. (1998). *Reading Comprehension Battery for Aphasia.* Austin, TX: PRO-ED.

Levin, H. S., O'Donnell, V. N., & Grossman, R. G. (1979). The Galveston orientation and amnesia test: A practical scale to assess cognition after head injury. *Journal of Nervous Mental Disorders, 167,* 675–684.

Logemann, J. A. (1998). *Evaluation and treatment of swallowing disorders* (2nd ed.). Austin, TX: PRO-ED.

Lomas, J., Pickard, L., Bester, S., Elbard, H., Finlayson, A., & Zoghaib, C. (1989). The communicative effectiveness index: Development and psychometric evaluation of a functional communication measure for adult aphasia. *Journal of Speech and Hearing Disorders, 54,* 113–124.

Love, R. J., & Webb, W. G. (1986). *Neurology for the speech–language pathologist.* Boston: Butterworths.

Lubinski, R. (1995). *Dementia and communication.* San Diego, CA: Singular Publishing Group.

Murdoch, B. E., & Theodoros, D. G. (2001). *Traumatic brain injury: Associated speech, language and swallowing disorders.* Albany, NY: Thomson Learning.

Myers, P. S. (1999). *Right hemisphere damage.* Albany, NY: Thomson Learning.

Nolte, J. (2002). *The human brain: An introduction to its functional anatomy* (5th ed.). St. Louis, MO: Mosby.

Paradis, M. (1987). *The assessment of bilingual aphasia.* Hillsdale, NJ: Lawrence Erlbaum.

Paradis, M. (1998). Aphasia in bilinguals: How atypical is it? In P. Coppens, Y. Lebrun, & A. Basso (Eds.), *Aphasia in atypical populations* (pp. 67–116). Malhwa, NJ: Lawrence Erlbaum Associates.

Payne, J. C. (1994). *Communication Profile: A Functional Skills Survey.* Tuscon, AZ: Communication Skill Builders.

Payne, J. C. (1997). *Adult neurogenic language disorders: Assessment and treatment.* San Diego, CA: Singular Publishing Group.

Perlman, A. L., & Schulze-Delrieu, K. (1997). *Deglutition and its disorders.* San Diego, CA: Singular Publishing Group.

Pimental, P. A., & Kingsbury, N. A. (1989). *Neuropsychological aspects of right brain injury.* Austin: PRO-ED.

Porch, B. E. (1981). *Porch Index of Communicative Ability* (3rd ed.). Palo Alto, CA: Consulting Psychologists Press.

Rappoport, M., Hall, K. M., Hopkins, K., and Associates (1982). Disability rating scale for severe head trauma. *Archives of Physical Medicine and Rehabilitation, 63,* 118–123.

Reisberg, B., Ferris, S. H., DeLeon, M. J., & Crook, T. (1982). The global deterioration scale for assessment of primary degenerative dementia. *American Journal of Psychiatry, 139,* 1136–1139.

Reitan, R. M. (1991). *Aphasia Screening Test* (2nd ed.). Tucson, AZ: Reitan Neuropsychology Laboratory.

Ripich, D. N. (1995). Differential diagnosis and assessment. In R. Lubinski (Ed.), *Dementia and communication* (pp. 188–222). San Diego, CA: Singular Publishing Group.

Robey, R. R. (1998). A meta-analysis of clinical outcomes in the treatment of aphasia. *Journal of Speech, Language, Hearing Research, 41,* 172–187.

Rosenbek, J., LaPointe, C., & Wertz, T. (1989). *Aphasia: A clinical approach.* Austin, TX: PRO-ED.

Sarno, M. T. (1969). *The functional communication profile: Manual of directions.* New York: New York University Medical Center, Institute of Rehabilitation Medicine.

Sarno, M. T. (Ed.). (1981). *Acquired aphasia.* New York: Academic Press.

Schuell, H. M. (1972). *The Minnesota Test of Differential Diagnosis of Aphasia.* Minneapolis: University of Minnesota Press.

Shadden, B. B., & Toner, M. A. (Eds.). (1997). *Aging and communication.* Austin, TX: PRO-ED.

Shekim, L. O. (1997). Dementia. In L. L. LaPointe (Ed.), *Aphasia and related neurogenic language disorders* (2nd ed., pp. 238–249). New York: Thieme Medical Publishers.

Shewan, C. M. (1979). *Auditory Comprehension Test for Sentences.* Chicago: Biolinguistics Clinical Institutes.

Sklar, M. (1983). *Sklar Aphasia Scale.* Los Angeles: Western Psychological Services.

Spreen, O., & Benton, A. L. (1977). *Neurosensory Center Comprehensive Examination for Aphasia.* Victoria, BC: University of Victoria.

Stanczak, D. E., & Associates (1984). Assessment of level of consciousness following severe neurological insult. *Journal of Neurosurgery, 60,* 955–960.

Tanner, D. C. (2003). *The psychology of neurogenic communication disorders: A primer for health care professionals.* Baltimore: Brookes Publishing.

Tanner, D. C., & Culbertson, W. (1999). *Quick Assessment for Aphasia.* Oceanside, CA: Academic Communication Associates.

Teasdale, G., & Jennett, B. (1976). Assessment and prognosis of coma after head injury. *Acta Neurochirargica (Wien), 34,* 45–55.

Tompkins, C. A. (1995). *Right hemisphere communication disorders: Theory and management.* San Diego, CA: Singular Publishing Group.

Vogel, D., & Cannito, M. P. (2001). *Treating disordered speech motor control* (2nd ed.). Austin, TX: PRO-ED.

Wallace, G. L. (1997). *Multicultural neurogenics.* Austin, TX: PRO-ED.

Wallace, G. L. (1998). Neurogenic disorders in adult and pediatric populations. In D. E. Battle (Ed.), *Communication disorders in multicultural populations* (2nd ed., pp. 309–333). Newton, MA: Butterworth-Heinemann.

Webster, D. W. (1999). *Neuroscience of communication* (2nd ed.). Albany, NY: Thomson Learning.

West, J. F., Sands, E. S., & Ross-Swain, D. (1998). *Bedside Evaluation Screening Test–Second Edition.* Austin, TX: PRO-ED.

Whurr, R. (1996). *The Aphasia Screening Test* (2nd ed.). San Diego, CA: Singular Publishing Group.

Wilson, B. A., Cockburn, J., & Halligan, P. (1987). *Behavioral Inattention Test.* Suffolk, England: Thames Valley Test Company.

Wirz, S., Skinner, C., & Dean, E. (1990). *Revised Edinburgh Functional Communication Profile.* Tuscon, AZ: Communication Skill Builders.

Yorkston, K. M., & Beukelman, D. R. (1981). *Assessment of intelligibility of dysarthric speakers.* Tigard, OR: C. C. Publications.

Yorkston, K. M., Miller, R. S., & Strand, E. A. (2003). *Management of speech and swallowing in degenerative diseases* (2nd ed.). Austin, TX: PRO-ED.

Yorkston, K. M., Beukelman, D. R., Strand, E. A., & Bell, K. R. (1999). *Management of motor speech disorders in children and adults.* Austin, TX: PRO-ED.

Study & Review
Answers

6. C. A patient with a history of heavy drinking who presents with memory problems, difficulty processing abstract information, and visual-spatial deficits probably has Wernicke-Korsakoff syndrome.

7. B. Conduction aphasia is caused by lesions in the region between Broca's area and Wernicke's area, especially in the supramarginal gyrus and the arcuate fasciculus.

8. B. Among the specified standardized tests of aphasia, the one that samples speech and language skills to only a limited extent is the *Porch Index of Communicative Ability*.

9. E. Fran probably has Parkinson's disease.

10. D. Because Fran has Parkinson's disease, you would expect her speech to be characterized by monopitch, a harsh and breathy voice, short rushes of speech, imprecise consonants, and respiratory problems.

11. C. Patients with Parkinson's disease usually present with a mask-like face, slow voluntary movements, tremors in resting muscles, and disturbed posture.

12. A. Functional communication tests seek to assess communication in natural or everyday situations.

13. A. Apraxia of speech is often associated with lesions in Broca's area.

14. D. Dysarthria is a speech disorder associated with muscle weakness or paralysis.

15. C. Of the stated disorders, the one associated with dysarthria is forced inspirations and expirations that interrupt speech.

16. D. Dick C. probably has apraxia of speech, which is characterized by general awareness of his speech problems, significant articulation problems, problems with volitional speech with relatively intact automatic speech; more difficulty with consonants than vowels; intonation and fluency problems; and trial-and-error groping and struggling associated with speech attempts.

17. A. Dysarthria, confused language (e.g., confabulation), auditory comprehension problems, confrontation naming problems, perseveration of verbal responses, pragmatic language problems, and reading and writing difficulties are typical of patients with TBI.

18. E. Characteristics of DAT include poor judgment; impaired reasoning; disorientation in new places; widespread intellectual deterioration; empty speech; jargon; incoherent, slurred, and rapid speech; and problems in comprehending abstract messages.

19. C. Rev. Johnson probably has right hemisphere syndrome, which is characterized by left side neglect, difficulty recognizing people until they begin to speak, and difficulty detecting sarcasm and humor in other people's speech.

20. B. It would be inaccurate to state that manometric assessment can assess the preparatory phase of the swallow using posterior and lateral plane examinations.

CHAPTER **9**

COMMUNICATION

DISORDERS

IN MULTICULTURAL

POPULATIONS

The United States has been likened to a

kaleidoscope that is constantly changing colors and becoming more and more diverse. The U.S. Bureau of the Census (2000) reported that ethnic and racial minorities accounted for up to 80% of the nation's growth in the 1990s. In the year 2000, there were nearly 87 million persons from minority backgrounds living in the United States, up 43% from 1990. With increasing numbers of culturally and linguistically diverse (CLD) adults and children in the United States, the number of those who have disorders of communication is also increasing. Clinicians frequently find themselves attempting to effectively serve an increasingly diverse client group, but find that they do not have the appropriate tools—especially assessment tools (Roseberry-McKibbin, Brice, & O'Hanlon, 2005). Research is scarce; an empirical foundation upon which to build assessment and treatment is lacking. But the field of communication disorders must do its best, with its current knowledge and tools, to effectively and knowledgeably serve CLD adults and children with communication disorders.

In this chapter, we begin by presenting foundational issues concerning the serving of CLD clients. We then describe the speech–language characteristics of African American, Hispanic, and Asian clients and the ramifications for assessment and treatment. Next, we discuss the differentiation of language differences and language disorders in children. Included in this discussion are issues of second-language acquisition and bilingualism. Knowledge of second-language acquisition and bilingualism is critical to a fair and unbiased assessment of CLD children. We describe considerations in the use of standardized tests, alternatives to standardized tests, and important concepts in working with interpreters in the assessment process. In our section on treatment considerations, we discuss issues related to treatment of CLD children with language-learning disabilities, as well as assessment and treatment considerations for CLD adults with neurologically based disorders of communication.

FOUNDATIONAL ISSUES

INTRODUCTION

There is an increasing number of CLD people living in the United States. Speech–language pathologists need to understand basic cultural characteristics that can impact service delivery to these persons. The American Speech-Language-Hearing Association has developed policies and position statements that provide guidance for clinicians who work with CLD clients.

Demographic Data

- The increasing diversity in the United States comes primarily from two sources: increases in birth rates among CLD groups and immigration trends. In 1820, 92% of immigrants were of European background; in 1990, 7% of immigrants were of European descent (U.S. Bureau of the Census, 1992).

- As previously stated, the U.S. Bureau of the Census (2000) reported that in the decade of the 1990s, ethnic and racial minorities accounted for up to 80% of the nation's population growth.

- The number of CLD children increases constantly. Since the 1990–1991 school year, the population of children with limited English proficiency has grown 105%, whereas the general school population nationwide has only grown 12% (Kindler, 2002).

- Some states have especially great diversity. In the school year 2000–2001, California had the largest enrollment of students with limited English proficiency: 1,511,646. California's limited English proficient students alone represented one third of the nation's population of this type of student (Kindler, 2002).

- The population of CLD elderly is also growing, and consequently it is anticipated that there will be an increased demand for services to elderly CLD clients with neurogenic and swallowing disorders (Tonkovich, 2002).

- With the growing number of CLD children and older adults, it is logical that there are more and more CLD clients who have communication disorders. Clearly, there is a great need for information about effective service delivery to the country's increasing culturally and linguistically diverse population.

General Cultural Considerations

Basic Principles

- When working with CLD clients of all ages, it is important to have a basic understanding of what culture is (Coleman, 2000). Although there are probably hundreds of definitions, it can be agreed that culture is a dynamic, multifaceted phenomenon that is influenced by many variables.

- *Culture* can be viewed as a framework through which actions are filtered as individuals go about the business of daily living. Culture includes the beliefs, behaviors, and values of a group of people (Battle, 2002). At the heart of culture are values; thus, when we study other cultures, it is important to examine that culture's underlying values.

- Speech–language pathologists must develop cultural competence. This can be done in many ways. The culturally competent SLP is one who (a) is actively in the process of becoming aware of his or her own assumptions, (b) actively attempts to understand the worldview of his or her culturally diverse clients and families, and (c) is actively developing and practicing culturally relevant, sensitive, and appropriate service delivery skills and practices (Sue & Sue, 2003).

- It is important for speech–language pathologists to develop as much cultural sensitivity as possible (Kritikos, 2003). This can be done through a variety of activities that focus on continually learning more about the cultures of the clients served.

- Reading literature, conducting home visits, and talking to families and community members about the cultures in question will help clinicians become sensitive to and aware of cultural variables that can impact service delivery.

- A danger of attempting to understand any cultural group is that stereotyping and overgeneralizing may occur. *Stereotypes* can be viewed as a means of categorizing others based upon perceptions that are incomplete.

- Ideally, speech–language pathologists should understand *tendencies* of various cultural groups so that students and families may be viewed as individuals within the general framework of their community and culture.

- Professionals must keep in mind the great heterogeneity within cultural groups. It is optimal to take a situational approach, wherein each individual is viewed as unique, with shifting needs, characteristics, and strengths.

- One way to view each individual as unique is to learn the name of the individual geographic or cultural group given by its members and use this name. For example, if a client is from Mexico, this client may be described as Mexican or Mexican American, not Hispanic. A client from the Philippines may be described as Filipino, not Asian. This shows respect for individuals and acknowledgment of their unique heritage (Battle, 2002).

Variables Influencing Individual Behavior Within a Culture

- A number of variables influence the behavior of individuals within a culture. The combination of general cultural practices and individual characteristics of people within cultures influences service delivery to those clients and their families (Huer & Saenz, 2003; Madding, 2002). Potential variables of influence upon individuals include (Roseberry-McKibbin, 2002):

  - *educational level,* which may be quite basic (e.g., several years of schooling) or sophisticated and extensive

- *language(s) spoken,* including the prestige of the language(s) in the area of residence and the level of skill in each language
- *length of residence* in an area
- *country of birth* (foreign born or native born), which relates to immigrant or refugee status versus being born in the United States
- *urban versus rural background*
- *gender*
- *religion*
- *age*
- *generational membership*
- *socioeconomic status or upward class mobility*
- *neighborhood and peer group*
- *degree of acculturation into mainstream American life*
- *outmarriage* (marriage to people from different ethnic backgrounds)
- *individual choice* within the intrapersonal realm

- Immigrants who come to the United States are incorporated into society by the processes of acculturation and assimilation. *Acculturation* refers to the process by which immigrants assume American cultural attributes (e.g., cultural norms and values). *Assimilation* is the process of their incorporation into the cultural and social networks of the host society (e.g., place of residence, family, leisure activities, work). It refers to the situation where immigrants give up their cultures and take on the characteristics of the new culture (Battle, 2002).
- There are various levels of acculturation. Immigrants who are *bicultural* are fully involved in both their own and the host culture. They maintain their native language and become fluent in the new language, too. They maintain many of their own cultural practices and adopt the host culture's practices as well. They are comfortable going back and forth between their own and the host culture.

CONCEPTS TO CONSIDER

Discuss the issue of culture in service delivery to CLD clients and their families. What is culture? What specific variables influence an individual's behavior within a culture?

_____

_____

_____

_____

_____

ASHA Guidelines Regarding Multicultural Issues

- Due to the increasing cultural and linguistic diversity in the United States, ASHA has developed policies, position statements, and guidelines regarding service delivery to CLD clients.

■ ASHA's Office of Multicultural Affairs and its Multicultural Issues Board are active in creation and implementation of these guidelines. Copies of guidelines and policies are available; interested readers can contact the national office in Rockville Pike, MD. ASHA has also created Special Interest Division 14 (SID #14), Communication Disorders and Sciences in Culturally and Linguistically Diverse Populations.

■ It is important to have a basic knowledge of the various position statements in order to provide effective service delivery that is consistent with ASHA's policies. ASHA has published various position statements and technical reports about service delivery to people from diverse backgrounds.

■ ASHA (1998; Joint Subcommittee of the Executive Board on English Language Proficiency) states that it is discriminatory not to accept individuals into the professions or into higher education programs solely on the basis of an accent or dialect. Speech pathologists with accents or dialects can provide effective services as long as they have the expected level of professional knowledge and can model target behaviors for clients.

■ ASHA has continuously attempted to address the issue of effective service delivery to members of various cultural and linguistic groups. For example, ASHA (2001a) developed a focused initiative relevant to improving services to members of culturally and linguistically diverse populations. ASHA (2002), in its Omnibus Survey, devoted a portion of this survey to measuring behaviors and attitudes with regard to improving responsiveness to serving members of culturally and linguistically diverse groups.

SUMMARY

✓ The increasing number of multicultural people living in the United States makes it imperative for clinicians to be sensitive to cultural issues that impact service delivery. Clinicians must become culturally competent.

✓ A number of variables, such as age and generational membership, impact the behavior of individual clients from various cultures.

✓ ASHA has published guidelines regarding effective service delivery to clients from linguistically and culturally diverse backgrounds.

SPEECH–LANGUAGE CHARACTERISTICS OF CLD CLIENTS

INTRODUCTION

When attempting to ascertain whether clients are manifesting language differences or language disorders, it is important to have a basic understanding of how various dialects and languages influence the production of Standard American English (SAE). It is also critical to remember that within each language group, there is great diversity. For example, the Philippines, a country the size of Arizona, has more than 87 mutually unintelligible languages.

Unfortunately, it is common for adults and especially children to be labeled as having a "disorder" when, in fact, they are merely manifesting language differences that are attributable to their primary language or dialect. For example, clients whose first language is Spanish, African American English, or an Asian language manifest characteristics of articulation, morphology, and syntax that differ from patterns of SAE. Clients who speak a dialect of American English may also manifest such characteristics (Goldstein,

2000). In this section, we discuss dialects of American English, African American English (AAE), Spanish-influenced English, and English influenced by Asian languages.

Dialects of American English

- In the United States, Standard American English, or SAE, is used in government communications, printing, national television newscasts, and many businesses. Many consider SAE to be the official language of the United States.

- Every language is spoken somewhat differently by different subgroups of a linguistic community. SAE has several dialects; each one has characteristic sound patterns, including typical expressions and unique accents.

- Dialectal differences are due to several interrelated factors, including geographic region, socioeconomic level, speaking situation, and subgroup membership.

- With regard to geographic region, people living in different parts of the United States develop variations of language use and production. Based on geographic regions, specialists have identified 10 major dialects of SAE: New York City, Eastern New England, Western Pennsylvania, Appalachian, Southern, Middle Atlantic, Central Midland, Southwest, Northwest, and North Central (see Figure 9.1).

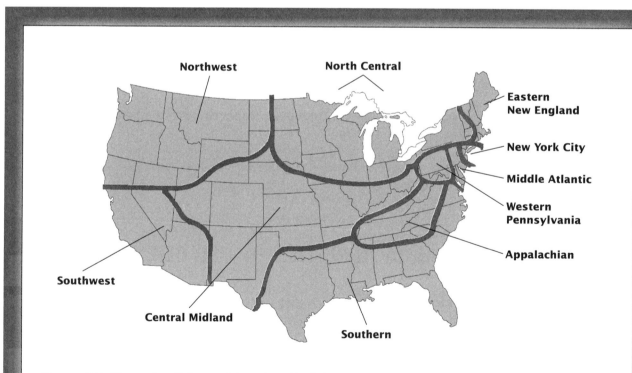

Figure 9.1. The major dialects of American English. *Note.* From *Introduction to Communicative Disorders*, 2nd ed. (p. 434), by M. N. Hegde, 2001, Austin, TX: PRO-ED. Copyright 2001 by PRO-ED, Inc. Adapted with permission.

African American English

General Background

- African American English (AAE) has undergone many changes in nomenclature over the years. It has been called Black Dialect, Black English, Black English Vernacular, African American Language, and Ebonics. The changes in nomenclature have been due in part to increasingly sophisticated understanding of AAE and to changes in sociolinguistic theory.
- Experts today consider AAE to be a dialect of mainstream American English. Battle (2002) defines a *dialect* as a rule-governed variation in a language used by a racial, ethnic, geographic, or socioeconomic group. She states that dialects of the same language may differ from each other in vocabulary, pronunciation, and grammar; however, they are enough alike to be mutually understood by speakers of different dialects of the same language.
- Use of AAE is influenced by a number of factors, including retention of some African language patterns, geographic region, socioeconomic status, education, gender, age of the speaker, and bonding between members of the African American community (Terrell, Battle, & Grantham, 1998; van Keulen, Weddington, & DeBose, 1998).
- A number of West African languages have impacted modern-day African American English: Bambara, Ewe, Fanta, Fon, Fula, Ga, Ibo, Ibibio, Kimbundu, Longo, Mandinka, Mende, Twi, Imbundu, Wolof, and Yoruba (Willis, 2004).

Misconceptions About AAE

- There are some widespread assumptions and misconceptions about AAE and its speakers, and these are listed below. It is important to be aware of these misconceptions so that AAE speakers are not be mistakenly identified as having disorders.
- *All African Americans speak AAE.* Some African Americans speak AAE; some do not. Some codeswitch back and forth between SAE and AAE depending on variables such as changes in topic, listener, and communicative intent. African Americans who are socialized primarily with Anglos generally speak SAE.
- *AAE is spoken only by African Americans.* AAE may be spoken by people of any ethnic and linguistic background. Non-African Americans may speak AAE if their primary peer group is composed of African Americans. For example, some Puerto Rican students in New York City speak AAE. Some Anglo students in Oakland, California, speak AAE.
- *AAE is a substandard form of mainstream American English.* Some people historically took a "deficit perspective"; a major premise of this view was that African Americans were cognitively unable to learn SAE. The *ethnolinguistic theory* of today states that AAE is a dialect in its own right; its roots can be traced to many languages of West Africa as previously stated.
- *AAE does not have a regular, predictable system.* In previous decades, it was believed that AAE was unpredictable and not rule governed. Today, it is widely known that AAE is a rule-governed system in which patterns can be predicted based on rules.
- *If children speak AAE, their use of AAE must be discontinued.* Some experts believe that speakers of AAE should become "bilingual" or "bidialectal" so that they can fluently speak both AAE and SAE (Campbell, 1993; van Keulen, Weddington, & DeBose, 1998). In this optimal situation, students preserve their culture, heritage, and community dialect as well as learning a style of speaking that is required in some daily situations, school learning experiences, and future places of employment.
- *Use of standardized language tests with AAE speakers is a nonbiased indicator of actual lan-*

guage knowledge and skill. Many currently used assessment instruments in schools are normed and standardized on Anglo, middle-class, monolingual English speakers. These tests have been criticized by many experts as being inappropriate for use with African American children (Craig, Thompson, Washington, & Potter, 2004; Hammer, Pennock-Roman, Rzasa, & Tomblin, 2002; Thomas-Tate, Washington, & Edwards, 2004; Wyatt, 2002).

- Many standardized tests of morphosyntactic skill, especially in the field of speech–language pathology, are biased against AAE speakers (and students from other non-English backgrounds, also). Table 9.1 shows examples of bias against speakers of AAE on formal, standardized language tests.

- It is recommended that when students who speak AAE are assessed, alternative forms of assessment be used. These alternative forms of assessment, including language sample analysis, contrastive analysis, and description of children's functional communication skills (Bliss, 2002; Campbell, 1996; McGregor, Williams, Hearst, & Johnson, 1997; Seymour, Roeper, & DeVilliers, 2002; Smith, Lee, & McDade, 2001; Stockman, 1996), should be used when assessing children who speak AAE. It is also recommended that standardized tests of aphasia be appropriately modified for adults who speak AAE.

Characteristics of AAE Morphology, Syntax, and Articulation

- When AAE speakers are tested, it is critical to know which aspects of their speech and language are reflective of AAE rules and which aspects are indicative of a disorder. Many speech–language pathologists take children who speak AAE in the public schools onto their caseloads for "remediation" of AAE. Not only is this illegal, it is often unsuccessful as well.

- However, some adult speakers of AAE may elect to become bidialectal in that they become proficient in SAE as well as AAE. Being bidialectal enables these speakers to maintain their use of AAE while also being able to use SAE for purposes such as conducting business with non-AAE speakers.

- When speech–language pathologists are aware of the normal characteristics of AAE, they can distinguish between a language difference and a language disorder in children who speak AAE. Table 9.2 shows the characteristics of AAE morphology and syntax, while Table 9.3 shows the characteristics of AAE articulation and phonology. Table 9.4 shows some examples of acceptable utterances by speakers of AAE.

Spanish-Influenced English

General Background

- The term *Hispanic* is a label of convenience used to refer to people who were born in or trace the background of their families to one of the Spanish-speaking Latin American nations or to Spain, and reside in the United States. Hispanics may also come from Carribean countries such as Puerto Rico and Cuba (Brice, 2002).

- *Hispanic* is used as an ethnic label by the Bureau of the Census; it does not denote a race, because most Hispanics are racially mixed, including combinations of American Indian, African Black, and European white. The majority are Mestizo, having both a European and an

(Text continues on p. 464)

Table 9.1   EXAMPLES OF BIAS AGAINST SPEAKERS OF AFRICAN AMERICAN ENGLISH ON FORMAL LANGUAGE AND INTELLIGENCE TESTS

1. Grammatical judgment items.
   - Examiner: Tell me whether the following sentences are correct or incorrect:

   Them girls is having a good time.

   The boys is going to the party.

   We don't have no time to talk to you.

2. Sentence repetition tasks.
   - Examiner: Repeat these sentences after me. Remember to say them EXACTLY as I say them!

   Neither of the children are using the swings.

   They had been hungry.

   She looks at the big, brown dog.

3. Grammatic closure tasks.
   - Examiner: I am going to say some sentences. I want you to fill in the word that is missing. For example, "A rose is a flower and a daisy is a flower. Daisies and roses are both _____ ." Now you do some:

   Today I play the marimba; yesterday I _____ the marimba.

   I have a cat, and you have a cat; we have two _____ .

   Today Sue <u>is</u> going to the store; yesterday she _____ going to the store.

4. Receptive grammatical tasks.
   - Examiner: We are going to look at some pictures. Each page has three pictures. When I say a sentence, you point to the picture that goes with the sentence I say. Here's the first picture.

   Show me "The cat<u>s</u> are playing in the garden."

   Now, show me "He play<u>ed</u> baseball."

   Point to "They <u>have been</u> painting the fence."

5. Articulation and phonological tasks. Most tests of articulation and phonology are normed on Anglo children. The speech–language pathologist must remember to take into account the unique characteristics of AAE when assessing articulation and phonology.

Note. From *Multicultural Students with Special Language Needs: Practical Strategies for Assessment and Intervention,* 2nd ed. (pp. 60, 65), by C. Roseberry-McKibbin, 2002, Oceanside, CA: Academic Communication Associates. Copyright 2002 by Academic Communication Associates. Reprinted with permission.

Table 9.2 CHARACTERISTICS OF AFRICAN AMERICAN ENGLISH MORPHOLOGY AND SYNTAX

AAE Feature/ Characteristic	Mainstream American English	Sample AAE Utterance
Omission of noun possessive	That's the woman's car. It's John's pencil.	That *the* woman car. It *John* pencil.
Omission of noun plural	He has two boxes of apples. She gives me five cents.	He got two box of *apple*. She give me five *cent*.
Omission of third-person singular present-tense marker	She walks to school. The man works in his yard.	She *walk* to school. The man *work* in his yard.
Omission of *to be* forms such as *is, are*	She is a nice lady. They are going to a movie.	*She* a nice lady. *They* going to a movie.
Present-tense is used regardless of person/number	They are having fun. You are a smart man.	*They is* having fun. *You is* a smart man!
Lack of person-number agreement with past and present forms of *to be*	You are playing ball. They are having a picnic.	You *is* playing ball. They *is* having a picnic.
Present-tense forms of auxiliary *have* omitted	I have been here for two hours. He has done it again.	I been here for two hours. He done it again.
Past-tense endings omitted	He lived in California. She cracked the nut.	He *live* in California. She *crack* the nut.
Past *was* used regardless of number and person	They were shopping. You were helping me.	They *was* shopping. You *was* helping me.
Multiple negatives (each additional negative form adds emphasis to the negative meaning)	We don't have any more. I don't want any cake. I don't like broccoli.	We don't have *no more*. I don't never want *no cake*. I don't *never* like broccoli.
None substituted for *any*	She doesn't want any.	She don't want *none*.
Perfective construction; *been* used to indicate that an action took place in the distant past.	I had the mumps when I was 5. I have known her for years.	I *been had* the mumps when I was 5. I *been* known her.
Done combined with a past-tense form to indicate that an action was started and completed	He fixed the stove. She tried to paint it.	He *done fixed* the stove. She *done tried* to paint it.
The form *be* used as the main verb	Today she is working. We are singing.	Today *she be* working. *We be* singing.
Distributive *be* used to indicate actions and events over time	He is often cheerful. She's kind sometimes.	*He be* cheerful. *She be* kind.
Pronoun used to restate the subject	My brother surprised me. My dog has fleas.	My brother, *he* surprise me. My dog, *he* got fleas.
Them substituted for *those*	Those cars are antiques. Where'd you get those books?	*Them* cars, they be antique. Where you get *them* books?
Future-tense *is, are* replaced by *gonna*	She is going to help us. They are going to be there.	She *gonna* help us. They *gonna* be there.
At used at the end of *where* questions	Where is the house? Where is the store?	Where is the house *at*? Where is the store *at*?
Additional auxiliaries often used	I might have done it.	I *might could* have done it.
Does replaced by *do*	She does funny things. It does make sense.	She *do* funny things. It *do* make sense.

Note. From *Multicultural Students with Special Language Needs: Practical Strategies for Assessment and Intervention*, 2nd ed. (pp. 61-62), by C. Roseberry-McKibbin, 2002, Oceanside, CA: Academic Communication Associates. Copyright 2002 by Academic Communication Associates. Reprinted with permission.

Table 9.3 CHARACTERISTICS OF AFRICAN AMERICAN ENGLISH, ARTICULATION, AND PHONOLOGY

AAE Feature/Characteristic	Mainstream American English	African American English
/l/ phoneme lessened or omitted	tool always	too' a'ways
/r/ phoneme lessened or omitted	door mother protect	doah mudah p'otek
f/voiceless th substitution at end or middle of word	teeth both nothing	teef bof nufin'
t/voiceless th substitution in beginning of a word	think thin	tink tin
d/voiced th substitution at the beginning, middle of words	this brother	dis broder
v/voiced th substitution at the end of words	breathe smooth	breave smoov
consonant-cluster reduction	desk rest left wasp	des' res' lef' was'
differing syllable stress patterns	*gui*tar po*lice* *Ju*ly	*gui*tar *po*lice *Ju*ly
Verbs ending in /k/ are changed	liked walked	li-tid wah-tid
Metathesis occurs	ask	aks ("axe")
Devoicing of final voiced consonants	bed rug cab	bet ruk cap
Final consonants may be deleted	bad good	ba' goo'
I/E substitution	pen ten	pin tin
b/v substitution	valentine vest	balentine bes'
diphthong reduction	find oil pound	fahnd ol pond
n/ng substitution	walking thing	walkin' thin

Note. Characteristics may vary depending on variables such as geographic region. From *Multicultural Students with Special Language Needs: Practical Strategies for Assessment and Intervention,* 2nd ed. (pp. 63–64), by C. Roseberry-McKibbin, 2002, Oceanside, CA: Academic Communication Associates. Copyright 2002 by Academic Communication Associates. Reprinted with permission.

Table 9.4   EXAMPLES OF ACCEPTABLE UTTERANCES BY SPEAKERS OF AFRICAN AMERICAN ENGLISH

Standard American English	African American English
That boy looks like me.	That boy, he look like me.
If he kicks it, he'll be in trouble.	If he kick it, he be in trouble.
When the lights are off, it's dark.	When the lights be off, it dark.
It could be somebody's pet.	It could be somebody pet.
Her feet are too big.	Her feet is too big.
I'll get something to eat.	I will get me something to eat.
She is dancing and the music's on.	She be dancin' an' the music on.
What kind of cheese do you want?	What kind of cheese you want?
My brother's name is Joe.	My brother name is Joe.
I raked the leaves outside.	I rakted the leaves outside.
After the recital, they shook my hand.	After the recital, they shaketed my hand.
They are standing around.	They is just standing around.
He is a basketball star.	He a basketball star.
They are in cages.	They be in cages.
It's not like a tree or anything.	It not like a tree or nothin'.
He does like to fish.	He do like to fish.
They are going to swim.	They gonna swim.
Mom already repaired the car.	Mom done repair the car.

Note. From *Multicultural Students with Special Language Needs: Practical Strategies for Assessment and Intervention,* 2nd ed. (p. 67), by C. Roseberry-McKibbin, 2002, Oceanside, CA: Academic Communication Associates. Copyright 2002 by Academic Communication Associates. Reprinted with permission.

Indian heritage. Most Hispanics prefer to be referred to according to their country of origin (e.g., Cuban American, Mexican American).

- Hispanics are the fastest-growing racial/ethnic group in the United States. In the decade of 1990–2000, the Hispanic population in the U.S. grew by 58%. In the year 2000, Hispanics comprised 12.1% of the U.S. population and 35% of Hispanics were under 18 years of age (U.S. Bureau of the Census, 2000).

Spanish-Language Characteristics and Considerations

- The diversity among Spanish speakers is great. Although Spanish is spoken in Spain, all of Latin America, and most of South America, there are variations, which are reflected mostly in pronunciation and some vocabulary (Goldstein, 2000).
- Spanish speakers in the United States may speak different dialects or varieties of Spanish. The two major Spanish dialects in the United States are southwestern (e.g., Mexican) and Carribean (e.g., Puerto Rican). Thus, clinicians must consider the individual client's background and origins, which are reflected in the variety of Spanish used, and not assume that each Spanish-speaking student can be viewed in the same way.
- Spanish-speaking students who learn English as a second language may manifest differences with SAE in articulation of sounds and in morphosyntactic structures. There are many structural differences between English and Spanish, especially with respect to morphology.
- These differences are not indicative of a disorder requiring intervention, but are differences that are normal and to be expected. It is important for professionals who work with Spanish-speaking clients to understand foundational information regarding Spanish-influenced English (Goldstein, 2004). Table 9.5 describes the articulation characteristics of Spanish and the possible influences on pronunciation of English. Table 9.6 describes the morphosyntactic characteristics of Spanish and possible influences on English production.

CONCEPTS TO CONSIDER

List two articulation differences that Spanish and African American English speakers might manifest that could be misinterpreted as signs of an articulation disorder (e.g., d/th). List two differences for each language background.

_____

_____

_____

_____

_____

English Influenced by Asian Languages

General Background

- Asians originate from three primary geographic regions:

  - *Southeast Asia:* the Philippines, Laos, Cambodia, Thailand, Indonesia, Singapore, Burma, Vietnam, and Malaysia

Table 9.5 ARTICULATION DIFFERENCES COMMONLY OBSERVED AMONG SPANISH SPEAKERS

Articulation Characteristics	Sample English Patterns
/t, d, n/ may be dentalized (tip of tongue is placed against the back of the upper central incisors).	
Final consonants are often devoiced	dose/doze
b/v substitution	berry/very
Deaspirated stops (sounds like speaker is omitting the sound because it is said with little air release).	
ch/sh substitution	Chirley/Shirley
d/voiced th, or z/voiced th (voiced *th* does not exist in Spanish).	dis/this, zat/that
t/voiceless th (voiceless *th* does not exist in Spanish).	tink/think
Schwa sound inserted before word-initial consonant clusters	eskate/skate espend/spend
Words can end in 10 different sounds: a, e, i, o, u, l, r, n, s, d	may omit sounds at the ends of words
When words start with /h/, the /h/ is silent	'old/hold, 'it/hit
/r/ is tapped or trilled (tap /r/ might sound like the tap in the English word *butter*)	
There is no /dʒ/ (e.g., judge) sound in Spanish; speakers may substitute y	Yulie/Julie yoke/joke
Frontal /s/ (Spanish /s/ is produced more frontally than English /s/)	Some speakers may sound like they have frontal lisps
The ñ is pronounced like a y (e.g., baño is pronounced bahnyo).	
Spanish has 5 vowels: a, e, i, o, u (ah, E, ee, o, u) and few diphthongs. Thus, Spanish speakers may produce the following vowel substitutions:	
i/ɪ substitution	peeg/pig, leetle/little
ε/æ, ɑ/æ substitutions	pet/pat, Stahn/Stan

Note. From *Multicultural Students with Special Language Needs: Practical Strategies for Assessment and Intervention,* 2nd ed. (pp. 61-62), by C. Roseberry-McKibbin, 2002, Oceanside, CA: Academic Communication Associates. Copyright 2002 by Academic Communication Associates. Reprinted with permission.

Table 9.6 LANGUAGE DIFFERENCES COMMONLY OBSERVED AMONG SPANISH SPEAKERS

Language Characteristics	Sample English Utterances
Adjective comes after noun.	The *house green.*
s is often omitted in plurals and possessives.	The *girl* book is ... Juan *hat* is red.
Past-tense *ed* is often omitted.	We *walk* yesterday.
Double negatives are required.	I don't have *no more.*
Superiority is demonstrated by using *mas.*	This cake is *more* big.
The adverb often follows the verb.	He drives fast his motorcycle

Note. From *Multicultural Students with Special Language Needs: Practical Strategies for Assessment and Intervention,* 2nd ed. (p. 84), by C. Roseberry-McKibbin, 2002, Oceanside, CA: Academic Communication Associates. Copyright 2002 by Academic Communication Associates. Reprinted with permission.

- *South Asia:* Sri Lanka, Pakistan, and India
- *East Asia:* Japan, Korea, and China

- Many Asians originate from countries in the Pacific Rim. The Pacific Rim includes all nations and regions touching the Pacific Ocean.
- Between 1990 and 2000, using the category of "race alone," the number of Asians in the United States increased by 48.3%. If one uses the figures from the category of "race alone or in combination," the number of Asians in the United States grew by 72.2% between 1990 and 2000, reaching a total of 11,898,828 in the United States in 2000 (U.S. Bureau of the Census, 2000).

Speech–Language Characteristics and Considerations

- Some of the most widely spoken Asian languages in the United States include Chinese, Filipino, Vietnamese, Japanese, Khmer, and Korean (Cheng, 2002).
- Many Asian languages have numerous dialects that may or may not be mutually intelligible (Hwa-Froelich, Hodson, & Edwards, 2002). For example, there are over 87 mutually unintelligible dialects in the Philippines.
- Some groups have no written language and rely on oral traditions.
- Vietnamese, Chinese, and Laotian are tonal languages; each tone change (toneme) is phonemic in nature and represents a meaning change. For example, in Mandarin, "ma" can mean *mother, horse, scold, flax,* or *curse* depending on the tone used in pronouncing it.
- Mandarin has four tonemes; Cantonese has seven tonemes; Northern Vietnamese has six tonemes; Central and Southern Vietnamese each have five tonemes.
- Japanese, Khmer, and Korean are not tonal languages.
- Chinese, Vietnamese, and Laotian are basically monosyllabic.
- Chinese and Vietnamese have no consonant blends.

- Many languages, such as Chinese, do not have inflectional markers.
- Some languages (e.g., Indonesian, Japanese, and Tagalog) do not have specific gender pronouns (do not differentiate between *he, she, it*).
- Asian speakers' prosody or intonation in English may sound very "choppy" and monotonous to native English speakers.
- Some Asian speakers may sound hypernasal in English.
- It is difficult to provide generalities about Asian speakers' English patterns due to the vast variety in Asian languages and dialects. Thus, the examples in Tables 9.7 and 9.8 may or may not be representative of various students; each must be assessed on an individual basis.

SUMMARY

✓ Knowledge of the influence of a primary language or dialect on English production is critical for differentiating language differences from language problems in CLD speakers.

✓ Speakers of African American English, Spanish, and Asian languages have unique and predictable characteristics, based on primary-language influence, that are signs of differences and not disorders.

✓ These differences do not need to be remediated; however, some speakers may seek elective intervention so that their productions may more closely approximate Standard American English.

LANGUAGE DIFFERENCES AND LANGUAGE-LEARNING DISABILITIES

INTRODUCTION

Clinicians around the United States are continually confronted with the need to distinguish language differences from language-learning disabilities (LLD). This challenge is impacted by the unique processes of second-language acquisition and by the nature of bilingualism and language proficiency. Knowledge of basic facts about acquiring a second language can help clinicians make accurate decisions in distinguishing language differences from LLDs in CLD children (Roseberry-McKibbin et al., 2005; Genesee, Paradis, & Crago, 2004).

Differentiating Language Differences from Language-Learning Disabilities

- When clinicians are confronted with CLD students who appear to be struggling in school, the first question they usually ask is: "Does this student have a language difference or an LLD?" (*Note:* Some clinicians refer to a language-learning disability as specific language impairment; see Chapter 4. In this chapter, the term language-learning disability is used.)

- In other words, can the problems be traced to cultural differences or the student's lack of facility with English, or is there an underlying language learning disability that requires special education intervention?

- Bloom and Lahey (1978) defined language as a system of symbols used to represent concepts that are formed through exposure and experience. Clinicians must ask about students' environmental and linguistic exposure and experience.

Table 9.7 LANGUAGE DIFFERENCES COMMONLY OBSERVED AMONG ASIAN SPEAKERS

Language Characteristics	Sample English Utterances
Omission of plurals	Here are two *piece* of toast. I got five *finger* on each hand.
Omission of copula	He *going* home now. They *eating.*
Omission of possessive	I have *Phuong* pencil. *Mom* food is cold.
Omission of past-tense morpheme	We *cook* dinner yesterday. Last night she *walk* home.
Past-tense double marking	He *didn't went* by himself.
Double negative	They *don't* have *no* books.
Subject-verb-object relationship differences/omissions	I messed *up it.* *He like.*
Singular present-tense omission or addition	*You goes* inside. *He go* to the store.
Misordering of interrogatives	You are going now?
Misuse or omission of prepositions	She is *in* home. He goes to school 8:00.
Misuse of pronouns	*She* husband is coming. She said *her wife* is here.
Omission and/or over-generalization of articles	*Boy* is sick. He went *the home.*
Incorrect use of comparatives	This book is *gooder* than that book.
Omission of conjunctions	You I going to the beach.
Omission, lack of inflection on auxiliary *do*	She not take it. He *do not* have enough.
Omission, lack of inflection on forms of *have*	She *have* no money. We been the store.

Note. From *Multicultural Students with Special Language Needs: Practical Strategies for Assessment and Intervention,* 2nd ed. (p. 108), by C. Roseberry-McKibbin, 2002, Oceanside, CA: Academic Communication Associates. Copyright 2002 by Academic Communication Associates. Reprinted with permission.

Table 9.8 ARTICULATION DIFFERENCES COMMONLY OBSERVED AMONG ASIAN SPEAKERS

Articulation Characteristics	Sample Utterances
In many Asian languages, words end in vowels only or in just a few consonants; speakers may delete many final consonants in English.	ste/step li/lid ro/robe do/dog
Some languages are monosyllabic; speakers may truncate polysyllabic words or emphasize the wrong syllable.	efunt/elephant *di*versity/diversity
Possible devoicing of voiced cognates	beece/bees pick/pig luff/love crip/crib
r/l confusion	lize/rise clown/crown
/r/ may be omitted entirely	gull/girl tone/torn
Reduction of vowel length in words	Words sound choppy to Americans
No voiced or voiceless *th*	dose/those tin/thin zose/those sin/thin
Epenthesis (addition of *uh* sound in blends, ends of words)	bulack/black wooduh/wood
Confusion of *ch* and *sh*	sheep/cheap beesh/beach
/ae/ does not exist in many Asian languages	block/black shock/shack
b/v substitutions	base/vase Beberly/Beverly
v/w substitutions	vork/work vall/wall
p/f substitutions	pall/fall plower/flower

Note. From *Multicultural Students with Special Language Needs: Practical Strategies for Assessment and Intervention*, 2nd ed. (p. 109), by C. Roseberry-McKibbin, 2002, Oceanside, CA: Academic Communication Associates. Copyright 2002 by Academic Communication Associates. Reprinted with permission.

- Some CLD students do not have the environmental and linguistic exposure and experience that are assumed by schools. They may come from nonliterate backgrounds, for example, or from backgrounds where the language is oral only and has not been put in written form.

- Some clinicians do not stop to ask themselves whether students have had any of the usual mainstream experiences that are inherently assumed, like exposure to literacy.

- This is often where deficits in students are created: When students' exposure and experiences are different than those expected in the mainstream school environment, clinicians may assume that there are deficits inherent in the students themselves.

- If students' background experiences and exposure to life situations and linguistic models are different from those expected by schools, it follows that their language, which represents their unique backgrounds, will not be consistent with that expected by the school.

- This difference in students' backgrounds and schools' expectations can lead to misdiagnosis of students and consequent inappropriate placement into special education. Historically in U.S. schools, disproportionate numbers of CLD children have been placed in special education unnecessarily.

- In the United States in the twenty-first century, increasing numbers of parents are adopting children from other countries such as Russia, Taiwan, China, and others. Many of these children live in orphanages in their home countries until they are adopted by their American parents. By some estimates, upon arrival in their adoptive homes, 20% of these children thrive, 60% experience delays in many areas with only partial improvement, and 20% show moderate to major developmental delays with little to no improvement (Pearson, 2001).

- Some of these children may show delays in their primary languages as well as English because of the environmental conditions in their home countries (Glennen, 2002). If a child is adopted from another country, the clinician must take this into account when assessing the child for the possible presence of a language learning disability.

- Children who speak more than one language can be properly diagnosed as having a language-learning disability only if they manifest language-learning difficulties *in both the primary language and in English*. Legally, it must be proven that the student in question has an LLD that underlies *both languages*.

- If a student has normal abilities in the primary language and is having difficulty with English, this student does not need special education remediation services such as speech–language therapy. Rather, the student needs other services, such as bilingual education, to facilitate English-language learning (see Figure 9.2).

Acquiring a Second Language

- In assessing any child to differentiate a language difference from an LLD, it is necessary to know what "normal" behavior is. A major challenge confronting clinicians is that normal behavior varies widely even among monolingual children. When one is attempting to work with CLD students, the picture becomes far more complex.

- Sometimes CLD learners who demonstrate normal second-language acquisition processes

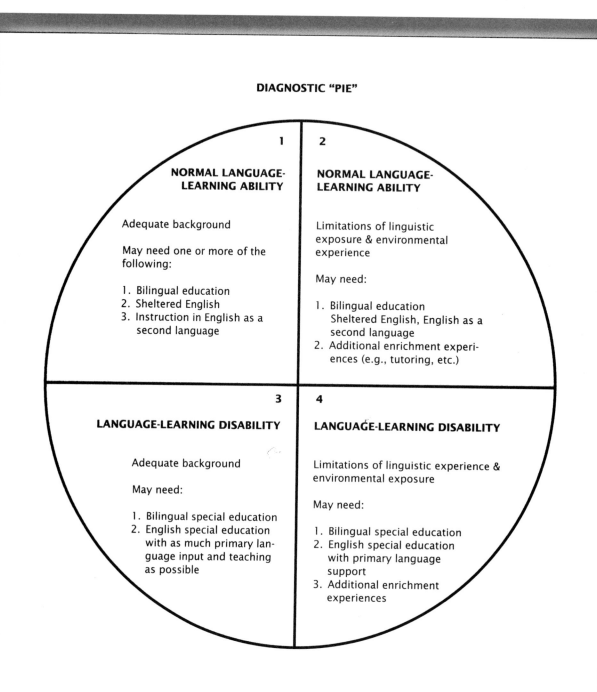

Figure 9.2. The diagnostic pie. *Note.* From *Multicultural Students with Special Language Needs: Practical Strategies for Assessment and Intervention*, 2nd ed. (p. 218), by C. Roseberry-McKibbin, 2002, Oceanside, CA: Academic Communication Associates. Copyright 2002 by Academic Communication Associates. Reprinted with permission.

can spuriously appear to have underlying language-learning disabilities. To avoid making inaccurate diagnoses of such learners, it is important to be familiar with normal processes of second-language acquisition (Genesee et al., 2004; Kayser, 2002).

Typical Processes of Second-Language Acquisition

- *Transfer or interference.* This refers to an error in a student's second language (L2) that is directly produced by the influence of L1 (the first or primary language). Interference can occur in all areas: syntax, morphology, phonology, pragmatics, and semantics. Researchers and practitioners disagree about the extent of L1 influence on L2 production; however, it seems safe to say that a percentage of errors produced by CLD students can be directly traced to the influence of L1.
- For example, a child from an Asian language background might say "The mom have two book." This would be an example of transfer, not an example of LLD.
- *Silent period.* Some students, when learning an L2, go through a "silent period," in which there is much listening and comprehension and little output. It is believed that children are using this time to comprehend the new language before producing it. The silent period can last anywhere from 3 to 6 months, although estimates vary.
- *Codeswitching.* Codeswitching can be defined as the alternating or switching between two languages at the word, phrase, or sentence level; this behavior is part of natural bilingual development and is used by normal bilingual speakers worldwide (Brice & Anderson, 1999).
- *Language loss.* If use of the L1 is discontinued or diminished, it is common for the second-language learner to lose skills in that first language. Because English is the dominant language of society in the United States, children often experience language loss of L1 and a gradual replacement of L1 with English, or L2.
- If a CLD student has experienced L1 loss and is still acquiring English, he or she may appear to be low functioning in both languages. Many clinicians might conclude that low functioning in L1 as well as L2 is indicative of a language-learning disability when it actually is a result of the loss of L1.

CONCEPTS TO CONSIDER

Summarize the reasons why it is challenging to differentiate language differences from language-learning disabilities in CLD students.

Basic Interpersonal Communication Skills and Cognitive–Academic Language Proficiency

■ A model of language proficiency that is useful in working with CLD children distinguishes basic interpersonal communication skills (BICS) from cognitive–academic language proficiency (CALP).

■ According to Cummins (1992, 2002), in CLD children BICS take approximately 2 years (in an ideal situation) to develop to a level commensurate with that of native speakers of L2. CALP takes 5–7 years to develop to a native-like level—and that frame is common for students from enriched backgrounds.

■ BICS involve face-to-face communication in which conversational participants can actively negotiate meaning and have a shared reality. BICS communication is typical of that found in the everyday world outside the classroom, where language is supported by a wide range of meaningful situational and paralinguistic gestures.

■ CALP, which involves grasping the fundamentals of written language and adopting key literacy habits, does not assume a shared reality. It may rely exclusively on linguistic cues for meaning and is more typical of the classroom.

■ CALP is characteristic of situations where knowledge is not automatized and the student must actively use cognitive strategies to perform a task (e.g., writing an essay in a foreign language).

■ Many professionals do not know the difference between BICS and CALP, and are unaware of the difference in the timelines for development of these types of language proficiency. Consequently, many students are misdiagnosed with language disorders because of the BICS-CALP gap (Roseberry-McKibbin, 2002; see Figure 9.3).

■ Many bilingual education programs help students who are "limited English proficient" (LEP) transition from English BICS to English CALP. Ideally, bilingual education would include maintenance of students' first languages and cultures and provision of second-language and culture instruction as well as subject matter (e.g., math, science). This scenario appears to promote the greatest linguistic, cultural, and cognitive benefits, especially when combined with active parent and community involvement.

■ Many European countries value multilingualism so much that they are now promoting a policy of trilingualism in schools. In Switzerland, for example, students cannot graduate from high school unless they speak three languages fluently.

■ Unfortunately, some United States citizens have a negative attitude toward bilingualism and believe that it has negative cognitive and social effects on children. Thus, the availability of strong, theoretically sound bilingual programs in the United States is limited. Some states, such as California, have even passed laws that almost entirely rule out bilingual education in any form.

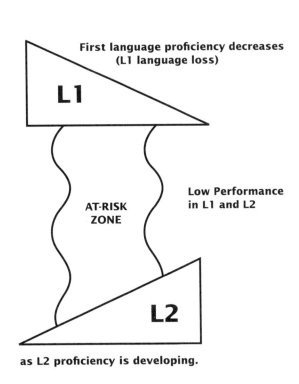

Figure 9.3. English-language learners at risk. *Note.* From *Multicultural Students with Special Language Needs: Practical Strategies for Assessment and Intervention,* 2nd ed. (p. 195), by C. Roseberry-McKibbin, 2002, Oceanside, CA: Academic Communication Associates. Copyright 2002 by Academic Communication Associates. Reprinted with permission.

Simultaneous and Sequential Bilingualism

- Researchers have broadly delineated two types of bilingualism: simultaneous and sequential. *Simultaneous bilingual acquisition* occurs when two languages are acquired simultaneously from infancy.
- Schiff-Myers (1992) has termed this phenomenon, in which two languages are spoken to a child beginning in early infancy, *infant bilinguality.* Such children acquire two languages simultaneously in natural communication situations, and this bilingual development closely parallels monolingual development. Children who acquire two languages simultaneously in naturalistic situations seem to do so with minimal interference.
- *Sequential bilingual acquisition* includes a greater diversity of rates and stages (Roseberry-McKibbin, 2003). Some students may acquire the second language with minimal interference; others may experience difficulties.
- If a student is introduced to an L2 before the L1 competency threshold has been reached, the development of L1 may be arrested or may regress while the child is focusing on L2 development.

- Since, as Cummins (1992) has stated, L2 proficiency is partially a function of L1 competence, a condition of "semilingualism" may occur, in which the student does not fully develop either language. For a period of time, these students may obtain low test scores in both L1 and L2 and consequently appear LLD.

- Thus, when clinicians are working with CLD students in the schools, it is necessary, when a student appears to be "low functioning," to ask how the student developed both languages—simultaneously or sequentially?

- If the languages were developed sequentially, was L1 stable and developed enough so that acquisition of L2 was beneficial? If not, the student's seemingly limited academic performance and limited skills in both languages could result from acquisition of L2 when the underlying system was not yet stable.

SUMMARY

✓ When clinicians attempt to distinguish a language difference from an LLD in CLD students, they must take into account factors of second-language acquisition and bilingual development.

✓ Normal processes of second-language acquisition include interference, the silent period, codeswitching, and language loss. BICS and CALP are two types of language proficiency that clinicians should be aware of in assessing students.

✓ In distinguishing language differences from disorders, it is critical to ask if a child has developed two languages simultaneously or sequentially.

✓ In many cases, errors in judgment and consequent inappropriate placement of CLD students can be avoided if clinicians are aware of second-language learning factors. The greater the understanding clinicians have of these factors, the more unbiased and appropriate will be the services provided to CLD students in the schools.

ASSESSMENT OF CLD CLIENTS

INTRODUCTION

Culturally fair and nonbiased assessment of CLD students is an issue impacting schools across the United States (Kohnert, Kennedy, Glaze, Kan, & Carney, 2003; Moore-Brown & Montgomery, 2001; Roseberry-McKibbin et al., 2005). A major consideration for all schools is state and federal mandates governing assessment of and intervention for CLD children. Clinicians must also look carefully at the typical practice of using standardized tests for assessment of LLD; most of these tests are biased against CLD students. Clinicians are increasingly using alternatives to standardized tests and working with interpreters from the clients' culture who can help ensure assessment is fair and unbiased (American Speech-Language-Hearing Association, 2001b; Jacobs & Coufal, 2001).

Legal Considerations

- A number of laws affect service delivery to CLD students. The key law currently in practice, the Individuals with Disabilities Education Act (IDEA, 1997), specifically mandates the following:

- All children, regardless of disability, are entitled to an appropriate and free education.
- Testing and evaluation materials and procedures must be selected and administered so that they are not racially or culturally discriminatory.
- Testing and evaluation materials must be provided and administered in the language or other mode of communication in which the child is most proficient.
- Tests must be administered to a child with a motor, speech, hearing, visual or other communication disability, or to a bilingual child, so as to reflect accurately the child's ability in the area tested, rather than the child's impaired communication skill or limited English-language skill.
- Multicultural education is to be considered in guaranteeing equal educational opportunities for minorities with handicaps.

Considerations in the Use of Standardized Tests

Foundational Concepts

- Many clinicians rely entirely on the use of standardized tests to evaluate CLD students' language abilities and to plan intervention, even though standardized tests are generally heavily biased against members of CLD populations (Roseberry-McKibbin, 2007; Wyatt, 2002).
- If clinicians continue to use these formal tests with CLD students, they should at least be aware of the tests' potential legal, psychometric, cultural, and linguistic limitations in terms of validity and reliability.
- It is important to be familiar with the assumptions underlying formal, standardized tests. When clinicians are familiar with these assumptions, they can modify standardized tests so the tests are less biased.

Formal Test Assumptions

- The development of formal tests has grown out of a framework that is Western, literate, and middle class. For these and many other reasons, formal tests are often very biased against CLD students.
- Formal tests are based on many inherent assumptions that clinicians may be only partially aware of. These assumptions are extremely important to consider when working with CLD students. These assumptions hold that test takers (students) will (Roseberry-McKibbin, 2002):

  - follow the cooperative principle, performing to the best of their ability and trying to provide relevant answers;
  - attempt to respond even when test tasks don't make sense;
  - understand test tasks (e.g., fill in the blank, point to the picture);
  - have been exposed to the information and experiences inherent in a test;
  - feel comfortable enough with the examiner in the testing setting to perform optimally.

- These assumptions cannot be made with regard to many CLD students. For example, some students come from cultural backgrounds where it is considered respectful to be silent in the presence of an unfamiliar adult. Cultural differences may cause students not to optimally display their competence and abilities when taking standardized tests.
- Clinicians must also remember that rules of interaction may differ from culture to culture. For example, in the African American speech community, several people may speak at once because there is greater tolerance for overlap during conversational exchanges (Wyatt, 1998).

- Thus, it would be important not to label an African American child as having "a deficiency in turn-taking skills" according to mainstream Euro-American standards.
- Many formal, standardized tests that involve storytelling assume that children come from a literate narrative tradition. In such a tradition, narratives are highly structured, decontextualized, and follow specific patterns. It is assumed that the speaker will provide explicit information for and *inform* the listener.
- However, some CLD children (e.g., African American and Native American children) come from *oral* narrative traditions where listener knowledge is assumed. The speaker's job is to *entertain* the listener; storytelling is not as structured (Klein & Moses, 1999). Clinicians must not mislabel these children as having language problems if they do not produce narratives according to a literate tradition.
- Most standardized tests that are normed on monolingual English-speaking children do not possess ecological validity. A test's *ecological validity* refers to the extent to which it reflects the child's actual, daily environment and life experience.

Translating Standardized Tests

- Translated versions of English tests are often used with CLD students. There are many difficulties with using translated English tests, so it is best to avoid this practice.
- Differences in structure and content between English and the primary language raise questions of comparability of scores. Many words cannot be translated directly from one language to another. For example, some Asian languages do not have pronouns; translating *she* or *he* versus *it* into those languages is impossible.
- Psychometric properties of tests, such as validity, reliability, sample sizes, and norming populations, do not carry over to translated versions.
- Translation assumes that CLD students have the same life experiences and background as the norming population, when they often do not.

Tests Developed in Primary Languages

- Many clinicians believe that they can obtain valid assessments of CLD students' language skills if they use tests specifically developed in the students' primary languages. For example, Spanish-speaking students can be given Spanish tests. There are some problems with this as well.
- One major problem is the great heterogeneity of various minority populations. For example, many dialects of Spanish exist, and Spanish-speaking children come from such different countries as Cuba, Mexico, Puerto Rico, the Dominican Republic, and Spain. Also, Spanish-speaking students raised in different parts of the United States use different vocabulary words for some items.
- A second difficulty is that there is little developmental data on languages other than English (Roseberry-McKibbin & Brice, 1999). Some Spanish norms for articulation have been developed, but few easily accessible, established language or articulation development norms exist for languages other than English.

Selecting, Administering, and Interpreting Standardized Tests

- When professionals are considering which tests to use with CLD students, they must keep in mind the following considerations:

    - *Purpose of the test.* Is it for screening or in-depth evaluation?
    - *Construct validity.* What theory was used in the test's creation? Is any theory mentioned?

Is it appropriate for this particular student?

- *Appropriateness of test content.* Professionals can have native speakers review the test; they also can get help in field-testing the assessment instrument so that they can change or delete items that most of the children miss.
- *Adequacy of norms.* How was the standardization sample selected? Are the students who are being tested represented in the norming and standardization processes?

- There are ways in which professionals can alter the administration of standardized tests so that CLD students will perform optimally in ways that reflect their true abilities (Roseberry-McKibbin, 2003):

  - Omit biased items that the student will probably miss.
  - Test beyond the ceiling.
  - Complete the assessment over several sessions.
  - Have a parent or another adult who is trusted by the child administer test items under the clinician's supervision.
  - Give instructions in both English and L1.
  - Rephrase confusing instructions.
  - Give extra examples, demonstrations and practice items.
  - Give the student extra time to respond.
  - Repeat items when necessary.
  - If students give "wrong" answers, ask them to explain and write down their explanations. Score items as correct if they are correct in students' cultures. Record all responses.

- There are also ways that professionals can interpret standardized tests to effectively reduce bias:

  - Review test results with family members and other people from the student's culture to gain additional insight into the student's performance.
  - Interpret overall test results in a team setting. If professionals review and interpret results alone, errors are more likely.
  - Don't identify a student as needing special education solely on the basis of test scores. Use informal measures to supplement standardized test scores.
  - Ascertain if students' errors are typical of other students with similar backgrounds.
  - When writing assessment reports, be sure to include cautions and disclaimers about any departures from standard testing procedures. In addition, discuss how the student's background may have influenced testing results.

Alternatives to Standardized Tests

Basic Principles

- Because the use of standardized tests poses many difficulties when professionals are evaluating CLD students, the use of nonstandardized, informal procedures and instruments for the assessment of CLD students has become increasingly frequent (Goldstein, 2004; Laing & Kamhi, 2003).
- A major advantage of informal testing is that it can be matched to students' curriculum. Another major advantage of informal testing is that it takes into account the fact that CLD students are often very capable in their own milieu and very functional in their own worlds.

Formal testing seldom taps these students' individualized, functional skills in their own environments.

- The assessment wheel of a team approach to comprehensive assessment (see Figure 9.4) illustrates the necessity of combining informal assessment strategies with more formal testing for CLD students. It is important to carry out thorough assessments that include a case history, language proficiency testing, environmental observations, and dynamic assessment.

- It is critical that any assessment measures used with CLD students have ecological validity

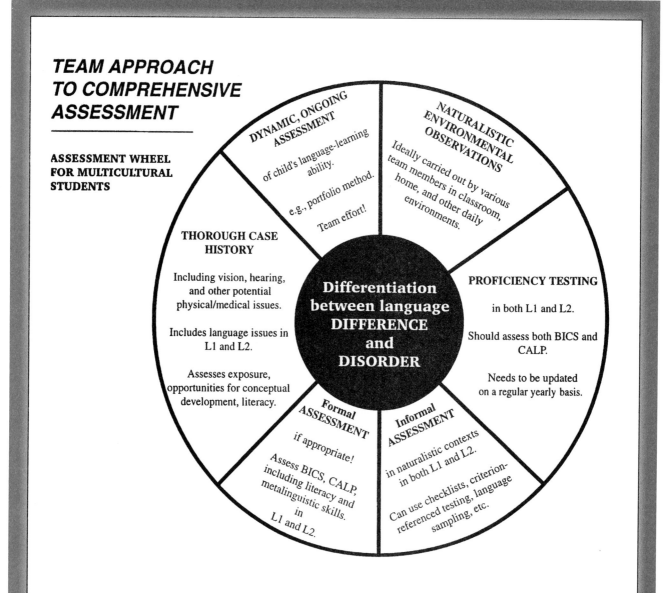

TEAM APPROACH TO COMPREHENSIVE ASSESSMENT

ASSESSMENT WHEEL FOR MULTICULTURAL STUDENTS

Differentiation between language DIFFERENCE and DISORDER

DYNAMIC, ONGOING ASSESSMENT of child's language-learning ability. e.g., portfolio method. Team effort!

NATURALISTIC ENVIRONMENTAL OBSERVATIONS Ideally carried out by various team members in classroom, home, and other daily environments.

THOROUGH CASE HISTORY Including vision, hearing, and other potential physical/medical issues. Includes language issues in L1 and L2. Assesses exposure, opportunities for conceptual development, literacy.

PROFICIENCY TESTING in both L1 and L2. Should assess both BICS and CALP. Needs to be updated on a regular yearly basis.

Formal ASSESSMENT if appropriate! Assess BICS, CALP, including literacy and metalinguistic skills. in L1 and L2.

Informal ASSESSMENT in naturalistic contexts in both L1 and L2. Can use checklists, criterion-referenced testing, language sampling, etc.

Figure 9.4. Team approach to comprehensive assessment: Assessment wheel for multicultural students. *Note.* From *Multicultural Students with Special Language Needs: Practical Strategies for Assessment and Intervention,* 2nd ed. (p. 246), by C. Roseberry-McKibbin, 2002, Oceanside, CA: Academic Communication Associates. Copyright 2002 by Academic Communication Associates. Reprinted with permission.

(mentioned earlier). These measures must reflect the child's unique environmental experience and daily life activities.

Specific Alternatives to Standardized Assessment

- Instead of relying exclusively on standardized tests for assessing CLD students, clinicians can (Roseberry-McKibbin, 2002, 2003):

  - *Obtain a thorough case history* of the child's development in all domains: linguistic, cognitive, physical, academic, and others. It is very important to ascertain the child's history of language exposure to the first language and English.
  - *Use observations in a variety of naturalistic contexts,* evaluating the student's ability to interact in various everyday situations. Use of multiple observations in naturalistic settings helps clinicians obtain information about the child's communication behavior in multiple contexts. Professionals can observe students in the classroom, at recess, at lunch, in the library, in the home, and in a variety of other settings.
  - *Use questionnaires* administered to teachers, parents, and others who interact with the student on a regular basis (Roseberry-McKibbin, 1993). Use of questionnaires gives a much broader picture of the student's communication functioning in daily contexts. It also helps the professionals doing the assessment to work as part of a team and not carry the entire responsibility for assessing the CLD student.
  - *Use authentic assessment,* which involves performances that have educational value in their own right; for example, clinicians can look at students' essays or portfolios of student work.
  - *Use a dynamic approach to assessment* in which a student is evaluated over time in a test-teach-retest format. Because so many students come from backgrounds of reduced exposure to mainstream school concepts and vocabulary, they do poorly in formal testing situations.

- A dynamic approach is highly preferable to a static approach in which the student is tested in one or two assessment sessions, because dynamic assessment evaluates a student's ability to learn when provided with instruction. If a child responds poorly to dynamic assessment, this may be a sign that she has a genuine language-learning disability (Long, 2005).

  - *Use narratives* appropriate to the student's background to assess the student's ability to construct narratives and remember stories she or he has heard.
  - *Use the portfolio method of assessment,* in which samples of the student's work are gathered over time. These work samples can be analyzed to see how much learning is taking place.
  - *Use language samples* to evaluate the student's communication skills in everyday contexts with various interlocutors.
  - *Use school records* of the student's achievement and performance. Cumulative files (permanent records kept for each student) often contain helpful information that allows the clinician to track a student's performance over time.

Working with Interpreters in the Assessment Process

- Due to the national shortage of trained professionals who speak a language other than English, schools are increasingly turning to interpreters for assistance in the assessment and treatment of CLD students. The clinician who is utilizing the services of an interpreter for assessment of

C O N C E P T S   T O   C O N S I D E R

Describe the problems inherent in using standardized tests to assess the language skills of CLD children. What can clinicians do to circumvent those problems?

_____

_____

_____

_____

_____

CLD students has ethical responsibilities to carry out. The clinician needs to make sure that he or she (Langdon & Cheng, 2002):

- makes sure that the permission for assessment form indicates that the services of an interpreter will be used during the assessment;
- makes clear in the assessment report that the services of an interpreter were used;
- recognizes the limitations of interpreted tests;
- allows interpreters to carry out only those activities for which they have been trained;
- involves others in training the interpreter when appropriate;
- gives the interpreter background information about the student who is to be tested;
- prepares the interpreter for each testing session and debriefs the interpreter afterwards;
- shows the interpreter how to use tests and makes sure the interpreter feels comfortable with the testing;
- allows the interpreter time, before the student arrives, to organize test materials, read instructions, and clarify any areas of question;
- ensures that the interpreter does not protect the student by hiding the extent of the student's limitations or disabilities;
- supervises the interpreter during the testing session and watches for possible inappropriate behaviors such as recording the assessment data incorrectly, prompting the student or giving clues, or using too many words;
- reminds the interpreter to write down all the student's behaviors seen during testing, even if the behaviors seem extraneous to the immediate task; and
- considers the interpreter's observations but does not place the responsibility for the placement decision on the interpreter.

SUMMARY

✓ **Federal law mandates nondiscriminatory, culture-fair testing for CLD students. However, many clinicians use standardized, formal tests that are biased against CLD students.**

✓ If clinicians use those tests, they must be aware of potential forms of bias and try to control for them as much as possible.

✓ Many clinicians are increasingly turning to nonstandardized, informal assessment, which is much more valid in assessing the true language-learning abilities and skills of CLD children. Interpreters can be a valuable part of this process.

TREATMENT CONSIDERATIONS IN SERVICE DELIVERY TO CLD CLIENTS

INTRODUCTION

CLD children with language-learning disabilities that underlie both the primary language and English can be served through different delivery models. Treatment should always be individualized and should be linguistically and culturally appropriate for the particular student involved. CLD adults who have neurologically based disorders of communication have unique needs that must be taken into consideration when providing services.

Children with Language-Learning Disabilities

Basic Principles

- As previously stated, students should not be diagnosed as having LLD if "problems" are observed only in English. If the student is truly LLD, problems in communication should be evident in both English and the primary language.
- An LLD affects a child's ability to learn any language. Exposure to two or more languages is not the cause of the disability. Bilingual children with underlying LLD will have difficulty learning any language.
- State and federal laws provide some specific guidelines for considering service options for CLD students. Many times CLD children do need assistance but do not qualify for special education.
- *It is illegal for clinicians in the public schools to place CLD students into special education to work on improving the students' English.* Thus, only a select number of CLD students are truly eligible for special education services, including speech–language therapy.
- If CLD students do not qualify for speech–language services but need support in learning English, clinicians can help teachers find other options, such as bilingual education, English as a Second Language (ESL) programs, and others.

Service Delivery Models

- If CLD students do qualify for special education services, including speech–language therapy, the following service delivery models can be considered (Roseberry-McKibbin, 2002):

  - a bilingual special education classroom
  - a monolingual, English, special education classroom with primary-language support through a bilingual teacher, tutor, or others

- pull-out services (speech–language therapy, resource support, or both) in the primary language
- pull-out services in English with primary-language support
- consultative, collaborative service provision in which the CLD child remains in the regular classroom and the teacher receives assistance from special education personnel or ESL or bilingual staff
- placement in a regular bilingual education or ESL classroom with support from special education

Treatment Principles

- If a student is more proficient in the primary language than in English, carrying out treatment in the primary language is usually much more efficient and effective (Kiernan & Swisher, 1990; Perozzi & Sanchez, 1992).
- If a CLD child is exposed to English in school, some professionals worry that conducting therapy in the child's stronger, primary language will have negative effects. However, research shows that CLD children with LLD can and do learn two languages effectively; being exposed to two languages is not a disadvantage and, in fact, is usually advantageous (Gutierrez-Clellen, 1999; Paradis et al., 2003; Restrepo & Kruth, 2000). If children are cut off from their primary language, this can have many negative effects (Kohnert & Derr, 2004).
- Ideally, intervention activities should (Roseberry-McKibbin, 2001):

  - focus on content rather than on mastery of specific grammatical forms;
  - include reading, writing, listening and talking; literacy should always be incorporated;
  - be built around whole themes, experiences, and events that have meaning to students;
  - promote effective communication and interaction among students;
  - be related to the classroom curriculum;
  - acknowledge students' cultural and linguistic backgrounds and experiences, and promote self-esteem; and
  - support students in learning the academic language that will help them be successful in the school setting

- It is critical for intervention to involve not just therapy in a pull-out model, but also intervention in the child's classroom setting. Clinicians must, as much as possible, see that they collaborate with classroom teachers to help children succeed in the academic and social setting of the classroom.
- Clinicians should work closely with children's families and include caregivers as collaborators in the development of treatment goals. It is also very helpful to work with people from the families' cultures in order to promote treatment success.

ADULTS WITH NEUROLOGICALLY BASED DISORDERS OF COMMUNICATION

Basic Issues

- The aging population is the most rapidly growing group in our country. Due to recent advances in health care, people are living longer. It is predicted that by the year 2025, approximately 60 million people in the United States will be over 65 years of age.

- As stated earlier, increasing numbers of CLD people are living longer. Members of CLD groups tend to have a higher prevalence of neurological impairments (typically found in older people) than is found in the general population. This is due to many factors, including lack of health insurance and preventive care (Galanti, 2004).
- The leading cause of neurological impairments is strokes. Strokes are associated with:

    - *hypertension,* which may result in hemorrhagic strokes. Hypertension is prevalent among many CLD adults, especially African Americans.
    - *arteriosclerosis,* a major etiological factor in strokes. In many CLD communities, arteriosclerosis is associated with high cholesterol levels. Also, foods that are high in salt and fat content (e.g., pork) are major causes of arteriosclerosis; these foods are popular in African American and Hispanic communities.
    - *sickle cell anemia,* which primarily affects people of African and Mediterranean descent. Areas of the brain supplied by small blood vessels don't get enough oxygen, which may cause a stroke.
    - *diabetes,* which affects Hispanics especially. Mexicans and Puerto Ricans have a rate of (adult onset) diabetes two to three times higher than the rate in the white population. Diabetes is associated with an increased risk of stroke .
    - *AIDS,* which is often associated with IV drug use, a pervasive problem in large urban areas.
    - *alcohol abuse,* which is a serious problem in many CLD groups because so often it begins in the early to middle teen years. This places abusers at high risk for neurological impairments, such as strokes, involving linguistic and cognitive deficits (Wallace, 1998).
    - *drug abuse,* which is very high in urban areas. Many inner-city residents have difficulties with drug abuse, and drugs such as crack (a vasoconstrictor) can cause strokes.

Theories Regarding Stroke Recovery in Bilinguals

- It is important to be aware of whether a stroke patient speaks more than one language. In one actual case, a bilingual English-Russian patient had a stroke and spoke only Russian after the stroke. The hospital staff, not having checked the patient's records, thought she was using jargon.
- Arambula (1992) has described four recovery theories, outlined below, for bilingual stroke patients.

Synergistic and Differential Recovery Theory

- According to this theory, both languages are impaired, but not necessarily to the same degree. One language may be more affected than the other.
- Both languages may eventually recover but not necessarily at the same rate.
- Synergistic and differential recovery is by far the most common type; 95–98% of bilingual patients manifest this type of recovery.

Antagonistic Recovery Theory

- According to this theory, one language returns at the expense of another previously recovered language. For example, a Spanish-speaking patient may recover Spanish and then English; however, when the English language returns, the Spanish language skills begin to disappear.
- There are few documented cases in which a patient has demonstrated antagonistic recovery.

Successive Recovery Theory

- According to this theory, one language returns only after another has been completely restored.
- There are few documented cases in which a patient has demonstrated successive recovery.

Selective Recovery Theory

- According to this theory, one of the patient's languages never recovers and remains impaired. This occurs even when the other languages have recovered.

Sociocultural Considerations in Rehabilitation: Implications for Assessment and Treatment

- It is important to consider individual patients' premorbid status as well as their functional needs within their personal life contexts. For example, many older African Americans have strong church connections (Andrews & Boyle, 2003); therapy activities could address daily communication skills that are centered around church activities.
- Clinicians must evaluate the family's culture in terms of the appropriateness of the rehabilitation goal of independence for the patient. Encouragement of independence may be offensive in some cultures (Galanti, 2004).
- For example, some Hispanic families believe it is their duty to take care of the neurologically impaired patient (Chong, 2002). Requiring the patient to attend rehabilitation and become independent would be looked on as disrespectful and would cause great shame to the family.
- Socioeconomic status has a great impact on CLD patients' potential for utilizing rehabilitation services. Unfortunately, many elderly CLD adults tend to have little money or insurance.
- For example, in 2003, 12.8% of native-born Americans were uninsured compared to 33.4% of immigrants (Camarota, 2003). Mexican Americans, who make up 58% of the Hispanic population in the United States, have especially low rates of health insurance because they are employed in low-paid sectors of the workforce that are not likely to provide insurance coverage as a benefit for their employees (Chong, 2002).
- Family relationships are an important consideration. For example, African Americans tend to be more involved than whites in providing help across the generations, and the extended family network is much greater for African Americans than for whites (Payne-Johnson, 1992). Asian families tend to be highly involved in caring for ill or infirm family members (Galanti, 2004). Clinicians can utilize family members for support.
- It is important to assess premorbid educational levels and vocational attainments of patients, because these impact assessment and treatment. For example, according to Reyes (1995), elderly Hispanics are six or seven times more likely to be functionally illiterate (have less than 5 years of schooling) than non-Hispanics. Approximately 73% of elderly Hispanics have an educational attainment of eighth grade or less, compared to 35% of all elderly individuals.
- Socioeconomic status and educational attainment impact patients' acceptance of and belief in conventional rehabilitation, especially that involving technology. For example, if an elderly Asian from a low-income Hmong refugee family needs to have a CT scan to determine if he has had a stroke, the family may resist the CT scan because they have not been exposed to "high-tech" neurodiagnostic procedures.
- Religion also may play a role in patients' and families' acceptance of rehabilitation (Andrews & Boyle, 2003; Galanti, 2004). Some families believe in folk healers, not traditional medicine. Other families believe that a disability caused by a stroke, for example, is the will of a Supreme Being, and thus rehabilitation would go counter to religious beliefs.
- When assessing bilingual patients, it is imperative that the clinician assess skills in both the

primary language and English. Assessment should be carried out as soon as possible and should focus on the most dominant language.

- Many standardized tests of aphasia are biased against CLD patients. Instead of using test norms, clinicians can evaluate a normal, healthy family member using a standardized test. That performance can then be used as an appropriate standard against which to compare the patient.

- Clinicians should ascertain which is the most appropriate language to use in rehabilitation of CLD clients. Factors impacting this decision include:

  - the patient's premorbid language history
  - the availability of an interpreter
  - the patient's abilities (both oral and written) in each language
  - whether the patient will return to a home or work setting

- For clients with swallowing disorders, clinicians must ascertain their food preferences and possible religious restrictions pertaining to consumption of food and beverages (Tonkovich, 2002). For example, during the month of Ramadan, many Muslims do not take food or liquid between sunrise and sunset.

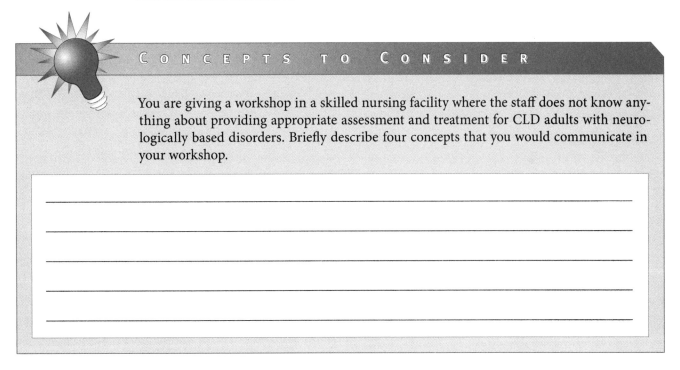

CONCEPTS TO CONSIDER

You are giving a workshop in a skilled nursing facility where the staff does not know anything about providing appropriate assessment and treatment for CLD adults with neurologically based disorders. Briefly describe four concepts that you would communicate in your workshop.

_____

_____

_____

_____

_____

SUMMARY

✓ A CLD child is considered to have an LLD only if he or she has language-learning difficulties that underlie both the primary language and English.

✓ CLD children in the schools who manifest LLD can be served through a variety of service delivery models. Treatment activities for these children should be culturally appropriate and should assist the children in becoming effective communicators in their environments. Family involvement is critical.

✓ Adults with neurologically based communication disorders, such as those resulting from strokes, may recover their languages in various ways after the stroke. Clinicians should be sensitive to these clients' bilingual status and the way it affects recovery.

✓ Assessment and treatment should occur in the patient's strongest language, if possible. Treatment must be functional for the individual patient's environment and appropriate for his or her cultural background.

CHAPTER HIGHLIGHTS

◆ **THE INCREASING NUMBERS OF** culturally and linguistically diverse (CLD) people in the United States have created a great need for speech–language pathologists to develop cultural sensivity and knowledge about how to best provide appropriate service delivery. ASHA has developed guidelines and policies regarding optimal service delivery to people from multicultural backgrounds.

◆ **SPEAKERS OF AFRICAN AMERICAN** English, Spanish, and the Asian languages manifest unique phonological, morphological, semantic, and syntactic characteristics and patterns that differ from those of Standard American English. These characteristics and patterns are indicative not of a disorder but of a difference.

◆ **IT IS IMPORTANT TO** take into account the influence of the primary language or dialect so that CLD clients are not misdiagnosed as having a language disorder. Some CLD individuals may choose to participate in elective speech–language therapy so that they may improve their Standard American English skills for vocational and other purposes.

◆ **A GREAT CHALLENGE FOR** speech–language pathologists is to differentiate between language differences and language-learning disabilities (LLDs) in children who speak more than one language. Frequently, there is a mismatch between the skills and abilities these children bring to the schools and the schools' expectations of these children. This mismatch often creates deficits in CLD students who have normal underlying language-learning ability.

◆ **PART OF ACCURATELY DIFFERENTIATING** between a language difference and an LLD is knowledge of normal second-language acquisition processes. The processes of interference, the silent period, codeswitching, and language loss can appear to be symptoms of an LLD; however, these processes are normal and common. The fact of whether children are developing a second language simultaneously with or sequentially to the first language also has an impact on development.

◆ **CLD CHILDREN LEARNING A** second language manifest different types of language proficiency. In ideal learning situations, basic interpersonal communication skills (BICS) take approximately 2 years to develop to a native-like level; cognitive–academic language proficiency (CALP) takes 5–7 years to develop to a native-like level. Awareness of the differences between these types of language proficiency can help clinicians not to misdiagnose CLD children as

CHAPTER HIGHLIGHTS

having underlying LLDs when, in fact, these children are following a normal time line of English-language development.

◆ **FEDERAL LAW MANDATES THAT** assessment of CLD children be fair, nondiscriminatory, and conducted in the children's most proficient language. Because most clinicians use standardized tests normed on English-speaking children, fair and nonbiased assessment of CLD children is a great challenge.

◆ **CLINICIANS CAN MAKE ALTERATIONS** in standardized testing to make testing less biased. Optimally, however, clinicians should use nonstandardized, informal assessment measures such as dynamic assessment, questionnaires administered to adults who are familiar with the child's daily communicative functioning, and language samples. Utilizing the services of well-trained interpreters can also be very helpful.

◆ **SOME CLD STUDENTS HAVE** underlying language-learning disabilities; they are not able to learn any language adequately. A number of service delivery options are available for these children. Treatment methods and activities should focus on improving functional communication, literacy, and knowledge of school curriculum and language, and should be culturally appropriate. It is imperative to include families in the treatment process.

◆ **CLD ADULTS TEND, AS** a group, to be more predisposed to strokes than the general population. This is due to such related factors as diabetes, hypertension, and arteriosclerosis. CLD adults may show various patterns of stroke recovery depending on which languages they speak. Assessment and treatment of CLD adults with neurologically based communication disorders must consider many variables, such as family support, religious beliefs, educational and vocational background, socioeconomic status, and other sociocultural variables.

✎ **ADD YOUR OWN CHAPTER HIGHLIGHTS HERE:**

_____

_____

_____

Study & Review Questions

Essay

1. Define the term *cultural competence*. How does a speech–language pathologist become culturally competent?

2. Describe three misconceptions about African American English and children who use African American English. How might these misconceptions impact assessment and intervention for these children?

3. What is the difference between BICS and CALP? What kinds of mistakes might a speech–language pathologist make if she assessed a CLD child for LLD without knowing the difference between these types of language proficiency?

4. Describe disadvantages of using standardized tests with CLD students who are suspected of LLD. What are some alternative forms of assessment that are more valid for these students?

5. Describe two principles of appropriate service delivery to older CLD patients with neurogenic or swallowing disorders.

Multiple Choice

6. Xu Fang is a 7-year-old girl in an all-English-speaking second-grade classroom. Xu's parents immigrated from mainland China 8 years ago; Xu was born in the United States. She came to an all-English kindergarten speaking only Mandarin; kindergarten was her first exposure to English on a regular basis. Xu had no prior preschool experience in either Mandarin or English. The second-grade teacher has referred Xu for a speech–language evaluation because he says that although she interacts well with her English-speaking classmates on the playground, she is "behind" her classmates in written language skills (e.g., spelling, reading). Based on Xu's background, you can state that:

   A. because basic interpersonal communication skills (BICS) take approximately 2 years to develop to a native-like level, Xu is developing on an appropriate time line.
   B. because cognitive–academic language proficiency (CALP) takes approximately 5–7 years to develop to a native-like level, it can be expected that Xu will lag somewhat behind English-speaking peers in written language skills.
   C. because Xu has been in an all-English-speaking classroom setting for at least 2 years, her written language skills should be more developed than they are. Her difficulties are a red flag, and a speech–language assessment should be conducted.
   D. A, C
   E. A, B

7. A teacher has referred Isaiah Brown to you for an evaluation. Isaiah is an African American kindergar-tener who is reportedly doing well in class academically. When you observe him on the playground with his peers, you see that he has many friends and does not appear to have problems interacting appropri-ately with other children. Isaiah's friends do not appear to have any difficulty understanding what he says. However, the teacher is concerned because "I think Isaiah pronounces some of his sounds wrong. I think he needs speech therapy." When you conduct a speech screening with Isaiah, you will remember: Which of the following are normal variations of African American English, not a sign of a disorder?

   A. f/th substitution in word-final position
   B. production of [æks] instead of [æsk]
   C. w/r substitution in all word positions
   D. A, B
   E. A, B, C

8. A classroom teacher refers a 9-year-old African American male student to you because she is concerned about his intelligibility. This teacher is anxious to avoid the mistake of mislabeling this student as having a "speech disorder" if he is merely manifesting characteristics of African American English. When you screen the boy, you find that he makes the following substitutions: d/m, t/n, f/n. You would:

   A. let the classroom teacher work with the student because this is such a mild problem.
   B. do nothing, knowing that boys mature more slowly than girls.
   C. do nothing, realizing that this is normal for speakers of African American English.
   D. treat the student, because this is a sign of an articulatory-phonological disorder involving denasalization of nasals.
   E. none of the above

9. In an adolescent speaker of African American English, which of the following utterances would be an example of the use of the perfective construction "been," indicating an action that took place in the distant past?

   A. "I been had a marble collection when I was 7."
   B. "Our family been gonna do it."
   C. "I might been coulda done it."
   D. "He been done it again."
   E. "They be cookin' a barbecue."

10. Consuela is a Mexican-American Spanish-speaking 6-year-old girl who is in the process of learning Eng-lish. Her parents immigrated from Mexico three years ago; thus, Consuela was exposed first to Spanish at home and was exposed to English in kindergarten at the age of 5 years and 3 months of age. Consuela's mother tells you that during the summer before kindergarten, Consuela attended an English-speaking preschool. The classroom teacher shares that she thinks Consuela may have an articulation disorder, but the teacher is not sure. The teacher provides you with some examples of things that Consuela has said in the past two to three weeks. As you look at these examples, which one of the following would NOT be typical for her in terms of predictable productions based on Spanish influence?

   A. t/th substitutions in word-initial positions (e.g., *tin/thin*)
   B. devoicing of final consonants (e.g., *beece/bees*)
   C. v/f substitutions in word-initial and word-final positions (e.g., *vine/fine; roove/roof*)
   D. y/j substitutions (e.g., *yava/java*)
   E. insertion of the schwa before word-initial s-clusters (e.g., *esleep/sleep*)

11. Which of the following is/are predictable productions for speakers of Asian languages?

    A. "He be going to bed now."   D. A, B
    B. "I see cat the little."   E. B, C
    C. "Yesterday she cook a pot of soup."

12. A 74-year-old bilingual Asian gentleman has had a stroke, and you are seeing him for therapy. He is recovering both his primary language and his English skills, but you are working only in English. There are no interpreters available, unfortunately, and the family has indicated that they would prefer treatment to be conducted in English anyway since many of the patient's grandchildren speak English fluently. Which of the following productions would be examples, on the patient's part, of English influenced by his primary language and not the stroke?

    A. "They coming over here now."
    B. "I done got to eat breakfast now."
    C. "She have no dollar in her purse."
    D. A, B, C
    E. A, C

13. A high school teacher refers a Japanese-speaking 10th grader, Kosuke, to you for an evaluation. Kosuke and his family have been in the United States for two years; the father was brought to the United States for a three-year computer project in a major American city. The family will be returning to Japan next year. Kosuke's teacher says that although he is doing well academically, he is "hard to understand sometimes." She says that the other students don't make fun of Kosuke, but they do seem to not always follow what he is saying. The teacher wonders if Kosuke could benefit from intervention for an "articulation disorder." You conduct a screening. Which of the following articulatory-phonological characteristics might be predictable based on Kosuke's first language of Japanese?

    A. substitution of a/ae (e.g., *sock/sack, fong/fang*)
    B. final-consonant deletion (e.g., *be-/bed, po-/pot*)
    C. r/l confusion (e.g., *laise/raise, clown/crown*)
    D. B, C
    E. A, B, C

14. Which one of the following is NOT TRUE according to the Individuals with Disabilities Education Act?

    A. Testing must be administered in a way that is not racially or culturally discriminatory.
    B. Testing and evaluation materials must always be provided and administered in the child's primary language.
    C. Testing must be administered to a bilingual child so as to reflect accurately the child's ability in the area tested, rather than reflecting limited English-language skill.
    D. Mandatory consent in the primary language is required.
    E. Multicultural education is to be considered in guaranteeing equal educational opportunities for minorities with disabilities.

15. A teacher has referred a third-grade boy to you for a speech–language assessment. She is concerned because she feels that he is academically "behind his peers." He and his family are Cambodian refugees, and they have been in the United States for eight months. Because the boy has been in refugee camps most of his life, his schooling in Cambodia was quite limited. His parents tell you that they estimate that he has had approximately 1.5 years of schooling in Cambodia. The teacher is concerned that the boy may have an underlying language-learning disability, and she wonders if he is eligible for speech–language services. What would be the best combination of assessment techniques to use with him?

A. dynamic assessment, language samples in Cambodian, and observations of his interaction with family members and other Cambodian children

B. use of the *Peabody Picture Vocabulary Test–Revised* and *Test of Language Development–P:3* translated into Cambodian, dynamic assessment, and language samples in Cambodian

C. use of a district-developed test for Cambodian students in your geographic area and administration of questionnaires to the boy's teachers and family

D. use of school records of the boy's achievement and performance so far in the English-speaking classroom and use of the *Language Processing Test* translated into Cambodian by an interpreter

E. use of formal, standardized tests in English combined with observations of the boy's interactions, in Cambodian, with peers and family members

16. You are working in a school district where there is an influx of immigrants from Russia. These immigrants have come to your area because there are Russian churches that have sponsored them. In the last few years, over 50,000 Russian families have moved in. Teachers are beginning to refer some Russian students to you for assessment for "language-learning disability," saying that the students are "not learning English fast enough." You consult with the pastor of a local Russian church. Pastor Soldantenkov is very highly regarded in his community, and you share with him the stories of some of the students who have been referred to you. As he listens, Pastor Soldantenkov tells you that many families in his church had difficulty leaving Russia and, though they now live in the United States, still want to limit their interactions with Americans as much as possible. Many parents wish to "preserve the Russian language and culture" and want to limit their children's exposure to English and American culture in general. Which of the following can you NOT conclude about the Russian students referred to you based on your conversation with Pastor Soldantenkov?

A. It is possible that instead of having language-learning disabilities, these students are normal language learners who have had limited assimilation into American mainstream society.

B. The families of these students who have been referred to you are bicultural, and this is part of the problem that the students are having in school.

C. The families of these students have limited acculturation into American life, and this factor may be influencing the students' performance in school.

D. The reluctance of the families to assimilate into American culture might be a factor that is influencing the students' interaction with other students who are native speakers of English, and this may be related to the Russian students' learning English more slowly.

E. The Russian families that these students come from prefer to not become bicultural, choosing instead to maintain as many aspects of their own language and culture as possible without assimilating into American culture.

17. A monolingual English-speaking speech–language pathologist is working in a Head Start in a city with many CLD children. In the last year, CLD children from over 15 different cultural and linguistic groups have come to the Head Start speaking only their primary languages. The ideal plan for dealing with the needs of these children is to:

A. encourage them not to speak their primary languages and to speak English as much and as quickly as possible.

B. tolerate the children's use of their primary languages and speak to them solely in English, hoping that they will eventually "pick up" English and discontinue using their primary languages.

C. hire bilingual aides from the neighboring communities and use them to help the children maintain their primary languages and learn English also.

D. hire aides who only speak the children's primary languages and not English so that the children will be in the ideal situation to maintain their primary languages.

E. assume that these children probably have language-learning disabilities in their primary languages and hire bilingual speech–language pathologists to assist in remediation.

18. A teacher refers Jose E. to you for a speech–language evaluation. Jose, a Puerto Rican American second grader who speaks both Spanish and English with equal fluency, transferred to your school district three months ago from another district in your state. In his previous district, Jose was in a bilingual classroom where his primary language of Spanish was maintained and he was exposed to English also. According to Jose's report card from the previous district, "Jose does well speaking both Spanish and English. I [the teacher] think he is beginning to show a preference for English. Jose is performing adequately in all academic areas." The second-grade teacher at your school, who teaches only in English, feels that after three months in her classroom, "Jose is catching on slowly. I wonder if he needs special education." Your best course of action would be to:

A. ask Jose's parents to sign a permission form so that he may be assessed immediately in English using only English tests since English is apparently beginning to be Jose's preferred language.

B. use a variety of English screening instruments to screen Jose's English ability because these instruments are ecologically valid for Jose.

C. do nothing at the present time and tell the teacher that you will wait for six months to see how Jose progresses in her classroom.

D. use a dynamic assessment model to evaluate Jose's language-learning ability and combine this with classroom observations over the next two to three months to evaluate his progress.

E. ask the district to send you a bilingual Spanish-speaking speech–language pathologist who can evaluate Jose because you are sure that he has a language disorder.

19. Mr. Nehru is a gentleman from India who has had a stroke and now has aphasia. His family reports that before the stroke, he spoke both Hindi and English fluently. In planning for therapy, you as a monolingual English-speaking speech–language pathologist think about the possibility of incorporating work on English idioms. Which of the following do you need to consider in terms of whether or not to make comprehension and expression of English idioms a treatment goal?

A. Mr. Nehru's oral and written abilities in both English and Hindi

B. your own interest in English idioms and whether or not you consider them important in therapy for a stroke patient

C. whether Mr. Nehru will return to his work setting, where his colleagues speak English, or whether he will now spend all of his time at home, where his family speaks primarily Hindi

D. A, B, C

E. A, C

20. A speech–language pathologist is new in a district that has a preponderance of CLD students. He finds that when he assesses the communication skills of these students, he will need to mostly work with interpreters because bilingual speech–language pathologists who speak the students' languages (e.g., Ukrainian, Tagalog, Farsi, Urdu, Ibo) are not available. What will this speech–language pathologist have to remember NOT to do when working with an interpreter in an assessment situation?

A. avoid giving the interpreter information about the student before the assessment session, because this might bias the interpreter in a negative or positive direction about the student's abilities

B. show the interpreter how to use the assessment instruments and make sure the interpreter is comfortable with using them

C. supervise the interpreter during the assessment session and watch for possible inappropriate behaviors such as prompting the student or giving too many clues

D. ask the interpreter to write down all behaviors observed, even if these behaviors appear extraneous to the immediate task

E. ensure that the interpreter does not overprotect the student by hiding the extent of the student's limitations (if they exist)

REFERENCES AND RECOMMENDED READINGS

American Speech-Language-Hearing Association Joint Subcommittee of the Executive Board on English Language Proficiency. (1998). Students and professionals who speak English with accents and nonstandard dialects: Issues and recommendations. Position statement and technical report. *Asha, 40* (Suppl. 18), 28–31.

American Speech-Language-Hearing Association. (2001a). Focused initiative: Culturally/linguistically diverse populations. *Asha* (Suppl. 21), 9.

American Speech-Language-Hearing Association. (2001b). *Guide to speech–language pathology assessment tools for multicultural and bilingual populations.* Rockville, MD: Author.

American Speech-Language-Hearing Association. (2002). 2002 omnibus survey. Rockville, MD: Author.

Andrews, M. M., & Boyle, J. S. (2003). *Transcultural concepts in nursing care* (4th ed.). Philadelphia: Lippincott Williams & Wilkins.

Arambula, G. (1992). Acquired neurological disabilities in Hispanic adults. In H. Langdon (Ed.) with L. L. Cheng, *Hispanic children and adults with communication disorders: Assessment and intervention* (pp. 373–407). Gaithersburg, MD: Aspen Publishers.

Battle, D. E. (Ed.). (2002). *Communication disorders in multicultural populations* (3rd ed.). Woburn, MA: Butterworth-Heinemann.

Bliss, L. S. (2002). *Discourse impairments: Assessment and intervention applications.* Boston: Allyn & Bacon.

Bloom, L., & Lahey, M. (1978). *Language development and language disorders.* New York: John Wiley.

Brice, A. (2002). (Ed.). *The Hispanic child: Speech, language, culture and education.* Boston: Allyn & Bacon.

Brice, A., & Anderson, R. (1999). Code mixing in a young bilingual child. *Communication Disorders Quarterly, 21,* 17–22.

Brice, A., & Roseberry-McKibbin, C. (1999). Turning frustration into success for English language learners. *Educational Leadership, 56,* 53–55.

Camarota, S. A. (2003). *Immigration in a time of recession: An examination of trends since 2000.* Retrieved July 23, 2004, from http://www.cis.org/articles/2003/back16003.html.

Campbell, L. R. (1993). Maintaining the integrity of home linguistic varieties: Black English vernacular. *American Journal of Speech–Language Pathology, 2,* 85–86.

Campbell, L. R. (1996). Issues in service delivery to African American children. In A. G. Kamhi, K. E. Pollock, & J. L. Harris (Eds.), *Communication development and disorders in African American children: Research and intervention* (pp. 73–94). Baltimore: Paul H. Brookes.

Cheng, L. L. (2002). Asian and Pacific American cultures. In D. E. Battle (Ed.), *Communication disorders in multicultural populations* (3rd ed., pp. 71–112). Woburn, MA: Butterworth-Heinemann.

Chong, N. (2002). *The Latino patient: A cultural guide for health care providers.* Yarmouth, ME: Intercultural Press.

Coleman, T. (2000). *Clinical management of communication disorders in culturally diverse children.* Boston: Allyn & Bacon.

Craig, H. K., Thompson, C. A., Washington, J. A., & Potter, S. L. (2004). Performance of elementary-grade African American students on the Gray Oral Reading Tests. *Language, Speech, and Hearing Services in Schools, 34,* 141–154.

Cummins, J. (1992). The role of primary language development in promoting educational success for language minority students. In C. Leyba (Ed.), *Schooling and language minority students: A theoretical framework* (pp. 3–50). Los Angeles: California State University.

Cummins, J. (2002). Foreword. In P. Gibbons, *Scaffolding language, scaffolding learning: Teaching second language learners in the mainstream classroom.* (pp. 2–4) Portsmouth, NH: Heinemann.

Galanti, G. (2004). *Caring for patients from different cultures* (3rd ed.). Philadelphia: University of Pennsylvania Press.

Genesee, F., Paradis, J., & Crago, M. B. (2004). *Dual language development and disorders.* Baltimore: Paul H. Brookes.

Glennen, S. (2002). Language development and delay in internationally adopted infants and toddlers: A review. *American Journal of Speech–Language Pathology, 11,* 333–339.

Goldstein, B. (2000). *Cultural and linguistic diversity resource guide for speech–language pathologists.* San Diego, CA: Singular/Thomson Learning.

Goldstein, B. (Ed.) (2004). *Bilingual language development and disorders in Spanish-English speakers.* Baltimore: Paul H. Brookes.

Gutierrez-Clellen, V. (1999). Language choice in intervention with bilingual children. *American Journal of Speech–Language Pathology, 8,* 291–302.

Hammer, C. S., Pennock-Roman, M., Rzasa, S., & Tomblin, B. J. (2002). An analysis of the *Test of Language Development-Primary* for item bias. *American Journal of Speech–Language Pathology, 11,* 274–284.

Huer, M. B., & Saenz, T. I. (2003). Challenges and strategies for conducting survey and focus group research with culturally diverse groups. *American Journal of Speech–Language Pathology, 12,* 209–220.

Hwa-Froelich, D., Hodson, B. W., & Edwards, H. T. (2002). Characteristics of Vietnamese phonology. *American Journal of Speech–Language Pathology, 11,* 264–273.

Individuals with Disabilities Education Act (IDEA; 1997). *Federal Register, Volume 62, No. 204 Part V.* Department of Education, 34 CFR parts 300, 303.

Jacobs, E. L., & Coufal, K. L. (2001). A computerized screening instrument of language learnability. *Communication Disorders Quarterly, 22,* 67–76.

Kayser, H. (2002). Bilingual language development and language disorders. In D. E. Battle (Ed.), *Communication disorders in multicultural populations* (3rd ed., pp. 205–232). Woburn, MA: Butterworth-Heinemann.

Kiernan, B., & Swisher, L. (1990). The initial learning of novel English words: Two single-subject experiments with minority-language children. *Journal of Speech and Hearing Research, 33*(4), 707–716.

Kindler, A. L. (2002). *Survey of the states' limited English proficient students and available educational programs and resources:*

2000–2001 summary report. Washington, DC: National Clearinghouse for English Language Acquisition and Language Instruction Educational Programs.

Klein, H. B., & Moses, N. (1999). *Intervention planning for children with communication disorders: A guide for clinical practicum and professional practice* (2nd ed.). Needham Heights, MA: Allyn & Bacon.

Kohnert, K. & Derr, A. (2004). Language intervention with bilingual children. In B.A. Goldstein (Ed.), Bilingual language development and disorders in Spanish-English speakers (pp. 311–338). Baltimore: Paul H. Brookes.

Kohnert, K. J., Kennedy, M. R. T., Glaze, L., Kan, P., & Carney, E. (2003). Breadth and depth of diversity in Minnesota: Challenges to clinical competence. *American Journal of Speech–Language Pathology, 12,* 73–91.

Kritikos, E. P. (2003). Speech–language pathologists' beliefs about language assessment of bilingual/bicultural individuals. *American Journal of Speech–Language Pathology, 12,* 73–91.

Laing, S. P., & Kamhi, A. (2003). Alternative assessment of language and literacy in culturally and linguistically diverse populations. *Language, Speech, and Hearing Services in Schools, 34,* 44–55

Langdon, H. W., & Cheng, L. L. (2002). *Collaboratiing with interpreters and translators: A guide for communication disorders professionals.* Eau Claire, WI: Thinking Publications.

Long, S. (2005). Language and linguistically-culturally diverse children. In V. A. Reed, *An introduction to children with language disorders* (3rd ed., pp. 301–334). Boston: Allyn & Bacon.

Lynch, E. W., & Hanson, M. J. (2004). *Developing cross-cultural competence: A guide for working with young children and their families* (3rd ed.). Baltimore: Paul H. Brookes.

Madding, C. C. (2002). Socialization practices of Latinos. In A. E. Brice (Ed.), *The Hispanic child: Speech, language, culture and education* (pp. 68–84). Boston: Allyn & Bacon.

McGregor, K., Williams, D., Hearst, S., & Johnson, A. C. (1997). The use of contrastive analysis in distinguishing difference from disorder: A tutorial. *American Journal of Speech–Language Pathology, 6*(3), 45–56.

Moore-Brown, B., & Montgomery, J. K. (2001). *Making a difference for America's children: Speech–language pathologists in public schools.* Eau Claire, WI: Thinking Publications.

Paradis, J., Crago, M., Genesee, F., & Rice, M. (2003). French-English bilingual children with SLI: how do they compare with their monolingual peers? Journal of Speech-Language-Hearing Research, 46, 113–127.

Payne-Johnson, J. (1992). Communications and aging: A case for understanding African-Americans who are elderly. *Asha, 34,* 41–44.

Pearson, C. M. (2001). Internationally adopted children: Issues and challenges. *The ASHA Leader, 6,* 4–13.

Perozzi, J., & Sanchez, M.L.C. (1992). The effect of instruction in L1 on receptive acquisition of L2 for bilingual children with language delay. *Language, Speech, and Hearing Services in Schools, 23*(4), 352–358.

Ray, J. (2002). Treating phonological disorders in a multilingual child: A case study. *American Journal of Speech–Language Pathology, 11,* 305–315.

Reyes, B. A. (1995). Considerations in the assessment and treatment of neurogenic disorders in bilingual adults. In H. Kayser (Ed.), *Bilingual speech–language pathology: An Hisopanic focus* (pp. 153–181). San Diego, CA: Singular Publishing Group.

Roseberry-McKibbin, C. (1993). *Bilingual classroom communication profile.* Oceanside, CA: Academic Communication Associates.

Roseberry-McKibbin, C. (2001). *The source for bilingual children with language disorders.* East Moline, IL: LinguiSystems.

Roseberry-McKibbin, C. (2002). *Multicultural students with special language needs: Practical strategies for assessment and intervention* (2nd ed.). Oceanside, CA: Academic Communication Associates.

Roseberry-McKibbin, C. (2003). *Assessment of bilingual learners: Language difference or language disorder?* [video] Rockville Pike, MD: The American Speech–Language-Hearing Association.

Roseberry-McKibbin, C. (2007). *Introduction to language disorders in children: A multicultural approach.* Boston: Allyn & Bacon.

Roseberry-McKibbin, C., & Brice, A. (1999). The perception of vocal cues of emotion by Spanish-speaking, limited English proficient children. *Journal of Children's Communication Development, 20*(2), 19–25.

Roseberry-McKibbin, C., Brice, A., & O'Hanlon, L. (2005). Serving English language learners in public school settings: A survey. *Language, Speech, and Hearing Services in Schools, 36,* 48–61.

Schiff-Myers, N. (1992). Considering arrested language development and language loss in the assessment of second language learners. *Language, Speech, and Hearing Services in Schools, 23,* 28–33.

Seymour, H. N., Roeper, T., & DeVilliers, J. (2002). *Diagnostic Evaluation of Language Variation.* San Antonio, TX: The Psychological Corporation.

Smith, T. T., Lee, E. & McDade, H. L. (2001). An investigation of T-units in African-American English-speaking and standard American speaking fourth grade children. *Communication Disorders Quarterly, 22,* 148–157.

Stockman, I. J. (1996). The promises and pitfalls of language sample analysis as an assessment tool for linguistic minority children. *Language, Speech, and Hearing Services in Schools, 27*(4), 355–366.

Sue, D. W., & Sue, D. (2003). *Counseling the culturally diverse: Theory and practice* (4th ed.). New York: John Wiley & Sons.

Terrell, S. L., Battle, D. E., & Grantham, R. (1998). African American cultures. In D. E. Battle (Ed.), *Communication disorders in multicultural populations* (2nd ed., pp. 31–72). Newton, MA: Butterworth-Heinemann.

Thomas-Tate, S., Washington, J., & Edwards, J. (2004). Standardized assessment of phonolgical awareness skills in low-income African American first graders. *American Journal of Speech–Language Pathology, 13,* 182–190.

Tonkovich, J. D. (2002). Multicultural issues in the management of neurgenic communication and swallowing disorders. In D. E. Battle (Ed.), Communication disorders in multicultural populations (3rd ed., pp. 233–266). Woburn, MA: Butterworth-Heinemann.

U.S. Bureau of the Census. (1992). *Statistical abstract of the United States, 1992.* Washington, DC: U.S. Government Printing Office.

U.S. Bureau of the Census. (2000). *Statistical abstract of the United States, 2000* (120th ed.). Washington, DC: U.S. Department of Commerce.

Van Keulen, J. E., Weddington, G. T., & DeBose, C. E. (1998). Speech, language, learning and the African American child. Boston: Allyn & Bacon.

Wallace, G. J. (1998). Adult neurogenic disorders. In D. E. Battle (Ed.), *Communication disorders in multicultural populations* (2nd ed., pp. 309–334). Newton, MA: Butterworth-Heinemann.

Walters, J. (2005). *Bilingualism: The sociopragmatic-psycholinguistic interface.* Mahwah, NJ: Lawrence Erlbaum Associates.

Willis, W. (2004). Families with African American roots. In E. W. Lynch & M. J. Hanson (Eds.), *Developing cross-cultural competence: A guide for working children and their families* (2nd ed., pp. 165–208). Baltimore: Paul H. Brookes.

Wyatt, T. (1998). Language structure and function. In C. M. Seymour & E. H. Nober, *Introduction to communication disorders: A multicultural approach* (pp. 43–58). Newton, MA: Butterworth-Heinemann.

Wyatt, T. (2002). Assessment of the communicative abilities of clients from diverse cultural and language backgrounds. In D. E. Battle (Ed.), *Communication disorders in multicultural populations* (3rd ed., pp. 135–178). Woburn, MA: Butterworth-Heinemann.

Study & Review Answers

6. E. Xu is developing according to an appropriate time line for BICS and CALP.

7. D. Many typically-developing speakers of African American English produce f/th substitutions in word-final position and show metathesis in productions like aks/ask. However, a w/r substitution is not common and probably indicates an articulation problem that is not related to the use of African American English.

8. D. The above-listed substitutions are not commonly found in speakers of African American English, so this student has a disorder involving denasalization of nasals.

9. A. In an adolescent speaker of African American English, the utterance "I been had a marble collection when I was 7" would be an example of the use of the perfective construction "been," indicating an action that took place in the distant past.

10. C. V/f substitions in word-initial and word-final positions (e.g., *vine/fine; roove/roof*) would NOT be typical for a Spanish-speaking 6-year-old girl who is in the process of learning English, in terms of predictable productions based on Spanish influence.

11. C. "Yesterday she cook a pot of soup" would be a predictable utterance for a speaker of most Asian languages. The other utterances would not be predictable based on the influence of any Asian language.

12. E. A 74-year-old Asian gentleman who has had a stroke and is receiving therapy in English could say "They coming over here now" and "She have no dollar in her purse" as English utterances influenced by his primary language and not the stroke.

13. E. Predictable utterances for a Japanese-speaking tenth grader, based on his primary language of Japanese, would be substitutions of a/ae (e.g., *sock/sack, fong/fang*), final consonant deletion (e.g., *be-/bed, po-/pot*), and r/l confusion (e.g., *laise/raise, clown/crown*).

14. B. Testing and evaluation materials must be provided and administered in the child's primary language *or other mode of communication in which the child is most proficient.*

15. A. Practices that are discouraged, in evaluating CLD children, include translated English tests and formal, standardized tests administered in English. A district-developed test for Cambodian students in the geographic location might or might not include subjects who recently immigrated from Cambodia.

16. B. You cannot assume this because immigrants who are *bicultural* are fully involved in both their own and the host culture. They maintain their native language and become fluent in the new language too. They maintain many of their own cultural practices and adopt the host culture's practices as well. They are comfortable going back and forth between their own and the host culture.

17. C. It would be ideal to hire bilingual aides from the neighboring communities and use them to help the children maintain their primary languages and learn English also. Research shows that with children, it is best to maintain and nurture their primary languages and also introduce English so that they (ideally) eventually become proficient bilingual speakers.

18. D. Use a dynamic assessment model to evaluate Jose's language-learning ability and combine this with classroom observations over the next two to three months to evaluate his progress. Assessing Jose in English only is not valid, and English screening instruments are not ecologically valid for Jose. It is inappropriate at this point to assume that Jose has a language disorder; thus, it is too soon to call a Spanish-speaking speech–language pathologist. It would be best to assess his ability to learn language and to observe him in the classroom for the next few months to see whether or not he progresses appropriately. If he does not, then the bilingual speech–language pathologist can undertake a formal evaluation of Jose's Spanish and English skills.

19. E. The answer is both A and C. You need to consider Mr. Nehru's Hindi and English oral and written abilities as well as whether he will return to his work setting, where his colleagues speak English, or whether he will now spend all of his time at home, where his family speaks primarily Hindi. Your own preferences as a monolingual English-speaking speech–language pathologist are secondary to Mr. Nehru's needs and individual situation.

20. A. It is very important for speech–language pathologists to give interpreters information about students before the assessment session so that the interpreters will be well prepared.

CHAPTER 10

AUDIOLOGY AND

HEARING DISORDERS

It is estimated that in the United States, the prevalence of hearing impairment is between 14 and 40 million, depending on the definition of hearing impairment that is used. There are estimated to be approximately 3–4 million children in the United States who are deaf or hard of hearing. *Audiology* is the study of hearing, its disorders, and the measurement and management of those disorders. The birth of the audiology profession occurred during World War II. Many servicemen had impaired hearing and needed rehabilitation; this need gave rise to the profession of audiology.

Audiologists are health-care professionals who provide a comprehensive array of services dealing with diagnosis, treatment, and prevention of hearing impairment and its associated communication disorders. Audiologists work in a variety of settings, such as hospitals or medical center facilities and school settings. Some audiologists work in residential health-care facilities, industry, universities, and other related agencies. Others work in nonresidential health-care facilities, such as physicians' practices, private clinics, and community speech and hearing centers (Stach, 2003).

Audiology as a profession has expanded into new areas of service. These areas include ear canal inspection and cerumen management, neonatal hearing screening, auditory electrophysiology (defined later), and multisensory modality monitoring in operating rooms where patients are undergoing tumor removal (especially nerve VIII tumors).

In the twenty-first century, many universities are offering a professional doctorate in audiology (Au.D.). In this model, students enroll in a 3–4 year program (similar to that required for dentistry and optometry). The early years are primarily devoted to academic training, and the later years to clinical training. At the end of the program, students receive the Au.D. and may practice independently.

The American Speech-Language-Hearing Association (ASHA) and the American Academy of Audiology (AAA) are working to make the Au.D. the entry-level degree for audiologists nationwide. However, across the United States, states vary in their requirements for the Au.D. as the entry-level degree. Most practicing audiologists who do not have the Au.D. are not required to obtain this degree to continue practicing audiology. However, they are not being "grandfathered" in terms of automatically receiving the Au.D. degree just because they are practicing audiologists. In the next 5–10 years, it will be interesting to see the degree to which individual state licensing agencies will comply with the new requirements of ASHA and AAA that the Au.D. be an entry-level degree for audiologists.

ANATOMY AND PHYSIOLOGY OF HEARING

INTRODUCTION

The ear is divided into three sections: the outer ear, the middle ear, and the inner ear. Efficient functioning of these sections of the ear is necessary for normal hearing. However, the auditory nervous system must also be intact in order for sound to be carried to its ultimate destination, the cortex, where it is interpreted.

The Outer Ear

- The outer ear is composed of two parts:

    - the *auricle* or *pinna,* which funnels the sound to the ear canal and helps localize sound (this is the most visible part of the ear and is composed primarily of cartilage)
    - the *external auditory canal* (also called the *external auditory meatus*), which goes from the pinna to the *tympanic membrane* or *eardrum*

- The external auditory canal is a muscular tube, made mostly of cartilage. The tube is not straight but curves slightly like an S. Thus, a specialist who examines the ear canal must first pull the pinna up and back to insert the *otoscope* (an instrument for examining the ear) into the canal.

- The external auditory canal is, on the average, approximately 2.5 cm (1 inch) long and resonates the sound that enters it. The canal ends at the tympanic membrane, or eardrum.

- The external auditory canal has special cells that secrete wax or *cerumen.* The functions of cerumen include lubricating and cleansing the canal, and protecting the ear from fungi, bacteria, and small insects (Gelfand, 2001).

The Middle Ear

■ The middle ear is an air-filled cavity. It is separated from the outer ear by the tympanic membrane.

■ The three small bones in the middle ear form the ossicular chain.

■ The eustachian tube connects the middle ear to the nasopharynx.

Tympanic Membrane

- The *tympanic membrane* is elastic, thin, and cone-shaped. It is flexible and tough and vibrates in response to sound pressure. The entire tympanic membrane responds to low-frequency sounds, but only certain portions respond to high-frequency sounds.
- It is easy to damage the tympanic membrane. It can be ruptured by a Q-tip, hairpin, or other object inserted into the ear. Explosions and sudden pressure changes can also rupture the tympanic membrane.
- A damaged or punctured tympanic membrane may heal spontaneously. However, repeated ruptures cause scar tissue, which reduces the tympanic membrane's mobility.

Ossicular Chain

- The *ossicular chain,* suspended in the middle ear by ligaments, is composed of three tiny bones: the malleus, incus, and stapes.
- The first and largest of the three bones is called the *malleus* (Latin for *hammer*) because it resembles a hammer. One end of the malleus is embedded in the tympanic membrane. Because of this attachment, the vibrations of the tympanic membrane are transmitted to the malleus.
- The malleus is attached to the second bone, which is called the *incus* (Latin for *anvil*). The malleus and incus are connected in a tight joint that permits very little movement.
- The incus is attached to the third bone, called the *stapes* (Latin for *stirrup*). The footplate, or other end of the stapes, is inserted into the oval window, a small opening that leads to the inner ear.
- The ossicular chain transmits sound efficiently and with no distortion. It also amplifies incoming sound by approximately 30 dB before transmitting it into the fluids of the inner ear.

Muscles and Reflexes

- Two small muscles in the middle ear dampen the vibrations of the tympanic membrane and the ossicular chain: the tensor tympani and the stapedius muscles.
- The *tensor tympani* is innervated by cranial nerve V (the trigeminal nerve). The *stapedius* muscle, the smallest in the body, is innervated by cranial nerve VII (the facial nerve).
- The stapedius muscle stiffens the ossicular chain so that its vibrations are reduced. The tensor tympani muscle tenses the tympanic membrane so that its vibrations are reduced.
- When a person hears very loud noises that could damage the ears, the middle ear muscles contract in a reflexive action called the *acoustic reflex.* The acoustic reflex stiffens the middle ear system, especially the tympanic membrane.

Eustachian Tube

- Also known as the auditory tube, the *eustachian tube* connects the middle ear with the nasopharynx. The eustachian tube goes from the anterior middle ear wall to the posterior wall of the nasopharynx.
- The eustachian tube helps maintain equal air pressure within and outside the middle ear. The nasopharyngeal end of the tube can be opened by yawning or swallowing. This ventilates the middle ear by letting in fresh air.
- The *tensor veli palatini,* along with the *levator veli palatini,* is one of two muscles of the nasopharynx responsible for opening the end of the eustachian tube (Stach, 2003).
- The eustachian tube can also allow germs and infections to spread into the middle ear, causing hearing problems. This is especially common in infants, whose eustachian tubes are more horizontal than those of adults.
- Infants with a cleft of the palate frequently have eustachian tube dysfunction, making them vulnerable to conductive hearing loss (described later).

CONCEPTS TO CONSIDER

List and briefly describe the key anatomic components of the middle and inner ear.

_____

_____

_____

_____

_____

The Inner Ear

- The *inner ear* is the most complex of the three divisions of the ear. It begins with the *oval window,* which is a small opening in the *temporal bone* that houses the inner ear. Through the movement of the footplate of the stapes in the oval window, the inner ear receives the mechanical vibrations of sound.

- The inner ear is a system of interconnecting tunnels called *labyrinths* within the temporal bone. The tunnels are filled with a fluid called *perilymph.*

- There are two major structures in the inner ear, each with separate functions. The first is the *vestibular system,* which contains three *semicircular canals.* The semicircular canals are responsible for equilibrium. Thus, the vestibular system is related to movement, balance, and body posture.

- The second major structure in the inner ear is the *cochlea.* The cochlea is snail-shaped and resembles a coiled tunnel. When stretched, the human cochlea measures about 3.8 cm (1.5 inches). It is filled with *endolymph,* a type of fluid.

- The floor of the cochlear duct is called the *basilar membrane,* which contains the *organ of Corti.* The organ of Corti is bathed in endolymph and contains several thousand hair cells or *cilia,* which respond to sound vibrations. Each ear contains approximately 15,500 hair cells.

- The vibrations created by the footplate of the stapes into the oval window create wavelike movements in the perilymph. Through *Reissner's membrane,* those movements are transmitted to the endolymph. The endolymph then transmits the movements to the basilar membrane.

- Different portions of the basilar membrane respond best to sounds of different frequencies. The tip of the membrane is thicker, wider, and more lax than the base.

- At the base, the membrane is thinner, narrower, and stiffer than at the tip. Low-frequency sounds stimulate the tip, and high-frequency sounds stimulate the base. The stimulating sound signals set off waves in the fluid, which in turn create movements of the membrane.

- The hair cells in the organ of Corti respond to the vibrations of the basilar membrane. The vibrations create a shearing force on those cells. At that point, the mechanical forces of vibrations are transformed into electrical energy, which can stimulate nerve endings.

- This energy transformation within the organ of Corti is critical, because the nerve fibers that carry the sound to the brain do not respond to mechanical vibrations—only to electrical impulses.

The Auditory Nervous System

- The nerve that picks up the neural impulses created by the movement of the hair cells in the cochlea is called the *acoustic nerve.* This nerve, also called *cranial nerve VIII,* is a bundle of neurons with two branches.

- The *vestibular branch* is concerned with body equilibrium or balance. The *auditory* or *acoustic branch* supplies many hair cells of the cochlea and conducts electrical sound impulses from the cochlea to the brain.

- The auditory division of the acoustic nerve has many endings in the cochlea. These nerve endings are in contact with the hair cells to pick up the sound vibrations that are transformed into neural impulses.

- Approximately 30,000 nerve fibers of the auditory nerve exist in the cochlea. The auditory nerve exits the inner ear through the *internal auditory meatus.*

- The nerve impulses carried by the right and left auditory pathways enter the brain stem. The auditory pathways up to this point (the brain stem) are considered *peripheral* (related to structures outside the brain). Beyond the brain stem, the pathways are considered *central* (within the brain).

■ At the *cerebellopontine angle,* the auditory nerve exits the temporal bone through the internal auditory meatus and enters the brain stem. At the brain stem level, most of the auditory nerve fibers from one ear *decussate* (cross over) to the opposite side, forming *contralateral* pathways.

■ Some, however, continue on the same side, forming ipsilateral pathways. This crossover of signals allows the brain to compare the sounds received from each of the two ears. It helps the brain localize and interpret sounds.

■ From the brain stem, the acoustic nerve fibers project sound to the temporal lobe of the brain. The temporal lobe contains the primary auditory area, which is responsible for receiving and interpreting sound stimuli. The temporal lobe, with its primary auditory area, is shown in Figure 10.1.

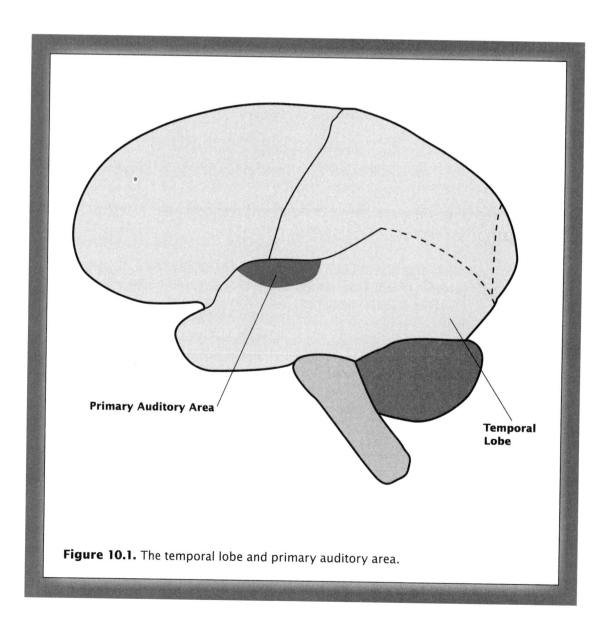

Primary Auditory Area

Temporal Lobe

Figure 10.1. The temporal lobe and primary auditory area.

SUMMARY

✓ The outer ear, composed of the auricle and the pinna, funnels sound to the middle ear. The tympanic membrane, which separates the outer ear from the middle ear, vibrates in response to sound.

✓ Sound is then responded to by the ossicles, which conduct the sound to the inner ear. The vestibular system and cochlea are the major structures of the inner ear. Energy is transformed, in the inner ear, to electrical impulses, which stimulate the acoustic nerve.

✓ The auditory branch of the acoustic nerve carries electrical sound impulses from the cochlea to the brain, where the sound is interpreted in the primary auditory area of the temporal lobe.

ACOUSTICS: SOUND AND ITS PERCEPTION

INTRODUCTION

Acoustics, a branch of physics, is the study of sound as a physical event. *Psychoacoustics* is the study of sound as the psychological experience of hearing. Speech is the most important acoustic signal for humans to perceive. (For a more in-depth discussion of acoustics, see Chapter 2.) Humans perceive sound in terms of frequency (pitch) and intensity (loudness). Hearing can be measured in terms of sound pressure or hearing level.

The Source of Sound

■ The source of sound is mechanical vibrations of an elastic object. The vibrations create waves of disturbance. The waves then travel through a gas, a liquid, or a solid—these are called *mediums.* The mediums must be elastic to carry sound. In order to be called a sound, the disturbance of the molecules must be audible.

■ There are many sources of sound: the vocal folds, the strings of an instrument, a tuning fork, and others. The vibrations of a tuning fork illustrate a source of sound. A tuning fork, when struck, vibrates at a single frequency.

■ Vibrations occur in *cycles,* or repeated patterns of movement that are measured per second. *Frequency* refers to the number of times a cycle of vibration repeats itself within a second. A tone of single frequency is called a *pure tone.* A tone of single frequency that repeats itself is called a *simple harmonic motion.* Two or more sounds of differing frequencies create a *complex tone.*

■ The vibrations that make up a complex tone may be periodic or aperiodic. As illustrated in Figure 10.2, *periodic* vibrations have a pattern that repeats itself at regular intervals. *Aperiodic* vibrations do not have such a pattern; they occur at irregular intervals (Stach, 2003).

Sound Waves

■ When an object such as a guitar string moves back and forth, it displaces nearby air molecules, causing them to move, too. This in turn causes movement in molecules lying farther and farther away from the vibrating object. These movements are called *sound waves.*

Figure 10.2 Periodic and aperiodic sound waves. *Note.* From *Introduction to Communicative Disorders,* 3rd ed. (p. 375), by M. N. Hegde, 2001, Austin, TX: PRO-ED. Copyright 2001 by PRO-ED, Inc. Reprinted with permission.

- The molecules near the vibrating object swing back and forth while remaining where they are (they do not move from one point to another). These swings disturb adjacent molecules, which then swing back and forth, thus disturbing the molecules next to them, and the process continues.

- The to-and-fro movements of the molecules change the air pressure, because the movements consist of an instance in which the molecules are compressed together (*compression*) and an instance in which they are farther apart (*rarefaction*). As Figure 10.3 illustrates, a single cycle consists of one instance of compression and one instance of rarefaction within a second.

- The term *hertz* (Hz) refers to cycles per second. For example, 200 Hz means that there are 200 cycles of compression and rarefaction in 1 second. It means the same thing as 200 cps, or cycles per second.

Frequency and Intensity

- The human ear is capable of responding to frequencies in the range of 20 Hz to 20,000 Hz. Some animals, such as dogs and dolphins, can hear sounds of much higher frequency.

- Variations in the frequency of vibratory cycles cause the sensation of different pitches. *Pitch* changes are basically changes in frequency. Pitch is the perceptual correlate of changes in frequency. Pitch is perceptual; frequency is physical.

- As well as varying in frequency, sounds vary in *intensity*. Changes in intensity are changes in the *loudness* of sounds. Loudness is a perceptual phenomenon; intensity is a physical phenomenon.

- Intensity is related to *amplitude,* which is the extent of displacement of the molecules in their to-and-fro motion. The greater the range of displacement, the greater the amplitude of the sound. And the greater the amplitude of sound, the greater the intensity of that sound. Tones of different amplitude in the context of different frequencies are illustrated in Figure 10.4.

- The human ear is sensitive to a wide range of intensity—perhaps 10 trillion units as measured on a linear scale that has an absolute zero point and equal numerical increments.

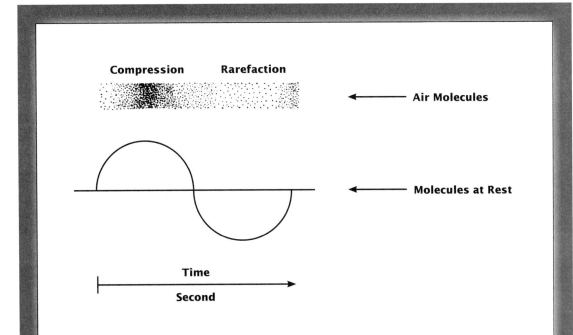

Figure 10.3. A tone of a single Hz (1 cps) containing one instance of rarefaction and one instance of compression of air molecules in 1 second. *Note.* From *Introduction to Communicative Disorders,* 3rd ed. (p. 376), by M. N. Hegde, 2001, Austin, TX: PRO-ED. Copyright 2001 by PRO-ED, Inc. Reprinted with permission.

■ Because measuring these large numbers is cumbersome, scientists use a *logarithmic scale.* On such a scale, one number is multiplied by itself a specified number of times.

■ On a logarithmic scale, the ear is sensitive to 130 units called decibels (dB). A decibel is 1/10 of a bel, the basic unit of sound pressure measurement named after Alexander Graham Bell.

CONCEPTS TO CONSIDER

Define the terms *frequency* and *intensity* as they apply to acoustics.

_____

_____

_____

_____

_____

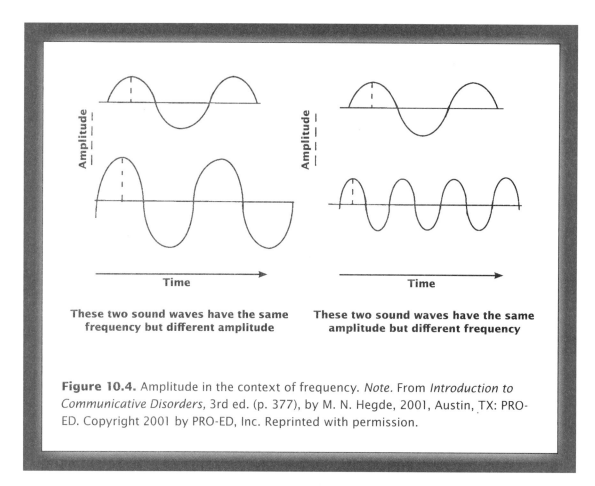

These two sound waves have the same frequency but different amplitude

These two sound waves have the same amplitude but different frequency

Figure 10.4. Amplitude in the context of frequency. *Note.* From *Introduction to Communicative Disorders,* 3rd ed. (p. 377), by M. N. Hegde, 2001, Austin, TX: PRO-ED. Copyright 2001 by PRO-ED, Inc. Reprinted with permission.

Sound Pressure Level and Hearing Level

- The decibel is a measure of sound pressure; it also measures the intensity of one sound against another.

- The value of *sound pressure* is the square root of power, which is measured in *watts.* The pressure is measured in terms of *pascals,* or pa. The intensity of a sound is expressed in terms of decibels at a certain *sound pressure level,* or SPL.

- For example, normal speech usually varies between 50 and 70 dB SPL. Very loud sounds, such as those of an airplane, may be as high as 100 dB SPL. People feel pain when sound level reaches 140 dB SPL.

- SPL is different from *hearing level* (HL), which is the lowest intensity of a sound necessary to stimulate the auditory system. Hearing level is the decibel level used on audiometers; it is the decibel level of sound referenced to audiometric zero (Stach, 2003).

- The auditory system is not equally sensitive to all frequencies at the same intensity. The human ear is most sensitive to sounds ranging between 1,000 and 4,000 Hz. Thus, to stimulate the auditory system, tones of 1,000–4,000 Hz can be less intense than tones of other frequencies. This differential sensitivity of the human ear to different frequencies creates complications in the measurement of hearing and hearing loss.

■ To deal with this problem, scientists first determined sound pressure levels necessary to stimulate the auditory system at different frequencies in a large number of people with normal hearing. Then those sound pressure levels were considered the 0-dB hearing level. For example, to stimulate the healthy normal ear of a young adult, a tone of 250 Hz must have a sound pressure level of 25.5 dB SPL. For the same purpose, a sound of 1,000 Hz needs only 7 dB SPL.

■ In measuring hearing with an audiometer, the actual SPL values needed to stimulate the auditory system of a normal person at those two frequencies were set at 0, although in the case of the 250 Hz tone, the SPL value is higher than in the other tone (1,000 Hz). Similarly, for all the frequencies that are tested on an audiometer, the amount of energy needed to stimulate the auditory system has been set at 0.

SUMMARY

✓ Sound must travel through a medium and create an audible disturbance of molecules in order to be heard. Sound occurs in cycles, each of which consists of one instance of compression and one instance of rarefaction.

✓ Humans hear sounds in various frequencies at various intensity levels and respond differentially to different frequencies. Human responses to sound can be measured by several means, including sound pressure level and hearing level.

THE NATURE AND ETIOLOGY OF HEARING LOSS

INTRODUCTION

The development of hearing begins in utero, where fetuses can respond to sound in the first trimester of development. Babies localize and discriminate sound with increasing skill as they grow older. Sound is conducted to the inner ear through either air or bone conduction. In people with hearing impairment, this process is disrupted through hearing loss of a conductive, sensorineural, or mixed nature. Some people also experience hearing loss due to auditory nervous system impairments.

Normal Hearing

Auditory Development

- Normal hearing is made possible by the complex working of the outer, middle, and inner ear as well as the auditory nerve and auditory areas of the brain. Normal hearing also involves a set of skills that develop over time.
- During the fetal development period, babies can hear in utero—in fact, a 20-week-old fetus responds to sound. Newborns can respond differentially to sounds of different intensity and frequency.
- By 3–4 months of age, babies turn their head toward sources of sound. Three-month-old babies respond to the mother's voice more consistently than to anyone else's voice.
- As babies grow older, they respond more precisely to auditory stimuli. Sounds are better discriminated and localized. By 6 months of age, an infant can localize speech that is very soft.

Young babies with normal hearing can hear better than adults.

Air and Bone Conduction of Sound

- In people with normal hearing, sound is conducted to the inner ear by two means: air conduction and bone conduction.
- In the process of *air conduction,* sound waves strike the tympanic membrane. The movement of the tympanic membrane causes the ossicles to move, creating movement of the fluids of the inner ear. These movements cause vibrations in the basilar membrane of the cochlea.
- The hair cells supplied by the acoustic nerve respond to these vibrations, and the sound is carried to the brain by the acoustic nerve. In this process, sound travels through the medium of air. Thus, the process is described as air conduction.
- The process of *bone conduction* is different. The fluids of the inner ear are housed in the skull. The larger bones of the skull conduct sound, as does the ossicular chain of the middle ear. The skull bones vibrate in response to airborne sound waves, causing movements in the inner ear fluids. Thus, bones have conducted the sound to the inner ear.
- Air and bone conduction result in the same kind of cochlear activity, in which the hair cells are displaced. Normally, air- and bone-conducted movements are integrated. It is only in certain kinds of hearing loss that the two can be distinguished.

Nature of Hearing Impairment

- Hearing impairment is an increasing health and educational problem. Many more people are living longer, manifesting hearing problems associated with the aging process (Tye-Murray, 2004).

- In addition, more newborn babies are at risk for hearing impairment. Advanced medical technology has enabled more fragile, high-risk, preterm infants to be saved; these infants are more vulnerable to hearing problems than healthy, full-term infants are.

- Factors that place a child at risk for hearing loss include anatomic malformations of the head and neck, maternal history of drug or alcohol abuse, certain maternal diseases such as rubella or syphilis during pregnancy, and a family history of childhood hearing impairment.

- Hearing impairment can be very mild, creating few or no problems in communication. It can also be severe to profound, causing major difficulties in articulation, resonance, and comprehension and reception of speech. The range of hearing loss in dB HL and the corresponding categories are shown in Table 10.1.

- The term *hearing impaired* refers to the condition of being hard of hearing or deaf.

- The child who is *hard of hearing* has a loss between 16 and 75 dB; children who are hard of hearing acquire speech and oral language with variable proficiency. The adult who is hard of hearing has a loss between 25 and 75 dB.

- Children and adults who are *deaf* are those who cannot hear or understand conversational speech under normal circumstances. Their hearing loss exceeds 75 dB, and in many cases is greater than 90 dB.

Table 10.1   RANGE AND CATEGORIES OF HEARING LOSS WITH THE CORRESPONDING dB HL

Hearing Loss	Characteristics
Up to 15 dB	Normal hearing in children. In adults the upper limit of normal hearing may extend to 25 dB.
16 to 40 dB	Mild hearing loss in children: difficulty hearing faint or distant speech; may cause language delay in children. In adults the range is between 25 and 40 dB.
41 to 55 dB	Moderate hearing loss: delayed speech and language acquisition; difficulty in producing certain speech sounds correctly; difficulty following conversation.
56 to 70 dB	Moderately severe hearing loss: can understand only amplified or shouted speech.
71 to 90 dB	Severe hearing loss: difficulty understanding even loud and amplified speech; significant difficulty in learning and producing intelligible oral language.
91+ dB	Profound hearing loss: typically described as deaf; hearing does not play a major role in learning, producing, and understanding spoken speech and language.

Note. From *Introduction to Communicative Disorders*, 3rd ed. (p. 385), by M. N. Hegde, 2001, Austin, TX: PRO-ED. Copyright 2001 by PRO-ED, Inc. Reprinted with permission.

■ The term *Deaf* with an upper-case D refers to deafness not as a disability but as a cultural identity (Helfer, 1998).

■ People who have a hearing impairment may have one of several kinds of hearing losses: conductive, sensorineural, or mixed. Some people also manifest central auditory or retrocochlear disorders, which are special categories.

Conductive Hearing Loss

■ In *conductive hearing loss* the efficiency with which the sound is conducted to the middle or inner ear is diminished. In pure conductive hearing loss, the inner ear, acoustic nerve, and auditory centers of the brain are all working normally. The person's bone conduction is also fairly normal (*normal bone conduction* refers to the skull bones, not the ossicular chain).

■ Even when the bones of the ossicular chain are not conducting sound, the bones of the skull do. Thus, conductive hearing loss is never profound; there is always some hearing left because of bone conduction created by the skull bones.

■ Consequently, people with conductive hearing loss can hear their own speech well. Thus, they tend to speak too softly, especially when there is background noise, which they cannot hear as well as their listeners can.

■ There are many causes of conductive hearing loss. These include abnormalities of the external auditory canal, the tympanic membrane, or the ossicular chain of the middle ear.

■ Birth defects, diseases, and foreign bodies can also block the external ear canal. Some children born with cleft palate or other craniofacial anomalies may have *aural atresia,* in which the external ear canal is completely closed. Atresia is often associated with *microtia,* in which the pinna is very small and deformed (Bess & Humes, 2003).

■ Another birth defect, *stenosis,* results in an extremely narrow external auditory canal. In these cases, most sound waves will not strike the tympanic membrane.

■ *External otitis,* caused by bacteria or viruses, is a fairly common infection of the skin of the external auditory canal; this is a cause of conductive loss. This infection, commonly found in swimmers, results in the swelling of the tissue of the external auditory canal. Consequently, sound transmission is reduced.

■ Foreign objects in the ear canal, such as beans, paper clips, and seeds, can block the ear canal and impede hearing. *Bony growths* and tumors may appear in the external ear canal, blocking the transmission of sound to the middle and inner ears.

■ *Otitis media,* also known as *middle ear effusion,* is an infection of the middle ear that is often associated with upper-respiratory infections and eustachian tube dysfunction. Figure 10.5 shows an audiogram representing a typical hearing loss seen in people with otitis media accompanied by effusion.

■ Otitis media occurs frequently in infants and children but rarely in adults. Differences in the incidence rate of otitis media have also been found among racial groups. African Americans have the lowest rate; the highest rates exist among Aborigines, Alaskan Eskimos, and Native Americans. These differences in incidence rates may be related to differences in the structure and function of the eustachian tube among various racial groups (Scott, 1998).

■ Otitis media usually creates a conductive hearing loss of 20–35 dB HL, which often goes undetected by regular pure-tone screenings, which are carried out at 25 dB HL. There are three types of otitis media: serous, acute, and chronic.

■ In *serous otitis media,* the middle ear is inflamed and filled with watery or thick fluid. The eustachian tube is blocked and thus does not allow fresh air to ventilate the middle ear. The middle ear thus becomes airtight; soon the air inside is thinned out and the pressure is reduced.

■ The increased air pressure outside the ear begins to push the tympanic membrane inward, reducing its mobility. The retracted membrane vibrates inefficiently, resulting in conductive hearing loss. Serous otitis media is frequently treated with antibiotics and *pressure equalizing*

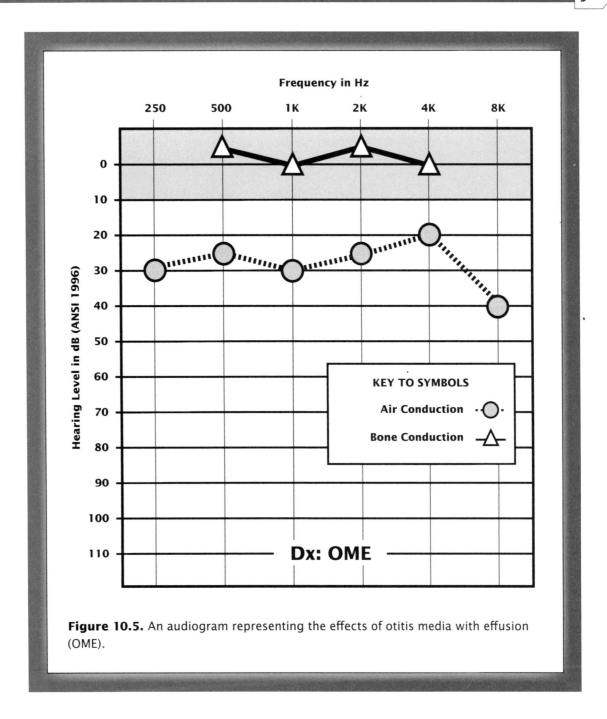

Figure 10.5. An audiogram representing the effects of otitis media with effusion (OME).

(PE) tubes. These tiny tubes are inserted through the tympanic membrane, ventilating the middle ear and restoring hearing.

- In a*cute otitis media,* there is sudden onset due to infection. A quick buildup of fluid and pus causes moderate to severe pain. The child has a fever and may experience vertigo. The buildup of pressure in the middle ear may rupture the tympanic membrane, giving instant relief as pus is discharged from the ruptured membrane.

- Acute otitis media is treated with medical and surgical procedures. In a surgical procedure known as *myringotomy,* small incisions are made in the tympanic membrane to relieve the pressure.

- In *chronic otitis media,* there is permanent damage to middle ear structures. This is frequently due to erosion of ossicles, cholosteotoma, or atrophy or perforation of the tympanic membrane.

- When the tympanic membrane is involved, it is permanently ruptured with or without associated middle ear diseases. Many patients may have a painless, foul-smelling discharge from the ear. Antibiotics may be prescribed if an infection is present. In a surgical procedure known as *myringoplasty,* the perforated tympanic membrane is surgically repaired.

- Mild and nonrecurrent otitis media generally does not cause permanent hearing loss. Permanent loss is more likely to result from chronic disease. However, even mild and fluctuating conductive hearing loss associated with prolonged middle ear infections in young children can adversely affect their speech and language development.

- *Otosclerosis* is another common cause of conductive hearing loss. It may be inherited and is more common in women than in men. It is found primarily among whites worldwide (Scott, 1998).

- In otosclerosis, a new, spongy growth starts on the footplate of the stapes. Consequently, the stapes becomes rigid, and the footplate does not move enough into the oval window to create pressure waves in the inner ear fluid. Figure 10.6 shows an audiogram representing the typical hearing loss seen in people with otosclerosis.

- *Carhart's notch,* frequently found in those patients with otosclerosis, is a pattern of bone-conduction thresholds characterized by reduced bone-conduction sensitivity predominantly at 2,000 Hz (Stach, 2003).

- A disease called *otospongiosis* causes the stapes to become too soft to vibrate. The diseased or fixated stapes is surgically removed in a procedure called a *stapedectomy.* A synthetic prosthesis of wire or Teflon replaces the removed stapes, often dramatically improving hearing postsurgically.

- Other causes of conductive hearing loss include collapsed ear canals, impacted cerumen, ossicular fixation, and disarticulation of the articulatory chain. Figure 10.7 shows an audiogram representing the typical hearing loss seen in people with disarticulation of the articulatory chain, also called *ossicular discontinuity.*

Sensorineural Hearing Loss

- In *sensorineural hearing loss,* the middle ear may conduct the sound efficiently to the inner ear, but damage to the hair cells of the cochlea or to the acoustic nerve prevents the brain from receiving the neural impulses of sound.

- Sensorineural loss is permanent because the damaged hair cells and the acoustic nerve are not repairable. The person with sensorineural loss experiences very mild to profound deafness.

- Bone as well as air conduction is impaired; thus, people with sensorineural loss have difficulty hearing themselves as well as others. This causes them to speak more loudly.

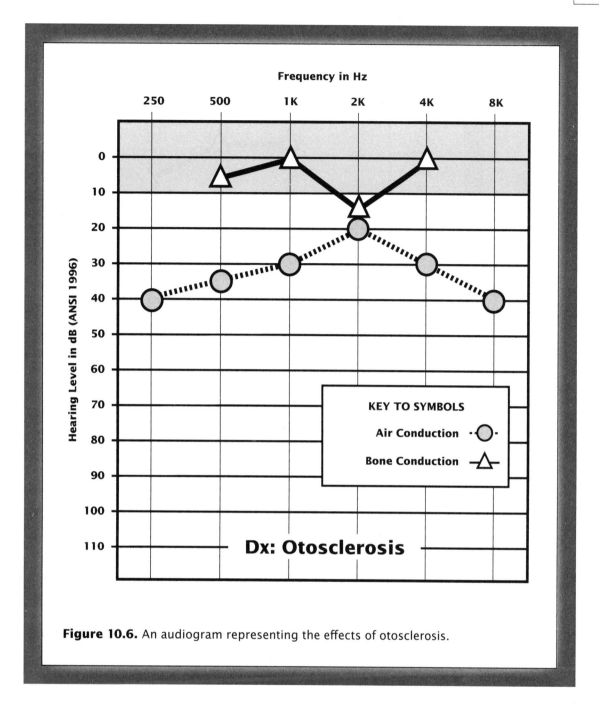

Figure 10.6. An audiogram representing the effects of otosclerosis.

■ Sensorineural loss is not the same across all frequencies; some frequencies are more adversely affected than others. The higher frequencies tend to be more profoundly affected by sensorineural loss than the lower frequencies.

■ A potential symptom of sensorineural hearing loss is recruitment. *Recruitment* refers to a disproportionate increase in the growth of perception of the loudness of sound when it is presented with linear increases in intensity. Recruitment makes a person hypersensitive to intense sounds and must be considered during hearing aid fitting.

■ People with sensorineural hearing loss may experience severe effects on their speech and

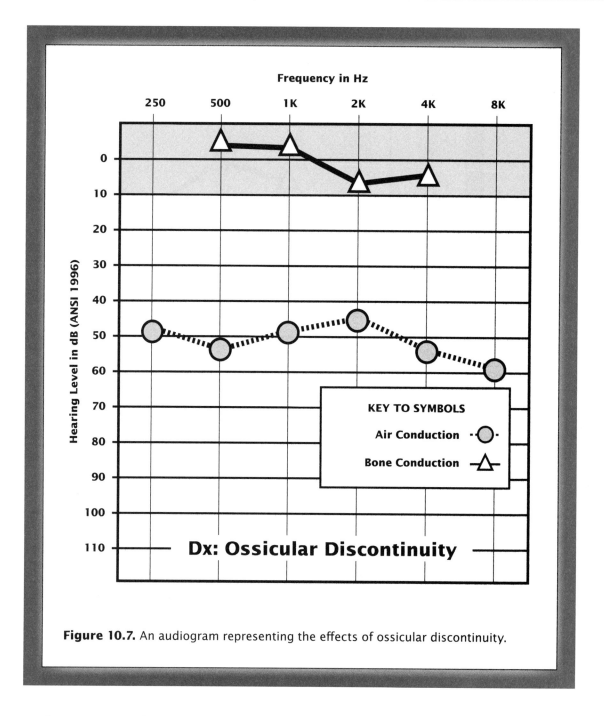

Figure 10.7. An audiogram representing the effects of ossicular discontinuity.

language. Articulation, resonance, and even voice may be affected. There are many causes of sensorineural hearing loss.

■ *Prenatal causes* of hearing loss include events that occur during pregnancy to damage the fetus's hearing. Certain drugs taken by the mother, especially during the 6th and 7th week of pregnancy, can cause cochlear damage in the fetus. In addition, children born to alcohol- and drug-addicted mothers may have sensorineural hearing loss.

■ *Ototoxic* drugs are drugs that reach the inner ear through the bloodstream and damage the cochlear hair cells or the acoustic nerve fibers in children and adults. Antibiotic drugs of the "mycin" family (kanamycin, meomycin, streptomycin) are especially ototoxic.

■ These powerful antibiotics should be used only in cases of severe, life-threatening infections such as those related to kidney malfunctioning. In such cases, profound hearing loss may be an undesirable and unavoidable side effect.

■ *Noise* is another factor that can induce sensorineural hearing loss. Prolonged exposure to intense noises (e.g., loud music, electric drills, airplanes, explosives) usually damages the cochlear hair cells. Noise-induced sensorineural hearing loss tends to be the worst from noise between 3,000 Hz and 6,000 Hz (see Figure 10.8).

■ A healthy, average person should hear normally up until about age 60 years if his or her unprotected ears have not been exposed to loud levels of noise. Unfortunately, it is estimated that between 5 and 30 million Americans are occupationally exposed to noise levels greater than 85 dB. It is estimated that one fourth of these workers will develop a permanent hearing loss that will probably be accompanied by tinnitus (a ringing or buzzing sound in the ears). It is very important for workplaces to help their employees protect their hearing when loud levels of noise are present (American Academy of Audiology, 2004).

■ *Birth defects* in some children may cause sensorineural hearing loss. For example, the auditory nerve or cochlea may not have developed normally by the time the baby is born, or portions of the inner ear may be missing.

■ Viral and bacterial diseases can also result in sensorineural hearing loss in children. Bacterial meningitis and mumps are two causes of sensorineural loss. The acronym STORCH refers to major causes of hearing loss in fetuses and newborns (Bess & Humes, 2003; Gelfand, 2001):

  - *Syphilis,* which some children contract from the mother at the time of birth, can cause inner ear damage.
  - *Toxoplasmosis,* a disease transmitted through the placenta, is often contracted when the pregnant mother handles cat feces or contaminated raw eggs and meat.
  - *Other.*
  - *Rubella,* or German measles, can be transferred to the fetus through the placenta.
  - *Cytomegalovirus,* the most common cause of viral hearing loss, is a herpes-type virus transmitted by close contact with infected children and also through sexual contact.
  - *Herpes simplex,* transmitted from the mother to the fetus, also can cause hearing loss.

■ A tumor called an *acoustic neuroma* can develop on the acoustic nerve and cause sensorineural loss by slowing nerve conduction of sound impulses to the brain.

■ *Presbycusis,* a hearing impairment in older people, is due to the effect of aging and is associated with sensorineural hearing loss. Presbycusis affects the high frequencies especially, resulting in a sloping, high-frequency loss (see Figure 10.9). Patients often have difficulty with recognition of speech, especially under challenging listening conditions such as noisy parties.

■ *Meniere's disease* is a condition that causes fluctuating sensorineural hearing loss, usually in adults. It is attributed to excessive endolymphatic fluid pressure in the membranous labyrinth, which causes Reissner's membrane to become distended (Gelfand, 2001).

■ Symptoms of Meniere's disease include hearing loss, spells of dizziness or vertigo, a sense of fullness in the ear, and *tinnitus,* a ringing or buzzing sound in the ears. Currently, no cure for this disease is available.

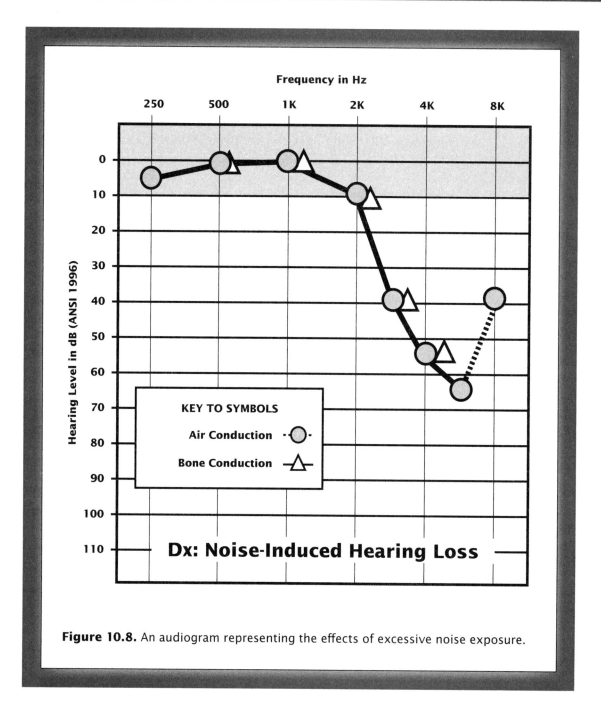

Figure 10.8. An audiogram representing the effects of excessive noise exposure.

- Some sensorineural hearing loss can be helped by medical and surgical intervention, but much cannot. Most people who have sensorineural hearing loss rely on a combination of early education (for children), amplification of sound, and speech–language therapy. These and other habilitative services are described later in the chapter.

Mixed Hearing Loss

- *Mixed hearing loss* occurs when neither the middle nor the inner ear is functioning properly. Any of the several conditions that cause conductive and sensorineural hearing loss can, in

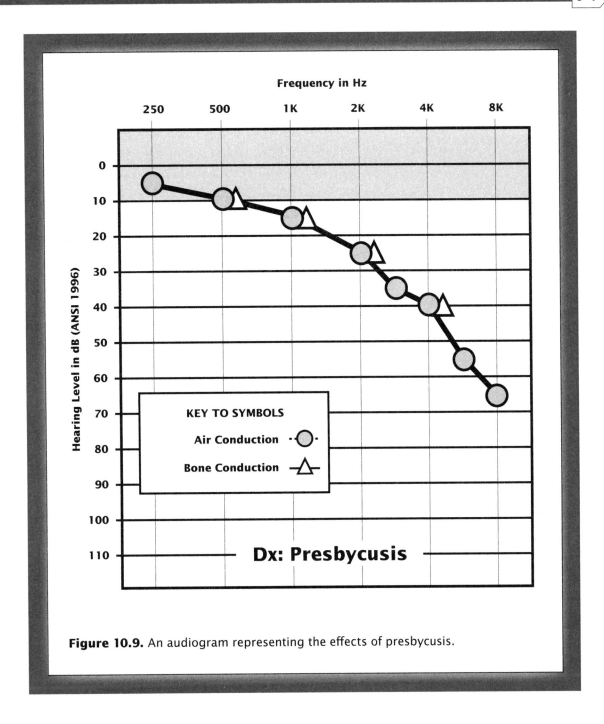

Figure 10.9. An audiogram representing the effects of presbycusis.

some combination, cause a mixed loss.

- Mixed losses may be caused by the presence of two separate disorders in the same ear. For example, a child could have a sensorineural loss *and* otitis media, which created a temporary conductive loss in the same ear.

- Another cause of mixed losses could be a single pathology, such as advanced otosclerosis or a head injury, that affected both sensorineural and conductive systems (Gelfand, 2001). A mixed loss affects both air and bone conduction. However, air conduction is affected more than bone conduction.

Define and describe the terms *conductive hearing loss* and *sensorineural hearing loss*. What are two causes of each type of loss?

_____

_____

_____

_____

_____

Auditory Nervous System Impairments

Central Auditory Disorders

- The *central auditory system* includes the brain stem, where the auditory nerve terminates, the fibers that project sound to the auditory centers of the brain, and those brain centers themselves.

- *Peripheral hearing problems* result from problems in the outer, middle, or inner ear (excluding the auditory nerve). *Central auditory disorders* refer to hearing losses due to disrupted sound transmission between the brainstem and the cerebrum as a result of damage or malformation. The temporal cortex of the brain may receive incorrect information, or the person may process information incorrectly (Tye-Murray, 2004).

- Central auditory disorders can be caused by tumors, traumatic brain injury, HIV, asphyxia during birth, various genetic disorders, infections such as meningitis and encephalitis, metabolic disturbances, cerebrovascular diseases, drug- or chemical-induced problems, central degenerative diseases such as Alzheimer's disease, and demyelinating diseases such as multiple sclerosis.

- There is great controversy in the literature about the existence, nature, and treatment of central auditory disorders. Empirical evidence is limited, and many researchers do not support "central auditory disorders" as a valid diagnostic label, although others do.

- People with central auditory disorders may have no significant peripheral hearing loss. Routine speech recognition tests in quiet environments and typical pure-tone threshold tests are not sensitive to central auditory disorders.

- Difficulty understanding distorted speech is a major symptom of central auditory disorders. In some of the central auditory tests, speech may be presented at low intensity, compressed in time, masked with noise, periodically interrupted, or filtered by eliminating certain frequencies of speech. *Dichotic listening* tasks, in which the listener must process different messages presented simultaneously to both ears, are also used.

- Although everyone has some difficulty understanding such distorted speech, those with central auditory disorders have great difficulty.
- For example, when there is a lesion in the temporal lobe of the brain, filtered-speech test scores may be poorer in the ear opposite the damaged side (contralateral) than in the ear on the side of the damage. People with central auditory disorders usually also have abnormal auditory discrimination because speech sounds are distorted at the cortical level (Mencher, Gerber, & McCombe, 1997).
- Patients with central auditory disorders typically have the following characteristics (Medwetsky, 2002; Mencher et al., 1997; Tye-Murray, 2004):

  - poor auditory discrimination (as stated)
  - poor auditory integration
  - poor auditory sequencing skills
  - poor auditory closure (e.g., recognizing that "_anta _aus" is "Santa Claus")
  - difficulty listening when background noise exists
  - poor auditory attention
  - poor auditory memory
  - poor auditory localization, or ability to locate a sound source in the environment
  - difficulty understanding rapid speech and other forms of auditory input that are characterized by reduced redundancy
  - difficulty following melodic and rhythmic elements of music
  - difficulty learning to read aloud due to inability to learn correct association of visual and auditory symbols

- Ferre (2002) describes behavioral intervention programs for children with central auditory processing disorders as tripods with three components: (a) direct intervention or remediation techniques aimed at improving audiotory skill, (b) helping the child use compensatory strategies to manage the deficit, and (c) modification of the environment to minimize adverse learning conditions. Sometimes FM systems (described later) are successful in helping children with central auditory processing disorders.

Retrocochlear Disorders

- People with *retrocochlear* pathology have damage to the nerve fibers along the ascending auditory pathways from the internal auditory meatus to the cortex (Bess & Humes, 2003). Thus, these disorders usually consist of pathology involving the cerebellopontine angle (described later) or cranial nerve VIII.
- Retrocochlear pathology is usually caused by unilateral tumors or *acoustic neuromas*. The patient often experiences a unilateral high-frequency hearing loss that may be accompanied by tinnitus and dizziness as well as a general feeling of disequilibrium (see Figure 10.10). When the affected ear is stimulated, acoustic reflexes are usually absent or present at elevated levels (Bess & Humes, 2003).
- Patients with acoustic neuromas may also experience alterations of facial sensation and movement because the facial and trigeminal nerves are compromised. There may be pain and headache in the ear and mastoid region, and a feeling of "fullness" in the affected ear. Due to compression of the brain stem and cerebellum, the patient may experience problems with balance.
- Symptoms of retrocochlear disorders are often subtle because patients have normal ability to detect pure tones as well as normal speech recognition in quiet. To help determine the presence of retrocochlear pathology, many audiologists use degraded speech signals, which

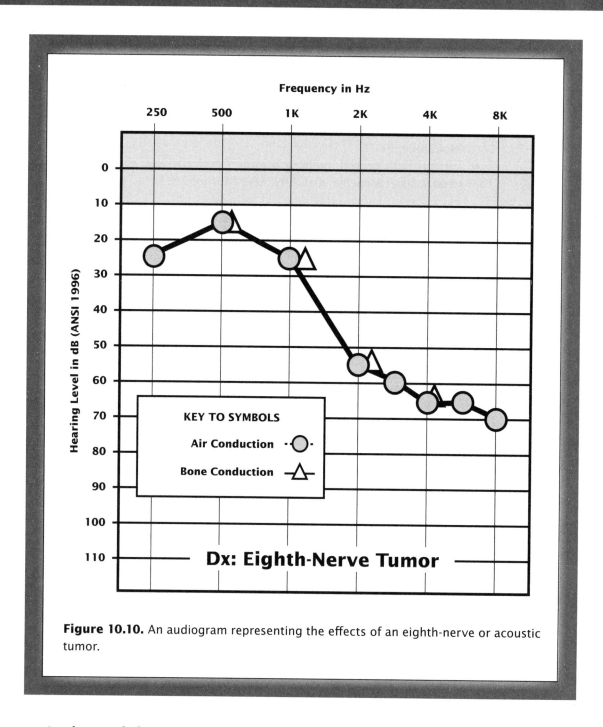

Figure 10.10. An audiogram representing the effects of an eighth-nerve or acoustic tumor.

involve speech that is interrupted, accompanied by noise, or filtered.

- An audiological diagnosis of acoustic neuroma is challenging to make. Because acoustic neuromas grow very slowly, the patient may not notice the ever-so-gradual loss of hearing until the acoustic neuroma is quite large and there is a serious hearing loss.

- It is not difficult to confuse the symptoms of acoustic neuroma with the symptoms of Meniere's disease. Auditory brain stem responses (described later) are a frequently used electrophysiologic measure because they are the easiest to obtain and interpret, and because they assist in differential diagnosis (Mencher et al., 1997).

- Retrocochlear disorders may be caused by *von Recklinghausen disease,* an inherited disease characterized by the presence of numerous small tumors that grow slowly and occur along various peripheral nerves. When they grow along cranial nerve VIII, they may initially be mistaken for acoustic neuroma. Patients with this disease may die if the tumors become malignant.

- Brain stem lesions, or tumors that appear in the brain stem at levels above cranial nerve VIII, are so rare that patients often die because the tumors are undiagnosed. Even if they are detected and surgery ensues, the surgery itself may create problems (e.g., facial paralysis). Some lesions are inoperable because they lie so deep in the brain stem.

SUMMARY

✓ Hearing is a phenomenon that begins even before babies are born and continues to develop throughout early childhood. Through air and bone conduction, sound reaches the inner ear and is sent to the brain for interpretation.

✓ However, some people have conductive, sensorineural, or mixed hearing losses, which disrupt the transmission of sound. People with auditory nervous system impairments such as central auditory and retrocochlear disorders also experience difficulties with sound transmission.

✓ It is important to accurately assess the type of hearing impairment so that appropriate treatment may be provided.

ASSESSMENT OF HEARING IMPAIRMENT

INTRODUCTION

Assessment of hearing impairment has been greatly improved by new technology and sophisticated instrumentation techniques that permit increasingly accurate diagnosis of hearing problems. An initial hearing screening rules out the need for more intensive testing for most people. For those who need such testing, pure-tone and speech audiometry are standard assessment procedures, as is acoustic immitance testing, which evaluates middle ear function.

Electrophysiological audiometry and medical imaging incorporate highly specialized diagnostic methods and instruments to evaluate auditory mechanism functioning. Children and infants may be tested by special methods appropriate for their age group. Once children and adults have been tested, the test results are interpreted and recommendations for treatment can be made.

Audiometry: Basic Principles

- An *audiometer* is an electronic instrument that generates and amplifies pure tones, noise, and other stimuli for testing hearing. Advanced audiometers are computerized.

- The audiometer generates tones at the frequencies of 125, 250, 500, 750, 1,000, 1,500, 2,000, 3,000, 4,000, and 8,000 Hz. The audiologist can select the frequency and vary the intensity of the sound stimulus through use of a dial that increases or *attenuates* (decreases) the intensity of the sound.

- The person to be tested sits in a specially constructed soundproof booth. This booth eliminates interference from ambient noise in the environment.

■ During air-conduction testing, the person wears earphones held in place by a steel headband fitting across the top of the head. The earphones deliver the sound stimulus directly to the ear. The person can respond by holding up a hand or by pressing a switch that lights up a small lamp on the audiometer.

Pure-Tone Audiometry

■ The *pure-tone* hearing test is carried out to determine the threshold of hearing for selected frequencies. A *threshold* is an intensity level at which a tone is faintly heard at least 50% of the time it is presented. Each tone is presented several times to reliably establish a threshold.

■ Audiologists test hearing at selected frequencies. Usually, a tone of 1,000 Hz is presented first because it is most easily detected. Next, tones of 2,000, 4,000, and 8,000 Hz are tested, in that order. Finally, the tones of 500 and 250 Hz are tested. All these frequencies are tested because they are the most important for human speech, which falls in the range of 100 to 8,000 Hz.

■ Both ears are tested, one at a time. The person is asked to listen and press the response switch immediately when even a faint sound is heard.

■ *Bone-conduction testing* assesses the sensitivity of the sensorineural portion of the auditory mechanism. The method is as follows. A bone vibrator is placed on the forehead or behind the test ear. When the sound strikes the bones of the skull, the bones vibrate and thus stimulate the fluid in both inner ears. Thus, it is difficult to determine which ear heard the sound and which did not.

■ To overcome this problem, the audiologist uses a procedure called *masking,* in which noise is sent through a headphone at a level that is strong enough to mask the tone heard in the opposite ear.

■ Even in *air-conduction testing,* masking is used when hearing in one ear is markedly better than hearing in the other ear. That is, the better ear is masked when the poorer ear is tested so that the person does not respond only because the sound is heard in the better, nontested ear.

Speech Audiometry

■ A person's pure-tone thresholds do not indicate how well he or she understands speech. *Speech audiometry* measures how well a person understands speech and discriminates between speech sounds.

■ The audiologist first determines a *speech reception threshold,* defined as the lowest level of hearing at which the person can understand 50% of the words presented. To make this determination, a list of *spondee words* is used; these words are two-syllable words with equal stress on each syllable (e.g., *baseball, hotdog*).

- The spondee words are either played through a tape recorder or spoken by the audiologist. When the person hears the words through the headphones, he or she writes them down or says them out loud.

- Another assessment made by an audiologist is based on a *word discrimination* or *word recognition* test. This test establishes how well a person discriminates between words by having the person correctly repeat monosyllabic words such as *cap* and *day*.

- Because the purpose of this test is to determine speech comprehension rather than speech threshold, the words are presented at a level of loudness that is comfortable for the person being tested.

- The speech discrimination score is the percentage of presented words that the person correctly repeats. This score helps identify people who can hear but not understand speech. People with sensorineural hearing loss are most likely to show this problem.

Acoustic Immitance

- *Acoustic immitance* refers to a transfer of acoustic energy. An energy transformation takes place when a sound stimulus reaches the external ear canal and strikes the tympanic membrane.

- The tympanic membrane and middle ear structures offer *impedance,* or resistance, to the flow of sound energy. *Admittance,* a counterpart of impedance, is a measure of the amount of energy that flows through the system.

- Both very low and very high impedance suggest pathology within the auditory system. For example, a child with middle ear fluid may demonstrate high impedance. An adult with a broken ossicular chain may show low impedance. Tympanometry and acoustic reflex thresholds are two common acoustic immitance measures.

- *Tympanometry* is a procedure in which acoustic immitance is measured with an electroacoustic instrument called an *impedance bridge* or *impedance meter.*

- This instrument allows the audiologist to place a sound stimulus in the external ear canal with an airtight closure and measure changes in the acoustic energy as the sound stimulates the auditory system. The instrument also helps create either negative or positive changes within the ear canal. Acoustic immitance is altered by such air pressure changes.

- The impedance meter can also measure *acoustic reflex,* a simple reflex response of the muscles attached to the stapes bone. The acoustic reflex is elicited in both ears by a relatively loud sound presented to either ear. The reflex response involves a stiffening of the ossicular chain, presumably to protect the ear from potential damage.

- Acoustic reflex testing is valuable in detecting middle ear diseases, including those that are not associated with hearing loss.

CONCEPTS TO CONSIDER

Briefly compare and contrast pure-tone audiometry, speech audiometry, and acoustic immitance. What is the purpose of each of these types of hearing testing?

_____

_____

_____

_____

_____

Other Methods

Electrophysiological Audiometry

- *Electrophysiological audiometry* is an objective measure of auditory mechanism functioning. In response to sound, the cochlea, acoustic nerve, and auditory centers of the brain generate measurable electrical impulses. These impulses are recorded as changes in the background electrical activity of the brain.

- Such electrical changes produced by sound stimuli are called *auditory-evoked potentials.* Usually, abnormal patterns of electrical activity in reaction to a sound stimulus indicate a hearing loss.

- *Electrocochleography* is the measurement of the electrical activity of the cochlea in response to sound. The electrocochleogram (ECoG) generated by this testing is a response consisting primarily of the compound action potential that occurs at the distal portion of cranial nerve VIII. Electrocochleography is most useful in monitoring cochlear function in operating rooms to simplify the placement of electrodes (Stach, 1998).

- *Auditory brain stem response* (ABR) is a technique used to record the electrical activity in the auditory nerve, the brain stem, and the cortical areas of the brain. It is useful in detecting brain stem diseases. It is also very helpful in testing the hearing of newborn infants.

- If the blood supply to the cochlea is interrupted or the nerve is severed or otherwise damaged when surgeons are operating on tumors or other masses near nerve VIII, either results in hearing loss for the patient.

- It is most helpful for an audiologist to be present during such surgeries. The audiologist uses auditory-evoked potential monitoring to measure the function of nerve VIII and provide feedback to the surgeon during the surgery (Stach, 1998).

Medical Imaging

- *Computerized axial tomography* (described further in Chapter 13) is an important tool in otological diagnosis. It can help detect small tumors as well as brain lesions (e.g., infections, strokes) that cause hearing impairment.
- *Magnetic resonance imaging* (also described in Chapter 13) is best for imaging the internal auditory canals, base of the skull, and pituitary gland regions to evaluate the possible presence of pathology affecting the auditory system. MRI is especially helpful in detecting acoustic neuromas or tumors.

Hearing Screening

- It is time consuming to test patients with a complete battery of hearing tests. However, it is important to identify people who may have a hearing problem. Hearing screening is a quick, preliminary way to determine whether the person being tested has normal hearing or may have a hearing problem and therefore need further, more in-depth testing.

- The three major groups of individuals who undergo hearing screening include newborns, schoolchildren, and adults in professions in which they are exposed to potentially hazardous levels of noise (Stach, 1998).

- In hearing screening, pure tones are presented at 20–25 dB. Only the frequencies of 500, 1,000, 2,000, and 4,000 Hz are tested. Testing usually takes place in a quiet room and may be done with individuals or groups.

- Some people undergo acoustic immitance testing as a part of the screening. In public schools, this is rare; usually, schoolchildren undergo pure-tone audiometric screening only.

Assessment of Infants and Children

- It is important to detect hearing loss in infants as soon as possible, because early intervention can reduce its effects on speech and language acquisition.

- Various committees and health boards such as the Joint Committee on Accreditation of Health Organizations and the Department of Health and Human Services are encouraging all hospitals to include universal newborn hearing screening programs.

- Because infants and some young children cannot give voluntary responses, hearing assessment procedures depend mostly on reflexive responses elicited by loud sounds. These sounds may include electronic instruments, toys, or bells. Testing of this type is most effective in eliciting reflexive responses from infants between birth and 6 months of age.

- *Localization audiometry,* often used with older infants, involves presenting a sound and seeing if the infant will turn his or her head toward the sound. This response is measured by presenting sound from different directions and noting the infant's response.

- In *operant audiometry,* a child's hearing is tested by conditioning voluntary responses to sound stimuli. Operant audiometry is best for children who are challenging to test using

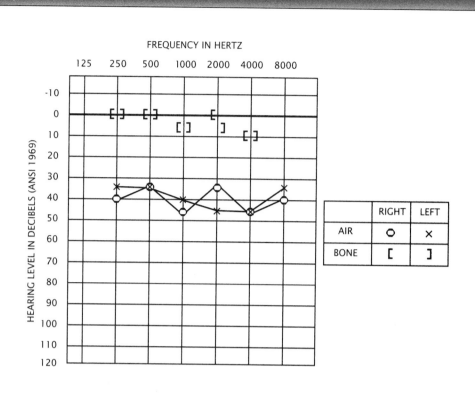

Figure 10.11. An audiogram illustrating conductive hearing loss. *Note.* From *Introduction to Communicative Disorders*, 3rd ed. (p. 396), by M. N. Hegde, 2001, Austin, TX: PRO-ED. Copyright 2001 by PRO-ED, Inc. Reprinted with permission.

traditional audiometric means. Children with mental retardation, attention-deficit disorder, and behavioral disorders often benefit from operant audiometry procedures.

Interpretation of Hearing Test Results

- Before audiologists make recommendations about the habilitation of a person with hearing impairment, they consider audiological test results and information gathered from a variety of sources. These sources include:

  - a case history and interview
  - a comprehensive speech and language assessment
  - otological records from the patient's otologist
  - any general medical reports that include information relative to the patient's hearing and overall health
  - for children, reports from regular and special education teachers

- Hearing losses can be judged as follows:

  - mild (16–40 dB)

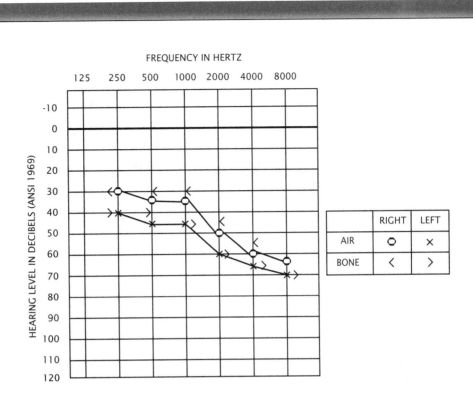

Figure 10.12. An audiogram showing a sensorineural loss. *Note.* From *Introduction to Communicative Disorders,* 3rd ed. (p. 396), by M. N. Hegde, 2001, Austin, TX: PRO-ED. Copyright 2001 by PRO-ED, Inc. Reprinted with permission.

- moderate (41–55 dB)
- moderately severe (56–65 dB)
- severe (66–89 dB)
- profound (90+ dB)

■ *Unilateral losses* are those found only in one ear, whereas bilateral losses affect both ears. The degree of loss may be the same in both ears, or there may be a difference between the ears.

■ *Audiograms* are graphs that display the results of air- and bone-conduction tests. A typical audiogram shows the hearing level in dB for both bone- and air-conducted tones for the tested frequencies.

■ Figure 10.11 shows an example of conductive hearing loss. The bone-conducted hearing is normal bilaterally because the sound is delivered directly to the inner ear through bone conduction. However, when sound is delivered to the outer ear, there is a hearing loss. The *air–bone gap* indicates that the loss is conductive.

■ An air–bone gap can be further described as the difference between a bone-conduction hearing threshold and an air-conduction hearing threshold for a given frequency in the same ear.

When the difference between the air- and bone-conduction frequencies averages 10 dB or more, this implies a conductive hearing loss (Nicolosi, Harryman, & Kresheck, 2004).

■ When the hearing is not significantly better in one ear, it is not necessary to use masking noise. Therefore, in Figure 10.12, unmasked bone-conduction thresholds are represented by different symbols. The audiogram shows that the person's hearing is better for some frequencies than others, which is typical of sensorineural hearing loss.

■ Figure 10.13 shows an audiogram representing a mixed hearing loss. A sensorineural component is evident because the thresholds are higher than normal when the sound is delivered directly to the cochlea via bone conduction. However, the air-conduction thresholds are also elevated. The difference between the air- and bone-conduction thresholds indicates a probable conductive hearing loss as well.

■ Figure 10.14 illustrates an audiogram of a noise-induced hearing loss. The difference in air- and bone-conduction thresholds indicates the sensorineural nature of the loss. There is also a notable diagnostic sign of noise-induced loss: a greater loss between 3,000 and 6,000 Hz.

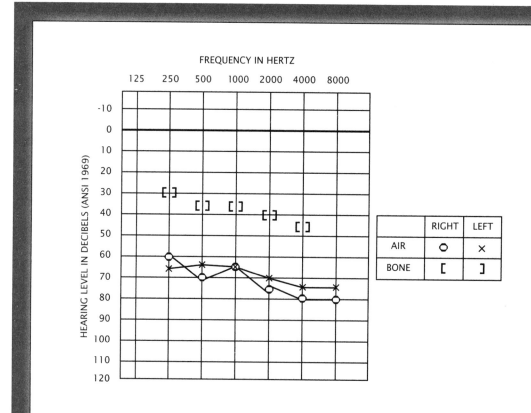

Figure 10.13. An audiogram showing a mixed hearing loss. *Note.* From *Introduction to Communicative Disorders*, 3rd ed. (p. 397), by M. N. Hegde, 2001, Austin, TX: PRO-ED. Copyright 2001 by PRO-ED, Inc. Reprinted with permission.

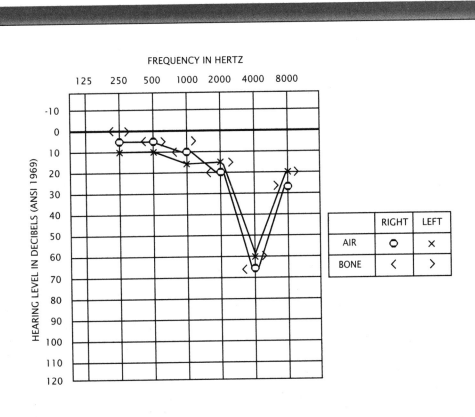

Figure 10.14. An audiogram showing a noise-induced hearing loss. *Note.* From *Introduction to Communicative Disorders,* 3rd ed. (p. 398), by M. N. Hegde, 2001, Austin, TX: PRO-ED. Copyright 2001 by PRO-ED, Inc. Reprinted with permission.

SUMMARY

✓ Primary methods of assessing hearing impairment include pure-tone and speech audiometry, acoustic immitance, and electrophysiological audiometry.

✓ Whether children or adults are assessed, it is important to accurately interpret the hearing test results so that appropriate management of the hearing impairment may be undertaken.

MANAGEMENT OF HEARING IMPAIRMENT

INTRODUCTION

Hearing impairments can range from mild to profound, and management of hearing impairment reflects this continuum. Depending upon the type and extent of the hearing loss, people with hearing impairment often manifest difficulties in articulation, language, voice, fluency, and resonance. Amplification devices such as hearing aids, cochlear implants, tactile aids, and assistive devices are often used in aural rehabilitation. Communication training may also be part of treatment, which involves methods such as auditory training, speech reading, cued speech, oral language training, and speech, rhythm, and voice training (Martin & Clark, 2003; Tye-Murray, 2004). There are two broad approaches to communication training: verbal approaches, which involve speech, and nonverbal approaches, which involve sign language.

Communication Disorders of People with Hearing Impairment

General Principles

- Without normal hearing, children may learn signs, gestures, and other modes of manual communication. However, spoken language is affected.
- Hearing supports the acquisition and production of speech and language in several ways. Hearing makes infants aware of environmental and speech sounds. Hearing also makes it possible to understand spoken language. Those who cannot hear and understand speech usually need special assistance.
- Hearing is also necessary in monitoring one's own production of speech and language. Self-monitoring enables people to monitor *how* they speak as well as what they say. People with hearing impairments have challenges in monitoring their speech, language, and voice productions.
- The extent of adverse effects of hearing impairment on speech, language, and voice depends on many variables—especially the *age of onset* of the hearing loss and the *degree of the loss.*
- *Congenital* hearing loss, or loss present at birth, has a greater impact than hearing loss acquired later in adult life. Children with *prelingual deafness* become deaf before they acquire speech and language, whereas children with *postlingual deafness* have a hearing impairment that occurred after age 5.
- Prognosis for speech and language improvement in hard-of-hearing and deaf children depends on several factors:

    - how early in life professional help is given
    - the quality and scope of services the child receives
    - the extent to which the parents help their deaf child
    - the presence of other disabling conditions (e.g., blindness, brain damage)

- In judging the impact of the hearing impairment on the patient's daily life, audiologists can have adults and older children carry out self-assessments. These typically involve questionnaires in which people evaluate the impact of the hearing loss on many aspects of their daily life and functioning.

Speech Disorders

- Children with hearing impairments have difficulty learning the speech sounds because they cannot hear these sounds well if at all. People who are profoundly deaf distort many vowels and almost all consonants. Omissions, substitutions, and distortions of sounds are common.
- It is common for people with hearing impairment to manifest the following speech problems:

    - distortion of sounds, especially fricatives and stops
    - omission of initial and final consonants
    - consonant cluster reduction
    - substitution of voiced consonants for voiceless consonants (e.g., g/d)
    - omission of /s/ in almost all positions of words
    - substitution of nasal consonants for oral consonants (e.g., *mat/bat*)
    - increased duration of vowels
    - imprecise production of vowels (e.g., diphthongization of vowels)
    - epenthesis, or adding a schwa sound to consonant blends (e.g., sətap/stap)

Language Disorders

- Some individuals who are deaf use language well; for example, there are accomplished writers who are deaf. However, many prelingually deaf people are likely to exhibit problems with language.
- Language problems of many prelingually deaf people include:

  - use of a limited variety of sentence types
  - use of sentences of reduced length and complexity
  - difficulty comprehending and producing compound, complex, and embedded sentences
  - occasional irrelevance of speech, including non sequiturs (utterances that do not relate to the topic at hand)
  - providing insufficient background information to the listener
  - limited oral communication, including lack of elaborated speech and reluctance to speak
  - difficulty understanding proverbs, metaphors, and other abstract utterances
  - slower acquisition of grammatic morphemes
  - omission or inconsistent use of many morphemes including past tense and plural inflections, third-person singular –s, indefinite pronouns, present progressive –ing, articles, prepositions, and conjunctions
  - poor reading comprehension
  - writing that reflects oral language problems (e.g., deviant syntax, limited variety of sentence types, omission of grammatic morphemes)

Voice, Fluency, and Resonance Disorders

- Problems in voice, fluency, and resonance depend heavily on the degree of hearing loss and the amount of intervention a person has experienced.
- Voice, fluency, and resonance problems in many people who are deaf include:

  - hypernasal resonance on non-nasal sounds
  - hyponasal resonance on nasal sounds

C O N C E P T S   T O   C O N S I D E R

Describe two characteristics each of the speech, language, voice, and resonance of people who are deaf.

_____

_____

_____

_____

_____

- abnormal phrasing, flow, and rhythm of speech
- monotone speech with lack of appropriate intonation
- improper stress patterns, including excessive pitch inflections
- restricted pitch range
- inappropriately high pitch
- rate of speech that is too slow or too fast
- pauses at inappropriate junctures
- inefficient breathing, including breathiness
- deviations in voice quality, including hoarseness and harshness

Aural Rehabilitation: Basic Principles

- *Aural rehabilitation* is an educational and clinical program implemented primarily by audiologists. It is designed to help people with hearing losses achieve their full potential.

- Aural rehabilitation includes several key components (Brackett, 2002; Tye-Murray, 2004):

  - an evaluation of the hearing loss
  - an assessment of the communicative needs of the person (including the patient's self-assessment)
  - determination of the availability of human and financial resources to support hearing habilitation
  - prescription and fitting of a hearing aid
  - auditory training
  - use of amplification systems in communication and educational training sessions
  - focus on communication patterns in the environment
  - addressing the impact of social, vocational, psychological, and educational factors of the hearing loss
  - counseling the person with the hearing impairment and his or her family
  - recommending additional services if needed
  - periodic reevaluation of the client's status

- Many specialists are involved in aural rehabilitation. They include:

  - the *audiologist,* who is primarily responsible for the aural rehabilitation components listed above
  - the *otologist,* who monitors the health of the ear (this medical specialist performs such ear surgeries as stapedectomy and tympanoplasty and prescribes medication for middle ear diseases)
  - the *speech-language pathologist,* who provides treatment for articulation, language, resonance, voice, and fluency
  - in schools, the *educator of the deaf,* a special educator who teaches communication methods such as American Sign Language as well as academic subjects to children with hearing impairments
  - the *vocational counselor*

- Professionals carrying out aural rehabilitation have historically focused intensive efforts on speech reading and auditory training. Today, there is a greater focus on hearing aid fitting and orientation, the environment and communication patterns within the environment, and early identification and intervention (Martin & Clark, 2003; Schow & Nerbonne, 2002).

Amplification

■ An important part of aural rehabilitation of people with hearing impairment is amplification of sound and speech. Sound and speech can be amplified through several means, including hearing aids, cochlear implants, and auditory trainers.

■ When children and adults with hearing losses are considered as candidates for amplification, there are two major considerations. First, do they truly need the amplification? Second, are they motivated to use the amplification and care for any amplification devices properly? Patient motivation is a major factor in deciding upon appropriate amplification.

Hearing Aids

▪ Most *traditional hearing aids* are small, electronic devices that are worn inside the ear unilaterally or bilaterally depending upon the needs of the person. Hearing aids amplify sound and deliver it to the ear canal. An ear mold, though not part of the hearing aid itself, is necessary for using the aid.

▪ There are several basic types of hearing aids:

- the *eyeglass variety,* in which the hearing aid is built into the frame of the eyeglasses
- *body aids,* worn under a person's shirt or blouse
- the *behind-the-ear model,* which fits behind the ear and has an internal receiver
- the *in-the-canal model,* which fits in the ear canal and is less visible
- the *completely-in-the-canal model,* which is smaller and even less visible than the in-the-canal model, and terminates close to the tympanic membrane
- the *in-the-ear model,* a smaller unit which fits within the concha of the external ear
- the *disposable hearing aid,* which has a 40-day use-life, costs under $100 for a binaural set, and can be fit and dispensed in one office visit (no impression of the ear is necessary) (Martin & Clark, 2003)

▪ *Analog hearing aids,* a common type of aid, create patterns of electric voltage that correspond to the sound input. All analog hearing aids consist of the same basic components: a microphone, an amplifier, a receiver, a power source (batteries), and volume control.

▪ Hearing aid *transducers* include the *microphone,* which picks up sound, and the *receiver,* which delivers the sound to the ear. These transducers convert one form of energy into another.

▪ The microphone converts the sound energy into electrical energy; the receiver, housed in the ear mold, converts the electrical energy back into sound waves. The *amplifier,* to which the electrical signals are fed, amplifies those signals and delivers them to the receiver.

▪ The more recently developed *digital hearing aid* contains microcomputer technology. Whereas the microphone of a traditional analog hearing aid creates a continuously variable voltage pattern that is analogous (similar) to the sound input, a digital aid rapidly samples the input signal and converts each sample into a binary system of zeros and ones. Those numbers are then processed by a computer housed in a unit worn on the body.

▪ There are several advantages of digital aids:

- They are more flexible than the analog aids and can be modified to adapt to each patient's pattern of hearing loss and communicative needs.
- Digital processing helps amplify selected frequencies for which loss is greater.
- Digital aids are more effective than analog aids in reducing irritating loud noises, such as

dogs barking and vacuums running.

- Digital aids provide a better *signal-to-noise ratio;* that is, they are more effective than analog aids in clearly separating speech from background noise, which also is more effectively suppressed.

- Advances in technology have greatly improved the quality of hearing aids. Advances include highly sensitive microphones, ear molds that are custom made for each person, and amplifiers that amplify sound with minimal to no distortion.
- State-of-the-art hearing aids are *programmable,* in that they can be programmed to provide different types of amplification depending upon the setting. For example, the wearer could choose among different settings depending upon whether he or she was at a party (with background noise) or watching TV alone at home (Gelfand, 2001).
- A recent development in hearing aid technology is *computerization.* Hearing aid specifications, automated testing procedures, prescriptive fitting methods, and hearing aid selection formulas are now available from computer software.
- Most hearing aids (such as those previously described) are air-conduction hearing aids. *Bone-conduction hearing aids* amplify sound for the patient using a bone-conduction vibrator. The vibrator can be built into the temple portion of the patient's eyeglasses or held in place with a spring headband (Gelfand, 2001).
- Bone-conduction hearing aids are used in place of air-conduction aids when the patient manifests certain pathologies such as atresia of the ear canal or other physical problems that make an air-conduction aid inadvisable.
- Selection of a hearing aid is a process involving several steps:

  - an ear examination by an otologist to identify any physical condition of the ear that may contraindicate the use of amplification;
  - diagnostic tests administered by an audiologist to help determine the extent and type of hearing loss;
  - a hearing aid evaluation, conducted by an audiologist, in which various models are tested to determine the best aid for the individual's needs; and
  - evaluation of whether the patient needs *monaural* (one ear only) or *binaural* (both ears) amplification.

- Several decades ago, it was deemed unethical for audiologists to sell hearing aids for profit. ASHA did not permit audiologists to sell hearing aids until the 1970s. Today, a hearing aid can be purchased from several sources, including audiologists and hearing aid dealers.

Cochlear Implants

- Hearing aids are an invaluable tool for many people with hearing losses. However, some people with profound hearing losses cannot benefit from hearing aids. The recent technology of cochlear implants may profit those individuals (Tye-Murray, 2004).
- *Cochlear implants* are electronic devices. They are surgically placed in the cochlea and other parts of the ear, and deliver the sound directly to the acoustic nerve endings in the cochlea. Although the patient may be profoundly deaf, there is often a large residual population of primary cochlear neural elements; a cochlear implant can take advantage of those residual elements.
- Cochlear implants differ from hearing aids primarily in that the hearing aid delivers amplified sound to the ear canal, whereas cochlear implants deliver electrical impulses, converted from sound, directly to the auditory nerve. Basically, cochlear implants replace the nonfunctioning inner hair cell transducer system.

- Cochlear implants can be thought of as "prosthetic cochleas." They consist of four elements (Martin & Clark, 2003; Stach, 2003):

  - A *microphone* is mounted on an ear mold and worn in the ear canal or on the body. It picks up the sound and converts it into electrical impulses.
  - The microphone is connected to a *processor,* which is contained in a small box that can be worn on a belt or placed in a pocket. The battery-operated processor suppresses extraneous noise and selects sounds salient to comprehending speech.
  - Those sounds are then sent to an *external transmitter,* a magnetic coil worn on the skull (in a manner similar to that of an external hearing aid). Behind the external transmitter, directly under the skin, an internal magnetic coil is implanted. The two magnetic coils are attracted to each other.
  - A ground electrode is implanted in an area outside the cochlea; active electrodes are placed inside of it. Through the skin, the external transmitter sends a signal to the *implanted receiver* (the internal coil and the electrodes), which stimulates the auditory nerve.

- Unlike earlier cochlear implants that had only one channel (one active electrode), more recent implants have multiple channels or electrodes. Implants with multiple channels stimulate different areas of the cochlea and attempt to produce various tonal perceptions (Stach, 2003; Thedinger, 1996).
- As previously stated, cochlear implants today are used only with people who have minimal or no hearing and cannot profit from hearing aids. Cochlear implants enhance patients' speech-reading performance (see "Speech Reading" later in this chapter), give patients general sound awareness, and help patients recognize environmental sounds (Gelfand, 2001).
- Candidates for cochlear implants are selected after extensive examinations carried out by teams of specialists. These specialists include audiologists, speech pathologists, deaf educators, psychologists, and otologists.
- Because placing a cochlear implant is a surgical procedure involving general anesthesia, there is a minimal risk of postsurgical infection and nerve damage involving facial paralysis.
- Parents of pediatric patients as well as adult implant recipients are generally advised that the implant recipient may not be able to discriminate speech sounds. However, although frequency discrimination is imperfect, voices can be heard at normal conversational levels. This provides awareness of sounds as well as cues such as rhythm and rate that can assist the implant recipient in speech reading (Martin & Clark, 2003).
- Prelingual children who receive cochlear implants can make substantial progress. Cochlear implants help maximize these children's potential and may positively impact the auditory system's ability to mature. Recent research has shown that the earlier children receive cochlear implants, the higher their reading comprehension scores later (Connor & Zwolan, 2004). Recent research has also shown that some adults with severe to profound hearing losses may also benefit from cochlear implants (Zwolan, 2002).
- It must be noted that many members of the Deaf community have shown resistance to cochlear implants. Some question the ethics of having others make decisions for children who are too young to choose if they would like to reside in the Deaf community or try in interact in the hearing world (Helfer, 1998; Martin & Clark, 2003).
- The *central electroauditory prosthesis* (CEP) is a more current development in implant technology. The CEP directly stimulates the cochlear nucleus of the auditory nerve at the brain stem level.
- When the cochlea and its hair cells are damaged to such an extent that a cochlear implant will not work, implants of electrodes may carry the sound to the auditory nerve fibers at the brain stem. More research is needed to establish the usefulness of the CEP.

Tactile Aids

- Tactile aids are a type of *sensory substitution method* used for individuals who are deaf (Gelfand, 2001). These aids are devices or methods that promote the comprehension of speech by means of touch. Thus, tactile (touch) sense is substituted for hearing.
- Tactile aids are sometimes used for individuals with profound deafness; they may also be used for individuals who are both deaf and blind. They convert sound into vibration for tactual stimulation (Stach, 2003).
- Because the human skin does not respond well to sounds of different frequencies, tactile aids have vibrators that generate patterns of stimuli that represent different speech sounds.
- Simple tactile aids have a single channel that transforms acoustic signals into mechanical signals and stimulates the skin. These aids help their wearers to detect environmental sounds. More complex multichannel tactile aids have multiple stimulators that stimulate different body parts mechanically or electrically. For example, different stimulators may stimulate the arm, abdomen, or wrist.
- Tactile aids are cheaper than cochlear implants and do not involve surgery. However, a great deal of practice and training are needed to make optimal use of the tactile signals (Gelfand, 2001).
- The *Tadoma Method*, a manual system for people who are deaf and blind, involves them placing hands on the speaker's face to feel the vibrations of speech.
- The listener feels the vibrations of the lips, cheeks, jaws, and vocal folds of the speaker. The listener also feels nasal and oral airflow. This method can be used to teach speech production to children who are deaf or deaf and blind.

Assistive Devices

- New technologies have been created to support the communication needs of individuals who are deaf and hard of hearing. Some can be used alone, whereas others must be used in conjunction with interpreters, speech reading (discussed later in this chapter), or other support systems.
- *Safety alerting devices* help people with hearing impairments to gain information through flashing lights or vibrators on common devices. These devices help people know, for example, when the doorbell rings or a burglar alarm goes off.
- *Closed captioning* on television provides subtitles on the screen to help people who are deaf know what is happening in a TV program.
- *Telecommunication devices for the deaf* (TDDs) allow people who are deaf to use the telephone. The TDD is a portable terminal that both sends and receives typed messages via telephone (Gelfand, 2001).

Communication Training

General Guidelines

- It is important to consider the impact of hearing loss on all aspects of a patient's life. Hearing loss often creates educational challenges for children and vocational challenges for adults (Martin & Clark, 2003; Tye-Murray, 2004).
- Acceptance of a hearing loss can vary from culture to culture. It is important to be sensitive to culturally determined reactions such as embarrassment or the belief that God has given a family a deaf child as a cross to bear (Nuru-Holm & Battle, 1998).

CONCEPTS TO CONSIDER

Several types of amplification are available for people who are deaf. Describe two of these types of amplification (e.g., cochlear implants).

_____

_____

_____

_____

_____

- When working with children who have a hearing loss, it is important to begin speech and language training as early as possible. The family should be involved in speech and language training and stimulation activities (DeBonis & Donohue, 2004).
- The child must be under appropriate medical and audiological management, including being fitted with a customized hearing aid. The child and parents should be trained in proper care and use of the hearing aid.
- Clinicians who serve children should work closely with classroom teachers and with educators of the deaf. The development of auditory skills must be integrated into the child's educational and speech–language programs.
- Children must be placed in appropriate educational settings. Those settings exist along a continuum from full inclusion in the general education classroom to enrollment in a residential school for the deaf.
- For many adults, hearing problems account for various levels of psychosocial difficulty even after a hearing aid is acquired (Tye-Murray, 2004).
- Thus, when working with adults, clinicians frequently need to provide psychosocial counseling to help patients and their families deal with impacts of the hearing loss and attitudes toward aural rehabilitation.
- Older people with hearing losses may be served through clinics, senior citizen centers, and nursing homes and other long-term health-care facilities. The patient's living setting must be carefully considered as aural rehabilitation efforts are carried out.

Auditory Training

- _Auditory training_ is designed to teach a person with hearing impairment to listen to amplified sounds, recognize their meanings, and discriminate sounds from each other.
- Individuals who use hearing aids generally undergo a _hearing aid orientation,_ which is provided by an audiologist or sometimes by a hearing aid dealer. The person is instructed in use and care of the hearing aid.
- _Desktop auditory trainers_ are frequently more effective and powerful in amplifying speech

than hearing aids. One reason is that hearing aids pick up all noise, including background, or *ambient,* noise, whereas auditory trainers pick up and amplify only the signal of interest (the speech of a speaker).

- When auditory trainers are used, the person with hearing impairment wears headphones. The clinician's or teacher's speech is fed to an amplifier through a microphone, and the amplified sound is fed to the earphones and the person's ear.

- Auditory trainers can be used with adults who are receiving articulation training. They are also used with children in educational and therapy settings; prelingually deaf children may especially benefit.

- An *FM auditory trainer* is a wireless system that can be used in group or individual treatment sessions. In a classroom, for example, it allows the teacher and the child or children to move about within a certain range. The children and teacher both wear receiving and transmitting units so they can hear and talk with each other.

- Ambient or extraneous noise in school classrooms is approximately 60 dB. The signal-to-noise ratio (S/N ratio), or the difference in dB between the stimulus of interest (usually the teacher's voice) and competing background noise, is often negative; that is, the teacher's voice cannot be adequately heard due to the background noise (Crandell, Smaldino, & Flexer, 2005).

- This negative S/N ratio is very detrimental to children with hearing impairments, and auditory trainers are extremely beneficial in such situations. The Acoustical Society of America is currently working toward recommendations and an action plan to reduce ambient noise and other acoustical barriers in classrooms (Soli, 1998).

- Auditory training goals for children with hearing impairments include discrimination of environmental sounds, discrimination of speech sounds and word pairs, and discrimination of phrases and sentences. Use of a multimodal approach (e.g., mirrors, pictures, charts, and tactile cues such as feeling the throat and lips) is a necessary component of auditory training.

Speech Reading

- Previously known as lipreading, *speech reading* involves deciphering speech by looking at the face of the speaker and using visual cues to understand what the speaker is saying.

- In speech reading, the listener watches the movements of the lips, jaw, and tongue as well as the shape of the lips and mouth. The speaker's gestures, hand movements, and facial expressions are also observed to understand the total message being conveyed.

- In English, only 30% of sounds are visible on the face. These include the labials /v/, /f/, /m/, /p/, and /b/. The labials are *homophenous;* that is, they look the same and may be confusing. Other sounds are less visible and very difficult to read (Tye-Murray, 2004). Ideally, speech reading should be supplemented with other means of communication.

Cued Speech

- *Cued speech* is speech produced with manual cues that represent the sounds of speech. It may be used to supplement speech reading.

- Cued speech differs from sign language because it is composed of eight signs or hand configurations for consonants and four signs for vowels.

- The hand gestures that constitute cued speech are often helpful in assisting the person with hearing impairment to distinguish among homophenous sounds.

- Research has demonstrated that people with hearing impairment benefit when the speaker uses cued speech. Nicholls and Ling (1982) showed that correct speech reading of syllables increased from 30% without cues to 84% with cues. A challenge in using cued speech is that speakers must be able to speak and cue simultaneously.

Oral Language Training: General Principles

- The aforementioned communication methods help people who are deaf to understand speech that is spoken to them. To be fully successful communicators, however, these people benefit from also learning to express themselves to others. Successful expression requires training.
- Oral language training should begin as early as possible. Language stimulation programs are best carried out in both clinical and educational settings as well as the home. These programs should involve cooperative efforts of a team consisting of an audiologist, family members, a speech–language pathologist, and an educator of the deaf.
- Parents of infants who are deaf should speak to their children as much as possible, talking about and labeling things in the environment. Caretakers can integrate visual with auditory stimulation by showing objects and naming them simultaneously as well as demonstrating actions when they are described.
- Initially, it is best to select and teach functional words that children use in their daily environments. Subsequently, children can be taught phrase and sentence structures to express their individual ideas and needs more fully.
- Clinicians should also focus on other structures and concepts that are especially difficult for children with hearing impairment. These include:

    - grammatic morphemes such as past tense *–ed* and plural *–s*
    - terms with dual meanings (e.g., *rock, pound*)
    - antonyms (e.g., *up–down, light–dark*) and synonyms (e.g., *happy–joyful*)
    - proverbs (e.g., "A penny saved is a penny earned")
    - abstract terms (e.g., *lighthearted, flimsy*)

- Children with hearing impairment have challenges with pragmatic skills. Therefore, clinicians must provide training in specific skills such as turn taking, topic initiation, topic maintenance, and eye contact.
- It is important to use visual cues in therapy sessions. These visual cues can include hand gestures, facial expressions, toys and other manipulatives, pictures, printed letters, books, and other visuals to supplement auditory input.

Speech, Rhythm, and Voice Training

- In teaching speech sound production, it is important to give many visual cues. Clinicians can use charts, pictures, and other visuals to assist children in correct sound production.
- Clinicians must pay special attention to affricates, fricatives, and stops. These sounds are especially difficult for children with hearing impairment.
- The voice–voiceless distinction is also critical for children with hearing impairment to learn. Clinicians can contrast the cognates /p/ and /b/, for example, through visual and tactile means.
- Clinicians must address any voice abnormalities such as hoarseness, harshness, high pitch, and monotone. Clients must learn to speak with proper volume, especially avoiding excessive loudness. Work with proper respiration—especially proper breath support—can be helpful.
- Resonance problems such as hypernasality and hyponasality must also be addressed. Clinicians may need to help clients balance oral–nasal resonance, and avoid cul-de-sac resonance (defined in Chapter 7).
- Goals in the area of prosody may include teaching normal intonation, smooth flow of speech, and modifying pauses that are placed inappropriately or are of inappropriate length.
- It is very helpful to use mechanical feedback devices such as the Visi-Pitch (described in Chapter 7) in working with voice and resonance problems.

Approaches to Training

Aural/Oral Method

- The aural/oral method is also called the *oral approach,* the *auditory-global approach,* and the *multisensory approach.* Users of this method attempt to use amplification methods such as hearing aids or cochlear implants to tap children's residual hearing.
- Children undergo intensive auditory training and speech reading instruction. It is expected that they will eventually learn to speak and will fit into mainstream social, vocational, and educational settings.

Manual Approach

- The manual method is a means of nonverbal communication that involves signing and finger-spelling (Nicolosi et al., 2004). Proponents of the manual approach believe that early in life, children who are deaf must be taught a comprehensive sign language system. The sooner the child learns this system, the better.
- The sign language system is viewed as part of the Deaf culture and is the standard means of communication in the community of people who are deaf. Therefore, children who are deaf learn not only a means of communication, but also a way of integrating into that community.

Total Communication

- Total communication, advocated by some experts, involves teaching both verbal and nonverbal means of communication. Signs and speech are used simultaneously. People who are deaf are taught speech and language along with a sign system. There is no attempt to tap residual hearing through amplification.
- Although critics believe that it is unrealistic to expect children to follow signs, read lips, and sign simultaneously, total communication is a popular current teaching method for children with hearing losses in the profound–severe range (Martin & Clark, 2003; Tye-Muray, 2004).

CONCEPTS TO CONSIDER

What are the basic differences between speech reading, cued speech, and total communication? In what situations might each of these communication methods be appropriate?

Nonverbal Communication: Sign Language

American Sign Language

- American Sign Language, or ASL, is the best known of the sign language approaches. Because there are many variations of ASL, there is no single definition.
- ASL is widely used in the United States and Canada. It is not considered a manual version of English, but is viewed as a separate language.
- In ASL, signs are used to express ideas and concepts through complex hand and finger movements. Each sign expresses a different idea.
- Different signs are made in quick succession, much like spoken words are put into sentences. The syntax of ASL differs from that of spoken Standard American English.

Seeing Essential English

- Seeing Essential English (SEE 1) primarily employs ASL. It breaks down words into morphemes and uses written English word order.
- SEE 1 uses some markers to help identify number and tense, and also uses specific signs for some verbs and articles (e.g., *the, an*).

Signing Exact English

- Signing Exact English (SEE 2) is similar to SEE 1. However, it is used more widely than SEE 1 and is more flexible about precise word order in sentences.
- SEE 2 breaks down words into morphemes that are words when they stand alone (e.g., *hot–dog*).

Fingerspelling

- In fingerspelling, ideas are communicated through quick, precise movements made by the fingers.
- Fingerspelling may be used alone or in conjunction with other methods such as ASL. Sometimes fingerspelling is used for unusual words that do not lend themselves to standard signs.

Rochester Method

- The Rochester method uses a combination of oral speech and fingerspelling. Signs are not used in this method. The oral aspect of the Rochester method is traditional English.

SUMMARY

✓ There are many approaches to the habilitation of people with hearing impairment. These people frequently have disorders of speech, language, voice, fluency, and resonance.

✓ People with hearing losses can be helped by amplification devices such as hearing aids, cochlear implants, tactile aids, and various assistive devices.

✓ These people may also receive communication training, which can consist of auditory training; speech reading; cued speech; oral language training; training in speech, rhythm, and voice; and various verbal and nonverbal approaches to communication.

◆ **AUDIOLOGY IS THE STUDY** of hearing, its disorders, and the measurement and management of those disorders. Audiologists identify, evaluate, and rehabilitate people with hearing losses due to peripheral or central auditory impairments.

◆ **THE EAR CONSISTS OF** three basic parts: the outer, middle, and inner ear. These parts must function normally in order for sound to be converted to electrical impulses within the cochlea and then sent to the brain via the auditory nervous system. Cranial nerve VIII, the acoustic nerve, sends sound impulses to the brain, where the sound is interpreted.

◆ **ACOUSTICS, A BRANCH OF** physics, involves the study of sound as a physical event. The human ear perceives sound in terms of pitch or frequency, and loudness or intensity. Frequency is measured in hertz, or cycles per second, while intensity is measured in decibels.

◆ **HEARING IS A MIRACULOUS** ability that depends on the intricate, precise, and accurate workings of the auditory system. When the outer or middle ear malfunctions, a person may manifest conductive hearing losses. Sensorineural losses reflect malfunctioning of the inner ear, and mixed losses reflect both conductive and sensorineural components. People with central auditory and retrocochlear disorders manifest auditory nervous system impairments, which are challenging to assess.

◆ **ASSESSMENT OF HEARING IMPAIRMENT** depends upon the nature of the problem. Standard procedures in assessment include pure-tone and speech audiometry, which can be carried out through air- or bone-conduction testing. Acoustic immitance testing, involving tympanometry or acoustic reflex testing, is used to assess middle ear function.

◆ **ELECTROPHYSIOLOGICAL AUDIOMETRY AND MEDICAL** imaging are often employed when retrocochlear damage is suspected. This damage is usually caused by tumors, which can grow slowly and make diagnosis very challenging. New, sophisticated techniques such as electrocochleography and magnetic resonance imaging help teams of specialists assess possible pathology of the auditory mechanism.

◆ **HEARING SCREENINGS QUICKLY IDENTIFY** people with normal hearing and people who need more in-depth testing due to possible hearing losses. Infants and children who have

CHAPTER HIGHLIGHTS

hearing losses often need to be assessed with special techniques that allow for reflexive responses if necessary.

◆ **PEOPLE WITH HEARING IMPAIRMENT** manifest a range of communicative disorders. The severity of these disorders depends on the age of onset of the hearing loss as well as the degree of the loss. People with hearing losses may manifest problems in one or more of the areas of articulation, fluency, voice, resonance, and language.

◆ **AURAL REHABILITATION INVOLVES AN** educational and clinical program implemented by teams to help people with hearing losses achieve their full potential. Aural rehabilitation usually includes several key components. Amplification, one component, can involve hearing aids, cochlear implants, tactile aids, and assistive devices.

◆ **COMMUNICATION TRAINING, A SECOND** component of aural rehabilitation, may involve one or more of several methods. These methods include auditory training; speech reading; cued speech; and training in oral language, speech, voice, fluency, and resonance. Various approaches to training may include a verbal emphasis (e.g., total communication and the aural/oral approach) or a nonverbal emphasis, which involves use of a form of sign language.

✎ **ADD YOUR OWN CHAPTER HIGHLIGHTS HERE:**

_____

_____

_____

_____

_____

_____

_____

Study & Review Questions

Essay

1. Describe the outer, middle, and inner ear. What are key anatomical components of each?

2. What are the differences between conductive, sensorineural, and mixed hearing losses? Discuss these differences and their causes.

3. What types of speech and language problems might a child manifest if she had a severe hearing loss?

4. Describe the types of hearing aids that are currently available.

5. What are the primary differences between auditory and oral training for persons with hearing losses? In what circumstances might you use each one?

Multiple Choice

6. A 51-year-old woman comes to an audiologist and states that she feels like she is losing her hearing in her left ear. The woman says that she generally feels healthy, but has noticed that she now uses her right ear exclusively when talking on the telephone. She states: "Sometimes the left side of my face tingles. It doesn't bother me much, but I do notice it sometimes." She also reports that she feels slight dizziness, and has noticed some mild balance problems. For example, when she is on an escalator, she has to "hang on more." She says that "sometimes my left ear rings." Her preliminary audiological results show that she has normal ability to detect pure tones, and that she has normal speech recognition in a quiet room. The most probable diagnosis of this woman's problem is:

    A. central auditory processing disorder.
    B. Meniere's disease.
    C. acoustic neuroma.
    D. otosclerosis.
    E. presbycusis.

7. A person with otosclerosis often has an audiogram reflecting *Carhart's notch*. Carhart's notch is:

    A. a specific type of sensorineural hearing loss characterized by a "dip" at 1,000 Hz.
    B. a specific loss at 4,000 Hz as indicated by both air- and bone-conduction testing.
    C. specific losses at both 2,000 and 4,000 Hz as indicated by bone-conduction testing.
    D. a specific loss at 2,000 Hz as indicated by bone-conduction testing.
    E. a specific loss at 2,000 Hz as indicated by air-conduction testing.

8. A mother brings her 3-year-old Sasha for a hearing screening. She shares that Sasha has had many middle ear infections, which have been treated with antibiotics. These middle ear infections started when Sasha was 9 months old. The mother has been told by a friend that "middle ear tubes" might be a good option for Sasha, but the mother states that she is afraid of the surgery that this would entail. After all, Sasha is only 3 years old, and her mother does not want her to be traumatized. The mother tells you: "Even though Sasha ignores me sometimes, I think everything will be OK. I just wanted her to get checked out to be sure." The audiologist assesses Sasha, with the resulting audiogram shown below. What type of hearing loss does Sasha have based on this audiogram?

A. mixed loss
B. retrocochlear loss
C. sensorineural loss
D. noise-induced loss
E. conductive loss

9. Key parts of the auditory nervous system include cranial nerve VIII, which has two branches: the _____ branch and the _____ branch, which carries the electrical sound impulses from the cochlea to the brain.

A. retrocochlear, vestibular
B. vestibular, auditory-acoustic
C. auditory-acoustic, retrocochlear
D. cochlear, auditory-acoustic
E. retrocochlear, auditory

10. Sensorineural hearing loss can be caused by many things. _____, a hearing impairment in older people, results in a sloping, high-frequency loss. _____ which also causes sensorineural hearing loss, is accompanied by vertigo and tinnitus.

A. Presbycusis, Meniere's disease
B. Meniere's disease, otosclerosis
C. Presbycusis, otosclerosis
D. Central auditory processing disorder, presbycusis
E. Otosclerosis, presbycusis

11. A patient has her hearing tested, and the resulting audiogram has the configuration below.

You can assume that this patient has:

A. a mixed hearing loss.
B. a conductive hearing loss.
C. sensorineural hearing loss.
D. noise-induced hearing loss.
E. a central auditory disorder.

12. A 65-year-old man with presbycusis comes to you complaining that when he is in social situations such as parties, people don't speak loudly enough. He says that the noise creates a problem for him in hearing what people are saying. This client has difficulty with:

A. signal-to-noise ratio.
B. auditory discrimination.
C. figure-ground discrimination.
D. pragmatic skills.
E. auditory memory.

13. Which one of the following is a homophenous pair?

A. *sheep–beep*
B. *man–ban*
C. *pan–fan*
D. *honey–money*
E. *list–gist*

14. The muscle that exerts the pull that allows the eustachian tube to open during yawning and swallowing is the:

A. tensor palatini.
B. levator palatini.
C. tensor tympani.
D. stapedius muscle.
E. levator veli palatini.

15. An infant with cleft palate will most likely have hearing problems because of:

A. aural atresia.
B. an incompletely formed cochlea.
C. eustachian tube dysfunction.
D. malformed ossicles.
E. tympanic membrane dysfunction.

16. A sensorineural hearing loss is related to damage in which area?

   A. the external auditory meatus
   B. the vestibular system
   C. the tympanic membrane
   D. hair cells of the cochlea
   E. the ossicular chain

17. Speech reception thresholds (SRTs) are:

   A. determined by the patient's response to a list of monosyllabic words presented at a low level of hearing.
   B. determined by looking at the patient's pure-tone test results at the frequencies most important to speech.
   C. the lowest level of hearing at which a person can understand 100% of the words presented.
   D. the lowest level of hearing at which a person can understand 50% of the words presented.
   E. the highest level of hearing at which a person can understand 50% of the words presented.

18. Popular forms of amplification today include hearing aids and cochlear implants. Which one of the following is NOT TRUE about these devices?

   A. Cochlear implants may be used with children and also some adults who have sensorineural hearing loss.
   B. Digital hearing aids provide a better signal-to-noise ratio than analog aids.
   C. Cochlear implants can help prelingual children to make substantial progress through maximizing their potential.
   D. A consideration in fitting clients with hearing aids is whether the clients are motivated to use and properly care for the aids.
   E. Cochlear implants deliver amplified sound to the ear canal, while hearing aids deliver electrical impulses (converted from sound) directly to the auditory system.

19. A father comes to you regarding his daughter, who is 8 months old. When the baby was 4 months old, he and his wife noticed that she did not respond to noise. Even when the dog barked loudly or the TV was turned up, the baby did not respond. They took her to an audiologist, and found out that the baby had a bilateral hearing loss and that she was profoundly deaf. The father states that he wishes for his daughter, as she grows older, to "fit in with children with normal hearing." He is interested in any possible amplification and says that he wants his daughter to lead a life that is "as normal as possible." Which training approach would best fit this father's wishes?

   A. total communication
   B. aural/oral method
   C. manual approach
   D. Rochester method
   E. intensive training in American Sign Language and fingerspelling

20. Which of the following are likely to characterize the speech and language of people who are deaf?

I. Omission of /s/ in almost all positions of words
II. Consonant cluster reduction
III. Occasional irrelevance of speech, including non sequiturs
IV. Improper stress patterns, including excessive pitch inflections
V. A voice that sounds strained and strangled

   A. I, II, III, IV
   B. I, III, V
   C. I, II, IV, V
   D. II, III, IV, V
   E. I, II, III, V

REFERENCES AND RECOMMENDED READINGS

American Academy of Audiology. (2004). Position statement: Preventing noise-induced occupational hearing loss. *Audiology Today, 16*(1), 13–16.

Bess, F. H., & Humes, L. E. (2003). *Audiology: The fundamentals* (3rd ed.). Baltimore: Lippincott Williams and Wilkins.

Brackett, D. (2002). Management options for children with hearing loss. In J. Katz (Ed.), *Handbook of clinical audiology* (5th ed. pp. 758–766). Baltimore: Lippincott Williams & Wilkins.

Connor, C. M., & Zwolan, T. A. (2004). Examining multiple sources of influence on the reading comprehension skills of children who use cochlear implants. *Journal of Speech, Language, and Hearing Research, 47,* 509–526.

Crandell, C. C., Smaldino, J. J., & Flexer, C. (2005). *Sound field amplification: Applications to speech perception and classroom acoustics* (2nd ed.). Clifton Park, NY: Delmar Learning.

DeBonis, D. A., & Donohue, C. L. (2004). *Survey of audiology: Fundamentals for audiologists and health professionals.* Boston: Allyn & Bacon.

Erdman, S. A., & Demorest, M. E. (1998). Adjustment to hearing impairment I: Description of a heterogeneous clinical population. *Journal of Speech, Language, and Hearing Research, 41*(1), 107–122.

Ferre, J. (2002). Behavioral therapeutic approaches for central auditory problems. In J. Katz (Ed.), *Handbook of clinical audiology* (5th ed. pp. 525–531). Baltimore: Lippincott Williams Wilkins.

Gelfand, S. A. (2001). *Essentials of audiology* (2nd ed.). New York: Thieme Medical Publishers.

Helfer, K. S. (1998). In C. M. Seymour & E. H. Nober (Eds.), *Introduction to communication disorders: A multicultural approach* (pp. 277–305). Newton, MA: Butterworth-Heinemann.

Katz, J. (Ed.). (2002). *Handbook of clinical audiology* (5th ed.). Baltimore: Lippincott Williams & Wilkins.

Martin, F. N., & Clark, J. G. (2003). *Introduction to audiology* (8th ed.). Boston: Allyn & Bacon.

Mencher, G. T., Gerber, S. E., & McCombe, A. (1997). *Audiology and auditory dysfunction.* Needham Heights, MA: Allyn & Bacon.

Moller, A. R. (2000). *Hearing: Its physiology and pathophysiology.* San Diego, CA: Academic Press.

Nicholls, G. H., & Ling, D. (1982). Cued speech and the reception of spoken language. *Journal of Speech and Hearing Research, 25,* 262–269.

Nicolosi, L., Harryman, E., & Kresheck, J. (2004). *Terminology of communication disorders: Speech-language-hearing* (5th ed.). Baltimore: Lippincott Williams Wilkins.

Nuru-Holm, N., & Battle, D. E. (1998). Multicultural aspects of deafness. In D. E. Battle (Ed.), *Communication disorders in multicultural populations* (2nd ed., pp. 335–378). Newton, MA: Butterworth-Heinemann.

Rose, S., McAnally, P. L., & Quigley, S. P. (2004). *Language learning practices with deaf children* (3rd ed.). Austin, TX: PRO-ED.

Schow, R. L., & Nerbonne, M. A. (2002). *Introduction to audiologic rehabilitation* (4th ed.). Boston: Allyn & Bacon.

Scott, D. M. (1998). Multicultural aspects of hearing disorders and audiology. In D. E. Battle (Ed.), *Communication disorders in multicultural populations* (2nd ed., pp. 335–354). Newton, MA: Butterworth-Heinemann.

Seikel, J. A., King, D. W., & Drumright, D. G. (2000). *Anatomy and physiology for speech, language, and hearing* (2nd ed.). San Diego, CA: Singular/Thomson Publishing Group.

Soli, S. (1998). Classroom acoustics workshop. *Audiology Today, 10*(1), 27.

Stach, B. A. (1998). *Clinical audiology: An introduction.* San Diego, CA: Singular/Thomson Publishing Group.

Stach, B. A. (2003). *Comprehensive dictionary of audiology* (2nd ed.). Clifton Park, NY: Delmar Learning.

Thedinger, B. S. (1996). Cochlear implants. In J. Northern (Ed.), *Hearing disorders* (3rd ed., pp. 291–298). Needham Heights, MA: Allyn & Bacon.

Tye-Murray, N. (2004). *Foundations of aural rehabilitation: Children, adults, and their family members* (2nd ed.). Clifton Park, NY: Delmar Learning.

Zwolan, T. A. (2002). Cochlear implants. In J. Katz (Ed.), *Handbook of clinical audiology* (5th ed. pp. 740–757). Baltimore: Lippincott Williams & Wilkins.

Study & Review
Answers

6. C. These symptoms are typical of a patient with an acoustic neuroma.

7. D. Carhart's notch reflects specific loss at 2,000 Hz as indicated by bone-conduction testing.

8. E. This child has a conductive hearing loss.

9. B. Key parts of the auditory nervous system include cranial nerve VIII, which has two branches: the vestibular branch and the auditory-acoustic branch; it carries the electrical sound impulses from the cochlea to the brain.

10. A. Sensorineural hearing loss can be caused by many things. Presbycusis, a hearing impairment in older people, results in a sloping, high-frequency loss. Meniere's disease, which also causes sensorineural hearing loss, is accompanied by vertigo and tinnitus.

11. C. A sensorineural loss is usually characterized by an audiogram reflecting a sloping, high-frequency loss.

12. A. People who have difficulty separating the signal of interest (speech) from background noise have difficulty with the signal-to-noise ratio.

13. B. Homophenous pairs are those words that look the same on the lips. *Man* and *ban* begin with bilabials; thus the words look similar to listeners with hearing losses.

14. A. The muscle that exerts the pull that allows the eustachian tube to open during yawning and swallowing is the tensor palatini.

15. C. Infants with cleft palate frequently have eustachian tube dysfunction because of the oral–facial anomalies inherent within the cleft palate condition.

16. D. A sensorineural hearing loss is related to damage in the hair cells of the cochlea.

17. D. Speech reception thresholds (SRTs) are the lowest level of hearing at which a person can understand 50% of the words presented.

18. E. Hearing aids deliver amplified sound to the ear canal, whereas cochlear implants deliver electrical impulses (converted from sound) directly to the auditory system.

19. B. The aural/oral method emphasizes: (a) making use of residual hearing through amplification, and (b) helping people with hearing impairment learn to communicate so that they are comfortable in mainstream settings with hearing people.

20. A. People with hearing impairment do not typically have a strained-strangled voice quality unless they also have a concomitant voice disorder.

CHAPTER 11

ASSESSMENT AND TREATMENT: PRINCIPLES OF EVIDENCE-BASED PRACTICE

Assessment and treatment of clients with

communicative disorders are the primary activities of speech–language pathologists. In this chapter, we discuss the principles of and procedures of assessment and treatment that are evidence based. The principles and procedures discussed are foundational, or standard, across most types of communication disorders. Specific information about assessment and treatment of various types of communication disorders may be found in chapters dealing with those specific disorders.

There is a difference between assessment and diagnosis. *Assessment* (also called *evaluation*) refers to the process of arriving at a diagnosis. A *diagnosis* is an understanding of the problem, or the identification of a disorder by analysis of the symptoms presented and, in some cases, analysis of their underlying causes (Haynes & Pindzola, 2004; Tomblin, Morris, & Spriestersbach, 2000). To assess clients and arrive at a diagnosis, clinicians optimally use standard assessment procedures and a combination of standardized and client-specific, nonstandardized assessment measures that are culturally and linguistically appropriate for individual clients.

Treatment in communicative disorders involves several common concepts and procedures. Although treatment is conceptualized in different ways, it essentially involves changing an existing, perhaps nonfunctional, pattern of communication. It requires working not only with clients, but also with the family members, teachers, and others who routinely interact with them. And it requires sensitivity to relevant cultural and linguistic variables. Designing effective treatment procedures requires an accurate assessment of the client's problem. In this chapter, we summarize the basic principles, procedures, and concepts relative to assessment and treatment. Consistent with the current trends in speech–language pathology, our emphasis in selecting and describing treatment procedures will be treatment efficacy evidence.

EVIDENCE-BASED PRACTICE IN SPEECH–LANGUAGE PATHOLOGY

Currently, in medicine, speech–language pathology, and all health-related professions, the emphasis is on evidence-based practice. *Evidence-based practice* ensures that the clients receive services that are known to be based on reliable and valid research and sound clinical judgment. As currently defined (and often debated), evidence-based practice has different connotations (Hegde, 2003; Lohr, Eleazer, & Mauskopf, 1998; Sackett, Rosenberg, Gray, Hayes, & Richardson, 1996; Sackett, Straus, Richardson, Rosenberg, & Hayes, 2000).

■ Most experts consider efficacy for treatment procedures a significant part of evidence-based practice. It is unethical to use treatment procedures that have not been supported by experimental research (see Chapter 12 for details on this kind of research). Only treatment procedures that have been shown to be better than no treatment and have been replicated in different settings, with different clients, and by different investigators may be recommended for general practice (Hegde, 2003). Evidence that supports treatment procedures is classified in somewhat different ways. See Chapter 12 for a summary of *levels of evidence* that help guide the selection of clinical procedures.

■ In a broader sense, evidence-based practice requires an integration of best research evidence for clinical methods with clinical expertise and sound judgment. Evidence-based practice is always client centered. That is, in selecting assessment and treatment procedures, the clinician takes into consideration not only the research evidence, but also what is best for an individual patient and his or her preferences (Sackett et al., 1996; Sackett et al., 2000). In case of children, the child and the family are all involved in making clinical decisions that affect them. This is because a method supported by evidence may be unacceptable to clients, their families, or both.

■ Evidence-based practice also means that the clinician would not use procedures unsupported by evidence, contradicted by evidence, or known to produce negative effects (Lohr et al., 1998). Before selecting clinical methods, especially treatment procedures, the clinician must critically analyze the quantity and quality of evidence supporting the use of advocated treatment techniques and consider the characteristics of the individual client seeking the services. The clinician also should critically examine his or her own training, expertise, and experience in advanced procedures before offering to use them.

■ Finally, evidence-based practice is ethnoculturally sensitive. Selection of assessment and treatment procedures should be made on the basis of not only the experimental evidence supporting them, but also the relevance of procedures to the ethnocultural and family background of the client. See Chapter 9 for more on ethnocultural issues that affect service delivery in communicative disorders.

■ In health-related professions today, the emphasis is on evidence-based practice. Evidence-based practice ensures that services provided for clients are based on sound clinical judgment and reliable and valid research.

■ Evidence-based practice is client-centered and is based on treatment procedures that have been supported by experimental research.

■ Evidence-based practice is also ethnoculturally sensitive; it is appropriate for the client's ethnic, linguistic, and cultural background.

STANDARD ASSESSMENT PROCEDURES

INTRODUCTION

Certain *standard assessment procedures* are used across types of communication disorders. These procedures usually include a screening, a case history, a hearing screening, an oral–peripheral examination, an interview, a speech and language sampling, and related assessment data (Hegde, 2001a; Shipley & McAfee, 2004).

Screening

■ A *screening* is a brief procedure that helps determine whether a client should undergo further, more detailed assessment.

■ Clients who pass screening procedures are judged to have normal skills in the area screened, and thus are not assessed at length. Clients who fail screening procedures are scheduled for comprehensive assessments because they may have communication disorders.

■ Screening procedures are used in many facilities, such as public schools, to determine who should receive full assessments and who should not.

Case History

■ The *case history* yields detailed information that helps the clinician understand the client and his or her communication disorder and associated variables. The case history involves gathering information about the family, health, education, occupation, and other variables such as cultural and linguistic factors.

■ The emphasis of the case history depends upon the age of the client and the nature of the disorder. Typically, a printed case history form and interview of the client, family, or both help obtain information.

■ The clinician should get identifying information (e.g., the client's name, date of birth, address, and phone number) as well as other information summarized below (see Hegde, 2001a; Shipley & McAfee, 2004, for more detail).

Description of the Communication Disorder

Clinicians ask adult clients or parents of child clients the following questions:

- What do you think is the problem?
- When and under what circumstances did you first notice the problem?
- What were the early signs of the problem?
- How has the problem progressed? Has it changed over time or remained the same?
- In your cultural community, are the difficulties you describe viewed as a problem?

Prior Assessment and Treatment of the Disorder

Clinicians ask adult clients or parents of child clients the following questions:

- Have you seen any specialists before this evaluation?
- What did these specialists recommend? Did you follow up on their recommendations?
- Did you (or the child) receive treatment?
- If so, what were the results of treatment?

Family Constellation and Communication

Clinicians ask adult clients or parents of child clients the following questions:

- Is there any family history of communication disorders?
- Who currently lives in the home? What is their relationship to you (your child)?
- How many sisters and brothers do you (does the child) have?
- Does the child communicate with other family members?
- Does the child play with other children? How does the child play with others? How does the child communicate with peers?
- What language(s) do you speak at home? What is your (your child's) first or primary language? Do you (does your child) fluently speak, read, or write in the primary language and English?

Prenatal, Birth, and Developmental History

These questions are usually asked if the client is a child:

- How was the mother's health during the pregnancy? Did she have any major accidents or illnesses? Did she take any drugs?
- What were the birth condition and birth weight of the child?
- Was the child premature or full term? Were there any complications at birth? What type of delivery occurred (feet first, head first, breech, Cesarean)?
- Did the child have any feeding or nursing problems?
- How would you describe your child's physical development? If it seemed normal, what were the specific problems?
- Have you ever noticed any signs of hearing loss? If so, what were those signs?
- How would you describe your child's speech and language development?
- Were you ever concerned about your child's speech and language development? If so, why?

Medical History

Clinicians can ask adult clients or parents of child clients the following questions:

- During the early childhood years, did the child (did you) have any illnesses? What kinds of illnesses?
- Did the child (did you) have any major traumas or accidents of any kind?
- What kinds of surgical and medical treatment did you (your child) have?
- Are you (is your child) currently taking any medications? What medications are they? How long have you (he or she) been taking them?

Educational History

Clinicians can ask adult clients or parents of child clients the following questions:

- What level of education have you completed?
- What grade is the child in? Has the child been held back or advanced a grade?
- Has the child received any special education services? What kinds of services has he or she received?

Occupational History

Clinicians can ask adult clients the following questions:

- What is your current occupation? What types of tasks do you do on your job? Does your communication problem negatively affect your job performance?
- How is your relationship with your colleagues and supervisors? How do they react to your communication problem? Are you concerned about their reactions?
- Do you think you are unable to get a job or receive a promotion because of your communication problem? Why do you think so?
- What is your occupational goal in seeking treatment at this time?

Prognosis

- Frequently, clients and their families wish to know the prognosis for improvement of a communication disorder. A *prognosis* is a professional judgment made about the future course of a disorder or disease. It is a predictive statement about what might happen under various future circumstances. For example, a clinician might predict what might happen if a disorder of fluency remains untreated in a 4-year-old child versus what might happen if the child receives treatment. Or a clinician might predict whether a client who has sustained a stroke will possibly be able to return to his or her previous job.
- Clinicians must be extremely careful in making statements of prognosis. The "Code of Ethics" delineates the parameters of what is considered ethical in making prognostic statements to clients.
- Factors influencing the prognosis for a client include:

  - the severity of the disorder
  - the client's general health
  - the physiological course of an underlying disease
  - the time of intervention (e.g., whether therapy occurred after a child had been stuttering

for 2 years, or when the child first began to stutter)
- the quality and intensity of treatment offered
- the consistency with which treatment is received
- family support for the client and participation in the treatment process
- the client's motivation to work hard in treatment and outside the treatment setting
- social reinforcement for maintaining gains made in treatment
- the client and family's religious and cultural beliefs about the necessity for and efficacy of treatment

Hearing Screening

- A *hearing screening* is a quick procedure to determine whether a client can be assumed to have normal hearing or needs to be more thoroughly evaluated by an audiologist.

- Clinicians should:

  - screen the hearing of all clients whom they assess
  - use a screening procedure adopted at their clinical sites
  - make sure the ambient noise in the screening situation does not compromise validity and reliability of screening results
  - generally, screen hearing at 20 or 25 dB HL for 500, 1,000, 2,000, and 4,000 Hz; screen at 25 dB HL for 500 Hz;
  - screen younger children at 15 dB HL for 500, 1,000, 2,000, 4,000, and 8,000 Hz;
  - refer the client who fails the screening test to an audiologist for a comprehensive hearing evaluation

Oral–Peripheral Examination

- This involves an examination of the oral and facial structures to evaluate their structural and functional integrity from the standpoint of speech production.

CONCEPTS TO CONSIDER

Standard components of any assessment include a case history, hearing screening, and oral–peripheral examination. What are two important facets of each of these components?

_____

_____

_____

_____

_____

■ The *oral–peripheral examination* helps identify or rule out obvious structural abnormalities that may require medical attention.

■ The oral–peripheral examination is an important standard and common assessment procedure that is used with a variety of clients, including children and adults with articulatory-phonological disorders, cleft palate, neurological problems, and others that affect speech production. (For more detailed information on the components of an oral–peripheral examination, see Hegde, 2001a; Shipley & McAfee, 2004.)

Interview

■ An *interview* involves a face-to-face exchange with the client, family members, or both to obtain additional information and to clarify and expand upon the information given on the printed case history form.

■ There are three basic purposes of interviewing (Haynes & Pindzola, 2004; Shipley & Roseberry-McKibbin, 2006):

- to obtain data or information
- to inform the clients and their families
- to provide support

■ An important component of the interview is for the clinician to establish rapport with the client and any family members present. Rapport involves respect, trust, and a harmonious relationship between the clinician and the family.

■ Establishing trust between the clinician and the clien's family involves (Shipley & Roseberry-McKibbin, 2006):

- orienting the interviewees to the nature of the interview
- explaining why certain information is requested
- not making the client feel rushed
- listening
- using appropriate verbal and nonverbal communication
- assuring the client of (and maintaining) confidentiality

■ Maintaining rapport and establishing trust also involve recognizing and accounting for cultural and linguistic variables that might influence the interview. For example, the family might need an interpreter present to assist in the process. Or the family might come from a culture where it is considered inappropriate to reveal personal details. Clinicians must be sensitive to these issues (Roseberry-McKibbin, 2002).

■ During the interview process, it is important to occasionally reflect or report to clients and family members what they have been saying. In this way, clinicians can make sure that they are recording accurate information.

Speech and Language Sample

Nature and Purposes

- The *speech and language sample* is the primary means of assessing a client's speech and language production. Many clinicians record the sample on audiotape for further listening, and some clinicians videotape the sample.
- Generally, a speech and language sample is more naturalistic than conducting standardized tests. Depending on a clinician's vewpoint, speech and language samples supplement the results of standardized tests or vice versa.
- The goal of speech and language sampling is to obtain a representative sample of the client's speech–language production in naturalistic contexts that reflect the client's everyday communication.
- Speech and language samples can be recorded during conversation between the client and the clinician, or between the client and a caregiver or other conversational partners. It is best to obtain speech and language samples that reflect the client's interactions with several different interlocutors.
- Clinicians can allow the sample to be completely unstructured, or they can manipulate contexts and materials to varying extents to evoke specific productions from clients.
- Speech and language samples can be used when analyzing a client's articulatory-phonological skills, language skills, or both. With both adults and children, sometimes clinicians want to obtain information about production of speech sounds in naturalistic conversational contexts. Other times, clinicians want information about the client's syntactic, morphologic, pragmatic, and semantic skills.

Procedures for Obtaining the Sample

- Procedures for obtaining language samples may vary from clinician to clinician and from setting to setting. However, in most settings, the following procedures are recommended for obtaining a representative speech and language sample (Hegde, 2001a; Shipley & McAfee, 2004):
- Tape-record the entire sample in stereo for an optimal dynamic range. Be sure that the presence of the tape recorder does not cause the client to be self-conscious, thus interfering with the naturalness of the sample obtained.
- Obtain 50–100 utterances. This may take at least 30 minutes.
- Observe carefully and take notes on the context of the utterances that may not be clear from the audiotaped sample. For example, when working with a 3-year-old child, the clinician might want to take notes on what books, toys, and other manipulatives are being used at certain times when recording the sample.
- Use a quiet room and avoid noisy stimulus materials. Some clinicians, when using toys, cover the table with a soft cloth to prevent additional noise on the audiotape.
- Carefully select stimuli that are appropriate for the client's cultural-linguistic background, educational level, occupation, and age.
- In the case of most adults, use objects and pictures only when necessary. In most cases, clinicians can converse with adults about relevant topics specific to the client. However, when evaluating adults with neurogenic disorders, clinicians may need to use pictures and objects.
- In the case of children, use procedures appropriate to the child's age. For most young children, it is best to have parents bring several favorite books and toys from home. Many young chil-

dren react best to interesting, attractive games, toys, and books that are appropriate to their age level.

- Use age-appropriate conversational topics (e.g., movies, sports) with older children. If necessary, use pictures with older children who are reluctant to converse.

- When appropriate, especially with young children, begin by having the child interact with one or more family members such as a parent or sibling. As the child's comfort level increases, the clinician may interact alone with the child.

- Do not bombard a child or adult client with questions. Let the client initiate the conversation sometimes, and allow enough periods of silence to encourage the client to initiate speech.

- With an unintelligible client (especially a child) who is being audiotaped, repeat what the client says so that the utterance can be understood on the audiotape.

- Ask as few yes–no questions as possible. Ask primarily open-ended questions; this usually involves wh- questions such as "What is …?" or "Why do …?"

- Obtain a home language sample if the family is willing to tape-record the client at home. The home sample would supplement the sample collected in the clinic and can give the clinician additional information about the client's speech–language skills in different settings.

- The language sample may be analyzed for various aspects of languge and communication. For example, speech sound production and production of various words, phrases, sentences, and different types of sentences may be analyzed. With younger children, the clinician can calculate the mean length of utterance. The clinicians can note such pragmatic skills as turn taking, topic initiation and maintenance, narrative skills, and eye contact during conversation. Clinicians may also use computer software to analyze certain aspects of language production.

Obtaining Related Assessment Data

- Clinicians need to obtain assessment data related to the communication disorder. Such data contribute to an overall understanding of the client as a whole person.

- When working with children, clinicians may want to obtain information related to:

  - hearing evaluations
  - behavioral evaluations
  - medical evaluations and current medications and their side effects
  - educational psychological evaluations
  - regular and special education evaluations (e.g., from teachers, resource specialists)

- When working with adults in medical settings, clinicians may want to obtain information related to:

  - the patient's current medical diagnosis, prognosis, and the current medications and their side effects
  - medical personnel's current and future medical treatment plans for the patient
  - brain imaging and radiologic data that might be related to diagnosis of the communication disorder (especially in older patients with neurological disorders)
  - audiologic findings that might be related to or integrated with the communication assessment
  - physical rehabilitation plans that might affect treatment of the communication disorder

- Clinicians may work on teams with other professionals. Westby, Stevens-Dominguez, and Oetter (1996) have described three kinds of teams:

- *Multidisciplinary teams:* Team members represent multiple disciplines, but each member conducts his or her individual evaluation, writes a separate report, and has little interaction with other team members.
- *Transdisciplinary teams:* Multiple specialists work together in the initial assessment, but only one or two team members provide services.
- *Interdisciplinary teams:* Team members from multiple disciplines interact and use each other's suggestions and information in interpreting data. The team collaboratively writes the evaluation report and intervention plan.

SUMMARY

✓ Most clinicians use standard, common assessment procedures when working with clients who exhibit a wide range of communication disorders. These procedures should be based on established evidence that demonstrates that the procedures are effective.

✓ These common procedures include screening, obtaining a case history, conducting a hearing screening and oral–peripheral examination, conducting an interview, obtaining a speech and language sample, and obtaining related assessment data.

✓ After these standard assessment procedures are completed, most clinicians administer standardized tests as the next step of the evaluation process.

PRINCIPLES OF STANDARDIZED ASSESSMENT

INTRODUCTION

Standardized, norm-referenced assessment is commonly used in speech–language pathology. It offers a number of advantages to clinicians: ease of test administration, ease of test scoring, and some assurance of reliability or stability when the test is readministered. For clinicians in the public schools, standardized test scores comply with legal requirements for determining children's eligibility for treatment. Standardized tests yield quantitative scores and can be judged according to their validity and reliability as measures of appropriateness for use with specific populations.

Nature and Purposes of Standardized Assessment

- A *standardized test* is one that is *systematic.* Standardized tests have explicit directions and strict controls about what the examiner must say and do; specific stimuli are used, and there are explicit rules for scoring the test (Klein & Moses, 1999; Tomblin et al., 2000).

- The goal of having such explicit rules in standardized testing is to ensure that the behaviors being measured not be influenced by the examiner's biases. In addition, the creators of standardized tests hope to ensure that the measurement process will be uniform across examiners (Tomblin et al., 2000).

- The results of standardized tests yield quantitative information (scores or numbers). These scores (described later) allow the client's performance to be compared to the performance of peers.

■ A standardized test is not the same as a *norm-referenced test*. A test can be standardized without being norm-referenced; however, many tests are frequently norm-referenced as well as standardized.

■ In creating norm-referenced tests, the authors select tasks that they believe are valid in measuring certain behaviors and administer those tasks to groups of subjects who are thought to be representative of the population. The performance of the large sample is analyzed, resulting in normative data for specific age groups (Haynes & Pindzola, 2004). Thus, *norms* represent the average performance of a typical group of people (typically children) at different age levels on a test in its process of standardization.

■ The primary purpose of norm-referenced tests is to compare the individual client's score to the average score of the norming group. In that comparison, the clinician determines: (a) if the client has a problem, (b) if the problem is clinically significant, and (c) whether the problem warrants intervention.

■ Ideally, the client is represented in the norming sample. For example, if a white, middle-class, 8-year-old girl is being tested, other white, middle-class, 8-year-old girls should be included in the norming sample.

■ As discussed in Chapter 12, clients tested are often not represented in the norming sample. This is a major problem when clinicians attempt to assess culturally and linguistically diverse children. Research shows that many clincians around the United States continue to use standardized tests to assess these children, even though this is not best practice (Roseberry-McKibbin, Brice, & O'Hanlon, 2005).

■ Use of standardized tests with diverse children is problematic because, for example, a test might have been normed on middle-class, monolingual, English-speaking, white children in Utah, Arizona, and Illinois. Such a test would be invalid for use with a bilingual, Spanish-speaking child who immigrated from Cuba at age 5 years and lives in Louisiana.

■ Unfortunately, many clinicians do not carefully examine the norming samples of tests they use, and thus norm-referenced tests are used inappropriately (Roseberry-McKibbin, 2003).

■ Ideally, in standardizing norm-referenced tests (hereafter referred to as *formal tests*), the authors select children from varied ethnocultural and socioeconomc groups so that the sample is representative of the clients who are tested. In addition, the sample should represent both the genders, all (relevant) age groups, and geographic regions.

■ However, many formal tests are not diverse enough to represent all segments of the society. In addition, many of these tests have small sample sizes. If a test has subgroups, there should be at least 100 subjects per group (Haynes & Pindzola, 2004). This is frequently not the case.

■ Another disadvantage of formal tests is that, although administration and scoring procedures are fairly similar across examiners and are thus repeatable or replicable, tasks are so highly structured that they are usually not representative of the client's behavior in natural environments. In addition, standardized tests rarely give information about how clients arrived at answers or the strategies they used to complete the activities (Westby et al., 1996).

■ Further, many formal tests sample behaviors inadequately, which helps keep the length of the test manageable. For example, in a test of child language, there may be only two or three items that sample the child's production of the plural morpheme.

■ A major problem in speech–language pathology testing is that many clinicians use the results of formal tests to create treatment goals. These treatment goals are based on a limited sampling of specific behaviors, and thus the goals have poor validity.

■ Because the goal of formal testing is to sample a broad range of behaviors, clinicians should take the items that the client answered incorrectly on the formal test and create informal probe measures that sample the behaviors of interest in much greater depth. For example, if the test results show a potential difficulty with the plural morpheme, the clinician can assess their production with words and phrases she creates.

■ Formal tests do not give clinicians specific guidance for planning treatment or evaluating treatment progress. It is critical for clinicians not to use formal tests for those purposes.

■ Thus, the optimal use of formal tests is as follows:

1. After administering a formal test (e.g., the *Orangevale Child Language Test*), examine incorrect items and record them. For example, "The child missed 3/4 items assessing the use of *is–verbing*, and 2/4 items assessing the use of regular past tense *–ed*."
3. Use informal probe tasks to assess the production of language skills in more depth. For example, use conversational speech and structured tasks with words, phrases, and sentences to assess the child's production of *is–verbing* and regular past tense *–ed*.
4. Document the accuracy of production of the skills during such probes. For example, "The child was 40% accurate for production of *is–verbing* in response to looking at pictures and being asked 'What is _____ doing?'" and "The child was 20% accurate for production of plurals during a board game when asked 'What are these?'"
5. Create treatment goals based upon these probe measures. For example, "The target is to have the child produce *is–verbing* with 80% accuracy when shown action pictures and asked 'What is _____ doing?'"
6. Measure treatment progress by assessing accuracy of the child's production of the target skills using tasks similar to the probe tasks (see "Treatment of Communication Disorders" later in this chapter for more details).

■ This is an appropriate and valid use of formal test results for creating treatment goals and assessing treatment progress. Formal test results should always be validated by the results of in-depth, client-specific, assessment.

Types of Scores in Standardized Assessment

■ As stated earlier, the goal of standardized testing is to yield scores or quantitative measures that compare the client's performance to that of a normative group—a group in which the client is represented.

■ A test administration yields a *raw score* for a client. Raw scores are the actual scores earned on a test. For example, on an aphasia test, a patient might receive a raw score of 55, indicating that he or she answered 55 items correctly. The raw score is converted so it can be viewed on a distribution.

C O N C E P T S   T O   C O N S I D E R

Describe why the use of formal (standardized, norm-referenced) tests for creation of treatment goals and assessment of treatment progress is inappropriate and should be avoided.

_____

_____

_____

_____

_____

■ To compare the client's performance to that of a normative group, test makers use *distributions*. Distributions yield measures of the client's performance compared to the performance of the norming sample.

■ Two statistical measures of a distribution are the mean and the standard deviation. The mean is the arithmetic average of the scores of the norming sample. The *standard deviation* is the extent to which scores deviate from the mean or average score. It reflects the variability of all the measures or scores of the norming sample. The larger the standard deviation, the more variable the scores and vice versa.

■ Among scores that have a normal distribution, 34.13% fall within one standard deviation above the mean and 34.13% fall within one standard deviation below the mean (Tomblin et al., 2000). In other words, if scores are normally distributed in a bell-shaped curve, 68% of the sample will have scores between 85 and 115 (assuming 100 is the average score). The standard deviation is 15 points.

■ A client's score enables the clinician to see where the client performs in relation to the mean. The client's score(s) may be expressed in terms of its standard deviation from the mean. Scores may also be expressed in terms of percentile ranks.

■ *Percentile ranks* are converted scores that show the percentage of subjects who scored at or below a specific raw score. Percentile ranks use percentile points to express a client's score relative to the norming sample. For example, if a child's score is at the 25th percentile, 75% of children will do better on the test than that child did.

■ The 50th percentile is equivalent to the mean and *median*. The median is the score in the exact middle of the distribution; it divides the distribution into two parts so that an equal number of scores fall to the right and to the left of it.

- Usually, clients whose scores place them one standard deviation below the mean score slightly below the 16th percentile. People whose scores are two standard deviations below the mean score close to the second percentile (Tomblin et al., 2000).

- Formal tests often yield age-equivalency and grade-equivalency scores. Scores indicating *age equivalency* show the chronological age for which a raw score is the mean or average score in the standardization sample. Scores indicating grade equivalency show the grade placement for which a raw score is the mean or average score. For example, a 6-year-old's score on a test might be typical of a 4-year-old's score in the norming sample. Or a fifth grader's score might be typical of the average score of the third-grade children in the norming sample.

- Because age- and grade-equivalency scores are easier for parents and clients to understand than percentile ranks and standard deviations, many clinicians use them to explain test performance. However, experts do not recommend this practice (see Haynes & Pindzola, 2004, and Tomblin et al., 2000, for further discussion of this issue).

Foundations of Measurement: Evaluating Psychometric Properties of Formal Tests

When clinicians select formal (standardized) tests to use with certain populations, they can evaluate those formal tests according to the broad parameters of validity and reliability.

- Recent research indicates that many clinicians express a low level of concern with these psychometric characteristics of tests (Huang, Hopkins, & Nippold, 1997); thus it becomes even more important to understand and apply the concepts of validity and reliability to the evaluation of tests.

Validity

- Validity refers to the degree to which a measuring instrument or test measures what it purports to measure. For example, for many years, the *Peabody Picture Vocabulary Test–Revised (PPVT–R)* purported to measure intelligence. This was not valid, however, because the PPVT–R measured only a single skill: that of receptive vocabulary. Receptive vocabulary is one very small part of the broad construct of intelligence. Thus, the PPVT–R came to be viewed as *invalid* for measuring intelligence. However, the PPVT–R did measure receptive one-word vocabulary skills; thus, it was and is considered to be a valid measure of receptive one-word vocabulary skills (Tomblin et al., 2000). Today, the PPVT–3 continues to be a *valid* measure of one-word receptive vocabulary skills.
- There are several kinds of validity that clinicians can look for when selecting tests and evaluating their appropriateness for use with given populations. These kinds of validity include *concurrent, construct, content,* and *predictive* validity.

Concurrent Validity

- This refers to the degree to which a new test correlates with an established test of known validity. For example, many new intelligence tests are evaluated against the well-known, trusted, and established *Stanford-Binet Intelligence Test.* If the new intelligence test correlates well with the *Stanford-Binet,* then concurrent validity is established for the new test (Tomblin et al., 2000).

- Too high a correlation suggests that the new test may be as valid as the old one and that the two tests are too similar, raising the question of the need for the new test. The right level of concurrent validity can be challenging to establish.

Construct Validity

- This refers to the degree to which test scores are consistent with theoretical constructs or concepts. Construct validity includes any qualitative or quantitative information that supports the test maker's theory or model underlying the test (Hutchinson, 1996). For example, a language test that shows higher scores for older children compared to younger children is consistent with the theoretical construct that language changes (improves) with age.
- Construct validity is challenging to establish because it requires that measurements be based on a theory. The test must then be developed in a way that is consistent with the theory. Next, the test creator(s) must demonstrate through supporting research that the test indeed conforms to the predictions of the theory (Tomblin et al., 2000).

Content Validity

- This is a measure of validity of a test based on a thorough examination of all test items to determine if the items are relevant to measuring what the test purports to measure, *and* whether the items adequately sample the full range of the skill being measured.
- For example, a test of articulation should include all speech sounds in all word positions and in phrases and sentences. Omission of sounds or inclusion of items not relevant to measuring articulation reduces the content validity of the test.

Predictive Validity

- This refers to the accuracy with which a test predicts future performance on a related task. For example, a test of language competence may be shown to predict academic performance. Many universities use *Graduate Record Examination* (GRE) scores as a criterion for admission into their master's degree programs. This practice is based on the belief that GRE scores have predictive validity—that the scores predict how well students will perform academically in the graduate program.
- Predictive validity is also known as *criterion-related validity* because future performance is the criterion used to evaluate the validity.

Reliability

- *Reliability* means the *consistency* or *stability* with which the same event is repeatedly measured. Scores are *reliable* if they are consistent across repeated testing or measurement of the same skill or event.
- In assessment, reliability of the test is influenced by several factors (Silverman, 1998; Tomblin et al., 2000):

  - fluctuations in examinee's behavior—the examinee may behave differently during various parts of a test due to factors like fatigue, attention span, the presence of medications in his or her system, and environmental distractions
  - examiner error—the examiner may be tired or distracted and thus misuse a test by not

administering it according to the standardized procedures dictated in the manual

- instrumentation or equipment errors—equipment might not be calibrated, or might malfunction

- Most reliability measures are expressed in terms of a *correlational coefficient*. The correlational coefficient is a number or index that indicates the relationship between two or more independent measures. It is usually expressed through Pearson Product Moment *r*.
- The highest possible positive value is $r = 1.00$; the lowest possible negative value is $r = -1.00$. An *r* value of 0.00 indicates that there is no relationship between the two measures. The higher the correlational coefficient, the greater the reliability of a test or measurement.
- Different types of reliability are associated with measurement. These types of reliability are *interjudge reliability, intrajudge reliability, alternate form reliability, test-retest reliability,* and *split-half reliability.*

Interobserver (Interjudge) Reliability

- This refers to how similarly a subject's performance is independently rated or measured by two or more observers (Hegde, 2003). The observers independently score the same set of behaviors, and then their scores are calculated in terms of how well they relate.
- The more similarly the observers independently rate the same skill or event, the higher the *interjudge reliability coefficient*. Optimally, there will be interjudge reliability coefficients of .90 or above to show good agreement among the examiners. The closer the coefficient is to 1.0, the more reliable the scoring (Haynes & Pindzola, 1998).

Intraobserver (Intrajudge) Reliability

- This is the consistency with which the same observer measures the same phenomenon on repeated occasions (Hegde, 2003). For instance, the same clinician measures the frequency of dysfluencies in the same speech sample of a client two or more times to establish her own consistency in measuring dysfluencies.
- If the repeated measures are similar, the clinician will have established intraobserver reliability.

Alternate Form Reliability

- Also known as *parallel form reliability, alternate form reliability* refers to the consistency of measures when two forms of the same test are administered to the same person. To establish alternate form reliability, a test must have two versions that sample the same behaviors.
- For example, the PPVT–R has two forms: A and B. One could use forms A and B of the PPVT–R with the same child and compare scores. Similar scores on the two forms demonstrate the parallel form reliability of PPVT–R.

Test-Retest Reliability

- This refers to consistency of measures when the same test is administered to the same person twice. The results of the two test administrations are compared for consistency. Thus, for example, if a child is given a specific test and receives a score of 96, he or she should receive a similar score if the test is readministered.
- Test-retest reliability suggests stability of scores over time.

Split-Half Reliability

- This refers to a measure of the internal consistency of a test. One can determine split-half reliability by showing that the responses to the items on the first half of the test are correlated with responses given to the items on the second half of the test. Or, one could compare answers on the even-numbered items of a test to answers on the odd-numbered items and see if those answers are correlated.

- To derive split-half reliability, the first and the second half of a test should measure the same skill. Split-half reliability generally overestimates reliability, as it does not measure stability of scores over time.

SUMMARY

✓ Many clinicians use formal (standardized, norm-referenced) tests to assess clients. There are both advantages and disadvantages to using formal tests.

✓ Formal test results alone should never be used to establish treatment goals or measure treatment progress.

✓ Clinicians can analyze formal tests to determine how reliable and valid the tests are, especially for the specific populations the clinician serves.

✓ Clinicians are increasingly using formal tests in conjunction with nonstandardized, client-specfic assessment tools to obtain the most complete profile of clients' skills.

PRINCIPLES OF NONSTANDARDIZED ASSESSMENT

INTRODUCTION

Because of some of the limitations inherent in standardized assessment tests, many clinicians supplement formal test results with those of nonstandardized assessment measures. Nonstandardized, informal assessment measures have the advantage of being flexible, adaptable to individual clients, and valid as a basis for planning treatment (Klein & Moses, 1999). However, behaviors, qualities, or skills as measured informally may be poorly defined and subject to examiner bias. For example, the quality of vocal hoarseness may be subjectively defined differently by various examiners. The skill of cohesive adequacy in narratives is difficult to operationalize, thus making it subjective. A major challenge with informal assessment is to make it reliable and valid for optimal use with clients (Haynes & Pindzola, 2004). Clinicians have attempted to establish validity and reliability by using various types of nonstandardized or informal assessment measures, including measurement scales, structured interviews or questionnaires, functional assessment, criterion-referenced testing, and dynamic assessment.

Measurement Scales

- Sometimes clinicians use rating scales to document observations. These scales are typically *nominal* or *ordinal* in nature.

- In a *nominal scale,* a category (e.g., hoarseness, hyponasality) is present or absent. Items or observations are classified into discrete groups (called groupings) that do not have numerical relationships to one another. For example, a client might be rated as a *mild, moderate,* or *severe* stutterer. Or a questionnaire might ask a stutterer, for a particular item, to circle *always, sometimes,* or *rarely.*

- An *ordinal scale* is a numerical scale that can be arranged according to rank orders or levels. For example, if a clinician is rating voice quality, an ordinal scale might look thus:

Breathiness	1	2	3	4	5	6
Harshness	1	2	3	4	5	6

Structured Interviews and Questionnaires

- *Questionnaires* may be administered personally to clients or sent to clients, who fill them out and then bring them to the clinician. Clinicians who work with children often administer questionnaires to adults, such as parents and teachers, who are familiar with the child in question.

- Questionnaires may be more valid with some populations than formal tests. For example, formal tests are generally inappropriate for use with culturally and linguistically diverse children and adults. Using questionnaires that account for linguistic and cultural background, clinicians can obtain information that more validly reflects clients' actual skills in natural, daily life settings (e.g., Brice & Montgomery, 1996).

- Interviews may stand alone or be used in conjunction with questionnaires. Interviews are generally carried out for the purpose of getting information about a particular client. Interviews have the advantage of being more personalized than questionnaires used alone.

- The use of questionnaires and interviews can yield quantitative data, qualitative data (verbal descriptions), or both. For example, a clinician working with an adult who stutters might ask the client to circle numbers on a scale reflecting attitudes toward stuttering, and also might record the client's verbal descriptions of his or her own attitudes toward stuttering.

Functional Assessment

- The purpose of *functional assessment* is to evaluate a client's day-to-day communication skills in naturalistic, socially meaningful contexts.

- Speech–language pathology is increasingly turning to functional assessment because reimbursers and third-party payers are requiring documentation of functional outcomes of treatment. Many clinicians target clients' functional communication skills during traditional assessments. Functional assessment requires the clinician to make targets, procedures, and settings of assessment as naturalistic and "real life" as possible.

- To target a client's functional communication during an assessment, clinicians may (Brice, 2002; Hegde, 2001a):

  - Observe the client's communication with family members and peers if appropriate.

- Arrange a child–caretaker interaction that approximates their typical, everyday interaction. In this way, it is possible to observe naturalistic communication rather than artificial communication, which frequently results during testing.

- Arrange for various peer interaction situations for children and adolescents and observe communication patterns within those situations. Talk with two or three peers about how the client communicates in social contexts.

- Obtain several home speech and language samples. Tell the family to record natural, everyday communication interactions.

- Observe the child in the classroom, in the cafeteria, on the playground, and in other settings with peers in school (educational) settings. Obtain information from teachers and other professionals about the child's communication skills as observed in everyday settings such as the playground and classroom.

- Observe the patient's interaction with health-care providers and family members while assessing clients in medical settings,. Interview them as to when and how the patient communicates with them (e.g., How does the patient communicate with the physician? With the nurses? With the physical therapist?).

- Interview at least one person with whom an adult client regularly interacts (e.g., colleague, significant other, friend).

- Emphasize conversational interaction. Do not make clinical judgments based solely on purely imitative or picture naming tasks (although use of those tasks, in conjunction with analysis of conversational interaction, may be necessary with some clients).

- Observe and record conversational speech in naturalistic situations outside the clinic room with various conversational partners.

- Create and structure assessment tasks that are meaningful to the individual client. This is especially important with linguistically and culturally diverse clients who do not relate well to the stimuli and pictures in standardized tests that are geared toward white, monolingual, English-speaking clients.

- Use sentences that include names of family members, activities the client enjoys, interests that the client has, and so forth, when carrying out meaningful assessment tasks.

- Document variations in the disorder in natural settings. For example, in assessing the fluency of a person who stutters, document the person's degree of fluency in such naturalistic contexts as talking on the telephone, ordering in a restaurant, or purchasing items in a store.

- Examine the effect the client produces when he or she attempts to communicate. Instead of emphasizing the language structures the client produces in response to the administration of standardized tests, assess communication that has an effect on others. For example, whether a patient with Alzheimer's dementia can communicate his or her basic needs effectively may be, at a certain stage, more important than the syntactic structure the patient uses to communicate those needs.

C O N C E P T S   T O   C O N S I D E R

Why are more clinicians turning to nonstandardized, informal assessment measures? Summarize advantages and disadvantages of those measures.

_____

_____

_____

_____

_____

Criterion-Referenced Testing

- *Criterion-referenced testing* is a form of assessment in which the examiner selects target behaviors to be assessed and uses stimulus materials that are effective for and individualized to the particular client.

- Some level of performance is viewed as minimal for being deemed "acceptable." For example, when assessing swallowing, the clinician needs a standard defining unacceptable level of aspiration. Thus, criterion-referenced testing involves a qualitative evaluation of what is acceptable and what is unacceptable performance (Tomblin et al., 2000).

- An example of criterion-referenced testing would be the clinician formulating specific questions and seeking answers to those questions. For example, the clinician might pose the question, "Does Susie use regular plural –s accurately in conversational speech?" Then the clinician might select ten pictures with plurals in them and ask Susie, "What do you see here?" The clinician, using a predetermined passing criterion of 80% accuracy (for example), would judge whether Susie "passed" for correct production of regular plurals.

- In standardized norm-referenced testing, a client's performance is explicitly evaluated against age-based norms. The purpose of norm-referenced testing is to rank individuals (McCauley, 1996). In criterion-referenced testing, the results are not compared against norms derived from the performance of a representative sample. Rather, skills are defined and individual performance is emphasized.

- Criterion-referenced measures may prove to be especially helpful when the norms of standardized tests do not apply to a particular client (e.g., a culturally and linguistically diverse client) or when the available standardized tests do not assess specific client skills of interest to the clinician (McCauley, 1996).

- Thus, criterion-referenced testing may assess aspects or skills that standardized tests do not include, and may assess those skills in greater depth than standardized tests do. Also, criterion-referenced testing is helpful in assessing a client's progress in treatment.

Dynamic Assessment

- Clinicians frequently use *static assessment,* or assessment that measures a client's abilities at one point in time. Static assessment accepts a client's current level of functioning as a predictor of how well the client will function in the future.

- Because clients learn, change, and grow, static assessment is not optimal. Increasingly, clinicians are using dynamic assessment. *Dynamic assessment* (also referred to in Chapter 9) measures a client's ability to learn over time when provided with instruction (Roseberry-McKibbin, 2002). In dynamic assessment, the question asked is: What is the child's underlying language-learning *ability?* What is the child's ability to learn when provided with instruction or intervention?

- Dynamic assessment typically occurs in a test-teach-retest paradigm. The client (usually a child) is tested, and his or her skills are measured. Then the child is taught the skills that he or she did not manifest during testing. Finally, the child is retested to assess how quickly and well he or she learned the material presented. A unique feature of dynamic assessment, then, is the incorporation of intervention into the assessment process (Lidz & Peña, 1996).

- Because many children come from backgrounds where they are not exposed to the information assumed by formal tests, they score poorly on formal tests even if their language-learning ability is normal. Dynamic assessment controls for this mismatch between children's backgrounds and formal test assumptions. Again, the child's capability for learning and changing in response to intervention is evaluated as opposed to the child's knowledge of given skills at a certain time without intervention.

SUMMARY

- ✓ Informal, nonstandardized measures include measurement scales, structured interviews and questionnaires, functional assessment measures, criterion-referenced measures, and dynamic assessment.

- ✓ These measures have many advantages for use with clients. Informal measures allow clinicians to tailor assessment to individual clients, create treatment goals, and monitor treatment progress.

- ✓ Clinicians must take precautions to ensure that informal assessment measures are reliable and valid.

TREATMENT OF COMMUNICATION DISORDERS: BASIC CONCEPTS

INTRODUCTION

Treatment, remediation, and *therapy* are all terms used to refer to ways of modifying communication disorders to achieve patterns of normal, functional, or socially more acceptable patterns of communication. Treatment follows a comprehensive assessment, which results in a diagnosis of a communicative disorder. We have summarized treatment procedures specific to given disorders in their respective chapters. In this section, we will define treatment, describe a treatment paradigm for communication disorders, and offer definitions of some basic treatment terms and techniques. The techniques defined in this section are applicable in treating a variety of communication and swallowing disorders.

Treatment: Definition

- *Treatment* may be broadly defined as "teaching, training, any type of remedial or rehabilitative work, and all attempts at helping people by changing their behaviors or teaching new skills" (Hegde, 1998a, p. 12). Treatment also involves working with family members of the client, teachers, peers, and institutional caretakers (e.g., the staff at a rehabilitation facility) to support and sustain communication skills in all natural and institutional settings.

- A more strict definition of treatment is that it is a procedure in which contingent relations between antecedents, responses, and consequences (described later) are managed by a clinician to effect desirable changes in communication behaviors.

- Communication behaviors are considered disordered when they attract negative attention, create difficulty in interactions, and cause speakers to sound different than other people in their speech communities (Locke, 1998). Communicative disorders also create academic, social, and occupational limitations for the invdividual.

- Success in treatment of communication disorders depends upon how effectively the clinician is able to change the way speakers and their listeners react to each other (Hegde & Davis, 2005).

- The clinician rearranges listener–speaker relations by first organizing his or her interaction with the client. Eventually, as the client learns new behaviors, the clinician must rearrange the communicative relations between the client and the client's family, friends, and other important people in the client's environment.

- Historically, speech–language pathologists have focused upon the clinician–client relationship within the therapy room. Although clients have learned to produce appropriate communication behaviors in the clinic, generalized production in the environment has been limited. Today's clinicians implement special procedures to have the child produce clinically learned skills in natural environments.

- That goal can be accomplished in several ways. Clinicians can spend increased time working with the client in interactions with significant others as well as in situations outside the therapy room. In public schools, for example, clinicians can collaborate with classroom teachers and carry out therapy in classroom settings (Brice & Roseberry-McKibbin, 1999; Roth & Worthington, 1996).

A Treatment Paradigm for Communication Disorders

- Clinicians identify target behaviors for a client, arrange stimulus conditions for those behaviors, select materials and procedures to evoke responses, evoke the responses, and apply consequences to the responses. In this way, clinicians manipulate the environment to positively affect the client's behaviors.

- Clinicians' manipulation of the environment to positively affect clients' behaviors should be based on a particular scientific philosophy (Hegde, 1998a; Roth & Worthington, 1996). This philosophy states that all concepts and procedures used must be empirically validated; that is, procedures should be experimentally demonstrated to be effective.

■ Unfortunately, many treatment concepts and procedures are not empirically validated. They are based upon speculation, anecdotal evidence, or opinions of "experts" who have not empirically tested their ideas. Many mistakes are made when clinicians "jump on a bandwagon" and vigorously use and promote treatment ideas that have never been subjected to scientific scrutiny.

■ Ideally, treatment procedures should be objective, measurable, empirical, and reliable. Clinical procedures should include methods that help document the effectiveness of treatment.

■ To help meet this need, the American Speech-Language-Hearing Association Task Force on Treatment Outcomes and Cost Effectiveness, created in 1993, has worked toward the goal of creating an outcomes database for speech–language pathology and audiology.

■ This database is currently composed of data gathered by clinicians participating in various projects that reflect the ages and types of communication disorders manifested by clients. The data have been and will be used, in part, to create functional communication measures (FCMs) (ASHA, 1997).

■ For example, FCMs for cognitive communication include seven levels. Level 1 is "No meaningful cognitive communication," and Level 2 is "Cognitive communication is limited to brief episodes of appropriateness with minimal cueing; client is unaware of deficits" (ASHA, 1997, p. 27). Level 7 is "Normal cognitive communication in all situations."

■ Ideally, FCMs involve treatment procedures and measures that are empirically valid as well as effective in helping clients communicate to the best of their potential in their everyday living environments.

C O N C E P T S T O C O N S I D E R

Define the term *treatment*. Summarize the above-described treatment paradigm for communicative disorders.

_____

_____

_____

_____

_____

Basic Treatment Terms

There are some common terms that most clinicians use in describing general treatment and specific techniques. An understanding of these terms helps clarify the treatment of specific disorders described in other chapters.

■ *Antecedents or treatment stimuli:* Various objects, pictures, instructions, modeling, prompts, and other stimuli the clinician uses to evoke target responses from clients.

■ *Aversive stimuli:* Events people tend to avoid; events people describe as unpleasant and hence work hard to avoid. For example, a person who stutters might try to avoid speaking on the telephone when possible; speaking on the telephone is an aversive event.

■ *Avoidance:* An action that results in not coming in contact with an aversive event and hence is repeated in the future when such contact seems imminent (e.g., avoiding an aversive person by not going to a place at a time when he or she is likely to be there). Avoidance is a behavior exhibited by many clients (e.g., stutterers who avoid specific speaking situations). It is a behavior that needs to be reduced in some cases.

■ *Escape:* A behavior that reduces or terminates an aversive event after having come in contact with that event; a behavior that increases in frequency because it helped to reduce or terminate an aversive event (e.g., a stutterer's response of terminating a conversation with a hostile listener). Escape is a behavior to be reduced in some clients.

■ *Baselines:* Measured response rates in the absence of treatment; the natural rate of a response when nothing special is done to affect its frequency. Baselines help establish that the client did not produce the target behaviors and hence the treatment was necessary; reliable baselines are a part of evidence-based practice.

■ *Booster treatment:* Treatment given any time after the client was dismissed from the initial treatment. It is an important maintenance strategy and may involve the original or a new form of treatment.

■ *Constituent definitions:* Definitions of target behaviors in dictionary terms; defining concepts with the help of other conceptual (not procedural) terms (e.g., *Language* is the mental capacity to communicate). Constituent definitions are not helpful in measuring what is being defined in contrast with operational definitions.

■ *Operational definitions:* Definitions that describe how what is defined is measured (e.g., *morphologic skills* include production of plural morphemes in words, phrases, and sentences with 90% accuracy). Operational definitions, in contrast with constituent definitions, are helpful in quantitatively measuring changes in target behaviors during treatment.

■ *Criteria:* Guidelines for making such clinical decisions as when to judge whether a response is trained, when to move on to another target, and when to dismiss the client from treatment.

■ *Corrective feedback:* Information given to the client on incorrect or unacceptable responses in an effort to decrease those responses (e.g., saying "no" or "wrong" when an incorrect response is given).

■ *Direct methods of response reduction:* Reducing behaviors by immediately providing a corrective feedback (e.g., reducing stuttering or asking inappropriate questions during treatment by saying "no"); contrasted with indirect methods of response reduction.

■ *Indirect methods of response reduction:* Reducing undesirable behaviors by positively reinforcing, and thus increasing, desirable behaviors. For example, reinforcing quiet sitting and other cooperative behavior during treatment with verbal praise and a token but ignoring uncooperative behaviors. Note that nothing is done directly to decrease the undesirable behaviors.

■ *Trial:* A structured and discrete opportunity to produce a response. A trial may involve showing various kinds of stimuli, asking questions, modeling, or prompting. The response given to each trial is scored separately.

■ *Discrete trials:* Treatment methods in which each opportunity to produce a response (e.g., individual words in learning correct articulation; specific sentences) is counted separately. Each opportunity is clearly separated in time (e.g., by pausing for a few seconds after each attempt and scoring each response as correct or incorrect). Discrete trials are helpful in establishing target behaviors but are less efficient in promoting generalization to natural settings than spontaneous productions.

■ *Evoked trial:* Clinical procedure in which no modeling is given; pictures, questions, and other stimuli are used to provoke a response (e.g., asking the client to name a picture or asking such questions as "Johnny, what is this?" while showing a picture or an object). Evoked trials follow modeled trials.

■ *Modeled trial:* A discrete opportunity to imitate a response when the clinician models it. A modeled trial is typically preceded by a question (e.g., "What is this? Say ...").

■ *Modeling:* The clinician's production of the response the client is expected to learn. Modeling is used to teach imitation and is effective in establishing target behaviors. It is used in the initial stages of treatment.

■ *Exemplar:* A specific target response that illustrates a broader target behavior. Exemplars are individual items trained in therapy sessions (e.g., the word *soup* in teaching the /s/ or the phrase *two cups* in teaching the regular plural inflection).

■ *Extinction:* Simply withholding such reinforcers as attention to reduce a response. Extinction is appropriate in reducing such behaviors as crying and interfering questioning in treatment.

■ *Fading:* A treatment procedure in which the controlling power of a stimulus is gradually reduced while the response is maintained (e.g., making modeling less and less audible to the client until finally only an articulatory posture is modeled and then withdrawn).

■ *Follow-up:* An assessment procedure designed to find out if clients have maintained their treatment gains. In most cases, follow-up involves recording a conversational speech sample to evaluate the continued use of clinically established communicative behaviors. Follow-up may involve a regular schedule (e.g., semiannual or annual assessments following dismissal from treatment).

■ *Functional outcomes:* Effects of treatment that are generalized, broader, and socially and personally meaningful to clients, their families, caregivers, and others. Functional outcomes are qualitative effects (e.g., a treated stutterer's social communication) that go beyond quantitative changes in traditionally measured behaviors (e.g., reduction in the number of stuttering behaviors).

■ *Generality of treatment:* Evidence that a treatment found effective in one situation, by one clinician, with some clients, is effective in other situations, when used by other clinicians, and with other clients. Generality is important in recommending a treatment for general practice.

■ *Generalized production:* Production of a clinically established behavior in natural settings with no particular or systematic reinforcement. Generalized production may be temporary unless reinforced.

■ *IEPs:* Individual educational programs for children with disabilities or special needs. IEPs are legally mandated in public school settings.

■ IFSPs: Individualized family service plans are legally mandated for infants and toddlers with disabilities or special needs and their family members. The goal is to involve the family members in the treatment process.

■ *Imitation:* A process of learning in which the learner reproduces what is modeled by an instructor or clinician.

■ *Informative feedback:* Telling clients how well they are doing in treatment sessions; giving specific quantitative information on performance to motivate the client (e.g., telling the client, "During the last sessions, you were 70% correct; this time, you are 85% correct").

■ *Intermediate response:* A response that helps move toward the final target in a shaping procedure (e.g., vocalizing the /m/, opening the mouth while vocalizing, and closing the mouth in saying the word *mom*). An intermediate response is not stabilized by excessive reinforcement.

■ *Initial response:* The first, simplified component of a target response the client can imitate while shaping a target response (e.g., putting the lips together for production of the word *mom*).

■ *Maintenance strategy:* Various methods used to help maintain treatment gains in natural settings. These methods include training family members and others in evoking and reinforcing target behaviors and the client's self-monitoring of communicative skills.

■ *Manual guidance:* The use of physical guidance in a shaping process (e.g., moving a client's tongue with a tongue blade to a correct articulatory position; taking a child's hand and pointing to the correct picture).

■ *Mode of responses:* Manner or method of a response; typical modes include imitation, oral reading, and conversational speech.

■ *Peer training:* Training peers of clients to identify, prompt, evoke, reinforce, and record target behaviors in natural settings. Peer training is a response maintenance strategy.

■ *Physical setting generalization:* Production of clinically established responses in environments such as the home, school, and office that are outside the therapy room.

■ *Physical stimulus generalization:* Production of clinically established responses to stimuli that were not used in training but are similar to stimuli that were used in training.

■ *Post-reinforcement pause:* Absence of responses following the delivery of a reinforcer. These pauses are more commonly observed under fixed-interval schedules of reinforcement.

■ *Pretests:* Procedures to measure target behaviors before starting treatment. Pretests are necessary to justify the need for treatment and to document changes under treatment. Pretests are compared with the results of posttests.

■ *Posttests:* Procedures designed to measure target behaviors after treatment to document changes from the pretests.

■ *Prompts:* Additional verbal (e.g., "The word starts with a *t*..." in teaching naming to aphasic patients) or nonverbal stimuli (showing an articulatory posture in the absence of voicing) that increase the probability of a target response. Prompts are useful with most clients.

■ *Probes:* Procedures to assess generalized production of responses without reinforcing them. Probes involve a criterion to be met before training advances to a more complex level or to another target behavior.

■ *Pure probes:* Procedures for assessing generalized production when only untrained stimulus items are presented.

■ *Intermixed probes:* Assessment of generalized production of trained responses by alternating trained and untrained stimulus items.

■ *Procedures of treatment:* Methods of treatment (e.g., modeling, instructions, verbal praise, prompting). Procedures are what the clinician does to teach target behaviors in clients.

■ *Punishment:* Procedures of reducing undesirable behaviors by response-contingent presentation or withdrawal of stimuli. Punishment includes corrective feedback, time-out, and response cost.

■ *Time-out:* A brief period of silence, inactivity, and lack of reinforcement imposed on a response to be reduced (e.g., a silent period of 5 seconds imposed on every instance of stuttering).

■ *Response cost:* A method of reducing responses by withdrawing reinforcers contingent on each response (e.g., taking a token away from the client for every incorrect production of a phoneme).

■ *Response generalization:* Production of new (untrained) responses that are functionally similar to those that have been trained.

■ *Response mode generalization:* Production of new (untrained) responses in a mode not involved in training (e.g., spontaneous production of untrained words after correct and reinforced imitation training).

■ *Stimulus generalization:* Evocation of established responses by stimuli not involved in training. For example, a child might have been trained to produce /s/ correctly in the words *see, sun,* and *saw.* If the clinician holds up a (untrained) picture of soup and says, "What's this?" and the child correctly says, "Soup," that is stimulus generalization.

■ *Self-control:* Deliberately maintaining, increasing, or decreasing specific behaviors of oneself. Self-control is useful in a response maintenance strategy and includes such procedures as self-monitoring correct responses and self-recording undesirable behaviors.

■ *Shaping:* A method of teaching nonexistent responses that are not even imitated. A target response is broken down into initial, intermediate, and terminal components and those are then taught in an ascending sequence. Shaping is also known as *successive approximation.*

■ *Targets of treatment:* Skills and behaviors a client is taught.

■ *Terminal response:* The final target behavior in a shaping procedure. For example, with a nonverbal child, the final target might be production of selected words in conversational speech the child produces in the home or other situations.

■ *Tokens:* Objects that are given for correct responses and later exchanged for backup reinforcers. Tokens require learning to be effective, and they are powerful because a variety of reinforcers can be used as backups. Tokens also help in resisting the satiation effect.

■ *Satiation:* An internal body state that renders primary reinforcers (such as food) temporarily ineffective. For example, a client might feel full and thus not desire the food reinforcers offered.

Reinforcers and Reinforcement: Basic Definitions

Clinicians shape and change clients' behavior through procedures such as reinforcement. Reinforcement is a key component of treatment programs, and is used with clients who have a variety of communication disorders.

Reinforcement

Reinforcement is a method of selecting and strengthening behaviors by arranging immediate consequences under specific stimulus conditions. Types of reinforcement include those defined below.

- *Continuous reinforcement:* A method of reinforcing all correct responses in treatment sessions; this can be contrasted with intermittent reinforcement.
- *Intermittent reinforcement:* Reinforcement of only some responses or responses produced, with some delay between reinforcers.
- *Differential reinforcement:* Teaching a client to give different responses to different stimuli (e.g., teaching the plural response to plural stimuli and the singular response to singular stimuli). Differential reinforcement involves reinforcing the correct response while ignoring the incorrect response to the same stimuli.
- *Differential reinforcement of alternative behaviors (DRA):* Reinforcing a specified, desirable alternative to an undesirable behavior. DRA involves replacing undesirable behaviors with desirable behaviors that give the client access to the same effects or consequences (e.g., teaching a child to use words instead of whining to get attention).
- *Differential reinforcement of low rates of responding (DRL):* Decreasing undesirable behaviors gradually by reinforcing progressively lower frequencies of that behavior (e.g., reinforcing a

child for asking progressively fewer interfering questions during treatment until the frequency is reduced to zero or near zero).

- *Differential reinforcement of incompatible behaviors (DRI):* Reinforcing a desirable behavior that cannot coexist with the undesirable behavior to be reduced (e.g., heavily reinforcing a child to sit quietly when the target is to reduce restless in-seat behavior or off-seat behavior during treatment).
- *Differential reinforcement of other behaviors (DRO):* Specifying one behavior that will not be reinforced (e.g., leaving the chair in a group treatment session) while reinforcing many unspecified desirable behaviors (e.g., quiet sitting, coloring, reading, writing), any one of which is accepted.
- *Negative reinforcement:* Strengthening of behaviors by the termination of an aversive event. Negative reinforcement is involved in aversive conditioning (e.g., strengthening a stuttering person's avoidance of speaking situations because such avoidance also helps that person avoid or terminate aversive listener reactions).
- *Reinforcement withdrawal:* Prompt removal of reinforcers to decrease a response; includes such procedures as extinction, time-out, and response cost.

CONCEPTS TO CONSIDER

What is reinforcement? Describe three types of reinforcement clinicians use in treatment.

_____

_____

_____

_____

_____

Schedules of Reinforcement

Schedules of reinforcement are different patterns of reinforcement that generate different patterns of responses. Schedules of reinforcement include those described below.

- *Fixed-interval (FI) schedule:* A schedule of reinforcement in which an invariable time duration separates opportunities to earn reinforcers. FI schedules are a form of intermittent reinforcement schedule based on time lapsed between two reinforcements (e.g., in an FI 2-minute schedule, correct responses given after a 2-minute lapse following the previously reinforced response are reinforced and any responses within the interval are ignored).
- *Fixed-ratio (FR) schedule:* An intermittent schedule of reinforcement in which a certain number of responses are required to earn a reinforcer (e.g., reinforcing the fifth correct response during articulation training). The FR schedule helps fade or reduce reinforcement density.
- *Variable-interval (VI) schedule:* A reinforcement schedule in which the time between reinforc-

ers is varied around an average (e.g., reinforcing fluency on a VI 10 seconds means that the client is praised for fluent speech once in 10 seconds on the average, but from one instance of reinforcement to the other the duration will vary). The VI schedule is a form of intermittent reinforcement schedule; it generates a high and consistent response rate.

- *Variable-ratio (VR) schedule:* A reinforcement schedule in which the number of responses needed to earn a reinforcer is varied around an average (e.g., reinforcing correct production of phonemes on a VR 10 means that an average of 10 correct responses is required before praising the client, but from one instance of reinforcement to the next, the number of correct responses will vary). The VR schedule is a form of intermittent reinforcement schedule that generates a high and consistent response rate.

Reinforcers

Reinforcers are events that follow behaviors and thereby increase the future probability of those behaviors. Reinforcers may be verbal or nonverbal and are essential to establish target behaviors. Descriptions of types of reinforcers follow:

- *Automatic reinforcer:* Sensory consequences of a behavior that reinforce that behavior (e.g., the sensation associated with an autistic child's head banging that increases its frequency).
- *Backup reinforcer:* Reinforcer given at the end of a treatment session in exchange for tokens the client earned in the treatment session. For example, if a child earns 10 happy face chips during the session, he or she might get a sticker at the end of the treatment session.
- *Conditioned generalized reinforcer:* Reinforcer whose effect does not depend on a particular motivational state of the client. These reinforcers are effective in a wide range of situations and include tokens and money.
- *Conditioned or secondary reinforcers:* Events such as praise, smiles, and approval that strengthen a person's response because of past experience.
- *Negative reinforcers:* Events that are aversive and thus reinforce a response that terminates, avoids, or postpones them. For example, an aversive event (negative reinforcer) might be teasing endured by a boy who stutters. The teasing negatively reinforces the boy's response of being silent because by being silent, the boy may avoid being teased.
- *Positive reinforcers:* Events that follow a response and thereby strengthen them. Positive reinforcers are necessary in teaching any kind of skill to any client. They may be verbal (e.g., verbal praise) or nonverbal (e.g., the presentation of a token).
- *Primary reinforcers:* Events whose reinforcing effects do not depend on past learning or conditioning. Primary reinforcers are biologically determined because of their survival value (e.g., food and water). They are useful for establishing target responses although not for promoting generalized productions. Primary reinforcers are also known as unconditioned reinforcers.
- *Secondary reinforcers:* Social or conditioned reinforcers whose effects depend on past learning (e.g., social praise and tokens).

SUMMARY

✓ Treatment involves teaching new skills to people who manifest disorders of communication. To teach those new skills, the clinician manages contingent relations between antecedents, responses, and consequences.

✓ Ideally, selected treatment procedures are supported by experimental evidence for their effectiveness.

✓ Many terms are used in describing treatment. Some of these terms are used to describe treatment stimuli, reinforcement, various reinforcement schedules, and types of reinforcers.

AN OVERVIEW OF THE TREATMENT PROCESS

There are various approaches to selecting treatment targets: the normative strategy, client-specific strategy, functional communication strategy, and integrated approach. After selecting target skills, the clinician can sequence treatment and implement the procedures of follow-up and booster treatment.

Selection of Treatment Targets

Different approaches may be used to selecting treatment targets. It is possible to have an integrated approach to treatment selection. A few common approaches and an integrated approach are described as follows.

Normative Strategy

- This strategy is based on the notion that, especially for children, norms provide the best basis for selecting target behaviors. This approach is most frequently used in treating language and articulation disorders in children. Within this approach, age-based norms dictate the target behaviors.
- For example, target responses for a 4-year-old child with language delay would be those language behaviors that are considered appropriate for a normally developing 4-year-old child. Similarly, phonemes selected for treatment in the case of a child with an articulation disorder will be age-appropriate sounds based on articulation norms.
- Published norms are often limted to speech sound and language structure acquisition.

Client-Specific Strategy

- Within this strategy, behaviors that will improve the client's communication, that will help meet the social, academic, and other demands made on the client, will be selected. Some of these behaviors may be consistent with the normative strategy, but others may not be.
- For example, in selecting language treatment targets for a 10-year-old child, with developmental disabilities, one might consider the special education class she attends and make an analysis of the educational terms she needs to learn. Those terms and their use in phrases and sentences might be the selected targets instead of what might be appropriate for a typical 10-year-old.
- The client-specific strategy is suitable for selecting target behaviors that are appropriate for clients of varied ethnocultural backgrounds. Because the approach emphasizes the individual's needs and uniqueness, it allows for a consideration of the particular cultural and linguistic background of the client in selecting target behaviors.

Functional Communication

- This approach is similar to the client-specific approach. In both approaches, what is most useful, what kinds of skills enhance communication, and what kinds of skills help meet the social and other demands made on the client are the main considerations in selecting target behaviors.

- Within the functional approach, grammatical accuracy and speech production accuracy are less important than effective communication. For example, a clinician could choose one of two target behaviors for a client with aphasia. One target behavior might be the use of grammatically correct sentences, but another, more functional target behavior might be effective communication by means of phrases or sentences, gestures, signs, writing, or a combination of these and other means.
- Functional communication targets help improve naturalistic communication. This approach is based on the assumption that any mode of response is appropriate, provided it results in effective communication.
- Functional communication approach and the client-specific approach most often go together. What is best for a given client is often the most functional or useful for that client.

Integrated Approach to Target Behavior Selection

- Within this approach, treatment targets are appropriate for the client's age, ethnocultural background, individual uniqueness, and communication requirements. The targets should be functional and useful and should enhance natural communication in everyday situations.
- As such, the approach places a greater emphasis on the client and effective communication and does not totally negate the importance of age-appropriate targets, especially for children.

C O N C E P T S T O C O N S I D E R

Summarize the different approaches to selecting target behaviors. Which approach do you most favor? Why?

_____

_____

_____

_____

_____

Treatment Sequence

Treatment has a typical sequence although it is usually modified to suit an individual client. The sequence may be based on several factors: response complexity, degree of structure, response modes, multiple targets, training and maintenance, and shifts in treatment contingencies.

Response Complexity

- Generally, treatment starts at a simple level and proceeds to more complex levels. At each level, a performance criterion must be met before the client advances to the next level of response complexity. Typical levels of response complexity include syllables, words, phrases, and sentences.

- For example, a child with a w/r substitution who could produce the /r/ sound correctly in isolation might progress to correct /r/ production in syllables, followed by words, phrases, and then sentences.

- It is neither necessary nor desirable always to start at the simplest level. Clinicians are free to start at a more complex level to see if the client would still learn. For instance, one child may need training at the sound or syllable level whereas another child might learn the sound at the word or even phrase level to begin with.

Degree of Structure

- The sequence of treatment is partially based on the degree of treatment structure. Treatment is more structured in initial stages than in later stages. To establish the target behaviors, the clinician uses highly structured discrete trials in the initial stages of training and at the beginning of each new response topography.

- As the client becomes more proficient in producing the target behaviors, and the training is moved to more spontaneous kinds of productions, the treatment structure is loosened. The training environment becomes more similar to natural settings in which everyday communication takes place.

- For example, an adult who stutters might initially work on producing fluent phrases with 80% accuracy in a one-on-one situation with the clinician in the therapy room. Eventually, after more training on longer utterances in different situations, the client might go with the clinician to a restaurant and practice ordering a meal using fluent speech.

Response Modes

- Another factor influencing the sequence of treatment is the different response modes used in training. In most cases, the treatment starts with imitation. When the client reliably imitates target responses, modeling is withdrawn, and evoked trials are introduced. Thus, imitation and spontaneous production are taught in that order.

- Spontaneous productions may be more or less structured or controlled. This too, can create a sequence. Initial spontaneous productions may be more controlled and structured than the eventual naturalistic conversational speech. Reading, if it is a part of training, might introduce an additional sequence.

Multiple Targets

- Most clients need to attain multiple targets in treatment. This influences the treatment sequence as well. Clients with fluency disorders receiving fluency-shaping treatment, for example, are taught airflow management, gentle phonatory onset, and rate reduction by syllable prolongation roughly in that order, although those skills are all soon integrated and practiced.

- Clients with language targets need to learn various language structures that must be sequenced (Roseberry-McKibbin, 2001). For instance, such pragmatic skills as conversational turn taking and topic maintenance cannot be taught until the client is taught certain words, phrases, and sentences that make it possible for the client to talk on a topic.

- When specific morphologic features are targets, they, too, must be sequenced. For instance, the child must master the present progressive –*ing* before mastering the auxiliary or copula *is*.

Training and Maintenance

- A well-known sequence is based on initial training (establishment of target behaviors) and eventual maintenance of those behaviors in natural settings and over time. Although many maintenance strategies may be incorporated from the beginning of treatment, others are appropriately sequenced at later stages of treatment.
- For example, while parents may be trained in identifying target behaviors from the beginning of treatment, prompting and reinforcing target behaviors produced in conversational speech at home and other natural settings will have to wait until treatment has progressed to that stage.

Shifts in Treatment Contingencies

- *Treatment contingencies* refers to the pattern of reinforcement and corrective feedback given for correct and incorrect responses, respectively. Initially, the client is reinforced for every correct response. Soon, the reinforcement schedule is changed from continuous to intermittent.
- For instance, the clinician may shift from a continuous reinforcement schedule to a schedule based on a fixed ratio of 2. In gradually sequenced steps the ratio may be stretched. This is important because in natural settings, the target behaviors may not be reinforced as heavily or as systematically as in clinical settings. When treatment is shifted to conversational speech, reinforcement may be sporadic, as it is in everyday communicative situations.

Follow-Up

- *Follow-up* is a clinical procedure designed to find out if the client has maintained the target communicative skills and if he or she needs additional treatment. Follow-up involves assessment of communicative behaviors.

- Typically, an extended conversational speech is recorded to analyze the continued production of communicative behaviors that were initially established. The need for treating additional targets may also be assessed. Follow-up in schedules may vary across clinics and may depend on the type of disorder; some may need more frequent assessments than others.

- For example, successfully treated clients with fluency disorders need to be followed up for more than 2 years, whereas similarly treated children with articulation disorders may need to be followed up only for a year or less.

- A general follow-up schedule is as follows:

    - first follow-up assessment: 3 months postdismissal
    - second follow-up assessment: 6 months postdismissal
    - third follow-up assessment: 1 year postdismissal
    - subsequent assessments as necessary

Booster Treatment

- *Booster treatment* refers to treatment offered any time after the initial dismissal from services. Booster treatment is important for maintenance. Clients with certain disorders have a greater need for booster treatment than those with other kinds of disorders.

■ For example, successfully treated adults who stutter need more frequent booster treatments than similarly treated children with articulation disorders.

■ Booster treatment may be:

- identical to the original effective treatment
- a modified version of the original treatment
- a different form of treatment known to be more effective than the original
- much less extended than the original

SUMMARY

✓ Clinicians may select treatment targets using the normative, client-specific, functional communication, or integrated approach.

✓ Treatment sequence is based on factors such as response complexity, degree of structure, response modes, multiple targets, training and maintenance, and shifts in treatment contingencies.

✓ Follow-up and booster treatment are implemented to ensure that clients maintain skills taught in therapy and to assess whether they need additional treatment.

A GENERAL OUTLINE OF A TREATMENT PROGRAM

INTRODUCTION

Successful treatment is based upon a thorough, individualized assessment of a client's communication skills. After the assessment, the clinician selects target behaviors for training, establishes baselines of those behaviors, and plans and implements a comprehensive treatment program. Finally, the clinician implements maintenance, follow-up, and booster treatment.

General Outline

◆ **STEP 1.** Assess the client's communication behaviors.

◆ **STEP 2.** Select target behaviors for training.
Target behaviors are empirical response classes that are functional and useful to the client. When these response classes are taught or modified, they will reduce or eliminate the disorder.
Select short-term and long-term target behaviors. Make these target behaviors objective, measurable, and functional for each client.

◆ **STEP 3.** Establish baselines of target behaviors.
Baselines are measured response rates in the absence of treatment. Baselines are usually established before treatment is initiated.
Establish baselines of all relevant response modes: conversational, modeled, and evoked speech, as well as oral reading if appropriate.

◆ **STEP 4.** Plan a comprehensive treatment program.

A treatment program specifies what the client will be required to do, what the clinician will do, and how the two will interact.

Ideally, the program should be written after baselines are established and before treatment is started.

◆ **STEP 5.** Implement the treatment program.

Careful management of behavioral contingencies is the most important aspect of a treatment program.

Manage two types of contingencies: those that will decrease undesirable responses and those that will increase desirable responses.

◆ **STEP 6.** Implement a maintenance program.

Most clients need a maintenance program. Although some generalization of target behaviors may automatically take place, such generalization may not be maintained.

Select responses that are useful to the client. Teach the client to self-monitor and train the key people in the client's environment to prompt and reinforce those responses. Arrange for booster treatment.

◆ **STEP 7.** Follow up on the client's progress.

Follow-up (previously described) is a procedure designed to assess response maintenance across time and in the natural environment. Responses are measured in the absence of treatment variables.

As previously stated, follow-up should be scheduled at regular time intervals to ensure that treatment gains are maintained.

◆ **STEP 8.** Arrange for booster treatment.

Booster treatment (previously described), or treatment offered any time after initial dismissal from services, is very beneficial for many clients.

Conduct booster treatment sessions after a client has been dismissed from the program in order to help promote maintenance of target behaviors taught in treatment.

SUMMARY

✓ Based on the results of an assessment, the clinician selects both short-term and long-term target behaviors for training. Before treatment is initiated, the clinician gathers baselines or measured response rates in the absence of treatment.

✓ After baselines are established, the clinician plans a comprehensive treatment program. This program is implemented through management of contingencies designed to decrease undesirable responses and increase desirable responses.

✓ To help clients maintain target behaviors over time, the clinician implements a maintenance program. The clinician ideally follows up on the client's progress and, when necessary, arranges for booster treatment.

CULTURAL-LINGUISTIC CONSIDERATIONS IN ASSESSMENT AND TREATMENT

INTRODUCTION

Due to the increasing numbers of culturally and linguistically diverse (CLD) clients with communication disorders, clinicians must be aware of special considerations that apply to CLD populations. Those considerations include prevalence and incidence of medical conditions and communicative disorders in various ethnocultural groups, potential sociocultural and linguistic barriers to service delivery, and the need for individualizing assessment and treatment.

Prevalence and Incidence Rates of Medical Conditions and Communication Disorders

- Clinicians must be aware that some CLD groups have higher prevalence and incidence rates of communication disorders or related medical conditions than others (Battle, 2002). (*Prevalence* refers to the current number of individuals; it is a head count. *Incidence* refers to the future occurrence of such an event in a population.)

- Each client should always be treated as an individual. Clinicians must be careful not to stereotype clients from specific cultural-linguistic groups.

- The presence of communication disorders and related medical conditions is related to several variables. These variables include, but are not limited to, lack of health insurance, low income, diet, and lack of access to medical services.

- Hispanics tend, as a group, to have:

  - low prevalence of esophageal cancer
  - high prevalence of cardiovascular disease
  - higher prevalence of strokes and diabetes (especially adult-onset diabetes) than whites
  - overall low smoking rate

- African Americans tend, as a group, to have:

  - high prevalence of traumatic brain injury, especially due to gunshot wounds in youth
  - high prevalence of strokes and hypertension
  - high prevalence of multi-infarct dementia
  - high prevalence of laryngeal, esophageal, and lung cancers
  - low incidence of cleft palate, especially cleft lip
  - overall low smoking rate

- Asian Americans, as a group, tend to have:

  - high prevalence of cleft palate, especially in Japanese and Chinese Americans

- high prevalence of nasopharyngeal cancer, especially in Chinese Americans
- high prevalence of strokes
- low prevalence of Alzheimer's disease, especially in Chinese Americans
- overall low rates of alcoholism and smoking

■ Native Americans, as a group, tend to have:

- generally low prevalence of lung cancer
- high prevalence of cleft palate
- high prevalence of otitis media
- generally high rate of smoking
- high prevalence of alcoholism and fetal alcohol syndrome

■ Awareness of the above-listed tendencies can help clinicians be sensitive to the needs of clients from various ethnocultural groups, thus increasing the efficacy and thoroughness of the assessment and treatment processes.

Potential Sociocultural and Linguistic Barriers to Service Delivery

■ When working with CLD clients and their families, it is important to recognize any barriers to full utilization of clinical services. Such barriers might include:

- the overclassification of CLD children as needing special education services
- client health-care access problems (e.g., lack of health insurance), leading to underdiagnosis of problems such as middle ear infections
- client presenting with more advanced states of communication disorders and related medical problems, caused by lack of health care and thus opportunities to prevent problems or treat them at an early stage
- client's and family's lack of English proficiency, and a lack of interpreters to serve as liaisons with the health-care system
- client's and family's distrust of of traditional, Western medicine and rehabilitation;
- lack of transportation to and from health-care facilities

CONCEPTS TO CONSIDER

CLD clients often experience barriers that prevent them from receiving optimal services. How might clinicians help clients overcome such barriers?

_____

_____

_____

_____

_____

The Need for Individualized Assessment and Treatment

While it is important to keep general ethnocultural and linguistic tendencies in perspective, all clinicians should also be aware of individual factors that might affect service delivery to CLD clients and families. Clinicians must be careful to:

- explore to what extent a member of a cultural group is different from the majority of that group (e.g., an African American who does not speak African American English or a southern rural white person who does);

- understand how refugee or immigrant status affects CLD people, and how CLD people born and raised in the United States differ from immigrants and refugees of the same cultural background (Roseberry-McKibbin, 2002);

- select standardized tests that have, in their standardization process, sampled the ethnocultural group to which the client belongs;

- avoid testing information about practices or events that may be culturally inappropriate (e.g., Christmas for Muslims);

- consider the client's home environment and past experiences (e.g., exposure to certain kinds of television shows, books, or toys) before selecting stimulus items to be used during assessment;

- consider the bilingual or multilingual status of the client, and select assessment tools that reflect that status;

- use trained interpreters to assess CLD clients who speak two or more languages;

- determine whether an underlying communication disorder exists that affects English, the primary language, or both (Roseberry-McKibbin, 2001);

- avoid diagnosing a communication disorder based solely on English production influenced by the primary language (e.g., labeling a Yugoslavian client who makes a d/th substitution in all word positions as having a disorder); and

- be aware of the great heterogeneity of language patterns and dialects among members of the same general language group (e.g., the Hmong language includes the different dialects of Green Hmong and White Hmong).

SUMMARY

✓ The increasing numbers of CLD clients in our society make it important for assessment and treatment to reflect sensitivity to the needs of those clients.

✓ Clinicians should be aware of the prevalence and incidence of medical conditions and communication disorders within certain groups. Clinicians must also recognize and help overcome potential sociocultural and linguistic barriers to service delivery.

✓ It is critical to individualize assessment and treatment for each client and family served.

◆ **WHEN ASSESSING CLIENTS WHO** present a wide range of communication disorders, clinicians generally carry out a number of standard assessment procedures. These procedures include a general screening, gathering a case history, a hearing screening, an oral–peripheral examination, an interview, obtaining a speech and language sample, and obtaining of related assessment data. Assessment procedures must be evidence-based in order to be optimal for use with clients.

◆ **THE VAST MAJORITY OF** clinicians then use standardized, norm-referenced tests to assess the communication skills of their clients. Standardized tests include systematic procedures for administration and scoring. Norm-referenced tests allow the clinician to compare the client's score to the average score of the test's norming group, thus yielding information (scores) about how the client's performance compares with that of the norming group. Most standardized tests are also norm-referenced, and vice versa, and are frequently called formal tests.

◆ **FORMAL TESTS CAN BE** evaluated according to their reliability and validity for use with specific client populations. Reliability refers to replicability, or a test's ability to yield scores that are consistent across repeated testing or measurement. Validity refers to the degree to which a test measures what it purports to measure. Even if they are both reliable and valid, formal tests should never be used to create treatment goals or assess treatment progress.

◆ **NONSTANDARDIZED ASSESSMENT MEASURES ARE** usually used to help create treatment goals, assess treatment progress, and provide functional descriptions of clients' communicative abilities in their daily environments. Commonly used nonstandardized, informal assessment measures include measurement scales, structured interviews and questionnaires, functional assessment tasks, criterion-referenced testing, and dynamic assessment.

◆ **TREATMENT INVOLVES CHANGING A** nonfunctional communication pattern and requires systematic work with clients and their families. Although there are many approaches to treating communicative disorders, certain common concepts, principles, and procedures apply. A mastery of these concepts, principles, and procedures will help clinicians effectively treat clients with varied disorders of communication.

◆ **TREATMENT TARGETS MAY BE** selected on the basis of the normative strategy, the client-specific strategy, the functional communication approach, or an integrated approach. Within the normative strategy, targets are created from age-based norms. Within the client-specific strategy, targets are based on the individual uniqueness and needs of and the communicative demands placed on the client. The functional communication approach requires the selection of targets based on effective and useful communication in natural settings. An integrated approach requires that the targets be age-appropriate and appropriate for the specific individual as well as functional.

◆ **TREATMENT IS SEQUENCED BASED** on response complexity, the degree of treatment structure, response modes, multiple targets, training and maintenance, and shifts in treatment contingencies. Based on these factors, various sequences are created: simpler responses are treated before complex responses, initial sessions are more structured than later sessions, imitation is used before spontaneous productions, certain targets are taught before certain other targets, certain maintenance procedures are implemented only in latter stages of training, and reinforcers are initially continuous and subsequently intermittent.

◆ **FOLLOW-UP IS AN IMPORTANT** procedure designed to assess maintenance of clinically established behaviors and the need for additional treatment. Typically a 3-, 6-, and 12-month follow-up schedule may be used; additional follow-up may be scheduled as necessary.

◆ **BOOSTER TREATMENT IS IMPORTANT** to help maintain communicative skills when a client's performance deteriorates. The booster treatment may be the same as the original treatment, a modified version, or a different form of treatment. In any case, booster treatment is typically brief unless the deterioration in skills is substantial.

◆ **WHEN WORKING WITH CULTURALLY** and linguistically diverse (CLD) clients, clinicians must consider issues such as the prevalence and incidence of certain medical conditions and communication disorders within specific ethnocultural groups. Clinicians must also deal effectively with potential barriers to service delivery, such as lack of transportation and health insurance and possible differences in attitude toward rehabilitation. Finally, it is important to avoid stereotyping CLD clients; this can be managed by individualizing assessment and treatment for each client and his or her family.

CHAPTER HIGHLIGHTS

ADD YOUR OWN CHAPTER HIGHLIGHTS HERE:

Study & Review Questions

Essay

1. Discuss the concept of *evidence-based practice*. What does this mean? What characterizes evidence-based practice?

2. What is a language sample? What is its purpose, and what are some procedures for gathering a language sample from a child?

3. Discuss the term *functional assessment*. Because this type of assessment is becoming increasingly important, it is important for clinicians to know how to carry out this type of assessment. How can a clinician target a client's functional communication behaviors during an assessment?

4. Describe a general outline of a treatment program. What steps are involved in most treatment programs for individuals with communcative disorders?

5. When clinicians use formal, standardized tests, they assume that the tests have various kinds of validity. Discuss the four types of validity that a clinician must be aware of when administering a standardized test.

Multiple Choice

Questions 6–8 *refer to the following scenario:*

> A new test is being published, and the publisher is excited about having the test become available to speech–language pathologists who work with children who have language disorders. This is a norm-referenced, standardized test.

6. If the test is being evaluated for internal consistency and whether responses to the items on the first half of the test correlate with responses to the items on the second half, then that test is being evaluated for:

   A. test-retest reliability.
   B. interjudge reliability.
   C. split-half reliability.
   D. parallel form reliability.
   E. predictive validity.

7. If this test has adequate construct validity, then:

   A. several judges have agreed that the test has been constructed appropriately and measures what it purports to measure.
   B. test items are relevant to measuring what the test purports to measure.

    C.   the test accurately predicts future performance on a related task.

    D.   test scores are consistent with theoretical concepts or constructs.

    E.   if a test is new, it correlates highly with an established test of known validity.

8. Which one of the following would NOT be a feature of this norm-referenced, standardized test?

    A.   the provision of systematic procedures for administration and scoring of the test

    B.   the comparison of a client's score to that of a norming sample

    C.   ideally, the ensuring of consistency of administration and scoring across examiners

    D.   the provision of information that can be used to create treatment goals and assess treatment progress

    E.   ideally, ensuring that the behaviors being measured are not influenced by the examiner's personal or subjective biases

9. A clinician was working with a 4-year-old boy, Emile, who stuttered. Unfortunately, the clinician found that every time she asked Emile to imitate a long phrase or sentence, he got up out of his chair and tried to wander around the room. He would not look at stimulus items. He would complain and say "That's too hard!" Within 2 weeks, Emile's uncooperative behavior increased and he seemed to be getting worse. To control Emile's undesirable behaviors, the clinician simplified the target skill; she modeled simpler, shorter sentences with the goal of increasing the utterance length more gradually and slowly than she had done previously. Fortunately, Emile's undesirable behaviors decreased and were eventually eliminated. This shows that Emile's undesirable behaviors were:

    A.   being effectively punished.

    B.   being positively yet indirectly reinforced during treatment sessions.

    C.   being reinforced on an intermittent, variable ratio schedule.

    D.   being negatively reinforced in treatment sessions.

    E.   being differentially reinforced with primary reinforcers.

10. Which of the following are TRUE, and thus important for clinicians to remember, with regard to appropriate assessment for culturally and linguistically diverse clients?

    I. Some groups demonstrate tendencies toward certain conditions; for example, Hispanics tend to have a higher prevalence of adult-onset diabetes than whites.

    II. A potential barrier for CLD clients to take full advantage of service delivery is that CLD children tend to be underclassified as needing special education services.

    III. Some families may not believe in traditional, Western concepts of medicine and rehabilitation.

    IV. A client who makes errors in English, due to the influence of a primary language or dialect other than English, should be diagnosed as having a communication disorder and consequently undergo remediation.

    V. There can be great heterogeneity of language patterns and dialects among members of the same general language group.

    A.   I, III, V

    B.   I, II, III, V

    C.   II, III, IV

    D.   I, III, IV

    E.   III, V

11. A 7-year-old boy, Cameron, has been diagnosed with a language disorder and you are seeing him for language therapy. Among other things, you are working on the goals of helping Cameron accurately produce the forms plural –s and regular past tense –ed. You need to document his progress very specifically. The best way to document Cameron's ongoing progress in attaining these goals would be to:

I. use the pre- and posttest results of a standardized test administered at the beginning and conclusion of treatment.
II. use criterion-referenced measures.
III. use conversational speech samples.
IV. use informal probe measures specifically designed to assess production of these forms.
V. ask Cameron how he thinks he is doing in production of the forms on the playground and at home.

    A. I, II, III, IV
    B. III, IV, V
    C. I, III, V
    D. I, II, IV
    E. II, III, IV

12. Baselines:

    A. help establish the initial level of clients' behaviors.
    B. help establish the need for treatment.
    C. help compare changes from the initial to the terminal phase of treatment.
    D. A, B
    E. A, B, C

13. A clinician in a hospital setting is informed that insurance companies have begun to demand specific evidence that therapy for clients with neurologically based disorders are receiving intervention that encourages functional communicative behaviors. Functional communicative behaviors can be defined as:

    A. age and norm based.
    B. useful only for adult clients.
    C. behaviors that promote communication in natural settings.
    D. useful only for clients with language disorders.
    E. behaviors that are displayed in the therapy setting but not in the client's natural environment.

14. Negative reinforcement:

    A. is involved in avoidance conditioning.
    B. is reinforcement that results from termination of aversive events.
    C. neither A nor B
    D. both A and B
    E. A only

15. A student is observing a hospital-based clinician who is treating a 65-year-old man who has aphasia. The treatment target that the student is observing in this part of the therapy session is correct naming of pictures of objects. The clinician uses phonological cues to prompt correct naming of objects. For instance, the clinician shows a picture of a dog and asks "What is this?" then gives the cue "It starts with a *D*." When the patient responds correctly, the clinician positively reinforces correct naming. After obtaining correct responses for a series of trained stimuli, the clinician shows ten untrained stimuli and asks "What is this?"

for each picture/stimulus item. However, the clinician does not give any cues or reinforce the patient when he names the pictures correctly. In this latter procedure, the clinician is:

A. fading the cues and reinforcers, but differentially applying indirect reinforcement.
B. treating the client without cues.
C. fading the cues and reinforcers.
D. assessing whether the client has learned to name the treatment stimuli.
E. measuring generalized production with a probe.

16. The difference between modeling and imitation is that:

A. modeling is clinician's behavior, and imitation is client's behavior.
B. modeling is a treatment target, and imitation is a target behavior.
C. imitation is usually superior to modeling as a treatment strategy.
D. A, B
E. A, B, C

17. IEPs and IFSPs differ in terms of:

A. the emphasis placed on the family involvement in IFSPs.
B. the need to write measurable treatment targets in IEPs.
C. the need to make a thorough assessment of communicative behaviors in IFSPs.
D. the need for IFSPs to be more highly individualized than IEPs.
E. the need for IEPs to conform exactly to federal mandates.

18. A clinician working in a public school was asked to assess the language skills of Rica, an 8-year-old speaker of Cantonese. Rica could speak both Cantonese and English. In the assessment, the clinician obtained extensive Cantonese and English language samples with the help of a Cantonese interpreter. The clinician also consulted with the teacher about what kinds of vocabulary words were being targeted in the classroom and what kinds of language skills would enhance Rica's academic performance. The clinician and interperter conducted an extensive interview with Rica's parents. After this interview, the clinician selected additional vocabulary items and common expressions to be included in systematic assessment. This type of assessment is known as:

A. functional and criterion-referenced assessment.
B. norm-referenced and criterion-referenced assessment.
C. standardized assessment without being norm-referenced.
D. functional and standardized assessment without being norm-referenced.
E. criterion-referenced assessment accompanied by standardized, norm-referenced assessment.

19. A clinician is working with a 3-year-old girl, Josie, who has a severe articulatory-phonological disorder. During the first few therapy sessions, Josie is very uncooperative. She hides under the table, throws therapy materials, and cries. The clinician tries to ignore the behaviors; this does not work. The clinician then firmly tells Josie to sit quietly; this does not work either. Then the clinician decides to implement a different strategy. She begins to praise Josie for sitting quietly for one minute and naming pictures; she also gives Josie a sticker for being a "good girl" during the preceding one minute. The clinician makes sure that she does not reinforce Josie for undesirable behaviors, but the clinician also does not do or say anything when those behaviors are exhibited. In gradual steps, the clinician extends the duration between verbal praise and presentation of stickers and eventually praises Josie only occasionally. The clinician has just used a procedure known as:

A. corrective feedback.
B. indirect method of response reduction.
C. time-out.
D. extinction.
E. punishment.

20. A clinician in private practice is assessing the language skills of Brett R. His parents brought him for an evaluation because they were concerned that he had some language deficiencies that might be impacting his performance in fifth grade. At the second trimester meeting with Brett's teacher to discuss Brett's report card, the teacher said that Brett was "low" in oral and written language skills. The parents request that Brett's language be thoroughly assessed. The clinician gathers a language sample and also administers several standardized tests of language skills. On one of those tests, the *Language Achievement Test* (**LAT**), Brett's overall score falls in the 25th percentile rank. This means that:

A. out of 100 children, 75 did better than Brett on the LAT and 25 children did worse.

B. 75% of the children upon whom the LAT was normed did better on that test than Brett did.

C. 75% of children upon whom the LAT was normed performed about the same as Brett did, but they scored 2–3 points higher on the test overall.

D. Brett scored about the same as 75% of fifth graders upon whom the LAT was normed.

E. Brett scored 25 points lower than the average fifth grader upon whom the LAT was normed.

REFERENCES AND RECOMMENDED READINGS

American Speech-Language-Hearing Association (1997). Treatment outcomes data for adults in health care environments. *Asha, 39*(1), 26–31.

Battle, D. (2002). *Communication disorders in multicultural populations* (3rd ed.). Boston, MA: Butterworth-Heinemann.

Brice, A. E. (2002). *The Hispanic child: Speech, language, culture and education.* Boston: Allyn & Bacon.

Brice, A., & Montgomery, J. (1996). Adolescent pragmatic skills: A comparison of Latino students in English as a second language and speech and language programs. *Language, Speech, and Hearing Services in Schools, 27*(1), 68–81.

Brice, A., & Roseberry-McKibbin, C. (1999). Turning frustration into success for English language learners. *Educational Leadership, 56*(7), 53–55.

Haynes, W. O., & Pindzola, R. H. (1998). *Diagnosis and evaluation in speech pathology* (5th ed.). Englewood Cliffs, NJ: Prentice-Hall.

Haynes, W. O., & Pindzola, R. H. (2004). *Diagnosis and evaluation in speech–language pathology* (6th ed.). Boston: Allyn & Bacon.

Hegde, M. N. (1998a). *Treatment procedures in communicative disorders* (3rd ed.). Austin, TX: PRO-ED.

Hegde, M. N. (1998b). *Treatment protocols in communicative disorders.* Austin, TX: PRO-ED.

Hegde, M. N. (2001a). *Hegde's pocketguide to assessment in speech–language pathology* (2nd ed.). Albany, NY: Singular Thomson Learning.

Hegde, M. N. (2001b). *Hegde's pocketguide to treatment in communicative disorders* (2nd ed.). Albany, NY: Singular Thomson Learning.

Hegde, M. N. (2003). *Clinical research in communicative disorders* (3rd ed.). Austin, TX: PRO-ED.

Hegde, M. N., & Davis, D. (2005). *Clinical methods and practicum in speech–language pathology* (4th ed.). Albany, NY: Singular Thomson.

Huang, R. J., Hopkins, J., & Nippold, M. (1997). Satisfaction with standardized language testing: A survey of speech–language pathologists. *Language, Speech, and Hearing Services in Schools, 28*(1), 12–29.

Hutchinson, T. A. (1996). What to look for in the technical manual: Twenty questions for users. *Language, Speech, and Hearing Services in Schools, 27*(2), 109–121.

Klein, H. B., & Moses, N. (1999). *Intervention planning for children with communication disorders: A guide for clinical practicum and professional practice* (2nd ed.). Needham Heights, MA: Allyn & Bacon.

Leith, W. R. (2002). *Clinical methods in communication disorders* (3rd ed.). Austin, TX: PRO-ED.

Lidz, C. S., & Peña, E. D. (1996). Dynamic assessment: The model, its relevance as a nonbiased approach, and its application to Latino American preschool children. *Language, Speech, and Hearing Services in Schools, 27*(4), 367–372.

Locke, J. (1998). Where did all the gossip go? Casual conversation in the information age. *Asha, 40*(3), 26–31.

Lohr, K. N., Eleazer, K., & Mauskopf, J. (1998). Health policy issues and applications for evidence-based medicine and clinical practical guidelines. *Health Policy, 46,* 1–19.

McCauley, R. (1996). Familiar strangers: Criterion-referenced measures in communication disorders. *Language, Speech, and Hearing Services in Schools, 27*(2), 122–131.

Paul, R. (2002). *Introduction to clinical methods in communication disorders.* Baltimore: Paul H. Brookes Publishing.

Peterson, H. A., & Marquardt, T. P. (1994). *Appraisal and diagnosis of speech and language disorders* (3rd ed.). Englewood Cliffs, NJ: Prentice-Hall.

Roseberry-McKibbin, C. (2001). *The source for bilingual students with language disorders.* East Moline, IL: LinguiSystems, Inc.

Roseberry-McKibbin, C. (2002). *Multicultural students with special language needs: Practical strategies for assessment and intervention* (2nd ed.). Oceanside, CA: Academic Communication Associates.

Roseberry-McKibbin, C. (2003). *Assessment of bilingual learners: Language difference or language disorder?* [Video] Rockville, MD: The American Speech-Language-Hearing Association.

Roseberry-McKibbin, C., Brice, A. E., & O'Hanlon, L. (2005). Serving English language learners in public school settings: A national survey. *Language, Speech, and Hearing Services in Schools, 36,* 48–61.

Roth, F. P., & Worthington, C. K. (1996). *Treatment resource manual for speech language pathology.* San Diego, CA: Singular Publishing Group.

Sackett, D. L., Rosenberg, W.M.C., Gray, J.A.M., Hayes, R. B., & Richardson, R. B. (1996). Evidence-based medicine: What it is and what it isn't. *British Medical Journal, 312,* 71–72.

Sackett, D. L., Straus, S. E., Richardson, W. S., Rosenberg, W., & Hayes, R. B. (2000). *Evidence-based medicine: How to practice and teach EBM.* London: Churchill Livingstone.

Shipley, K. G., & McAfee, J. G. (2004). *Assessment in speech–language pathology: A resource manual* (3rd ed.). Albany, NY: Singular Thomson Learning.

Shipley, K. G., & Roseberry-McKibbin, C. (2006). *Interviewing and counseling in communicative disorders: Principles and procedures* (3rd ed.). Austin, TX: PRO-ED.

Shipley, K. G., & Wood, J. M. (1996). *The elements of interviewing.* San Diego, CA: Singular Publishing Group.

Silverman, F. H. (1998). *Research design and evaluation in speech–language pathology and audiology* (4th ed.). Needham Heights, MA: Allyn & Bacon.

Tomblin, J. B., Morris, H. L., & Spriestersbach, D. C. (Eds.). (2000). *Diagnosis in speech–language pathology* (pp. 1–28). Albany, NY: Singular Thomson Learning.

Westby, C. E., Stevens-Dominguez, M., & Oetter, P. (1996). A performance/competence model of observational assessment. *Language, Speech, and Hearing Services in Schools, 27*(2), 144–156.

Study & Review
Answers

6. C. If a test is being evaluated for internal consistency and whether responses to the items on the first half of the test correlate with responses to the items on the second half, then that test is being evaluated for split-half reliability.

7. D. The concept of adequate *construct validity* means that test scores are consistent with theoretical concepts or constructs.

8. D. Norm-referenced, standardized tests are NOT meant to provide information that can be used to create treatment goals and assess treatment progress. These tests are meant to provide systematic procedures for administration and scoring, an opportunity to compare a client's score to that of a norming sample, and, ideally, the ensuring of consistency of administration and scoring across examiners, as well as ensuring that the behaviors being measured are not influenced by the examiner's personal biases.

9. D. Emile's undesirable behaviors were being negatively reinforced in treatment sessions.

10. A. With regard to appropriate assessment for culturally and linguistically diverse clients, clinicians need to remember that some groups have tendencies toward certain conditions (e.g., some families may not believe in traditional Western concepts of medicine and rehabilitation), and that there can be great heterogeneity of language patterns and dialects in the same language group.

11. E. The best way to document the Cameron's ongoing progress in attaining those goals would be to use criterion-referenced measures, conversational speech samples, and informal probe measures specifically designed to assess production of those forms.

12. E. Baselines help establish the initial level of clients' behaviors, help establish the need for treatment, and help compare changes from the initial to the terminal phase of treatment.

13. C. Functional communicative behaviors are behaviors that promote communication in natural settings.

14. D. Negative reinforcement is involved in avoidance conditioning and is reinforcement that results from termination of aversive events.

15. E. The clinician is measuring generalized production with a probe.

16. D. Differences between modeling and imitation are that modeling is clinician's behavior, and imitation is client's behavior; and also that modeling is a treatment target, and imitation is a target behavior.

17. A. IEPs and IFSPs differ in terms of the emphasis placed on the family involvement in IFSPs.

18. A. The clinician is using functional and criterion-referenced assessment.

19. B. The clinician has used the indirect method of response reduction.

20. B. Brett's overall score falls in the 25th percentile rank. This means that 75% of the children upon whom the LAT was normed did better on that test than Brett did.

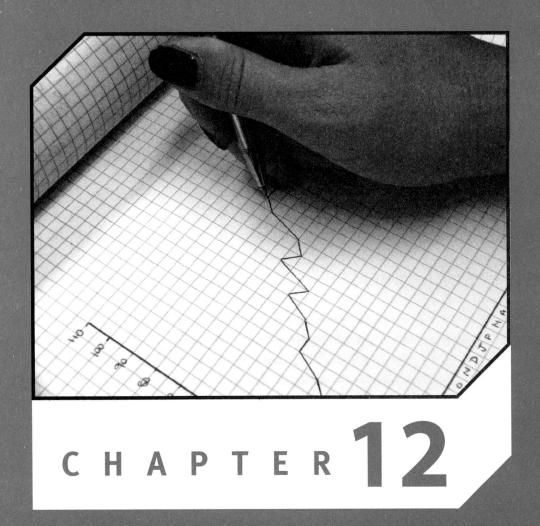

C H A P T E R **12**

RESEARCH DESIGN

AND STATISTICS:

A FOUNDATION

FOR CLINICAL SCIENCE

All professional practices are built upon

a foundation of basic and applied research. The current emphasis on *evidence-based practice* in medicine and all health-care professions, including speech–language pathology, underscores the importance of understanding the philosophy of science, methods of basic and applied research, techniques of data analysis, and the constraints on drawing valid conclusions from data. Speech–language pathology and audiology are clinical sciences that build upon research evidence gathered by scientistis in several disciplines. Today's clinicians are expected to be critical consumers of research so that the methods of assessment and intervention they select for their clients are based on scientifically replicated evidence for their usefulness and effectiveness.

In this chapter, we discuss basic concepts of science, principles of research design, and statistical analysis of research data. We assume that readers have completed coursework that has given depth of knowledge in the areas covered; thus, we seek to refresh readers' knowledge and strengthen their understanding of some important concepts they have already learned. We discuss the essentials of the scientific method, characteristics of experimental and descriptive research, evaluation of research, and data organization and analysis (statistics). (A few of the ideas in this chapter are also covered in Chapter 11, on assessment and treatment. For the reader's convenience and ease of learning the material, the repeated ideas are worded almost exactly the same in both chapters.)

ESSENTIALS OF THE SCIENTIFIC METHOD

INTRODUCTION

Scientists use objective, experimental methods to systematically investigate questions. Research methods are means of answering research questions. These methods involve observation, measurement, and manipulation of some variables to produce valid and reliable data from which objective conclusions may be drawn.

The Philosophy of Science: Basic Precepts

- Science was born out of curiosity and a need to understand the world around us. The beginnings of science were in the philosophical inquiry into truth. Therefore, philosophy, especially empirical philosophy, is the basis of modern science (Hegde, 2003; Maxwell & Satake, 1997).

- Sometimes the terms *research* and *science* are used interchangeably. However, although their meanings overlap, they have different connotations. Science is a philosophy of events and nature that values evidence more than opinions. The scientist uses objective, experimental methods to systematically investigate research questions and produce valid and reliable results that help answer them.

- *Research* is what scientists do as they practice science. Research is the process of asking and answering questions; it includes steps scientists take as they search for uniformity and order in nature. Science is conceptual and philosophical; research is methodological. Basically, research is science in action.

- The two philosophical hallmarks of science are empiricism and determinism. *Empiricism* is the philosophical position that statements must be supported by experimental or observational evidence.

- According to the empiricist, sensory experience is the basis of knowledge. This sensory experience (the touching, seeing, tasting, smelling, and hearing of phenomena) must be objectively verifiable. In other words, events must be experienced in such a way as to permit *observation* and *measurement*.

- *Determinism* means that events do not happen randomly or haphazardly; they are caused by other events. Scientific activity based on determinism is a search for causes of events.

- The goals of science are to (Hegde, 2003; Maxwell & Satake, 1997):

  - *describe* natural events or phenomena;
  - *understand* and *explain* natural phenomena, especially in terms of cause–effect relationships;
  - *predict* occurrences of events; and
  - *control* natural phenomena by understanding the causes of events and predicting their occurrence.

- Scientists frequently conduct research with the goal of explaining events and effects. An explanation of an event specifies its causes, and an event is scientifically explained when the scientist experimentally demonstrates its cause(s). As scientists attempt to explain events, they can use one of two approaches: the inductive method or the deductive method.

■ The *inductive method* is an experiment-first-and-explain-later approach. The researcher starts by conducting a series of experiments, and then he or she proposes a theory based on the results of those experiments. In using the inductive method, a scientist would first observe events, then experiment with them, and later arrive at some general conclusions regarding the nature and causation of those events. In sum, a scientist who is using inductive reasoning first experiments and then proposes a theory based upon the results of the experiments.

■ The *deductive method* is an explain-first-and-verify-later approach. In this method, the investigator explains an event and then attempts to verify the explanation through the results of experiments. In using the deductive method, a scientist would first make a series of proposals or statements—based on initial observations—but without conducting crucial experiments. Then the scientist would conduct experiments to generate evidence to test those proposals. In sum, a scientist using deductive reasoning first proposes a theory and then verifies it.

■ Scientists use inductive and deductive reasoning to build theories. A *theory* is a systematic body of information concerning a phenomenon, describing an event, explaining why the event occurs, and specifying how the theory can be verified. A theory specifies causal variables; a theory states that X causes Y.

■ While a theory is usually a comprehensive description and explanation of a total phenomenon, a *hypothesis* is concerned with a more specific prediction stemming from a theory. In less technical terms, a hypothesis is a proposed answer to a specific question. Hypotheses are testable propositions derived from a theory. As such, hypotheses are limited in scope compared to theories.

■ For example, the *behavioral theory* of language learning (see Chapter 3) explains the process of language learning in all children around the world. A *hypothesis* might address language learning in children with autism.

■ Hypotheses are usually formulated prior to an investigation and are predictive statements of cause–effect relationships between certain variables. For example, a hypothesis might state, "When people who stutter are put in highly stressful speaking situations, their amount of stuttering will increase." In other words, the hypothesis is that *stressful speaking situations will cause the effect of increased stuttering.*

■ Hypotheses may be labeled either *null* or alternative hypotheses. The term null means zero, and a *null hypothesis* states that two variables are not related. An alternative hypothesis states that the two variables are indeed related; perhaps one is the cause of the other.

■ In the above example, the null hypothesis would be that stressful situations and stuttering are *not* related, that when people who stutter are placed in highly stressful speaking situations, the amount of stuttering does not increase. The alternative hypothesis is that there is indeed a cause–effect relationship between stressful situations and stuttering. That is, highly stressful speaking situations do cause people who stutter to become more dysfluent.

■ The researcher hopes to *reject the null hypothesis* and *accept the alternative hypothesis,* because the researcher often believes in the alternative hypothesis. The *alternative hypothesis* holds that there is a relationship between the variables specified.

- To test their hypotheses, scientists gather data. *Data* are the result of systematic observation, and in many cases, experimentation. Scientists observe events and record some measured values of those events (e.g., the actual number of dysfluencies when stress was increased). Scientific data are empirical; they are based upon actual events that resulted in some form of sensory contact.

- *Qualitative data are verbal descriptions* of attributes of events, whereas *quantitative data are numerical descriptions* of attributes of events. Qualitative data involve words; quantitative data involve numbers.

- For example, a clinician might state, "The client has a severe articulation disorder characterized by multiple omissions of phonemes" (qualitative data). The clinician might further state, "In a 5-minute spontaneous speech sample, the client omitted word-final phonemes 75% of the time" (quantitative data).

- Scientific data should meet two criteria of *validity* and *reliability.* Validity and reliability are critical aspects of any type of scientific measurement. Measures in speech–language pathology, whether they apply to research studies or clinical measurement of clients' skills, need to be valid and reliable, as defined in the next section.

CONCEPTS TO CONSIDER

Describe basic precepts of the philosophy of science. What are the goals of science? What methods do scientists use to arrive at conclusions?

_____

_____

_____

_____

_____

Validity of Measurements

- *Validity* is the degree to which an instrument measures what it purports to measure. For example, a valid child language test should measure language skills, not auditory memory.

- There are different kinds of validity.

    - *Predictive validity,* also called *criterion validity,* is the accuracy with which a test predicts future performance on a related task. For example, a graduate student's score on comprehensive examinations might predict whether or not he or she will be a competent clinician. Thus, future performance is the criterion used to evaluate the predictive validity of a measure: the comprehensive examination in this case.

- *Concurrent validity,* considered a form of criterion-related validity, is the degree to which a new test correlates with an established test of known validity. For example, a new receptive vocabulary test might be correlated with the well-established *Peabody Picture Vocabulary Test–Revised* (Dunn & Dunn, 1981) to demonstrate the concurrent validity of the new test. A moderate, positive correlation is good for the new test; if the correlation is too high, however, there may be a question of the need for the new test.

- *Construct validity* is the degree to which test scores are consistent with theoretical constructs or concepts. For instance, a test of language development in children should meet the theoretical expectation that as children grow older, their language skills improve.

- *Content validity* is a measure of test validity based on a systematic examination of all test items to determine if they adequately sample the full range of the skill being tested and if they are relevant to measuring what the test purports to measure. Content validity is based on expert judgment that a particular test measures what it purports to measure.

Reliability of Measurements

- *Reliability* refers to the *consistency* with which the same event is measured repeatedly. Scores are reliable if they are consistent across repeated testing or measurement. For example, a clinician, Susan Smith, measures a child's dysfluencies on Monday, April 15, 2006. She states that the child is 35% dysfluent in a 100-word sample. Susan becomes ill, and a substitute clinician named Donald Jones calculates the child's dysfluencies on Wednesday, April 17, 2006. Donald states that the child, in a 100-word sample, is 37% dysfluent. There is good reliability of these dysfluency scores; they were consistent across repeated testing or measurement. If the two scores were too far apart (e.g., 35% and 10%), however, the measurement of dysfluencies would be unreliable. The concept of reliability applies to any kind of measure, including standardized tests (Hegde, 2003).

- Most measures of reliability are expressed in terms of a *correlational coefficient.* The correlational coefficient is a number or index that indicates the relationship between two or more independent measures. It is usually expressed through Pearson Product Moment r (often referred to as Pearson r).

- An r value of 0.00 indicates that there is no relationship between two measures. The highest possible positive value of r is 1.00. Conversely, the lowest possible negative value of r is −1.00. The closer r is to 1.00, the greater the reliability of the test or measurement. There are several types of reliability of a measure or a test:

  - *Test-retest reliability* refers to consistency of measures when the same test is administered to the same people twice. When the two sets of scores are positively correlated, the stability of the scores over time is assumed.

  - *Alternate form reliability* (also known as *parallel form reliability*) is based on the consistency of measures when two parallel forms of the same tests are administered to the same people. For example, the *Test of Nonverbal Intelligence–Third Edition* (TONI–3; Brown, Sherbenou, & Johnson, 1997) includes Form A and Form B. If both those forms are administered to an adult client and the scores are very similar, then the TONI–3 has alternate form reliability.

- *Split-half reliability* is a measure of internal consistency of a test. Split-half reliability is determined by showing that the responses to items on the first half of a test are correlated with responses given on the second half. Or the responses to even-numbered items should correlate with responses to odd-numbered items. Split-half reliability generally overestimates reliability because it does not measure stability of scores over time.

- *Interobserver* or *interjudge reliability* refers to the extent to which two or more observers agree in measuring an event. For example, if three judges independently rate the fluency of a subject, there is high interjudge reliability if there is good agreement between judges. Optimally, good agreement results in an interjudge reliability coefficient of .90 or more.

- *Intraobserver* or *intrajudge reliability* refers to the extent to which the same observer repeatedly measures the same event consistently. For example, if the same clinician rates a child's intelligibility over several sessions, those ratings should be consistent if there is good intraobserver reliability (assuming, of course, the child's speech intelligibility has not changed).

SUMMARY

✓ Science is based on certain philosophical assumptions including *empiricism* (knowledge based on sesory experience or objective observations) and *determinism* (events have causes, nothing happens without a cause).

✓ People who use the scientific method may use either inductive or deductive reasoning to create theories and test hypotheses.

✓ Validity and reliability of measurements are important aspects of good scientific measurement.

EXPERIMENTAL RESEARCH

INTRODUCTION

The hallmark of experimental research is the investigation of cause–effect relationships. Experimenters manipulate independent variables to assess the effect of these variables upon dependent variables. Group designs, the most popular type of experimental design in medicine and speech–language pathology, usually involve control and experimental groups. Single-subject designs, which usually involve 1–6 subjects, are experimental designs that help establish cause–effect relations based on individual performance as opposed to group averages.

Foundational Concepts

- An *experiment* is a means of establishing *cause–effect* relationships. Experiments test *if-then* relationships. For example, *if* a person who stutters is put into a highly stressful situation, *then* will he or she stutter more? Does the highly stressful situation *cause* the *effect* of increased stuttering?

- An experiment involves a controlled condition in which an independent variable is manipulated to produce changes in a dependent variable (Hegde, 2003). An *independent variable* is directly manipulated by the experimenter. This manipulation causes changes in the dependent variable. In treatment research, for example, all treatments are independent variables.

■ A *dependent variable* or *effect* is the variable that is affected by manipulation of the independent variable. In treatment research, all disorders are dependent variables. Manipulation of treatment (independent variable) changes or affects the dependent variable (disorder or a pariticular skill). Dependent variables must be defined very specifically so that they are measurable. Table 12.1 contains examples of independent and dependent variables.

■ Good experiments involve conditions that are carefully controlled to eliminate *extraneous* or *confounding* variables. When establishing a cause–effect relationship, the experimenter must ensure that only the independent variable of interest is affecting the dependent variable. In treatment research, the investigator should rule out the influence of extraneous variables that may also affect the disorder or the skill. For instance, in demonstrating that a langauge treatment is effective, the investigator must rule out the influence of maturation, and the effects of teachers' or parents' work on the child's language skills.

■ To give another example of ruling out an extraneous or confounding variable, an experimenter may want to find out if increased background noise (the independent, manipulated variable) causes persons to speak more loudly (the dependent variable). The experimenter arranges a party situation and begins to play music louder and louder while measuring the loudness of the speakers' voices.

Table 12.1 EXAMPLES OF INDEPENDENT AND DEPENDENT VARIABLES

Independent Variable	Dependent Variable
Stressful situation	Amount of stuttering
Amount of noise in environment	Amount of difficulty hearing speech
Length and complexity of reading passage	The number of errors a client with aphasia makes while reading it
Number of times client uses hard glottal attack	Amount of hoarseness present when client is speaking
Number of toys and games present in clinic room	Length of child's MLU as he or she interacts with the clinician
The clinician's modeling of a target skill	The client's imitation of the skill
Clinician's verbal praise for correct articulation	Increase in the client's correct phoneme production

Note. All things that cause disorders, and all things that are treatment procedures, may be classified as independent variables. All disorders themselves, and target skills that are treated, may be classified as dependent variables.

■ The experimenter finds that the speakers are indeed speaking louder as the music is played more loudly. However, the increased loudness of the subjects' voices (dependent variable) may be due to the alcohol (confounding independent variable), the louder music (the independent variable of interest), or both. Thus, the experimenter has not succeeded in determining whether progressively louder music alone caused the change in vocal intensity.

■ The types of experimental designs used in speech–language pathology can be placed in two broad categories: group designs and single-subject designs.

Group Designs of Research

Basic Principles

- Research involving a group design may be experimental or nonexperimental. If it is *nonexperimental,* it will consist of only one group; the research is then observational, or a case study if it is clinical. If it is *experimental,* it will consist of two or more groups (Hegde, 2003).
- True experimental designs using groups rule out the influence of confounding (extraneous) variables through the use of experimental and control groups. An *experimental group* contains participants who receive treatment and thus show changes in behaviors treated.
- A *control group* contains participants who do not receive treatment. The goal of having these two groups is to demonstrate that the experimental participants improved and the control participants did not, thus showing the efficacy of the treatment.
- In forming two or more groups, researchers use either randomization or matching. Using the first option, they randomly draw a *sample,* or a small number, of participants needed for the study from the population. A *population* is a large, defined group (e.g., patients scheduled for laryngectomy surgery, people who stutter) identified for the purpose of a study. Randomly *selected* participants are then randomly *assigned* to different groups. These two kinds of randomization—*random selection* and *random assignment*—are expected to result in groups that are equal to begin with. The selection is random when each potential participant in the population has an equal chance of being selected for the study. The assignment is random when each selected participant has the same chance of being selected to one or the other group. The two levels of randomization reduce experimenter bias in selecting participants and ensures that the sample is *representative* of the population.

Pretest-Posttest Control Group Design

- There are several group experimental designs (Hegde, 2003). Many advanced designs are variations of the basic designs. We will describe one basic design that helps evaluate the effects of a single treatment and the other basic design that helps evaluate more than one treatment.
- In the *pretest-posttest control group design,* there are two groups: an experimental group and a control group. This design helps evaluate the effects of a single treatment.
- The participants are randomly selected and assigned to groups. Each participant in each group undergoes a pretest and a posttest.
- *Pretests* are participants' existing behaviors or skills measured before starting an experimental treatment or teaching program. Posttests are measures of behaviors established after completing the treatment program. A comparison of pre- and posttest measures helps demonstrate the effects of treatment while ruling out the influence of confounding variables.
- The pretest-posttest design is based on the logic that to assess the effects of an independent variable (treatment), the only difference between groups must be that variable. To isolate the

effect of the independent variable, the two groups are, ideally, selected to be identical except for the independent variable.

- For example, an investigator might want to study the effects of enriched maternal speech on infant language development. She selects a control group and an experimental group of infant–mother pairs. The experimental group of mothers is taught specific strategies for enriching their infants' language; the control group of mothers is not taught those strategies. The vocalizations of babies in the experimental and control groups are measured before the experiment (pretest) and after the experiment (posttest).
- To isolate enriched maternal speech as the independent variable of interest, the investigator must match the mothers on such characteristics as age, socioeconomic status, language background, and educational level. If the mothers are not matched on such relevant variables, any increased vocalizations found in the experimental infants may or may not be due to the enriched maternal speech. The increased vocalizations may be due to the mothers' differential age or education, for instance.
- Figure 12.1 illustrates the pretest-posttest control group design.

Multigroup Pretest-Posttest Design

- Investigators use the multigroup pretest-posttest design to evaluate the relative effects of two or more treatments. A question of *relative effects* asks: Which treatment is more effective? Each additional treatment to be evaluated adds another group to the design.
- In evaluating the relative effects of three treatments, for example, the investigator randomly selectes a sample from the population and randomly assigns them to one of three groups. Each group receives a different treatment. All three treatments may be new, or one of them may be an established (previously evaluated) treatment. The investigator may include an optional control group; if a control group is included, the investigator will know whether treatments are better than no treatment and whether one treatment is better than the other. If no control group is included, the investigator cannot know whether treatments are better than no treatment; he or she can only answer the question: Whis is better?
- The multigroup pretest-posttest design with three treatments and an optional control group is illustrated in Figure 12.2.

Experimental Group	Pretest	Treatment	Posttest
Control Group	Pretest	—	Posttest

Figure 12.1. The pretest-posttest control group design. The participants are selected and assigned to the two groups randomly. Ideally, the pretest measures of the two groups are similar and if the treament was effective, the posttest measures will be significantly different.

Experimental Group	Pretest	Treatment 1	Posttest
Experimental Group	Pretest	Treatment 2	Posttest
Experimental Group	Pretest	Treatment 3	Posttest
(Control Group)	Pretest	—	Posttest

Figure 12.2. The multigroup pretest-posttest design. The illustrated design helps evaluate the relative effects of three treatments. The participants are selected and assigned randomly. Each group receives a different treatment. The control group in this design is optional; hence it is shown in parentheses.

Advantages and Disadvantages of Group Experimental Designs

- True experimental designs are the most powerful of the group design strategies. They are extremely useful in isolating cause–effect relationships between variables.
- Well-conducted experimental group designs have strong internal validity (described later), in that extraneous or confounding variables are ruled out. Thus, the experimenter can be confident that it was indeed the manipulation of the independent variable that caused the change in the dependent variable.
- From a clinical standpoint, a major limitation of true group experimental designs is that it is not always possible to randomly draw participants from specific clinical populations. To do this, one needs access to large populations of clients with specific disorders. Clinicians do not always have that access.
- Another limitation of group experimental designs is that they may not allow extension of the study's results to individual clients. Most practitioners are interested in studies whose results will allow application to individual clients with whom they are working.
- Group experimental designs thus yield helpful information for investigators and for the profession, but that information may have limited use for practitioners who seek application of results to individual clients. These practitioners may benefit from the results of single-subject design studies.

Single-Subject Designs

Basic Principles

- *Single-subject designs* (SSDs) are playing an increasing role in establishing efficacy of treatment procedures used in speech–language pathology. These designs help establish cause–effect relations based on individual performances under different conditions of an experiment.

- Unlike group designs, single-subject designs allow extended and intensive study of individual subjects and do not involve comparisons based on group performances.
- Instead of the pre- and posttests of group designs, SSDs measure the dependent variables continuously. Subjects are not necessarily randomly selected, and the results of SSDs are not always analyzed statistically.
- Although a SSD study may have only one participant, most studies have four to six participants. The data generated from each participant are not averaged as they are in group designs; rather, data for each individual are recorded and displayed separately (usually in graphic form).
- Most single-subject designs are experimental. However, as in the group design strategy, there is a single-subject design that is not experimental. Called an AB design, it is similar to the *case study* that is used also in group design strategy. The routine clinical work in which the baselines are established (A), treatment is offered (B), and the progress is summarized is a case study. Based on a case study results, the clinician only can claim improvement but not effectiveness for the procedure.
- The SSD experimental strategy involves methods of demonstrating treatment effects by showing contrasts between conditions of no treatment, treatment, withdrawal of treatment, and other control procedures. All of these conditions are applied to all participants; there are no control subjects who do not receive treatment.
- There are many types of single-subject designs (Hegde, 2003); we will describe the two basic types:

    - the ABA and ABAB designs
    - multiple-baseline designs and their variations

CONCEPTS TO CONSIDER

Compare and contrast group and single-subject experimental designs. What are their similarities and differences? When would you use each type of design?

_____

_____

_____

_____

_____

ABA and ABAB Designs

- The *ABA design* is the basic single-subject experimental design. The *ABAB design* is an extension of the basic design. Both are useful in establishing treatment efficacy. The letters designate the different conditions of an experiment. The first A condition refers to baselines. The next B condition refers to treatment. The third A condition refers to treatment withdrawal. Finally, the fourth B condition refers to the reinstatement of treatment.

- The ABA design consists of three conditions:

    - the first, A phase during which the skills are measured without intervention
    - the second, B phase during which the skills are taught (application of the independent variable)
    - the final, A condition in which the treatment is withdrawn

- The ABA design demonstrates that the skills were stable in the baseline, increased when the treatement was applied, and decreased when the treatment was reappplied. Such results demonstrate that it was the treatment, and no other variable, that was responsible for the increase in skill levels during treatment (see Figure 12.3 for a graphic representation of hypothetical results from an ABA design study). Although the design can establish treatment efficacy, it ends with no treatment, and hence no benefit to the participants. The next design avoids this problem.
- ABAB designs consists of four conditions:

    - The first, A phase in which the target skills are base rated without treatment

Figure 12.3. Hypothetical results of an ABA single-subject experimental study. A target behavior that is stable under the A condition (baseline, BL) increases in the A condition when treated (TR), and decreases in the final A condition when the treatment is withdrawn (WI). *Note.* From *Clinical Research in Communicative Disorders: Principles and Strategies,* 3rd ed. (p. 328), by M. N. Hegde, 2003, Austin, TX: PRO-ED. Copyright 2003 by PRO-ED, Inc. Reprinted with permission.

- The second, B phase in which the new treatment is offered
- The third, A phase in which the treatment is withdrawn
- The fourth and final, B phase in which the same treatment is reinstated

- The ABAB design, by adding the final treatment reinstatement condition, ends with treatment; clients benefit from the experiment. The final phase may be continued as long as it is necessary to stabilize the newly established skills. By showing the stable and low-level skills (A) increased markedly under the new treatment (B), but decreased when the treament was withdrawn (A) and increased again when the treatment was reapplied (B), we demonstrate that treatment was indeed effective (see Figure 12.4 for a graphic representation of the results of a hypothetical study using the ABAB design).

Multiple Baseline Designs

- A single-subject design that avoids the disadvantage of treatment withdrawal is the *multiple-baseline design,* in which the effects of treatment are demonstrated by showing that untreated skills did not change and only the treated skills did. The three variations of the multiple-baseline design are across subjects, across settings, and across behaviors (Hegde, 2003).

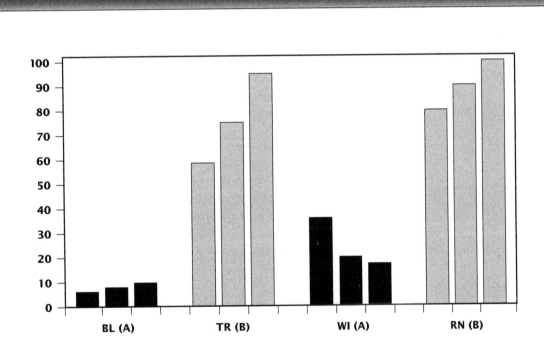

Figure 12.4. Hypothetical results of an ABAB single-subject experimental study. A target behavior that is stable under the A condition (baseline, BL) increases in the A condition when treated (TR), decreases in the final A condition when the treatment is withdrawn (WI), and increases again when the treatment is reinstated in the final condition (RN for reinstatement). The results demonstrate that the treatment was effective. *Note.* From *Clinical Research in Communicative Disorders: Principles and Strategies,* 3rd ed. (p. 332), by M. N. Hegde, 2003, Austin, TX: PRO-ED. Copyright 2003 by PRO-ED, Inc. Reprinted with permission.

- A *multiple-baseline-across-subjects design* involves several participants who are taught one or more behaviors sequentially (in a staggered fashion) to show that only the behaviors of treated participants change; those of untreated participants do not change. This outcome, too, demonstrates that the treatment was effective. The researcher:

  - selects a target behavior to be taught to three or more participants;
  - base rates the target behaviors in all participants;
  - treats one participant while repeating the base rates on the untreated participants;
  - treats the second participant while repeating the base rates on the untreated participants; and
  - alternates treatment and base rates until all participants are trained.

- A *multiple-baseline-across-settings design* involves a behavior being sequentially taught in different settings to demonstrate that the behavior changed only in a treated setting, and thus treatment was effective. The researcher:

  - base rates a target behavior in three or more settings (e.g., the hospital room, hospital lobby, parking lot, and home);
  - teaches the behavior in one setting;
  - repeats the base rates in the remaining untreated settings;
  - teaches the behavior in another setting; and
  - continues to alternate base rates and teaching in different settings until the behavior is trained in all settings.

- A *multiple-baseline-across-behaviors design* involves several behaviors that are sequentially taught to show that only treated behaviors change, untreated behaviors show no change, and thus the treatment was effective. The researcher:

  - selects three or more target behaviors;
  - establishes base rates on those target behaviors;
  - trains the first behavior to a training criterion (e.g., 80% accuracy over three sessions);
  - repeats the base rates on the remaining untreated behaviors;
  - trains the second behavior while repeating base rates on the remaining untreated behaviors; and
  - continues to alternate base rates and treatment until all the behaviors are trained.

Advantages and Disadvantages of Single-Subject Designs

- Single-subject designs are highly suitable for clinical research for many reasons (Hegde, 2003). First, clinicians can integrate research and clinical service by using the clients they serve as participants in experiments that attempt to answer significant clinical questions. Clients who serve as participants receive treatment; they are not denied treatment as clients in a control group might be if a group design is used.
- Another advantage of SSDs is that they help generalize from research studies to individual clients. Detailed descriptions of individual client characteristics and treatment effects can help establish generalizability of treatments across a wide variety of clients.
- Single-subject designs are much more easily replicated than group design studies. This is the case partially because clinicians do not need to seek unattainable random samples of clients. As stated, clinicians can use their own clients as subjects.
- A disadvantage of SSDs is that the results of one or a few studies cannot be generalized to the

population. However, the results may be extended to individual clients who have the same profile as those in the research study.

- Another disadvantage of single-subject designs is that they are not efficient to predict the behavior of groups of individuals; they are good at intensively studying individuals.

- To extend the conclusion of single-subject design studies, investigators need to replicate studies in different settings with different participants. Replications are needed to extend conclusions to the population even when group designs are used, however.

SUMMARY

✓ The goal of experimental research is to establish cause–effect relationships. In experiments, investigators inquire into whether certain variables have caused various effects.

✓ Investigators attempt to assess the effects of an independent variable on a dependent variable, and rule out confounding variables that might affect the dependent variable.

✓ To establish efficacy of new treatment procedures, it is necessary to use experimental research.

✓ Researchers may use group designs or single-subject designs to achieve that goal.

VARIETIES OF DESCRIPTIVE RESEARCH

INTRODUCTION

While the goal of experimental research is to establish cause–effect relationships between variables, the goal of descriptive research is to describe phenomena. There is no manipulation of variables (e.g., offering treatment) in descriptive research; descriptive research cannot demonstrate cause–effect relationships. There are several varieties of descriptive research, which include ex post facto research (retrospective research), survey research, comparative research (standard-group comparisons), and developmental (normative) research, correlational research, and ethnographic research (Hegde, 2003; Schiavetti & Metz, 2002).

Foundational Concepts

- In *descriptive research*, the researcher observes phenomena of interest and records his or her observations. The researcher does not want his or her presence to interfere with the natural phenomena that are being observed (Schiavetti & Metz, 2002).

- Unlike experimental research, no variety of descriptive research can lead to cause–effect statements (Hegde, 2003). This is the most important hallmark distinguishing descriptive from experimental research.

- There are two types of variables in some kinds of descriptive research. The *classification variable* is analogous to the independent variable in experimental research, and the *criterion variable* is analogous to the dependent variable in experimental research.

- For example, people with dementia might be compared to people without dementia on cognitive and linguistic measures. The classification variable would be group status (*dementia* as opposed to *without dementia*) and the criterion variable would be the performance on the cognitive and linguistic measures.

■ Although descriptive research cannot lead to cause–effect statements, it is useful when it would be unethical to use experimental methods. For example, researchers would not tell one group of women to drink alcohol daily during pregnancy, tell a second group of women not to drink alcohol during pregnancy, and measure the language skills of babies of the two groups during the first 5 years of life. However, researchers can observe and measure the language skills of babies born to women who consumed notable quantities of alcohol during pregnancy and *describe* those language skills.

■ Descriptive research is also useful in understanding a phenomenon. For instance, descriptive research helps us understand what are language disorders, what are the typical behaviors of children with autism, what is a stroke, what are the stages by which children acquire their speech sounds or language structures, and so forth. In essence, descriptive research helps us understand what it is, and experimental research helps us change it.

Ex Post Facto (Retrospective) Research

- *Ex post facto research* is after-the-fact research. The investigator begins with the effect of independent variables that have occurred in the past. Thus, the investigator is making a retrospective search for causes of events (Hegde, 2003). Therefore, this type of research is also called *retrospective research* and in most clinical disciplines, they also may be called *case studies*.
- Some case studies may try to establish *potential* causes of disorders. For example, one might investigate the potential causes of hearing loss in a child. In this case, both the causes and the effects have occurred in the past. A detailed history of the child may reveal that the mother, while carrying the child, had an infection that is suspected to cause middle ear damage. Potential causes of many disorders are suggested only through ex post facto case studies. The relationship between lung cancer and smoking, the relationship between various food habits and diseases in human beings, just to cite two examples, are retrospective case studies. Investigators have observed, using case studies, that smokers have a higher chance of developing lung cancer than nonsmokers or that among those who have had lung cancer, many smoked in the past. Similarly, among those who have had particular diseases, certain patterns of eating are common.
- Another example of ex post facto or retrospective research involves an attempt to find out how many children admitted to a children's hospital in the past five years had a swallowing disorder. Once again, the investigator would examine the case histories of children admitted and the number of children in whom a swallowing disorder was diagnosed.
- In contrast to retrospective research, one might design a study in which the children admitted to a hospital will be thoroughly screened for swallowing disorders for a period of five years. This type of study is called *prospective*.
- Retrospective cases studies also help study rare, individual cases of diseases and disorders in depth. For example, a child with Russell-Silver syndrome (a type of dwarfism) would be an ideal subject for a case study because the syndrome is rare and almost no literature exists that describes communication disorders in that population.
- It is important to recognize the weaknesses as well as the strengths of ex post facto research. First, retrospective studies can only suggest a potential cause; they cannot confirm them because there is no experimentation to rule out the extraneous variables. For instance, when a researcher claims that a certain diet is associated with lower incidence of heart attacks, it is possible that people who eat certain kinds of foods also are those who exercise regularly; one

would not know the relative contribution of diet and exercise in such a retrospective study. The results of case studies generally have limited generality.

- Retrospective studies are useful because in many cases, it is not possible to experiment. For example, researchers would not ask some people to smoke and others not to and then observe over the years to see if those who smoked developed lung cancer. Thus, in many cases, ex post facto research is all that is ethically possible.

Survey Research

- *Surveys* assess some characteristics of a group of people or a particular society. Surveys attempt to discover how variables such as attitudes, opinions, or certain social practices are distributed in a population (Hegde, 2003). The purpose of survey research is to generate a detailed inspection of the prevalence of phenomena in an environment by asking people as opposed to direct observation (Schiavetti & Metz, 2002).
- Because survey researchers cannot assess an entire population, they attempt to survey a randomly selected, representative sample of that population. Each person in the sample is asked a set of questions designed to evoke answers of interest.
- The two most common types of survey research tools are *questionnaires* and *interviews* (the two may also be combined). Many survey researchers use personal interviews when they want to obtain in-depth answers from survey participants. Questionnaires filled out by survey participants may yield a greater quantity of responses, but those responses may not contain the depth of those given in interviews.
- An advantage of surveys is the wide range of data that can be obtained. For example, one can literally sample thousands of people through a survey. The problems of surveys are that (a) they cannot be used to illustrate cause–effect relationships, and (b) their samples are often biased because those who return surveys are more likely to be people who have strong opinions about the issue surveyed.

Comparative Research

- The purpose of *comparative research* is to measure the similarities and differences of groups of people with defined characteristics (Schiavetti & Metz, 2002). This type of research is also known as standard-group comparisons (Hegde, 2003).
- Comparative research might be used, for example, to compare people with head injury to people without head injury on tests of attention and memory skills. The results of such tests would enable the researchers to draw conclusions about similarities and differences of head-injured and non-head-injured subjects in their attention and memory skills.
- A difficulty with comparative research is that the similarities and differences found between groups of subjects might be due to variables other than the classification variable. For instance, in the above example, clients with head injury might perform differently than non-head-injured clients due to educational or socioeconomic differences, not the presence or absence of head-injury.

Developmental (Normative) Research

- The purpose of *developmental research* is to measure changes in subjects over time as individuals get older. In developmental research, the presumed independent variable is maturation. That is, researchers choose this type of research when they tend to believe that age is the cause of changes seen in people, especially developing children. Developmental research has been used extensively to create developmental norms. Therefore, developmental research is also known as *normative research*.

- Normative research methods have been used extensively to study children's emerging phonological and language skill. The goal of this kind of research is to specify the skills at different age levels (norms). Developmental research has also been used to study the cognitive skills of older adults as they continue to age. Three methods are used in developmental or normative research: longitudinal, cross-sectional, and semilongitudinal.

  - In *longitudinal research,* the same participants are studied over time. The investigator follows participants and observes the changes that occur *within* them as they get older. An advantage of longitudinal research is that the investigator can directly observe changes in the behavior(s) of the same participants as they get older. For example, investigators might observe the fluency of a group of 10 children between 18 months and 3 years of age. This yields valuable information about the development of fluency skills. Disadvantages of longitudinal research are that it is (a) time consuming, (b) expensive, and (c) vulnerable to subject attrition. Thus, longitudinal studies often have small numbers of subjects, limiting the generalizability of the results.

  - In the *cross-sectional method,* researchers select participants from various age levels and observe the behaviors or characteristics of the groups formed on the basis of age. In essence, children of different age levels are observed simultaneously, or within a short duration of time. The cross-sectional method is cheaper, faster, and more practical than longitudinal research. For example, researchers might select a group of 3-year-olds, a group of 5-year-olds, and a group of 7-year-olds and observe the articulation characteristics of each group to establish age-based norms. A problem with cross-sectional studies is that investigators make observations of differences *between* subjects of different ages to observe differences that occur *within* subjects as they mature (Schiavetti & Metz, 2002). For example, the three groups of children in the developmental study of articulation might be observed in the year 2000. It would be assumed that in the year 2002, the children who were 5 years old would perform like the group of 5-year-olds did in 2000. That might not be the case.

  - In the *semilongitudinal procedure,* the total age span to be studied is divided into several overlapping age spans. The subjects selected are those who are at the lower end of each age span, and they are followed until they reach the upper end of their age span. For example, researchers might select three groups of subjects and study the language development of those groups for 1 year (2007–2008). The groups might be as follows: 3-year-olds followed

C O N C E P T S   T O   C O N S I D E R

How does descriptive research differ from experimental research? What is the basic purpose of each type of design?

_____

_____

_____

_____

_____

until the age of 4; 4-year-olds followed until the age of 5; and 5-year-olds followed until the age of 6. In the year 2008, the researcher would have made observations both *between* and *within* subjects as time passed.

Correlational Research

- In *correlational research,* the researcher investigates *relationships or associations between variables.* A critical distinction between experimental design and correlational design is that experiments lead to cause–effect statements; correlational studies never do. Correlation does not imply causation.
- Another important distinction between experimental designs and correlational designs is that in a correlational design, the word *effect* would never be used. Rather, when correlations are described, the words *relationship* and *related to* are often used.
- A correlation is a statistical method of data analysis suggesting that two or more events are somehow associated or related. It suggests the *direction* (positive or negative) and the *strength* (high or low) of the relationship.
- A *positive correlation* is found when high values of one variable predict high values of the other variable; when one event increases, the other event increases. For example, as the temperature rises on a hot July day, local grocery stores sell increased quantities of ice.
- A *negative correlation* is found when high values of one variable are associated with low values of the other variable. When one event increases, the other event decreases. For example, as a person who stutters experiences more pressure to communicate, her fluency decreases.
- As previously stated, to express the strength and direction of correlational relationships, the Pearson product moment correlation coefficient is used. This is usually abbreviated *Pearson r.* Pearson *r* is a number ranging from −1.0 to +1.0 (see Figure 12.5).
- The closer a number is to +1.0, the stronger and more positive the relationship. The closer a number is to −1.0, the stronger and more negative the relationship. The closer a number is to zero, the weaker the relationship.
- Thus, if a researcher says that a strong relationship of $r = .35$ was found, the reader knows that the relationship is actually weak because .35 is closer to zero than to +1.0. Conversely, a relationship of $r = .95$ would be considered to indicate a strong negative correlational relationship.
- In another example, a researcher might find that there is −.96 relationship between rate of speech and lack of intelligibility; the faster a person talks (high value of one variable), the more unintelligible he becomes (low value of another variable).

Figure 12.5. Positive and negative correlation coefficient 1 in relation to zero.

Ethnographic Research

- Ethnographic research involves observation and description of naturally occurring phenomena; thus, it is included under the aegis of descriptive research (albeit somewhat artificially). It is not an experimental type of research.

- *Ethnographic research* was originally designed by anthropologists as a means of conducting in-depth analytical descriptions of cultural scenes. The most common method of ethnographic research is for investigators to immerse themselves in the situation being studied. In this type of research, the investigators try to fully understand phenomena as they naturally occur in an environment. Ethnographic researchers do not create phenomena to study them, as do experimenters.

- The investigators conduct detailed observations, making copious notes and sometimes video and audio recordings of phenomena and people being studied. The investigators do not formulate hypotheses, but take an inductive approach in which observations eventually lead to conclusions. Unlike experimental research, ethnographic research is qualitative.

- In speech–language pathology, ethnographic research is advantageous for detailed study of clients, situations, and cultural groups when experimentation is not ideal or possible. Disadvantages of ethnographic research are that it is time consuming, often expensive, yields data that are difficult to quantify, and lacks the objectivity of experimental research. Ethnographic research is still relatively new in speech–language pathology.

SUMMARY

✓ A variety of descriptive research studies are used when investigators want to observe and describe phenomena that are naturally occurring in the environment. No cause–effect relationships can be inferred in descriptive research.

✓ Common descriptive research varieties include ex post facto (retrospective or case studies), survey, comparative or standard-group comparisons, developmental or normative, correlational research, and ethnographic research.

EVALUATION OF RESEARCH

INTRODUCTION

Research studies can be evaluated according to the parameters of internal and external validity. In evaluating internal validity, one asks, "Did the study demonstrate a cause–effect relationship?" In evaluating external validity, one asks, "To which people and situations can these results be generalized?" The answers to these two questions depend on the design of the study and whether factors that negatively affect validity (of both kinds) have been adequately controlled. In other words, investigators must attempt to control for *threats* to both the internal and external validity of a study.

Internal Validity

- *Internal validity* is the degree to which data in a study reflect a true cause–effect relationship (Hegde, 2003). A study with strong internal validity is one in which the dependent variable was affected only by manipulation of the independent variable. No confounding variable was present. In a treatment study, for example, an internally valid study can claim that *it was the treatment, and no other variable, that produced the positive changes in the clients who received it.*

- Certain factors can reduce the internal validity of a study. These *threats to internal validity* include instrumentation, history, statistical regression, maturation, attrition, testing, subject selection biases, and interaction of factors (Hegde, 2003; Schiavetti & Metz, 2002).

Instrumentation

- Instrumentation refers to problems with such measuring devices as mechanical and electrical instruments, pencil-and-paper instruments (e.g., questionnaires and tests), and human observers.
- Mechanical and electrical problems may occur with instruments that need regular calibration or that are defective; such problems affect validity.
- For example, if participants' hearing is tested at the beginning of a study, the audiometer is calibrated halfway through the study, and the participants' hearing is posttested at the end of the study, the study's outcomes may reflect the mid-study audiometer calibration, not true changes in the participants' hearing.
- Instrumentation problems also occur when investigators use inadequate or inappropriate pencil-and-paper instruments. For example, an investigator attempting to distinguish language differences from language disorders in Vietnamese refugee children who speak English as a second language may use standardized tests normed on monolingual, English-speaking, white children. This would be a serious threat to the internal validity of the study.
- Behaviors are often rated by observers or judges with varying degrees of objectivity and expertise. Judges may reduce validity in several ways. They may become more experienced in measuring the variable of interest (e.g., glottal fry in subjects' voices) during the study and thus score more instances of the variable occurring during the posttest than during pretest observations, in which they missed some instances of glottal fry. Or they may become bored during the posttest and fail to observe and score as vigilantly. Finally, criteria used by individual judges may become more or less stringent over the course of a study.

History

- History includes the subjects' life events that may be partially or totally responsible for changes recorded in the dependent variable after the independent variable is introduced. In other words, history involves events that occur, in addition to the experimental variable, between the first and second (or subsequent) measurements.
- For example, the first author once treated a preschool girl with a moderately severe phonological delay. After 8–10 weeks, great improvement in intelligibility (the dependent variable) was noted, apparently as a result of the clearly superior treatment (the independent variable) the girl was receiving.
- It was later discovered that during the second week of treatment, the child had received pressure-equalizing tubes in her ears. Thus, the life event for this subject (the tubes) might have made some or most of the difference in her intelligibility—not the treatment.
- Generally, the longer the time between measurements, the greater the chance of history having an effect on the study's results. Relevant events that occur outside the experimental setting, and thus outside the experimenter's control, have a greater chance of occurring in long-term

studies (Schiavetti & Metz, 2002). Most group and single-subject experimental designs adequately control for history.

Statistical Regression

- Statistical regression, also called *statistical regression to the mean,* refers to a behavior that goes from an extreme high or low point to an average level.
- In clinical research, many clients seek treatment when their problem is at its worst. For example, clients who abuse their voices may seek treatment when they are the most hoarse after cheering at a ballgame. Thus, though the voice is very hoarse, it will not remain at that level of hoarseness. The voice will eventually (in most cases) sound less hoarse.
- Participants selected for a voice experiment that begins when they are at the peak of their voice problems (such as hoarseness) may begin to sound less hoarse as the experiment continues. In this case, the improvement in voice quality may be incorrectly attributed to the treatment, instead of to statistical regression.

Maturation

- *Maturation* refers to biological and other kinds of changes within participants themselves; such changes can have an effect on the dependent variable. The experimenter is not able to control those changes.
- For example, an investigator may wish to study the effect of a language stimulation program on kindergarten children. The investigator measures the children's language skills in the fall of 2001, implements the stimulation program, and remeasures the language skills in May of 2002. Any improvement noted may be attributed to the language stimulation program. However, maturation might be a partial explanation for the children's improvement.

Attrition

- Also called *mortality, attrition* refers to the problem of losing participants as the experiment progresses. This has an effect on the final results the investigator interprets.
- Group designs, which depend heavily on analysis of results based on group averages, are very vulnerable to attrition. Attrition is a serious problem when the investigator uses statistical analysis based on group means and the attrition is *differential.* For example, if more severely affected participants drop out of the experimental group and less severely affected participants drop out of the control group, the pre- and posttest scores of the two groups may differ in favor of treatment, even if the treatment was ineffective.
- Attrition is not a threat in single-subject designs that include several participants. Subjects who drop out of those studies are typically replaced. Also, there are no groups of subjects to be statistically compared. A problem may be, though, that a single-subject design with few participants may lose all subjects, resulting in no study to report.

Testing

- *Testing* refers to a change that occurs in a dependent variable simply because it has been measured more than once. The dependent variable is affected because of repeated measurement (e.g., the administration of pre- and posttests). In such cases, the investigator may incorrectly conclude that the treatment variable was responsible for the change recorded. Some behaviors change when repeatedly measured or tested. *Reactive measures* are measures of behavior that change as a function of repeated testing.

- For example, attitude questionnaires filled out before and after treatment by clients who stutter are reactive. The clients may show significant attitude changes when they fill out the posttreatment questionnaire, even though their attitudes have not changed much.
- If possible, investigators should handle testing as a threat to internal validity by measuring behaviors directly, not through questionnaires and interviews.

Subject Selection Biases

- *Subject selection biases* are subjective factors that influence the selection of who participates in a study. A key feature of internally valid experiments is that differences found between experimental and control groups on posttests are attributable only to the treatment. However, if the two groups were different to begin with, differences in subjects themselves may account for the differences in posttest measures.
- To control for subject selection biases, it is best to use randomly selected and assigned groups. Another solution is to use groups that have very carefully matched subjects—that is, subjects who are similar on important variables.

Interaction of Factors

- Results of a study may be confounded by a combination of factors described so far. For example, a study involving the use of questionnaires to evaluate attitudes of spouses of people with aphasia might suffer from both testing and attrition.
- Interpretation of data may especially be confounded by the interaction between participant selection and some other factor such as maturation (Schiavetti & Metz, 2002).

CONCEPTS TO CONSIDER

Briefly define internal validity and give two examples of threats to internal validity.

_____

_____

_____

_____

_____

External Validity

- *External validity* refers to *generalizability*: to what settings, populations, treatment variables, and measurement variables the effect can be generalized (Campbell & Stanley, 1966; Hegde, 2003). External validity is a matter of the extent to which the investigator can extend or generalize the study's results to other subjects and situations.

- While the threats to the internal validity of a study result in a failure to establish a cause–effect relation between an independent variable (e.g., treatment) and a dependent variable (e.g., skills taught to clients), threats to *external* validity *limit the degree* to which internally valid results can be generalized (Hegde, 2003; Schiavetti & Metz, 2002). Most consumers of research do not expect that a single study—regardless of the design used—can be generalized to a wide variety of settings and subjects.

- External validity of a study can be threatened by several factors. These include the Hawthorne effect, subject selection, multiple treatment interference, and reactive or interactive effects of pretesting (Hegde, 2003).

Hawthorne Effect

- The *Hawthorne effect* is the extent to which the participants' knowledge that they are taking part in an experiment or that they are being treated differently than usual affects the results.
- For example, people who take part in research studies may know what is expected of them; this knowledge alone may influence how they respond under different experimental conditions.
- To illustrate, let's say that researchers are studying the efficacy of certain types of treatment methods for adults who stutter. The adults are given a questionnaire at both the beginning and end of treatment to assess their satisfaction with the treatment methods used. Because they know they are part of a research project, the adults might want to make the experimenters happy, and thus on the questionnaire at the end of treatment, they are especially positive about the impact of treatment. The experimenters then conclude that the treatment made a significant positive difference for these adults.
- Because the adults knew that they were part of a research project, the results of the study could not be generalized to a group of adult stutterers who did not know that they were part of a research project. The results would be limited to adult stutterers who knew that they were part of an experiment.

Multiple Treatment Interference

- In most research studies, investigators assess the effects of a single independent variable or single treatment. However, in some experiments, investigators assess the effects of multiple independent variables or treatments.
- *Multiple treatment interference* refers to the positive or negative effect of one treatment over another (Hegde, 2003). This is likely when two or more experimental treatments are administered to the same participants.
- For example, when people who stutter receive both counseling and time-out for stuttering, administered in a certain order, the overall outcome may be a result of one treatment influencing the other and one treatment following the other (called the *order effect*). The results may be generalized only to those clients who receive both treatments, administered in the same order, not to any one treatment.

Reactive or Interactive Effects of Pretesting

- The dependent variable in a study might be assessed through a pretest that might sensitize the participants to the treatment in such a way as to enhance the effect of the treatment variable. This is called *reactive or interactive effects of pretesting*.
- For example, people who regularly abused their voices through speaking loudly and using

hard glottal attacks might fill out a questionnaire before treatment that assessed the frequency with which they used such abusive vocal habits.

- The participants, thus sensitized to how often they abused their voices, might begin to modify their vocally abusive habits as a result of their increased awareness. At the end of treatment, the participants' improved vocal quality might be attributed to the treatment. However, the subjects' increased awareness affected the improvement. In such cases, results of the study cannot be generalized to subjects who have not been given a similar pretest.

Levels of Evidence for Evidence-Based Practice

- A critical examination of research evidence is the heart of evidence-based practice (see Chapter 11 for a description of evidence-based practice). After examining the internal and external validity of treatment research studies, clinicians may choose techniques that are supported by well-designed and well-executed treatment efficacy studies. Evidence to support a treatment procedure is often not categorical; it varies on a continuum. Often, the levels of evidence in medicine are classified into three major classes.

  - Class I evidence. Class I evidence is based on a randomized group experimental design study, often referred to as a *randomized clinical trial;* this is the best evidence supporting a procedure. To be classified as Class I, the evidence must come from at least one larger clinical trial with experimental and control groups as described earlier.

  - Class II evidence. Class II evidence is based on well-designed studies that compare the performance of groups that are not randomly selected or assigned to different groups. Because of lack of randomization, the groups may or may not be equal to begin with. Therefore, there is no assurance that differences noted on posttests are due to treatment.

  - Class III evidence. Class III evidence is based on expert opinion and case studies. As noted, case studies can claim improvement, but not effectiveness. Case studies do not include control groups. This is the weakest of the levels of evidence. Nevertheless, evidence based on case studies are preferable to that based on expert opinion.

- For these levels of evidence and any updated information, see the American Speech-Language-Hearing Association's website: http://www.asha.org/members/slp/topics/ebp/.htm.

One problem with the levels of evidence just described is that they ignore the single-subject designs that we described earlier. Also, they equate expert opinion with uncontrolled case studies. Results of case studies are better guidelines for treatment procedure selection than are expert opinions. An alternative way of classifying evidence for clinical procedures accepts all valid research designs and is based on research that is uncontrolled, controlled, and replicated by the same or different investigators. This hierarchy of evidence moves from the least desirable to the most desirable evidence (Hegde, 2003):

- *Level 1. Expert advocacy.* There is no evidence supporting a treatment; the procedure is advocated by an expert. Such a procedure is good only for research, not for routine clinical practice.

- *Level 2. Uncontrolled unreplicated evidence.* A case study with no control group or such single-subject control conditions as baseline, withdrawal, reinstatement, or multiple baselines has shown the procedure to produce improvement; there is no assurance of effectiveness. The procedure is acceptable only if one with better evidence is not available.

■ *Level 3. Uncontrolled directly replicated evidence.* A case study without controls has been replicated by the same investigator in the same setting and has obtained the same or similar levels of improvement. While there is better evidence than that in the previous two levels, still there is no assurance of effectiveness (we do not know if it is better than no treatment).

■ *Level 4. Uncontrolled systematically replicated evidence.* A case study has been replicated by another investigator in another setting with different clients and has obtained the same or similar levels of improvement reported by the original investigators. Although still uncontrolled, the evidence is getting stronger and is likely to show effectiveness in a controlled study.

■ *Level 5. Controlled unreplicated evidence.* The first level at which efficacy is substantiated for a treatment procedure. One of the group or single-subject designs is used to show that treatment is better than no treatment and that extraneous variables (such as maturation or parents' work at home) are not responsible for the positive changes observed. Not only improvement, but effectiveness is demonstrated for the procedure.

■ *Level 6. Controlled directly replicated evidence.* The same investigator who demonstrated the effectiveness for the first time has replicated the study with new clients and has obtained similar results to document effectiveness. The technique is now known to reliably produce the effects, at least in the same setting.

■ *Level 7. Controlled systematically replicated evidence.* This is the highest level of evidence. The effectiveness of a treatment technique has been replicated by other investigators, in different settings, with different clients, to show that the technique will produce effects under varied conditions. A technique that reaches this level may be recommended for general practice.

It is the reponsibility of the clinician who opts for evidence-based practice to evaluate treatment techniques in terms of the level of evidence they have attained. Generally, it is unethical to select a technique with a lower level of evidence when one that is supported by a higher level of evidence is available. This is why it is important to understand the research methods used in generating scientific evidence.

SUMMARY

✓ Investigators who conduct studies must control for threats to both the internal and the external validity of those studies.

✓ Threats to internal validity include instrumentation, history, statistical regression, maturation, attrition, testing, subject selection biases, and interaction of two or more of those factors.

✓ Threats to external validity include the Hawthorne effect, multiple treatment interference, and reactive or interactive effects of pretesting.

✓ A critical examination of research evidence is at the heart of evidence-based practice. Clinicians should choose techniques that are supported by well-designed and well-executed treatment efficacy studies.

DATA ORGANIZATION AND ANALYSIS: PRINCIPLES OF STATISTICS

Group design studies conducted in speech–language pathology use statistics to help organize, summarize, and analyze data. Dozens of statistical techniques are available. Commonly used techniques include measures of variability and measures of central tendency. Measurement scales are often involved, as they are closely related to statistical scaling techniques.

Foundational Concepts

- Data organization and analysis techniques are statistical tools. These tools aid the investigator in drawing conclusions and making inferences from a study. Because descriptive and experimental studies use the same statistical techniques to analyze data, one cannot tell from the techniques used whether the study is experimental or descriptive (Schiavetti & Metz, 2002).

- When used to refer to a body of knowledge, *statistics* refers to the field of study involved with the art and science of data analysis. Statistics deals with *probability,* or the chance of something occurring. For example, if the probability of rain is 0.75, there is a 75% chance of rain.

- When used in the plural form, *statistics* refers to specific pieces of data that will be or have been gathered. For example, baseball statistics might include a baseball player's number of home runs and strikeouts (Grimmett, 1995).

- A *statistic* can be defined as a measure calculated from a sample. This differs from a *parameter,* which refers to a population value. Examples of statistics, or summaries of samples, include percentages, means, variances, standard deviations, and other measures calculated from samples.

- There are several major purposes for statistics. The first purpose is to take large quantities of data and reduce them to manageable form. For example, if there are 100 individual scores on an examination, it is easier to calculate a mean and a standard deviation (defined later) than to look at and remember 100 individual scores.

- The second purpose of statistics is to aid the researcher in making inferences. An *inference* is a conclusion one arrives at through reasoning. Statistical inferences are frequently made from samples to populations. That is, researchers make observations on a sample, or small group of people, to make a decision about a larger group.

- For example, investigators have studied the effects of exercise on cholesterol levels in samples of subjects. They have discovered that in those subjects, cholesterol levels were decreased when the subjects increased their exercise levels. Thus, the investigators *inferred* that people not in the study, the larger population of people with high cholesterol, might benefit from increased levels of exercise.

Statistical Techniques for Organizing Data

- As stated earlier, data must be organized and summarized. Statistics help the investigator do that. Three measures help organize and summarize data: measures of central tendency, measures of variability, and measures of association.

- Measures of association (also called measures of correlation) have been described already. Thus, measures of variability and measures of central tendency will be briefly discussed.

Measures of Variability

- *Variability* refers to the dispersion or spread in a set of data. Common measures of variability include the range, interquartile range, semi-interquartile range, and standard deviation. For example, if an instructor administers an examination to fifty students and the highest score is 100 and the lowest score is 40, there is great variability in that set of scores. But if the lowest grade is 90 and the highest grade is 100, there is very little variability in that set of scores.
- The *range* is the difference between the highest and the lowest scores in a distribution or set of scores. For example, a test on which the highest score is 100 points and the lowest score is 40 points, the range is 60 points. One hundred (highest score) minus 40 (lowest score) yields the *range* in that set of scores. The range can be deceptive, however, because extremely high and low scores can make the range appear greater or more variable than it really is. For example, let us assume one student received a score of 40 on the examination. The next highest score was 70, and 49 out of the 50 students received scores between 70 and 100. The one student scoring 40 caused the class to have a 60-point range in scores instead of a 30-point range.
- To deal with this type of situation, the *interquartile range* and semi-interquartile range may be used. The interquartile range "cuts off" the highest and lowest 25% of the scores in a distribution. Thus, what is left is the middle 50% of the scores. The *semi-interquartile range* is the interquartile range divided by two. For example, if 100 students take an examination and the 25 highest scores range from 75 to 100 and the 25 lowest scores range from 0 to 25, the interquartile range of those scores is 50 because the lowest 25 scores and the highest 25 scores are disregarded. The semi-interquartile range is 25: 50 (the interquartile range) divided by 2.
- The *standard deviation* is the extent to which scores deviate from the mean or average score. The standard deviation reflects the variability of all measures or scores in a distribution. The larger the standard deviation, the more variable the scores. The smaller the standard deviation, the less variable the scores. For example, if an instructor gives an examination to a class and the highest score is 100 and the lowest score is 50, that 50-point difference in the highest and lowest scores results in a large standard deviation. If an instructor gives an examination on which the highest score is 100 and the lowest score is 85, that 15-point difference between the highest and lowest scores results in a relatively small standard deviation.

Measures of Central Tendency

- The *central tendency* of a distribution or set of scores is an index indicating the *average* or *typical* score for that distribution. There are three measures of central tendency: mean, median, and mode.
- The *mean* is the most commonly used measure of central tendency. To calculate a mean, the investigator adds up the scores and divides the total by the number of scores that were added together. For instance, 60 + 50 + 40 + 80 = 230. Next, 230 ÷ 4 = 57.5. Thus, the mean for this set of scores is 57.5.

- The *median* is the score in the exact middle of the distribution. The median divides the distribution into two parts so that an equal number of scores fall above and below it. The following illustrates a median score:

| 38 | 42 | 51 | 57 | 63 | **69** | 78 | 85 | 88 | 90 | 97 |

The *median* score is 69 because five scores fall below it, and five scores fall above it.

- The *mode* is the most frequently occurring score in a distribution. This is illustrated as follows:

| 22 | 29 | 34 | 46 | 57 | **63** | **63** | **63** | 78 | 85 | 100 |

The mode is 63, because 63 is the most frequently occurring score in this distribution.

- If distributions are relatively symmetrical, the three measures of central tendency should be the same. This would result in a *normal distribution* or *bell-shaped curve*.

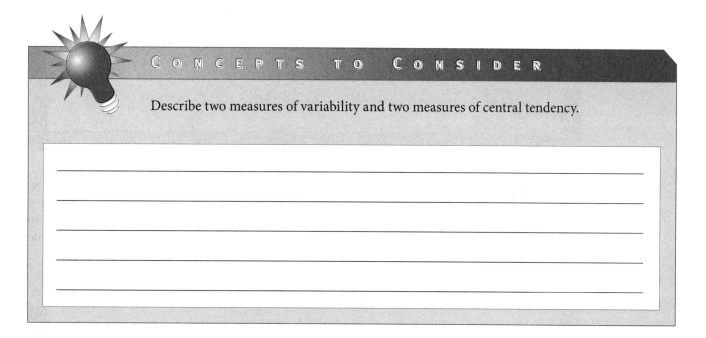

CONCEPTS TO CONSIDER

Describe two measures of variability and two measures of central tendency.

Types of Measurement Scales

- Psychological and social scientists typically describe what they term *levels of measurement*. Some of these levels of measurement are closely related to statistical scaling techniques. The four commonly used levels of measurement are represented by nominal, ordinal, interval, and ratio scales.

- In a *nominal scale*, a category is present (e.g., hypernasality) or absent (normal nasality). Items or observations are classified into named groupings or discrete categories that do not have a numerical relationship to one another. For example, in a survey of clinical practices, respondents might be asked if they "never," "sometimes," or "always" use a certain clinical practice. Or, a researcher might label diagnostic categories in a nominal way as "aphasia," "specific language impairment," "dementia," "dysphagia," and others.

■ An *ordinal scale* is a numerical scale that can be arranged according to rank orders or levels. Ordinal scales use relative concepts such as *greater than* and *less than*. The numbers in an ordinal scale and their corresponding categories do not have mathematical meaning. Also, the intervals between numbers of categories are unknown and probably not equal. Examples of ordinal scales of measurement are:

1 = strongly agree   2 = agree   3 = neutral   4 = disagree   5 = strongly disagree

1 = little hoarseness   3 = moderate hoarseness   5 = great hoarseness

■ An *interval scale* of measurement is a numerical scale that can be arranged according to rank orders or levels; the numbers on the scale must be assigned in such a way that the intervals between them are equal with regard to the attribute being scaled (Silverman, 1998). For example, in Figure 12.6, the attribute of distance is equal between one number and another.

1------2------3------4------5------6------7------8------9------10

Figure 12.6. Interval scale of measurement.

■ A *ratio scale* has the same properties as an interval scale, but numerical values must be related to an *absolute zero point*. The *zero* suggests an absence of the property being measured. An example of a ratio scale is one that involves frequency counts in stuttering; it is possible to have zero instances of stuttering in a speech sample. Figure 12.7 below illustrates a ratio scale for the attribute of distance (Silverman, 1998).

0-----1-----2-----3-----4-----5-----6-----7-----8-----9-----10

Figure 12.7. Ratio scale of measurement.

SUMMARY

✓ The use of statistical techniques enables investigators to organize, summarize, and analyze data in a useful way. These techniques include measures of variability and measures of central tendency.

✓ Measures of variability include the range, interquartile range, semi-interquartile range, and standard deviation from the mean.

✓ Measures of central tendency include the mean, median, and mode. Measurement scales used in studies include nominal, ordinal, interval, and ratio scales.

◆ **SCIENCE, A PHILOSOPHY BASED** on empiricism and determinism, uses objective experimental methods to systematically investigate research questions and produce valid and reliable results. Scientists may use either inductive or deductive reasoning to create theories and test hypotheses. Hypothesis testing is a major goal of science.

◆ **A RIGOROUS METHOD OF** hypothesis testing is experimental research. An experiment is a means of establishing cause–effect relationships between variables. An independent variable is directly manipulated by the experimenter to cause changes in the dependent variable being studied. Ideally, confounding variables are ruled out as potential causes of changes in the dependent variable.

◆ **THERE ARE MANY EXPERIMENTAL** group designs. In the basic experimental group design, there is at least one experimental group that receives treatment, and one control group that does not. These groups constitute the sample, a small number of subjects drawn from the population. The sample should be randomly selected and representative of the population.

◆ **THE PRETEST-POSTTEST DESIGN IS** a prototype of experimental group designs. In this design, the experimental and control groups are similar to begin with. They are different only after the experimental group receives treatment. Both groups are given a pretest, only the experimental group receives the treatment, and then both groups are given a posttest. This arrangement allows the researcher to evaluate the effect of the independent variable (treatment). This basic design may be extended to include additional groups to evaluate multiple treatments.

◆ **SINGLE-SUBJECT DESIGNS ARE EXPERIMENTAL** designs that demonstrate cause–effect relationships in small groups of subjects (usually 1–6 subjects) whose performance is recorded individually. ABA and ABAB designs are commonplace in single-subject design research. The A phase is the no-treatment phase, and the B phase is the treatment phase. Multiple-baseline designs are another common type of single-subject research designs.

◆ **SOMETIMES EXPERIMENTAL RESEARCH IS** not possible or desirable, so investigators use descriptive research strategies instead. In descriptive research, there is no demonstration of cause–effect relationships. Common types of descriptive research include ex post facto (retro-

CHAPTER HIGHLIGHTS

spective or case study), survey, comparative or standard-group comparison, developmental or normative, correlational, and ethnographic research.

◆ **RESEARCH MAY BE EVALUATED** in terms of its internal and external validity. Internal validity refers to the degree to which data in a study reflect a true cause–effect relationship. External validity refers to the generalizability of a study's results.

◆ **POSSIBLE THREATS TO A** study's internal validity include instrumentation, history, statistical regression, maturation, attrition, testing, subject selection bias, and interaction of two or more of those factors. Possible threats to external validity include the Hawthorne effect, multiple treatment interference, and reactive or interactive effects of pretesting.

◆ **WHEN CLINICIANS CHOOSE TREATMENT** techniques to use with their clients, they should ideally choose techniques that are supported by well-designed and well-executed treatment efficacy studies. This will help the clinicians to use evidence-based practice, or practice that is supported by research.

◆ **STATISTICS MAY BE DEFINED** as the field of study involved with data organization, summary, and analysis. Statistics is based on the theory of probability. Two foundational types of statistical analysis used for data organization and summary include measures of variability and measures of central tendency.

◆ **LEVELS OF MEASUREMENT USED** by scientists are related to statistical scaling techniques. Four commonly used levels of measurement include nominal, ordinal, interval, and ratio scales.

✎ **ADD YOUR OWN CHAPTER HIGHLIGHTS HERE:**

_____

_____

_____

Study & Review Questions

Essay

1. What is evidence-based practice? Why should clinicians use it when planning therapy for their clients?

2. Define the terms *reliability* and *validity.* What types of reliability and validity are evaluated when research is is being analyzed? List and describe these.

3. Compare and contrast group vs. single-subject experimental designs. What are advantages and disadvantages of each one?

4. What is the purpose of descriptive research? List and briefly describe three types of descriptive research designs.

5. Describe four types of measurement scales (e.g, nominal, etc.).

Multiple Choice

6. A measure of validity of the accuracy with which a test predicts future performance on a related task is called:

A. content validity.
B. concurrent validity.
C. construct validity.
D. predictive or criterion validity.
E. index validity.

7. *Reliability* means that a test or measure:

A. measures what it purports to measure.
B. has scores that are consistent across repeated testing or measurement.
C. has items that adequately sample the full range of the skill being tested.
D. correlates well with an established test of known validity.
E. is consistent with theoretical constructs or concepts.

8. An investigator carries out a study in which the effect of rate of speech upon stuttering during sibling interaction is being investigated. The investigator gathers conversational samples from children who stutter and their siblings. In the control group, siblings are asked to speak as they normally would at home. In the experimental group, siblings are asked to speak much more quickly than they would at home. The investigator wishes to measure the effect of rate of siblings' speech upon the amount of stuttering done by the children who stutter. In other words, the investigator is asking if increased rate of sibling speech causes children to stutter more. In the above study, the dependent variable is:

A. the amount of stuttering done by the children who stutter when the siblings increase their rate of speech.
B. the rate of speech of the siblings in the experimental group.
C. the rate of speech of the siblings in the control group.
D. the combined amount of stuttering done by the children in both the experimental and the control groups.
E. B and C

9. An experimental design involving one or a few subjects would be called a:

A. case study design.
B. ex post facto design.
C. single-subject design.
D. single correlational design.
E. single-subject case study design.

10. In a single-subject design, the following are true:

I. The A phase is the no-treatment or baseline phase.
II. The B phase is the treatment phase.
III. The A phase is the treatment phase.
IV. The B phase is the no-treatment or baseline phase.
V. There may be anywhere from 1 to 6 subjects.

A. III, IV
B. III, IV, V
C. I, II
D. I, II, V

11. A type of research in which independent variables have occurred in the past and the investigator is making a retrospective search for causes of events is called:

A. retrospective research.
B. ex post facto research.
C. historical research.
D. case study research.
E. survey research.

12. A difficulty with cross-sectional studies is that:

A. observations are made of differences *between* subjects of different ages to generalize about developmental changes that would occur *within* subjects as they mature.
B. observations are made of differences *within* subject groups of different ages to generalize about developmental changes that would occur *between* subjects as they mature.
C. the same subjects are studied over time, and this is expensive, time consuming, and difficult because subjects might drop out of the study.
D. the total age span of children to be studied is divided into several overlapping age spans, and it is difficult to follow subjects from the lower to the upper end of each age span.
E. the investigator is examining data already on file to answer questions about children in various age groups, and that data might not be reliable.

13. A measure of variability denoting the extent to which scores deviate from the mean or average score is called the:

A. deviant variability index.
B. standard deviation.
C. interquartile range.
D. semi-interquartile range.
E. standard variance squared.

14. A group of clinicians wishes to conduct research in a hospital setting. These clinicians work with clients who have voice disorders. Many of the clients are hoarse because they work in noisy factories where they shout a great deal during the work week. The clinicians devise a rating scale to evaluate the hoarseness of these clients during evaluation sessions. The scale looks like this:

1	2	3	4
almost no hoarseness	slight hoarseness	moderate hoarseness	great amount of hoarseness

This type of scale would be called a:

A. ratio scale.   D. logarithmic scale.
B. nominal scale.   E. ordinal scale.
C. interval scale.

15. The *range* in a distribution can be defined as:

A. the difference between the highest and the lowest scores in a distribution.
B. the middle 50% of scores of a distribution.
C. the middle 50% of scores in a distribution divided by 2.
D. the variance plus the difference between the highest and lowest scores in a distribution.
E. the lowest and highest 25% of a distribution.

16. A researcher is describing the speech of a group of children who have developmental apraxia of speech. She finds that the faster the children speak, the less intelligible they are. The researcher obtains a Pearson *r* correlational relationship of –.92. One could say that this shows that there is _____ between rate of speech and intelligibility.

A. a positive correlational relationship
B. a strong negative correlational (or inverse) relationship
C. a canonical correlational relationship
D. a cause-and-effect relationship
E. virtually no correlational relationship

17. A researcher wishes to assess the efficacy of the new Bloomberg method of training children to say /r/ accurately. He decides to use a single-subject design because he does supervision in a university clinic that serves a number of children who have w/r substitutions. The researcher needs to keep several concepts in mind as he begins his research. Which one of the following concepts is *false?*

A. ABAB designs rely upon two conditions: (a) the A phase or no treatment phase, where target behaviors are base rated with no treatment, and (b) the B phase or treatment phase, where the target behavior is treated
B. In a multiple-baseline-across-subjects design, there are several subjects who are taught a behavior sequentially to show that only treated subjects change, and thus the treatment was effective.
C. An example of a multiple-baseline-across-settings design would be having a behavior (correct /r/ production) being sequentially taught in different settings to demonstrate that the behavior changed only in a treated setting and thus treatment was effective
D. For this researcher, an advantage of using a single-subject design to evaluate the efficacy of the Bloomberg method of training children to say /r/ accurately is that he can integrate research and clinical service by using the clients he and his students serve as subjects in an experiment that attempts to answer a significant clinical question.
E. In the ABAB withdrawal design, a target behavior is base rated (e.g. /r/ in the A phase),

taught to the subject (accurately-produced /r/ in the B phase), reduced by teaching its counterpart or an incompatible behavior (teaching w/r in the A phase), and then taught again (accurately-produced /r/ in the B phase) to show that the treatment was effective.

18. In Middleton City, a speech–language pathologist has a thriving private practice comprised heavily of non-native speakers of English. This clinician, Richard W., works to help his clients increase their intelligibility in English for business purposes. One way that Richard evaluates the success of the accent training he provides for these clients is to rate their overall intelligibility of speech before they start accent training and after 10 weeks of training. He finds that the clients appreciate these "before and after" measures of their progress. After serving a number of accent clients, Richard realizes that a potential problem with his "before-and-after" intelligibility ratings is that he has become accustomed to the clients' speech as he has gotten to know them; this could be impacting the "after" intelligibility rating. Richard goes to a local university and selects four speech–language pathology graduate students to watch "before-and-after" videos of his accent clients and independently rate each client's intelligibility. He finds to his dismay that the four students vary greatly in their ratings of the same clients. For example, one student might rate Mr. Fong, a Chinese client, as "95% intelligible after 10 weeks of accent training." A second student might rate Mr. Fong as only 60% intelligible after 10 weeks of accent training, whereas a third student might rate Mr. Fong as 45% intelligible, etc. In this situation, one can say that:

   A. there is low interjudge reliability.
   B. there is high interjudge reliability.
   C. there is moderate interjudge reliability.
   D. there is low intrajudge reliability.
   E. there is high intrajudge reliability.

19. A hospital-based clinician is conducting an experiment with patients with aphasia. She is assessing the efficacy of the new, exciting Newton Aphasia Program (NAP) in increasing the word-retrieval skills of her patients. The experimental and control groups have been carefully matched on all variables. Halfway through the experiment, the clinician finds that many of the experimental subjects attend church each Sunday and go to Sunday school after church. In Sunday school, there is Bible study and a great deal of discussion. None of the control subjects attends church or Sunday school. At the end of the experiment, the clinician finds that the experimental group of subjects who received the NAP have improved significantly in their word-retrieval skills compared to the control subjects, who have been treated with more traditional word-retrieval therapy techniques. What can the researcher safely conclude from her study?

   A. The NAP was more successful in helping the experimental patients improve their word-retrieval skills than were the traditional methods in helping patients in the control group improve their word retrieval skills.
   B. The NAP was not successful in helping the patients in the experimental group improve their word-retrieval skills; the improvement was due to weekly church and Sunday school attendance.
   C. The fact that most experimental subjects attended Sunday school and church on a weekly basis was a possible confounding variable in the study, making it impossible to firmly conclude that the NAP alone caused the difference in the performance of the experimental and control groups.
   D. The NAP was only moderately successful in helping experimental group patients improve their word-retrieval skills.
   E. Traditional word-retrieval therapy techniques are the most reliable and valid; the clinician should not attempt to use the NAP again.

20. A clinician in private practice receives many referrals from local public school clinicians. The children being referred are those whose language test scores are too high to legally qualify them for therapy in the public schools. The parents of these children want services and are willing and able to pay for them out of pocket. The clinician in private practice often administers the *Word Abilities Keystone Evaluation–Upper Portion* (WAKE-UP) test to the children who are referred to her. One day, she becomes curious about the "typical score" of the children to whom she administers the WAKE-UP. The clinician takes the WAKE-UP scores of 17 children and lines them up in order from highest to lowest score:

33   33   46   48   51   55   60   69   73   82   85   89   91   93   95   95   95

The clinician concludes that the "typical" or average score on the WAKE-UP is is 73. In terms of measures of central tendency, the average score calculated by the clinician is the:

A. mean.
B. mode.
C. median.

D. standard deviation.
E. measure of central variability.

REFERENCES AND RECOMMENDED READINGS

Brown, L., Sherbenou, R. J., & Johnson, S. K. (1997). *Test of Nonverbal Intelligence* (3rd ed.). Austin, TX: PRO-ED.

Campbell, D. T., & Stanley, J. C. (1966). *Experimental and quasi-experimental designs for research.* Chicago: Rand McNally.

Doehring, D. G. (2002). *Research strategies in human communication* (3rd ed.). Austin, TX: PRO-ED.

Dunn, L. M., & Dunn, L. M. (1981). *Peabody Picture Vocabulary Test–Revised.* Circle Pines, MN: American Guidance Service.

Grimmett, D. R. (1995). *Statistics study cards.* Springfield, OH: Visual Education Association.

Hegde, M. N. (2001). *Hegde's pocketguide to treatment in speech–language pathology* (2nd ed.). Albany, NY: Thomson Learning.

Hegde, M. N. (2003). *Clinical research in communicative disorders: Principles and strategies* (3rd ed.). Austin, TX: PRO-ED.

Hegde, M. N., & Davis, D. (2005). *Clinical methods and practicum in speech–language pathology* (4th ed.). Albany, NY: Thomson Learning.

Kerlinger, F. N. (1973). *Foundations of behavioral research.* New York: Holt, Rinehart & Winston.

Maxwell, D. L., & Satake, E. (1997). *Research and statistical methods in communication disorders.* Baltimore: Williams & Wilkins.

Payne, K. T., & Anderson, N. B. (1991). *How to prepare for the NESPA national examinations in speech pathology and audiology.* San Diego, CA: Singular Publishing Group.

Schiavetti, N., & Metz, D. E. (2002). *Evaluating research in communicative disorders* (4th ed.). Needham Heights, MA: Allyn & Bacon.

Silverman, F. H. (1998). *Research design and evaluation in speech–language pathology and audiology* (4th ed.). Boston: Allyn & Bacon.

Study & Review
Answers

6. D. A measure of validity of the accuracy with which a test *predicts* future performance on a related task is called *predictive* or criterion validity.

7. B. *Reliability* means that a test or measure has scores that are consistent across repeated testing or measurement. The other answers in this item relate to validity, not reliability.

8. A. The dependent variable is the amount of stuttering done by the children who stutter when the siblings increase their rate of speech. The rate of speech of siblings in both groups is the independent variable, which is manipulated by the investigator.

9. C. Single-subject designs are *experimental* and may involve one or a few subjects. Case study designs are *descriptive*.

10. D. In a single-subject design, the A phase is the no-treatment or baseline phase, the B phase is the treatment phase, and there may be anywhere from 1 to 6 subjects.

11. B. A type of research in which independent variables have occurred in the past and the investigator is making a retrospective search for causes of events is called ex post facto research.

12. A. A difficulty with cross-sectional studies is that observations are made of differences *between* subjects of different ages to generalize about developmental changes that would occur *within* subjects as they mature.

13. B. A measure of variability denoting the extent to which scores deviate from the mean or average score is called the standard deviation.

14. E. An ordinal scale of measurement would be represented by numbers that can be arranged according to rank orders or levels, but the intervals between the numerals are unknown and probably not equal.

15 A. The *range* in a distribution can be defined as the difference between the highest and lowest scores in a distribution.

16. B. A researcher who finds that the faster the children speak, the less intelligible they are (Pearson r is −.92) has shown that there is a strong negative correlational (or inverse) relationship between speed and intelligibility; high values of one variable (speed) are associated with low variables of the other value (intelligibility).

17. E. It is not true that in the ABAB withdrawal design, a target behavior is base rated (A phase), taught to the subject (B phase), reduced by teaching its counterpart or an incompatible behavior (A phase), and then taught again (B phase) to show that the treatment was effective. This happens in the ABAB reversal design.

18. A. If judges who are measuring the same event markedly disagree with one another, then one can say there is low interjudge reliability.

19. C. The only thing the reseacher can accurately state from the results of this study is that the experimental subjects' weekly attendance at church and Sunday school was a possible confounding variable, making it impossible to firmly conclude that the NAP alone caused the difference in the performance of the experimental and control groups.

20. C. The clinician has just calculated the median score, which is the score in the exact middle of the distribution. An equal number of scores fall above and below it.

CHAPTER 13

SPECIAL TOPICS

IN SPEECH–LANGUAGE

PATHOLOGY

In the 21st century, the profession of speech–

language pathology has expanded to include service delivery to a greater number and variety of clients with communicative disorders and their families. Such expansion of service delivery is due to several variables; one of the most influential variables has been technological development. A major force behind technological development is the National Institutes of Health (NIH). NIH has received substantial increases in funding, and thus since the late 1990s, there have been advances in the following areas of medicine that impact the care of clients with communication disorders related to medical problems: the aging process, cancer therapy, antibiotics and resistant infections, brain damage, spinal cord injury, pharmacogenomics, and autoimmune disease (Sapienza & Casper, 2004). Because of the expansion of services to a greater number and variety of clients with communication disorders and their families, speech–language pathologists (SLPs) are more than ever in need of information regarding issues related to counseling, basics of medical speech–language pathology, and craniofacial anomalies and genetic syndromes. This chapter discusses these three areas and their implications as SLPs attempt to provide high-quality, appropriate service delivery to an ever-growing and changing population.

COUNSELING

INTRODUCTION

Speech–language pathologists and audiologists frequently find themselves in a position where clients and families need help and support with emotional issues related to communicative disorders and their effects. Such help and support can take place in the form of counseling. Counseling in the context of communicative disorders can be defined as creating an interpersonal, helping relationship whose goal is to support clients and families who experience emotional distress related to a communicative disorder (Shipley & Roseberry-McKibbin, 2006). Families and clients who feel supported emotionally frequently are more willing to cooperate with and carry out treatment recommendations. In many circumstances, SLPs and audiologists can successfully provide the support that clients and their families need.

However, SLPs and audiologists are not trained, qualified psychotherapists. It is imperative for professionals in communicative disorders to recognize their limitations and to be sensitive to instances when clients need referrals to trained mental-health professionals. Nevertheless, professionally appropriate counseling is often necessary as part of service provision. In this section, we discuss qualities needed to be effective in counseling activities, including various counseling approaches, special issues in counseling, reactions and emotions related to communicative disorders, and potential defense mechanisms to be aware of when working with clients.

Qualities Necessary for Effective Counseling

- In order for SLPs and audiologists to be most effective in counseling activities, they should possess the following qualities (Mosheim, 2004; Shames, 2000; Shipley & Roseberry-McKibbin, 2006):

  - objectivity
  - competence and knowledge
  - honesty and openness
  - flexibility
  - empathy
  - trustworthiness
  - emotional stability
  - ability to motivate clients to take action
  - a nonjudgmental attitude
  - ability to be positive yet realistic

- While the adoption and application of all these qualities may seem like a tall order to many professionals, it must be remembered that acquiring these traits is a lifelong process. The most important thing is to be constantly aware of and continually working toward developing the qualities that make counseling and therefore treatment maximally effective for clients and their families.

Approaches to Counseling

There are different theories of counseling and providing help and support for others. Most SLPs and audiologists find the greatest success using directive, behavioral approaches to counseling, in which the focus is on the problem and action steps that can be taken to solve the problem. Nevertheless, it is important to be aware of other major approaches that include elements relevant to particular situations.

Psychodynamic Theory

- Based on psychoanalytic theory and created by Freud, this approach views behavior as the product of conflictual interaction between three systems: the id, ego, and superego. Anxiety is created when emotions arising from the conflicts among these three systems are repressed.
- Freud also discussed five psychosexual stages that develop from birth through adolescence. According to him, a healthy personality cannot develop without the successful resolution of each stage.
- Adults who have neuroses or problems can solve those problems through resolving difficulties that occurred during the development of one or more of the psychosexual stages.
- The purpose of psychoanalytic treatment is to make clients conscious of repressed issues and help them to resolve those issues so that the personality can be healthy and whole.
- The psychoanalytic approach to counseling is best undertaken by trained mental health professionals who understand it and believe in its efficacy. Use of the psychoanalytic approach is outside of the realm of communicative disorders professionals who are not specifically trained in its use and application.

Client-Centered Theory

- Also called the *person-centered theory*, this approach was created by Carl Rogers in the 1930s and 1940s. It was in large part a reaction to the rigidity of the psychoanalytic school of thought that predominated during those decades (Okun, 2002).
- According to this theory, clients need acceptance and positive unconditional regard in order to develop congruence between their self-concept and their behavior (Flasher & Fogle, 2004). Thus, the foundation of client-centered therapy is an empathic relationship between client and therapist that allows the client to freely experience and express all his or her emotions in a completely accepting climate.
- In the nondirective client-centered approach, clients freely express their emotions while the clinician listens and responds to both the content and the feelings behind the words the client is saying. The clinician does not use specific techniques or recommend specific courses of action to change the client's behavior.
- Proponents of the client-centered theory believe that the self-exploration and growth that occur in the nondirective, listening context make the client open to change. Eventually, the client is expected to take responsibility for determining goals and then to take action toward achieving those goals.

The process can be expressed thus:

◆ STEP 1. The client is encouraged to freely express emotions. All these emotions are accepted and explored in a warm, empathetic climate of listening.

◆ STEP 2. The clinician responds to both the content and the feelings of what the client expresses. Again, listening, not giving advice, is critical in this nondirective approach.

◆ STEP 3. As a result of the warm, accepting relationship with the clinician, the client becomes open to change and self-growth.

◆ STEP 4. This openness leads the client to take responsibility for determining goals and then to take action toward achieving those goals.

- When confronted with emotional situations, many clinicians make the mistake of immediately trying to change clients' perceptions and behaviors by giving advice, information, and specific directions. But it is important not to get clients back into a "cognitive role" prematurely.
- Instead, clinicians should first accept and acknowledge the feelings being expressed. For most clients, being understood and listened to is a critical, foundational first step, that precedes listening to advice and taking action to constructively change a situation (Luterman, 2001).
- Many clinicians use elements of the client-centered theory in counseling clients with communicative disorders and their families. Elements of this approach can be helpful in the early stages of a clinician–client–family relationship, especially when the family is newly facing a major trauma with accompanying strong emotions such as shock and grief.

Behavioral Theory

- A major influence in the development of *behavioral theory* was that scientists could not measure and document outcomes of the psychoanalytic and client-centered approaches to helping clients. Scientists wanted to measure the outcomes of helping approaches, based on quantifiable, objective, and observable behaviors (Okun, 2002).
- Clinicians who use a behaviorist approach focus on what is observable, with an emphasis on environmental, external influences (Luterman, 2001). They believe that:

    - all behavior is caused by environmental stimuli;
    - human behavior is the product of external reinforcements;
    - behavior is shaped and maintained by immediate consequences;
    - reinforcement must be given immediately after a particular behavior has occurred; timing must be precise;
    - positive reinforcement increases the chance that a behavior will reoccur;
    - negative reinforcement, such as when a person's behavior causes an aversive stimulus to be removed, can also cause a behavior to reoccur;
    - the reinforcement must be aversive enough or desirable enough to the client to cause a behavioral change; and
    - behaviors that occur in the absence of reinforcement will be extinguished.

- In the behavioral approach, clinicians focus on specific outcomes of counseling and interacting. Rather than discussing thoughts and feelings, clinicians emphasize clients' identifiable attitudes or behaviors and strive to make positive changes in those variables through the use of operant conditioning methods (reinforcement, punishment, and others).
- Many SLPs and audiologists are comfortable with the behavioral approach because it:

    - focuses specifically on areas that affect the client's communicative abilities;
    - permits the creation of specific goals and objectives whose attainment can be objectively measured in a data-based manner;
    - allows clinicians to measure the success of the counseling relationship; and
    - allows for documentation of behavioral outcomes in a manner that is consistent with the demands of many of today's third-party payers, such as insurance companies.

- Some experts believe that a strictly behavioral approach is limited in scope. For example, Luterman (2001) states: "The 1970s, when behavior modification took hold in our field, seems to be what could be called the 'Fruit Loop' decade. One could rarely stick one's head into a therapy observation room without seeing a student clinician reinforcing a child's behavior with a Fruit Loop … The behavioral approach presupposes a very narrow view of the … clinician's role and responsibilities, reducing the clinical task to one of dispensing cereal. The mystery and art of client–clinician relationships are not developed" (pp. 11–12),

- Use of a behavioral approach may not be effective in the beginning of a client–clinician relationship, especially when there is an initial diagnosis of a communicative disorder, with accompanying strong emotions. In such situations, a behavioral approach is most successful subsequent to a client-centered approach, which allows clients to express feelings first so that they may then focus on positive behavioral changes.
- In all situations, it is the clinician's responsibility not only to listen empathetically but also to eventually provide specific guidance for behavioral changes that will make a measurable difference in clients' communication abilities (Shipley & Roseberry-McKibbin, 2006).

Cognitive-Behavioral Theory

- In this approach it is held that a client's *thoughts* are key to his or her feelings and actions. According to Albert Ellis, founder of the approach, the key variable is the *meaning* a person attributes to an event (Luterman, 2001).
- The clinician helps the client focus on the problem, specifically to identify the distorted thoughts or cognitions accompanying the problem, and replace the old distorted thoughts with newer, more rational thoughts that lead to behavioral changes. Clients are asked to assume responsibility for their behavior.
- Proponents of the cognitive-behavioral theory believe that counseling is a three-step process:

    - Change the client's thinking ➔ change the belief system ➔ change the behavior

- For example, a client with spasmodic dysphonia states that because of her voice, "Everyone looks down on me." She is resistant to therapy because of this belief, and is not making behavioral changes toward a better-sounding voice. Treatment is not succeeding. The clinician's job would be to:

    - *Help the client explore this thinking.* ("So you think that everyone looks down on you because of your voice. Does everyone look down on you, or just some people?")
    - *Challenge the client to test the validity of her old belief through experimentation.* ("When you go to the party tonight, observe people's reactions to you. Does everyone look down on you, or just some people?")
    - *Create a change in thinking through analyzing the data gathered through experimentation.* (Clinician: "What happened at the party?" Client: "Many people enjoyed talking to me at the party; several moved away and appeared uncomfortable.") Thus, after the party, the client and clinician would compare the client's old belief against the positive evidence gathered at the party.
    - *Create a change in behavior based on the new, positive evidence.* The clinician would use the positive evidence to motivate the client toward taking active steps to improve her voice through therapy techniques such as relaxation and easy onset.

- The cognitive-behavioral approach thus explores discrepancies between a client's thoughts and reality, and helps the client to adopt a new set of thoughts or cognitions so that he or she can deal with the problem situation in a constructive way.
- Many SLPs and audiologists are comfortable with the cognitive-behavioral approach and find it effective, because it deals with feelings and thoughts and helps the client change specific behaviors, which can then be directly measured and observed (Shipley & Roseberry-McKibbin, 2006).

- A limitation of the cognitive-behavioral approach is that it may, for certain clients, cut short the expression of legitimate strong emotions about a situation. Those emotions need expression and acknowledgment so that the counseling process can go forward.
- The cognitive-behavioral approach may be most helpful in dealing with adult clients who have such negative thoughts about their communicative disorder and its effects that treatment progress is hampered. If clinicians can help clients analyze, evaluate, and test their negative thoughts against reality, clients can move forward and take active steps to deal with their communicative disorder constructively.

Eclectic Approach

- There are many other theories and approaches to counseling. However, most clinicians find that a combination of the client-centered, behavioral, and cognitive-behavioral approaches is most useful for providing help and support for clients.
- Clients who are accepted and listened to nonjudgmentally, especially in the earliest stages of dealing with the impacts of a communicative disorder, become more ready to change their behaviors.
- If feelings are accompanied by negative thoughts that are preventing progress, clinicians can deal with those thoughts openly and constructively through helping clients test the validity of the thoughts.
- Finally, clinicians can recommend and help clients implement constructive behaviors that help them overcome the effects of the communicative disorder to the best of their potential. Those behaviors can be analyzed and measured so that both clients and clinicians can objectively, in a data-based manner, assess the progress being made.

CONCEPTS TO CONSIDER

How do the client-centered, behavioral, and cognitive-behavioral theories of counseling differ from one another?

_____

_____

_____

_____

_____

Special Issues in Counseling

Most SLPs and audiologists act in ways that are consistent with mainstream, Western beliefs. It is important, however, to be aware of the special, non-mainstream beliefs or practices that clients may bring to the counseling situation (Berman, 2005; Sue & Sue, 2003):

■ *Gender* can influence a counseling relationship between a clinician and client. For example, in some cultural groups, a woman client may not be alone in a room with a male therapist. A male family member must be present at all times.

■ *Age* is sometimes a factor in client–clinician relationships. Older people from some cultures might not respect a young clinician. Or, older patients might prefer to be referred to as "Mr." or "Mrs.," not by a first name as is common among younger Americans.

■ *Culture* can influence counseling activities. In the United States, for example, open expression of emotion and directness of expression are encouraged. But indirectness is the norm in many cultures, and clients may be offended if a clinician is too frank or pushes them to be too emotive (Sue & Sue, 2003).

■ *Time* can impact counseling with clients. In some cultures, being late is acceptable and common. In the United States, if clients are not prompt, professionals may be offended or angry. Clear communication about time expectations is necessary.

■ *Religion* can have an impact on the way families view services offered by communicative disorders professionals. Clients from some cultures, for example, believe in alternative methods of healing such as using herbs, massage, and religious rituals. Counseling clients to take advantage of therapy or rehabilitation opportunities might be unacceptable.

Reactions and Emotions Related to Communicative Disorders

Many clients and families experience strong emotions related to the communicative disorder and its effects, especially at the time of initial diagnosis. Clinicians should be able to recognize and deal with the following reactions:

■ *Shock and disbelief.* This is especially prevalent upon initial diagnosis of a communicative disorder. For example, a family who expected a healthy baby may undergo shock and disbelief when the doctor who delivers the baby reports that the infant has Down syndrome.

■ *Denial.* This can be seen when the client or family does not acknowledge the extent or implications of the communicative disorder—for example, when parents of a profoundly mentally retarded fifth grader continue to expect that he will be able to attend college someday. People who are in denial may become quite angry upon being confronted with reality. Clinicians must not take this personally, and must realize that acceptance is sometimes a long and multistage process.

■ *Anger.* This strong emotion can be composed of rage and hostility and actually be an attempt at self-protection. Clients and families may feel fear, powerlessness, and frustration; thus, anger ensues. This anger can be directed at the clinician and may even result in verbal abuse of the clinician.

■ *Grief.* This response involves sorrow and depression because of a loss, and it typically is experienced in stages. It is normal for clients and families to experience profound grief in response to diagnosis of a communicative disorder. Clinicians must allow clients to express their grief openly, for this will help clients move to a stage where they are ready to accept the situation and take constructive action.

■ *Guilt.* Sometimes clients or families believe that they have in some way caused or contributed to the communicative disorder; they blame themselves. They experience *personalization,* or the inappropriate assumption of responsibility for an event they did not cause. In addition, they may believe they are not "doing enough" to deal with the disorder. Clinicians need to gently and directly deal with guilt feelings expressed explicitly or implicitly, and allow open expression of those feelings. Giving information can be very helpful in alleviating feelings of guilt.

■ *Anxiety.* Clients may feel worry or apprehension because they are uncertain about a situation and its ramifications. Anxiety may be present throughout the therapeutic process and may arise in response to different situations (e.g., "How bad was my husband's stroke? The doctor didn't tell me anything." And later, "Will my husband be able to come home and go back to his job eventually?"). Clinicians can best deal with anxiety by encouraging open expression of questions and feelings, providing information and facts, and being willing to repeat information if it is not understood or heard the first time.

Defense Mechanisms

■ In order to deal with the strong emotions experienced in relation to communicative disorders, some clients and families may employ defense mechanisms.

■ Clients or their families who demonstrate prolonged use of one or more defense mechanism need to be served by professionals who are trained to deal with emotional issues. However, for many clients and family members, use of defense mechanisms is temporary and based upon the shock and trauma of dealing with a sudden blow, such as the diagnosis of a child with a severe disability or the profound changes brought about when a family member acquires a neurological problem.

■ Awareness of the defense mechanisms that clients and families may use can be most helpful to clinicians as they attempt to provide the most comprehensive and appropriate services possible (English, 2002; Shames, 2000, Shipley & Roseberry-McKibbin, 2006). Common defense mechanisms include:

- *Rationalization.* In this form of resistance, the client provides a logical but untrue explanation of why something has occurred. For example, a client who stutters may explain away his lack of a social life by saying, "No one will talk to me because I stutter."
- *Reaction formation.* Clients who experience this have thoughts or emotions that are shocking and unacceptable to them; thus, they react with opposite emotions. For instance, the husband of an elderly Alzheimer's patient secretly wishes his wife would die. In reaction formation, he sacrifices all his own needs and wants to care for his wife, telling the clinician he loves his wife dearly and could not live without her.
- *Displacement.* The client takes his or her feelings of hostility or anger about a situation and transfers them to a safe object or person. For example, recently the first author was involved with parents who spent several hours blaming and castigating her for, among other things, stating in a report that their severely mentally retarded teenage daughter had "profound cognitive and linguistic delays."
- *Projection.* Clients attribute their own emotions, thoughts, or actions to someone else. For example, a mother told the first author that the school personnel who served her son never communicated with one another. The school personnel shared with the first author that this mother rarely communicated with school personnel, creating problems for everyone.

- *Repression.* Clients keep their thoughts and feelings under very strict control, out of view of others. Clients themselves are not aware of these thoughts and feelings, which are below the conscious level.
- *Suppression.* This is similar to repression. Clients keep their feelings and thoughts highly controlled, but they are consciously aware of those feelings. Suppression is the norm in some cultures. It should be viewed as a difference, not a defense mechanism, in those situations.

SUMMARY

✓ Speech–language pathologists and audiologists sometimes have to deal with client emotions that arise in response to communication disorders and their effects. Some situations require a referral to a trained mental-health professional.

✓ In other situations, the clinician can successfully combine approaches to counseling to help clients and families take active steps to constructively deal with communicative disorders.

✓ Clinicians must be aware of phenomena that can impact counseling; these phenomena include special issues such as culture and gender, and clients' demonstration of emotional reactions and defense mechanisms. When clinicians are aware of and prepared for these phenomena, counseling and ultimately treatment efforts will prove much more successful.

MEDICAL SPEECH–LANGUAGE PATHOLOGY

INTRODUCTION

Thousands of SLPs work in a variety of medical settings. These settings provide unique challenges and require a specific set of skills, which differ from those needed in other settings. As speech–language pathology becomes more and more specialized, clinicians need more in-depth knowledge about service to specific kinds of patients who are seen in medical settings. In this section, we discuss the scope of practice and responsibilities of clinicians in medical settings, medical team specialists and their roles, infectious disease control, patients with HIV and AIDS, and medical imaging techniques.

Practice and Responsibilities of Speech–Language Pathologists

In the majority of medical settings, SLPs carry out the following duties (American Speech-Language-Hearing Association, 2001; Golper, 1998; Johnson & Jacobson, 1998):

■ *assessment and treatment of patients* in the areas of:

- mental or cognitive status (e.g., orientation, memory, attention)
- neurogenic speech and language disorders
- swallowing (dysphagia) and upper-aerodigestive disorders (e.g., infant feeding)
- sensory awareness related to communication or swallowing
- voice disorders
- speech and resonance problems concomitant with or secondary to laryngeal, velopharyngeal, or oral surgery

- communication problems due to nonvocal, tracheostomized, and ventilator-dependent status

■ *use of such instruments as videofluoroscopy, EMG, nasendoscopy, stroboscopy, and computerized instruments* to observe, collect, and analyze data relative to communication and swallowing functions

■ *selecting, fitting, and training in the use of prosthetic devices* for communication and swallowing (excluding hearing aids)

■ *participation on interdisciplinary teams,* including knowledge of the roles of each team member in the particular setting

■ *staff education* (inservicing colleagues and other staff about various aspects of speech–language pathology)

■ *providing counseling and education* to families of patients, including facilitating interaction between the patient, family, and other team specialists

■ *continuing education* (updating of one's own skills and competencies)

■ *participation in the medical facility's efforts to contain costs*

■ *participation in the facility's internal and external reviews,* including providing a record of clinical activities and treatment efficacy

■ *participation in quality management and quality assurance efforts* through monitoring and evaluating programs and resolving any problems in patient care, possibly including risk management, or identifying and reducing factors that put patients at risk in any way

■ *securing reimbursements,* including documenting assessment findings and treatment progress for insurance companies as well as Medicaid and Medicare (managed care companies, which provide health coverage at fixed costs, want to use facilities and providers that produce documented positive outcomes that directly impact patients' activities of daily living)

■ *documentation of assessment and treatment activities,* often carried out through SOAP notes:

- S = *subjective* (observations such as the patient's complaint, what the examiner notices about the patient; e.g., patient says, "I'm always forgetful.")
- O = *objective* (examiner's objective findings, facts and data; e.g., "The patient was 90% accurate in defining 10 common words.")
- A = *assessment* (examiner's interpretation of findings; e.g., "Patient appears more oriented today.")
- P = *plan* (plans for treatment, steps taken or recommended; e.g., "Tomorrow we will begin left-right orientation.")

Medical Team Specialists and Their Roles

In every medical facility, the medical team specialists and their roles are somewhat different. Speech–language pathologists tend to interact most with the following specialists, who usually perform the following services (Bzoch, 2004; Golper, 1998; Miller & Groher, 1990):

■ *Dieticians.* These nutrition specialists frequently interact with the medical team for patients with dysphagia. Clinicians consult often with dieticians about patients who need assistance with oral feeding.

■ *Infectious disease specialists.* These doctors are especially involved with patients who have AIDS and AIDS-related diseases; clinicians consult with them about patients who have speech, language, cognitive, and swallowing problems secondary to AIDS.

■ *Neurosurgeons.* These surgeons specialize in conducting surgery on the spinal cord, peripheral nerves, and brain; clinicians consult with them about speech–language disorders secondary to neurological problems.

■ *Nurses.* These specialists are directly involved in numerous aspects of patient care, and clinicians interact with them on almost a daily basis.

■ *Occupational therapists.* These specialists work with patients who need functional or adaptive restoration of upper-extremity disabilities. They may also help patients who have perceptual-motor and visual-perceptual disorders. Clinicians may work with them in providing assistance and adaptive devices for patients with dysphagia.

■ *Otolaryngologists or head and neck surgeons.* These doctors, who used to be called ear, nose, and throat (ENT) specialists, perform surgical services for patients with problems in the nasal, oral, laryngeal, pharyngeal, and esophageal structures. Clinicians consult with them about patients who have speech and swallowing problems.

■ *Pediatricians.* These physicians see children and youth (ages birth–21) who have medical diseases and developmental disorders. Pediatricians often refer to other specialists. Clinicians work with pediatricians regarding children who need early identification and treatment of communication disorders.

■ *Pharmacists.* These specialists dispense drugs. Clinicians work with pharmacists regarding patients whose medications may affect speech, language, cognition, or swallowing.

■ *Physical therapists.* These specialists carry out physical rehabilitation activities with patients who have physical disabilities due to disease or injury. Physical therapists help such patients to achieve adaptive and functional restoration of movement. Clinicians often work on rehabilitation teams with physical therapists.

■ *Plastic surgeons.* These surgeons provide reconstructive surgery to patients who have had parts or all of the mandible, maxilla, or tongue removed, for example, as well as patients who have velopharyngeal incompetence. Clinicians work with plastic surgeons in cases in which speech, resonance, or both are affected by the surgery.

■ *Prosthodontists.* These specialists construct prosthetic speech appliances for patients with such needs as obduration of clefts and fistulas and lifting of the velum for increased velopharyngeal closure, and patients who have had maxillary or mandibular surgery and need help in preserving their facial contours.

■ *Psychiatrists.* These doctors assess and treat patients with mental or emotional difficulties related to their medical problems. Treatment usually takes the form of psychotherapy, medication, or a combination of the two. Clinicians work with psychiatrists in cases in which patients have mental or emotional difficulties concurrent with a communication disorder.

■ *Pulmonary specialists.* These doctors manage patients with chronic and acute lung disorders. Clinicians may consult with them about patients who have speech, voice, or swallowing problems related to respiratory difficulties.

■ *Radiologists.* These doctors work with clinicians especially in dynamic evaluation of swallowing. Radiologists also carry out such diagnostic tests as magnetic resonance imaging (described later). Clinicians work with radiologists regarding patients who have swallowing problems and possible language and cognition problems secondary to diseases detectable through radiologic diagnostic tests.

■ *Social workers.* These professionals provide links between the hospital and the community, often helping meet patients' immediate social needs such as marital and psychological adjustments to disabilities, job placement, applying for benefits, obtaining family counseling, and others. Clinicians often work with social workers regarding patients and their families who have such social needs related to a communication disorder.

C O N C E P T S   T O   C O N S I D E R

Summarize the role of SLPs in the medical setting. List four other medical team specialists that SLPs might interact with.

_____

_____

_____

_____

_____

Infectious Disease Control

Speech–language pathologists are increasingly serving in roles in which they come into contact with patients' bodily fluids: blood, saliva, mucous, and cerumen. Many clinicians have limited knowledge and use of appropriate procedures for avoiding infectious diseases. It is important for clinicians not to expose themselves—and thus others—to those diseases.

■ Infections can have bacterial, viral, or fungal origins. Patients who may transmit infectious diseases to clinicians include but are not limited to those who:

- are referred after head and neck surgeries;
- are receiving dysphagia therapy;
- have uncovered tracheostomies;
- have HIV or AIDS;
- are prone to bite clinicians (e.g., young children with behavior problems); and
- are newborns who have infections acquired in utero or after birth.

■ Medical facilities requiring the use of *universal precautions* require that all personnel who engage in patient contact:

- wear gowns if clothes are likely to become soiled;
- wash hands before and after contact with patients;
- put sharp instruments and disposable needles and syringes in a labeled "sharps" disposal container;
- wear gloves if there is to be contact with broken skin, bodily fluids, or mucous membranes; and
- protect the eyes and mouth if any splashes containing bodily fluid are likely.

■ Hand washing should occur before and after patient contact, when coming on or off duty, after using the toilet, when the hands are dirty, and after wiping or blowing one's nose. Hand washing should include the use of hot water, antibacterial soap, and paper towels. All areas of the hands and forearms should be washed for 1–2 minutes.

■ Masks with clear plastic eye protectors should be worn when working with a patient who can transmit a disease through airborne means or through splashing; infections can enter through the eyes.

■ Sterile gowns should be worn in surgery or when required by isolation precautions (those precautions are usually posted on the patient's door).

■ Clinicians should use new gloves for each patient. Because latex and vinyl gloves are susceptible to tears and perforations, some clinicians wear two sets of gloves when working with especially high-risk patients.

■ Clinicians should take care to prevent bodily fluids (e.g., saliva) from contaminating things that cannot be disinfected (e.g., records, files).

■ It is wise to clean and disinfect all items and surfaces used if possible. This includes tables, equipment, toys, and other materials. Hospital supply stores often have powerful disinfectants that kill many microorganisms.

Working with HIV and AIDS Patients

■ Patients who are infected with the *human immunodeficiency virus* (HIV) experience depletions of *T lymphocytes*, a particular type of white blood cells. This eventually leads to extended, severe suppression of the immune system and consequent development of *acquired immune deficiency syndrome* (AIDS).

■ Patients may live for some years with a diagnosis of "HIV positive" before they develop AIDS.

AIDS refers to the later stages of HIV infection. The immune system's failure predisposes the patient to the development of malignancies and severe, life-threatening infections.

- Language, speech, and hearing problems often result because HIV attacks the central nervous system. Nearly 100% of its manifestations occur in the head and neck. Communicative disorders can occur as a result of treatment options used to treat opportunisitic infections (those which occur when a patient's resistance to disease becomes impaired).

- Frequently, treatments for patients with HIV, AIDS, and related opportunistic infections rely heavily on drugs that are potentially ototoxic (American Speech-Language-Hearing Association, 2004). Thus, communicative disorders professionals must be aware that drugs given to their patients may be compromising those patients' auditory function.

- As many as 75% of adults with AIDS experience auditory dysfunction, which can stem from opportunistic infections such as cytomegalovirus, herpes zoster oticus, and herpes simplex virus. Many adults with HIV and AIDS experience vertigo, tinnitus, and hearing loss (American Speech-Language-Hearing Association, 2004).

- Patients with AIDS may have additional symptoms and communication problems (American Speech-Language-Hearing Association, 2004; Benninger & Gardner, 1998; Golper, 1998; Vogel, Carter & Carter, 2000; Wallace, 1998):

  - AIDS dementia complex, with cognitive problems such as disorientation, confusion, loss of memory, loss of concentration
  - aphasia
  - motor-speech impairment (e.g., dysarthria, apraxia)
  - ataxia
  - dysphagia
  - articulation, swallowing, respiration, and voice problems due to candidiasis (yeast infections) that can occur in the mouth, esophagus, bronchial tubes, lungs, and trachea
  - apathy and social withdrawal
  - reduced verbal output
  - confabulations
  - language of confusion
  - stuttering
  - voice disorders
  - deterioration in handwriting
  - meningitis
  - encephalitis
  - Kaposi's sarcoma (cancer that arises first in skin and then progressively affects other body sites, possibly including major organs)
  - incontinence
  - in children, hearing impairment secondary to middle ear disease
  - in children, language delays (especially pragmatic problems), cognitive problems, and articulation disorders
  - in children, elective mutism, hysterical aphonia

- Speech–language pathologists may serve patients with HIV or AIDS who have communication problems, swallowing problems, or both (American Speech-Language-Hearing Association, 2004). Treatment may involve, among other things, the use of augmentative or alternative communication for patients who are deteriorating in speech, language, or cognitive function in the later stages of AIDS.

■ HIV has been found in certain human body tissues and in human excretions. When working with patients who are HIV positive or have AIDS, clinicians must be especially careful to observe universal precautions and to prevent transmission of the HIV virus.

Medical Imaging Techniques

While it is beyond the scope of this chapter to provide a detailed description of all available medical imaging techniques, we provide some basic definitions of imaging techniques that are commonly used with patients who have communication disorders. Speech–language pathologists who work in medical settings will encounter these techniques as used with patients, and should know the basics of what each involves (Bzoch, 2004; George, Vikingstad, & Cao, 1998; Golper, 1998; Hegde, 2001a; Nicolosi, Harryman, & Kresheck, 2004):

■ *Tomography.* Also called *laminography,* this is a computerized radiographic method of taking pictures of different planes of body structures. It is used to scan brain structures, and is frequently used as a neurodiagnostic method for people with communication disorders such as aphasia secondary to stroke.

■ *Computerized axial tomography (CAT) scan* (also known as *CT scan* or *computed tomography*). In this radiographic imaging procedure, x-ray beams circle through segments of the brain and pass through tissue. A camera takes pictures of sections of the structure being scanned. The scanner detects density differences, and a computer analyzes the images generated by the scanning machine and produces pictures of the scanned structures. CAT scans can detect hemorrhages, lesions, tumors, and other pathologies. CAT scans are often used in the diagnosis of neuropathology associated with strokes.

■ *Electroencephalography (EEG).* This neurodiagnostic method records and measures electrical impulses of the brain through small surface electrodes attached to the scalp. EEG can show different kinds of brain waves associated with different kinds of activity (e.g., talking, listening, thinking). EEG indicates cerebral pathology by abnormal electrical activity and is often used to detect seizures.

■ *Magnetic resonance imaging (MRI).* This neurodiagnostic imaging technique, in which the patient lies completely still in a cylinder container, is used to show fine detail in brain and spinal cord structure. MRI can also be used to provide images of the soft tissues, large blood vessels, and heart. The method is based on alignment and realignment of nuclei of atoms in the cell when a structure is placed in a strong magnetic field. Variations introduced in the amount of magnetic radiation will cause alignment and realignment of nuclei. Such changes produce electromagnetic signals, which a computer analyzes to produce images of the structure. MRI does not use x-rays and provides higher-resolution images than CAT scans, sometimes detecting lesions missed by CAT scans. However, MRI is expensive, and patients may have difficulty tolerating it.

■ *Positron emission tomography (PET).* This neurodiagnostic procedure is a type of emission-computed tomography that allows imaging of metabolic activity through measurements of radioactivity in the section of the body being viewed (e.g., the brain). The patient is injected with a radioactive substance that spreads throughout the brain; the amount of radioactivity is then scanned, and observed differences in the amount of radioactivity suggest different rates of cerebral metabolism. Lower than normal metabolic rate suggests neuropathology. If the patient is suspected of having cerebral dysfunction secondary to a stroke, for example, PET scans can be helpful by evaluating the function of blood flow and brain metabolism (whereas CAT and MRI scans evaluate only structure).

■ *Single-photon emission computed tomography (SPECT).* This neurodiagnostic procedure evaluates the amount of blood flowing through a structure. Also known as *regional cerebral bloodflow (rCBF),* SPECT helps assess cerebral metabolism. The patient inhales xenon 133, a radioactive gas that immediately spreads throughout the cerebral hemispheres and enters the bloodstream. A scanner detects radiation uptake in cerebral blood, and a computer calculates the amount of blood flow in given regions and displays variations in blood flow with different colors. SPECT is helpful in diagnosing cerebral lesions associated with various neuropathologies causing communication disorders.

■ *Videofluoroscopy.* This is a radiologic method of examining movement of internal structures and recording the movement patterns for assessment and diagnosis. It is useful in assessing the functions of the velopharyngeal mechanism, vocal folds, swallowing, and respiratory movement. X-rays are transmitted through the tissue under observation; the soft tissue is coated with barium with the help of a nasal spray, and observers can have multiple views of the structures (e.g., frontal, lateral, base, and oblique views of the velopharyngeal mechanism) and their movements. The images are shown on a phosphorescent screen and recorded on a videotape for later examination and diagnosis. Videofluoroscopy is often used to assess swallowing function in patients with confirmed or suspected dysphagia.

SUMMARY

✓ Clinicians who work in medical settings have specific responsibilities related to assessment and treatment of patients, as well as participation in professional and institutional activities.

✓ Speech–language pathologists work on interdisciplinary teams whose members have specific roles, which differ slightly from setting to setting. As part of their jobs in medical settings, clinicians must rigorously practice infectious disease control measures, particularly when working with patients who are HIV positive or have AIDS.

✓ Some patients are assessed with specialized imaging techniques, and clinicians often get medical reports that discuss findings of such procedures as CAT scans, videofluoroscopy, and others.

✓ When working with patients and with other medical professionals, clinicians should be familiar with imaging procedures as well as with their common abbreviations that are used in charts in medical settings.

CRANIOFACIAL ANOMALIES AND GENETIC SYNDROMES

INTRODUCTION

Craniofacial anomalies, mostly due to genetic factors, create many clinical conditions and syndromes, some of which are associated with communicative disorders. In this section, major craniofacial anomalies including clefts of the lip and palate and some major genetic syndromes that are associated with communicative disorders are reviewed.

Craniofacial Anomalies

- Craniofacial anomalies are abnormalities of the structures of the head and face. These abnormalities are congenital and in many cases due to genetic factors.

- A variety of factors have been demonstrated or hypothesized to cause craniofacial anomalies. Clefts of the lip and the soft palate are better known to SLPs, but there are hundreds of genetic syndromes with craniofacial anomalies that are associated with communicative disorders (Bzoch, 2004; Hegde, 2001a; Volden, 2004).

- Selected syndromes with significant association with communicative disorders are summarized in a later section of this chapter.

Cleft Lip

- A *cleft* is an opening in a normally closed structure. Cleft lip, therefore, is an opening in the lip, usually the upper lip. Lower lip clefting is very rare. Clefts of the lips alone are rare; they are usually associated with cleft of the palate.

- However, clefts of the palate are often not associated with cleft lips. Clefting is a congenital disorder; it is present at the time of birth. A congenital disorder may or may not be inherited.

- Cleft lips are more often unilateral than bilateral, and they occur more frequently on the left side than on the right side. Rare bilateral lip clefts have an even greater tendency to coexist with palatal clefts than unilateral left lip clefts do.

- Cleft lips alone rarely result in speech disorders and are less frequently associated with other genetic anomalies than palatal clefts.

Cleft Palate

General Facts

- *Palatal clefts* are various congenital malformations resulting in an opening in the hard palate, the soft palate, or both. These malformations are due to disruptions of the embryonic growth processes resulting in a failure to fuse structures that are normally fused.
- Cleft palates may be a part of a genetic syndrome with other anomalies. It is now believed that clefting of the lip and palate is etiologically different from clefting of the palate only (Shprintzen & Bardach, 1995).
- The incidence of palatal clefts in different populations varies. In the U.S. population, about 1 in 600 to 750 live births may be diagnosed with clefting. The highest to the lowest incidence rates are found among Native Americans, Japanese, Chinese, Whites, and African Americans, in that order.
- Generally, males tend to exhibit a higher frequency and greater severity of cleft lip (with or without cleft palate) than females, who tend to exhibit higher frequency of palatal clefts (without the cleft lip).

Overview of the Embryonic Growth of the Facial Structures

The most crucial period for genetic malformations is the embryonic period, which consists of the first seven to ten weeks of gestation. Most new organs emerge in the embryonic period. The 4th to the 6th week of pregnancy poses the greatest threat of embryonic disruptions, as it is the most sensitive period of growth. This period is characterized by:

- Multiplication of embryonic cells during the first few weeks.
- Development of three layers of cells from which different organs emerge.
- Development of a marked bend in the top portion of the embryo, creating a bulge that becomes the primitive forebrain by the end of the 3rd week.
- Development of a groove known as the *stomodeum,* which is the primitive mouth and nose.
- Development of the *frontonasal process,* which develops into the nose, the central part of the upper lip, and the primary palate.
- Development of two *maxillary processes,* which form most of the face, mouth, cheeks, and the sides of the upper lip; most of the hard palate; the alveolar ridge; and the soft palate.
- Development of the *upper lip* and the *primary palate* (by the end of the 7th week). The upper lip does not develop as a single structure, hence it is prone to clefting. The nose and the midline of the upper lip are formed out of one structure, and the two sides of the lip are formed out of another structure. As a result, the cleft of the lip typically appears at either the right or the left side of the nose.
- Development of the two *mandibular processes,* giving rise to the lower jaw (mandible), lower lip, and chin; these are formed and fused by the end of the 4th or 5th week.
- Development of the mandible, which moves to a lower and more normal position.
- Growth of the tongue, which initially lies higher, at the level of the nose; it drops down to its normal position when the jaw develops.
- Growth of the hard and the soft palates; this growth is identifiable at the 5th week of gestation. The two shelves of the maxillary bone that form the hard palate remain in a vertical position, on either side of the high-placed embryonic tongue; when the tongue drops, the palatal shelves move in an upward and lateral manner and toward each other to form the roof of the mouth.
- *Fusion* of the two shelves of the hard palate at the midline between the 8th and 9th weeks; this is a front-to-back fusion, a fact reflected in the clefting process. Also, fusion of the maxillary shelves with the triangular premaxillary bone (the primary palate) occurs, thus separating the mouth from the nose.
- Growth of the muscles of the soft palate, initially as two separate halves. Palatal bones, as they move toward the midline, also bring the two halves of the soft palate together. By the 12th week, the muscle mass from the two sides fuses to form the soft palate.

Etiology of Clefts

Clefts are related to a variety of genetic, chromosomal, environmental, and mechanical factors. Some of the more common factors are as follows.

Genetic Abnormalities

- autosomal dominant inheritance in some syndromes (e.g., Apert syndrome, Stickler syndrome, van der Wude syndrome, Waardenburg syndrome, and Treacher Collins syndrome)
- recessive genetic inheritance in some syndromes (e.g., orofacial-digital syndrome)
- x-linked inheritance in some syndromes (e.g., oto-palatal-digital syndrome)

CONCEPTS TO CONSIDER

Describe three critical anatomical structures that must develop intactly when a baby is in utero in order for the lip and palate to be normal. Which are the most critical weeks of gestation for the development of these structures?

- chromosomal abnormalities (e.g., Trisomy 13).

Environmental Teratogenic Factors

The following are external factors that affect the genetic material:

- fetal alcohol syndrome
- illegal drug use
- side effects of some prescription drugs (e.g., anticonvulsant drugs or thalidomide, a sedative)
- rubella

Mechanical Factors

- intrauterine crowding
- twinning
- uterine tumor
- amniotic ruptures

Classification of Clefts

- Clefts are classified in different ways. No system of classification captures the variations and combinations found in clefts. Therefore, none is universally accepted although today, there are several preferred classifications (see Bzoch, 2004, for more details). Clefts vary in extent, often measured in thirds ($\frac{1}{3}$, $\frac{2}{3}$, or $\frac{3}{3}$) and widths.
- The major types of clefts include the following:

  - cleft lip (complete or incomplete, unilateral or bilateral)
  - cleft of alveolar process (unilateral, bilateral, median, or submucous)
  - cleft of prepalate (combination of previous types with or without prepalate protrusion or rotation)

- cleft of the palate (of the soft palate, of the hard palate, or submucous)
- cleft of prepalate and palate (any combination of clefts of the prepalate and palate)
- facial clefts other than prepalate and palate (e.g., such rare forms as horizontal clefts, lower mandibular clefts, lateral oro-ocular clefts, and naso-ocular clefts)

- Children might also manifest *microforms,* which are minimal expressions of clefts, including a hairline indentation of the lip or just a notch on the lip. Microforms are revealed only through laminographic examination.
- Microforms include *submucous clefts* (also called *occult cleft palate*), in which the surface tissues of the soft or hard palate fuse but the underlying muscle or bone tissues do not (Nicolosi et al., 2004).

Congenital Palatopharyngeal Incompetence

- Congenital palatopharyngeal incompetence (CPI) is not a form of clefting, but rather is a related disorder. It refers to impaired velopharyngeal closing-valve functioning.
- CPI is characterized by significant impairment of velopharyngeal functions as revealed by videofluoroscopy or endoscopy (inadequate velopharyngeal closure), although the laryngeal structures appear normal.
- CPI may be caused by a short palate, reduced muscular mass of the soft palate, a deep or enlarged larynx, incorrect insertion of levator muscles (insertion to hard palate instead of the normal insertion to soft palate), or a combination of such factors.
- People with CPI typically have hypernasal speech, which ranges in nature from mild to severe. They can benefit from speech therapy, surgery, prostheses, or a combination of these.

Communication Disorders Associated with Clefts

Hearing Loss

- Children with clefts are prone to middle ear infections and hearing loss. The most common cause of hearing loss in children with cleft palate is otitis media. Otitis media with effusion compromises movement of the ossicular chain and the tympanic membrane.
- Eustachian tube dysfunction is also prevalent in children with clefts. This creates conditions conducive to conductive hearing loss especially. In babies with cleft palate, eustachian tube dysfunction is probably mostly related to the lack of contraction of the tensor veli palatini muscle and increased compliance of the tubal wall.
- After palatal reconstructive surgery, tensor veli palatini dysfunction improves but may never normalize. Chronic otitis media with effusion (COME) continues to be a problem after palatal surgery. The incidence of hearing loss in the cleft palate population is about 58%. Usually the hearing loss is bilateral and conductive, but not necessarily symmetrical (Kemker & Antonelli, 2004).

Articulation Disorders

Articulation disorders are more significant if the palatal cleft is not repaired early or the repair is inadequate. Articulation disorders include errors such as those described below:

- greater difficulty with unvoiced sounds than with voiced sounds, pressure consonants, audible or inaudible nasal air emission, and distortion of vowels
- compensatory errors including various types of substitutions that help compensate for the inadequate closure of the velopharyngeal mechanism, such as substitutions of stops, frica-

tives, and affricates with unusual (often posterior) movements and posture of the tongue to stop the air or to produce friction noise (e.g., substitution of glottal stops for stop consonants, substitution of laryngeal fricatives for fricatives, and substitution of pharyngeal affricates for affricates)

Language Disorders

Language disorders may not be as significant as articulation disorders unless other conditions are associated; language is normal in many cases. Common problems include:

- initially delayed language development, with significant improvement as the child grows older; normal language possible by age 4 or so
- significant language disorders in children whose clefts are a part of genetic syndromes that include hearing loss, developmental disabilities, sensory problems, and so forth
- relatively normal receptive language skills, with delays in expressive language

Laryngeal and Phonatory Disorders

Children with palatal clefts tend to exhibit a higher prevalence of laryngeal and vocal disorders, which may include:

- vocal nodules
- hypertrophy and edema of the vocal folds
- vocal hoarseness, reduced vocal intensity, reduced pitch variations, and strangled voice
- resonance disorders characterized by hypernasality, hyponasality, denasality, or a combination

Assessment of Children with Clefts

Assessment of children with cleft palate includes all the standard procedures (e.g., case history, interview of the parents and the child if appropriate). The main concern is to assess speech sound production and velopharyngeal adequacy. It is also important to screen hearing and assess language.

Assessment of Velopharyngeal Function

- Most SLPs work as part of a cleft palate team when they assess children. It is recommended that routine speech and language evaluations be a part of the cleft palate team evaluation for every child starting before the early postnatal period of treatment (Bzoch, 2004). SLPs should also routinely be involved with assessments as children grow older.
- Procedures for assessment of velopharyngeal function include judgments about hypernasality and hyponasality, whose presence indicates velopharyngeal inadequacy.
- Objective assessment of the velopharyngeal mechanism includes an endoscopic examination of the velopharyngeal mechanism (*nasopharyngoscopy*). In nasopharyngoscopy, a nasopharyngoscope is passed through the middle meatus and back to the area of velopharyngeal closure. The examiner can then observe the posterior and lateral pharyngeal walls, as well as the nasal aspect of the velum and the adenoid pad as the client produces sentences (Kummer & Marsh, 1998).
- Objective assessment also includes a videofluoroscopic examination of the velopharyngeal mechanism in order to observe the movements of the soft palate, the lateral pharyngeal wall,

the posterior pharyngeal wall, and the tongue as the client produces consonant–vowel combinations, voiced and voiceless fricatives, and selected phrases.

- When assessing velopharyngeal closure, an oral manometer can be helpful. The patient either sucks from or blows into a mouthpiece as forcefully as possible. The inhalation task gives a negative reading, while the exhalation task yields a positive pressure reading from manometer gauges. The clinician obtains a ratio by comparing pressures achieved in the nostrils-occluded and the nostrils-open conditions. A normal ratio of 1.00 suggests adequate velopharyngeal closure. Ratios less than 1.00 may indicate VPI, reduced intelligibility, and hypernasal speech in patients with cleft palate. Ratios less than 0.89 are especially indicators of these phenomena (Haynes & Pindzola, 2004).
- Kay Elemetrics sells the Nasometer, a computer-based system that measures nasalence. *Nasalence* is a ratio formed between oral and nasal sound pressures, which is expressed as a percentage. The patient speaks syllables or words, and the Nasometer measures nasalence during this task (Case, 2002; Haynes & Pindzola, 2004). Use of the Nasometer can be most helpful in objectively assessing velopharyngeal function.
- Assessment also includes an orofacial examination to take note of the clefts in the lip, the hard palate, and the soft palate as well as adequacy of the surgical repair of the cleft, facial abnormalities indicative of a genetic syndrome, and the velopharyngeal mechanism.

Assessment of Articulation Disorders

- Assessment of articulation and phonological disorders in children with clefts includes standard procedures used in assessing similar disorders in children without clefts.
- However, special considerations are given to assess the kinds of errors and compensatory error patterns that are typical of children with cleft palates (e.g., pressure consonants).
- Many clinicians administer the *Iowa Pressure Articulation Test* (a subtest of the *Templin Darley Test of Articulation*) as well as other standardized tests of articulation and phonological skills.

Assessment of Language Disorders

- Assessing language disorders in children with clefts includes standard procedures used in assessing both language comprehension and production.
- It is important to gather a comprehensive language sample to analyze the use of semantic, syntactic, morphologic, and pragmatic use of language.

Assessment of Phonatory Disorders

- Assessing phonatory disorders in children with clefts includes standard procedures used in assessing voice disorders in children with no clefts.
- The clinician makes clinical judgments about voice quality deviations (e.g., hoarseness, harshness, breathiness).
- He or she also assesses vocally abusive behaviors, evaluates pitch and loudness of voice, and may conduct an instrumental assessment of voice disorders (e.g., with the use of Visi-Pitch or the Phonatory Function Analyzer).

Assessment of Resonance Disorders

- This includes assessing hypernasality in conversational speech by making clinical judgments.
- Rating of hypernasality in connected speech by two or more clinicians may also take place, and assessing hyponasality may be necessary.

Treatment of Children with Clefts

Treatment of children with clefts is a team effort involving several specialists, including oral surgeons, pediatricians, orthodontists, otolaryngologists, psychologists, and speech–language pathologists. Often, the surgical repair of the palate is the major initial treatment implemented (Bzoch, 2004; Golding-Kushner, 2001; Hegde, 2001b).

Surgical Management of the Clefts

- *Primary surgery for the clefts* is the initial surgery, in which the clefts are closed.
- *Secondary surgeries for clefts* are done to improve appearance and functioning, after the initial closure of the clefts.
- *Lip surgery* is done to close unilateral or bilateral clefts of the lip; this is typically done when the baby is about 3 months old or weighs about 10 pounds.
- *Palatal surgery* is done to close the cleft or clefts of the palate; this is typically done when the baby is 9–24 months.
- *V-Y retroposition* or the *Veau-Wardill-Kilner* method of surgery is done to repair the cleft of the palate; single-based flaps of palatal mucoperiosteum are raised on either side of the cleft and brought together and pushed back to close the cleft; this push-back (retropositioning of the flaps) lengthens the palate and improves chances of velopharyngeal approximation.
- The *von Langenbeck surgical method* is performed to repair the cleft of the palate by raising two bipedicled (attached on both ends) flaps of mucoperiosteum, bringing them together and attaching them to close the cleft; this leaves denuded bone on either side and does not lengthen the palate.
- *Delayed hard palate closure* is a surgical procedure in which the cleft of the soft palate is closed first, and the cleft of the hard palate is closed later.
- *Pharyngeal flap* is a secondary palatal surgical procedure in which a muscular flap is cut from the posterior pharyngeal wall, raised, and attached to the velum; the openings on either side of the flap allow for nasal breathing, nasal drainage, and production of nasal speech sounds. The flap helps close the velopharyngeal port and thus reduce hypernasality.
- *Pharyngoplasty* is another surgical procedure in which such substances as Teflon, silicone, dacron wool/silicone gel bag, and cartilage may be implanted or injected into the posterior pharyngeal wall to make it bulge and thus help close the velopharyngeal port.

Treatment of Articulation and Phonological Disorders

- Treatment is sequenced from sounds, syllables, words, phrases, and sentences, in that order.
- More visible sounds are taught before less visible sounds except for the linguadentals.
- Stops and fricatives are taught before other classes of sounds.
- Training on /k/ and /g/ may be inappropriate if the child's velopharyngeal functioning is inadequate.
- If stimulable, fricatives, affricates, or both may be trained; in any case, they may be trained after stops are mastered.
- Linguapalatal sounds, lingua-alveolars, and linguadentals should be taught, in that order.
- Frequent presentation of auditory and visual cues and modeling may be helpful.
- Compensatory articulatory positioning, where appropriate, may be taught.
- The clinician may teach the child to avoid posterior articulatory placements and to articulate with less effort and facial grimacing.
- Tactile cues and instruction to improve tongue positioning may be useful.

Treatment of Language Disorders

- Early language stimulation by parents is needed in some cases.
- When necessary, formal language treatment may be offered if language stimulation is not sufficient.
- It may be especially important to stimulate expressive language, as it tends to be more delayed than receptive language.

Treatment for Resonance Disorders

- Hypernasality due to velopharyngeal incompetence should not be treated until: (a) there are surgical or prosthetic efforts to improve the physiological functioning, and (b) the child is capable of velopharyngeal closure but is using previously established inappropriate compensatory articulation that can be modified.
- Children with mild hypernasality may respond positively to behavioral exercises alone. However, children with more severe symptoms of velopharyngeal anatomical insufficiency or neuromuscular incompetency usually need surgical or prosthetic intervention, or both, before speech therapy can succeed (Dworkin, Marunick, & Krouse, 2004).
- Voice therapy techniques designed to reduce hypernasality may be used (e.g., increased loudness, discrimination training to distinguish oral and nasal resonance, lowered pitch, encouragement of increasing oral opening).
- It is often helpful to teach the child to decrease intra-oral breath pressure on stop consonants and fricatives, while simultaneously using loose articulatory contacts.
- Biofeedback instruments (e.g., Tonar II) to reduce hypernasality may also be useful.
- In order to successfully assess and treat children with velopharyngeal incompetence, clinicians need to be well trained and qualified. According to Pannbacker (2004, p. 198): "The consequences of improper or inadequate speech–language services and the effects of inappropriate decisions may be more harmful than no services at all … The risk of inappropriate decisions about diagnosis and treament of VPI would be greatly reduced if decisions were based on *both perceived speech symptoms and direct imaging techniques such as endoscopy or radiography* … [italics the authors'] Unfortunately, clinical decisions about VPI are too often based only on speech." Clinicians will usually work on teams with other professionals and

C O N C E P T S   T O   C O N S I D E R

Treatment for children with cleft palates can be surgical or traditional/therapy-based. Summarize two surgical and two traditional/therapy-based treatment methods.

_____

_____

_____

_____

_____

use appropriate instrumentation to adequately assess and treat persons with velopharyngeal incompetence.

Genetic Syndromes

■ A *syndrome* is a constellation of signs and symptoms that are associated with a morbid process; a genetic syndrome is such a constellation with a known genetic basis.

■ Many genetic syndromes are associated with communication disorders. Syndromes that involve the craniofacial complex and those that affect general intellectual functions tend to produce the most significant effects on communication. Some of the most common syndromes that affect communication include the following (Bzoch, 2004; Hegde, 2001a; Volden, 2004):

Apert Syndrome

- This may be caused by spontaneous autosomal dominant mutations. The gene and locus of Apert syndrome is FGR2 at 10q25-26 (Bzoch, 2004). Its transmission is limited because of low reproductive capacity of affected people.
- Its physical characteristics include syndactyly (digital fusion) involving the second, third, and fourth digits, cranial synostosis resulting in smaller anterior-posterior skull diameter, flat frontal and occipital bones and high forehead, increased intracranial pressure and compensatory growth in cranial structures.
- Other physical characteristics include midfacial hypoplasia (underdevelopment), an arched and grooved hard palate, conductive hearing loss in some individuals, class III malocclusion, irregularly placed teeth, thickened alveolar process, long or thickened soft palate, and cleft of the hard palate in 25–30% of cases.
- Communication problems include a tendency toward hyponasality, forward carriage of the tongue, and articulation disorders involving mostly alveolar consonants (e.g., /s/ and /z/) and labial dental sounds (e.g., /f/ and /v/). There may also be deficiency in language skills depending on the level of intellectual function and hearing (Hegde, 2001a).

Cri du Chat Syndrome

- This is caused by an absence of the short arm of the fifth chromosome (known as 5p). Its physical characteristics include a cry resembling that of a cat (hence the name) in the infant.
- Other physical characteristics include low-set ears, a narrow oral cavity, and laryngeal hypoplasia.
- Communication problems include articulation and language disorders typically associated with mental retardation.

Crouzon Syndrome

- This is caused by autosomal dominant inheritance, with varied expression in individuals. Its physical characteristics include *craniosynostosis* (fusion of the cranial suture, especially that of the coronal) and hypoplasia of the midface, maxilla, or both.
- Other physical characteristics include a small maxillary structure, sphenoethmoidal synchondroses, ocular *hypertelorism* (eyes that are far apart), a parrotlike nose, facial asymmetry and tall forehead, malocclusion Class III in some cases, a highly arched palate, shallow oropharynx, a long and thick soft palate, and *brachycephaly* (short head).

- Communication problems include conductive hearing loss in some individuals, articulation disorders associated with hearing loss and abnormalities of palatal oral cavity structures, hyponasality, and language disorders in the cases with hearing loss and cognitive deficits.

Down Syndrome

- This is caused by an extra whole number chromosome 21, resulting in 47, rather than the normal 46 chromosomes. Physical characteristics include generalized hypotonia; a flat facial profile; small ears, nose, and chin; and brachycephaly.
- Other physical characteristics include midface dysplasia, shortened oral and pharyngeal structures, a narrow and high arched palate, a relatively large and fissured tongue that tends to protrude, a short neck with excess skin on the back of it, hyperflexible joints, cardiac malformations in about 40% of cases, and short fingers.
- Communication problems include conductive loss in many cases and sensorineural loss in some. There may be language delays and disorders, especially deficient syntactic and morphologic features accompanied by relatively better vocabulary skills. Hypernasality and nasal emission, breathier voice, and articulation disorders may also be present.

Fragile X Syndrome

- *Fragile X syndrome* is the leading inherited cause of mental retardation in males. An expanded number of Cytosine-Guanine-Guanine (CGG) nucelic acid repeats on a specific gene on one of the distal ends of the X chromosome (Roberts, Mirrett, Anderson, Burchinal, & Neebe, 2002).
- Physical characteristics include a large, long, and poorly formed pinna, a big jaw, enlarged testes, and a high forehead.
- Most males with Fragile X syndrome have mental retardation. During childhood, this mental retardation is mild-moderate, becoming more severe in adulthood.
- Communication problems include jargon, perseveration, echolalia, inappropriate language or talking to oneself (more often in the male), lack of gestures and other nonverbal means of communication that normally accompany speech, voice problems, and articulation disorders.
- Males with Fragile X syndrome may avoid eye contact, withdraw socially, have limited attention spans, be hyperactive, and have autistic-like social deficiencies. Generally, adolescent and adult males with Fragile X syndrome have delays in pragmatic, semantic, phonologic, and syntactic aspects of language. Speech intelligibility may be compromised (Roberts et al., 2004).

Hurler's Syndrome

- Hurler's syndrome is a rare, congenital metabolical disease caused by autosomal recessive deficiency of X-L iduronidase. It occurs in approximately 1 out of 10,000 births and most children with Hurler's syndrome die in their early teens or sometimes even before they are 10 years old (Enerson, 2001).
- In the 1800s and early 1900s, Hurler's syndrome was called "gargoylism." The name changed around 1919–1920. Hurler's syndrome is characterized by: dwarfism, hunchback, mental retardation, short and thick bones, a "gargoyle-like face," sensorineural deafness, and noisy respiration. Children with Hurler's syndrome also usually have a protuberant abdomen, angina pectoris, frequent chest infections, decreased joint mobility, and thickening of the coronary arteries. Their hands may be short, wide, and thick.
- Children with Hurler's syndrome have thick, everted lips, a large tongue, and small, malformed teeth. Thus, they frequently have compromised intelligibility (Kahn, 2004).

Landau-Kleffner Syndrome

- The causes of *Landau-Kleffner syndrome* (LKS) are unknown. LKS is a form of aphasia whereby formerly healthy children between the ages of 3–7 years lose their ability to comprehend language and then to speak it. This change can occur suddenly or gradually.
- Some children are left with severe, permanent language disorders. Others regain many of their language abilities over a span of months or years. For some children, relapses and remissions occur.
- Abnormal brain wave patterns have been detected through EEG in persons with LKS. It is estimated that 70% of affected children develop epilepsy. They usually have infrequent seizures that may or may not be accompanied by convulsions (M.I.N.D. Institute, 2004).

Moebius Syndrome

- This has a heterogeneous causation including agenesis or aplasia of the motor nuclei of the cranial nerves. There is sporadic, unpredictable occurrence in most cases and autosomal dominant inheritance in some cases.
- Its physical characteristics include involvement of facial and hypoglossal nerves in most and of the trigeminal nerve in some cases.
- There is also bilabial paresis and weak tongue control for lateralization, elevation, depression, and protrusion, unilateral or bilateral paralysis of the abductors of the eye, limited strength, range, and speed of movement of articulators, feeding problems in infancy, and a masklike face.
- Communication problems include conductive hearing loss in only a few cases and delayed language in some cases, especially in children with frequent hospitalizations. There may also be articulation disorders ranging from mild to severe, with bilabial, linguadental, and lingua-alveolar sounds affected more than the others.

Pierre-Robin Syndrome

- This is caused by autosomal recessive inheritance in most cases. In some cases, this syndrome may be a part of Stickler syndrome, in which case autosomal dominant inheritance may be the genetic basis.
- Its physical characteristics include mandibular hypoplasia, *glossoptosis* (downward displacement of the tongue), a cleft of the soft palate (but typically not associated with cleft of the lips), velopharyngeal incompetence, a deformed pinna and low-set ears, and temporal bone and ossicular chain deformities.
- Communication problems include unilateral or bilateral conductive hearing loss associated with otitis media and cleft palate, delayed language and language disorders, hypernasality and nasal emission, articulation disorders, and hypercompensatory articulation.

Prader-Willi Syndrome

- This is suspected to be caused by autosomal dominant inheritance and deletion in the region of the long arm of chromosome 15 (15q11–15q13) in some cases.
- Its physical characteristics include low muscle tone, early feeding difficulties, failure to thrive initially, obesity after the first year, excessive eating, and underdeveloped genitals.
- Many children with Prader-Willi syndrome have imprecise articulation, oral motor difficulties that contribute to poor articulation, and hypernasality. Some also exhibit flat intonation patterns, a slow speaking rate, a harsh or hoarse vocal quality, and abnormal vocal pitch due

to clinical characteristics listed below.

- Children with PWS frequently also have developmental delays and mental retardation. Many have impaired expressive and receptive language skills, with expressive skills being more impaired than receptive skills. These speech–language characteristics can result from clinical features of Prader-Willi syndrome, which are described below. However, there is a continuum of abilities ranging from nonverbal individuals to those who develop normal speech and language skills by adulthood.
- Clinical characteristics of individuals with Prader-Willi syndrome that can contribute to speech and language problems include (Lewis, Freebairn, Heeger, & Cassidy, 2002):

    - *hypotonia:* slow movement of articulators, stretching of laryngeal muscles, and poor velopharyngeal movement, which can contribute to slow rate of speech, imprecise articulation, hyper- or hyponasality, and variations in vocal pitch and quality
    - *larynx:* altered growth as a result of endocrine dysfunction, which leads to pitch variations
    - *mouth:* narrow overjet, micrognathia, narrow palatal arch, which contribute to reduced intelligibility/articulation skills
    - *dentition:* decay due to reduced output of saliva and hypoplasia of the enamel, which contribute to reduced intelligibility/articulation skills
    - *cognitive:* sequencing problems and mental retardation, which contribute to delayed receptive and expressive language skills as well as poor narrative skills
    - *behavioral disturbances:* stubbornness, temper tantrums, emotional lability, compulsive behavior, argumentativeness, poor social relationships, and difficulty detecting social cues, which contribute to poor pragmatic skills

- At this time, new medical treatments are being utilized with individuals who have Prader-Willi syndrome. These include use of growth hormones as well as surgical procedures to reduce hypernasality

CONCEPTS TO CONSIDER

Many syndromes are associated with speech–language problems. Describe two of these syndromes and their associated speech–language difficulties.

Russell-Silver Syndrome

- This is suspected to be caused by genetic factors, although information about etiology is very scarce. Babies with Russell-Silver syndrome have low birthweight, are small for their gestational age, and are considered to have dwarfism.
- Physical characteristics include asymmetry of the arms or legs, a disproportionately large head, craniofacial disproportion, mandibular hypoplasia, a high, narrow palate, and *microdontia* (abnormal smallness of the teeth).
- Communication problems often include hypernasality, feeding problems in infancy, articulation disorders, expressive and receptive language disorders, and an abnormally high-pitched voice (Buckholz & Roseberry-McKibbin, 1997).

Tourette's Syndrome

- Tourette's syndrome is a neurological, inherited disorder. It is characterized by uncontrollable vocal sounds (tics) and repeated involuntary movements. Sometimes the tics include involuntary, inappropriate words and phrases such as swear words and other obscene language (coprolalia).
- An estimated 100,000 Americans have full-blown Tourette's syndrome, whereas others have a partial manifestation of the disorder (e.g., transient childhood tics, chronic multiple tics). Tourette's syndrome affects males 3–4 times more often than females, and affects persons from all ethnic backgrounds.
- No one knows what causes Tourette's syndrome; however, some researchers speculate it is due to an abnormality in the genes affecting the brain's metabolism of neurotransmitters such as serotonin, norepinephrine, and dopamine.
- Symptoms of Tourette's syndrome usually appear before 18 years of age. Usually, the first symptoms are facial tics such as eye blinking; however, tics can include grimaces or nose twitching. In time, other motor tics may appear, including neck stretching, head jerking, body twisting and bending, and floor stamping. Tics "go up and down" in terms of increasing and decreasing in frequency, location, and type; that is, symptoms may subside for weeks or months and then recur.
- As stated, people with Tourette's syndrome may utter unacceptable sounds, words, or phrases. Commonly, they clear their throats, grunt, sniff, cough, shout, yelp, or bark. Some persons may demonstrate echolalia and may repeat actions unncessarily and obsessively (M.I.N.D. Institute, 2004).

Treacher Collins Syndrome

- This is caused by autosomal dominant inheritance in most cases and spontaneous mutation in some. Its physical characteristics include underdeveloped facial bones, including mandibular hypoplasia (small chin) and malar (cheek) hypoplasia, dental malocclusion and hypoplasia, and downwardly slanted palpebral fissures.
- Other characteristics include *coloboma* (lesion or defect, usually a cleft) of the lower eyelid, stenosis or atresia of the external auditory canal, malformations of the pinna, and middle and inner ear malformations.
- There is usually a high hard palate, a cleft palate in about 30% of the cases, a submucous cleft in some cases, a short or immobile soft palate, and sucking and swallowing problems in infancy.
- Communication problems include congenital, bilateral, conductive hearing loss in many cases and sensorineural loss in some cases as well as language disorders typically associated with

hearing impairment.

- Other communication problems include hypernasality and nasal emission in cases with clefts and velopharyngeal incompetence, as well as articulation disorders consistent with hearing loss and gross oral structural deviations.

Turner Syndrome

- This occurs only in females and is caused by a missing or deformed X chromosome in most cases. A similar syndrome that occurs in both males and females is called *Noonan syndrome.*
- Its physical characteristics include ovarian abnormality, resulting in absence of menstruation and infertility, congenital swelling of the feet, neck, and hands, cardiac defects, webbing of the neck (excess skin over the neck), and a low posterior hairline.
- Other physical characteristics include a broad chest with widely spaced nipples, *cubitus valgas* (elbows bent outward or away from the midline), pigmented skin lesions, a narrow maxilla and palate, and *micrognathia* (abnormally small lower jaw).
- Further physical characteristics include anomalies of the auricle including low-set, elongated, and cup-shaped ears, thick earlobes, a high arched palate, a cleft palate in some cases, and evidence of right hemisphere dysfunction.
- Communication problems include sensorineural loss in many cases (usually noticed after the tenth year); middle ear infections during infancy and early childhood; conductive loss in some cases; language and articulation disorders consistent with hearing impairment; and visual, spatial, and attentional problems.

Usher Syndrome

- This is caused by autosomal recessive inheritance in most cases and is X-linked in rare cases. This syndrome may affect 50% of individuals who are deaf and blind.
- Its physical characteristics include night blindness in early childhood, limited peripheral vision as visual problems worsen, eventual blindness, and cochlear abnormalities.
- Communication problems include sensorineural loss, language and articulation disorders consistent with hearing impairment, and hypernasality and nasal emission.

Velocardiofacial Syndrome

- *Velocardiofacial syndrome, or VCFS,* is the syndrome most commonly associated with a cleft palate, usually a cleft of the soft palate. VCFS is also called *Shprintzen syndrome* after Dr. Robert Shprintzen, who first described this condition in 1978.
- Though the exact cause of VCFS is not known, it is known to be a genetic disorder. A small part of chromosome 22, known as 22q11.2, is missing in most people with VCFS. VCFS is an autosomal disorder; only one parent needs to have the gene in order to pass it on to the children. VCFS has also been called *DiGeorge sequence.*
- In addition to cleft palate, over 180 other anomalies are associated with VCFS (see Golding-Kushner, 2001, for a thorough listing). Not every child has all anomalies, nor is one anomaly present in all children with VCFS. Major anomalies include middle ear infections, learning problems, speech and feeding problems, and unique facial characteristics. Facial characteristics include a wide nose, small ears, almond-shaped eyes, and an elongated face (Cleft Lip and Palate Association of Ireland, 2005). There may also be significant verbal language difficulties (Volden, 2004).
- The neonatal period of babies with VCFS is especially challenging. Feeding problems and failure to thrive are common, and often doctors refer these infants to SLPs for feeding therapy. Feeding problems are frequently complicated by generalized and pharyngeal hypotonia, la-

ryngeal and vascular anomalies, and nasal regurgitation and nasal vomiting. Special feeding strategies that are carefully implemented can help to make gastrostomies and nasogastric tubes unnecessary (Golding-Kushner, 2001).

Williams Syndrome

- Williams syndrome (WS) is a rare genetic disorder that impacts an estimated 1 out of every 20,000 babies. Sometimes WS is called *elfin-face syndrome* because people with WS have a physical resemblance to elves. They are often small-boned and short, with a long upper lip, wide mouth, full lips, small chin, upturned nose, and puffiness around the eyes.
- WS is caused by an abnormality on chromosome 7, including a gene that makes the protein elastin. Elastin provides elasticity and strength to blood vessel walls. It is thought that developmental and medical problems are caused by deletions of additional genetic material near the elastin gene.
- Most people with WS have IQs between 50 and 70; however, they can show high intelligence in certain areas such as music, language, and interpersonal skills. Children with WS often have charming personalities; they are courteous, gregarious, and loving, and are unafraid of strangers (which worries their parents).
- WS causes a varied profile of medical and developmental problems; each child's profile is unique. Some children have an elevated blood calcium level, or hypercalcemia, which can cause extreme irritability. Sometimes it is necessary for these children to undergo medical or dietary intervention.
- Most children with WS have narrowed pulmonary arteries and a narrowed aorta. These problems can range from mild to severe, and may necessitate surgical intervention.
- Children with WS may also have abnormalities of dental occlusion or bite as well as small, widely spaced teeth. Usually these problems can be corrected with orthodontia (M.I.N.D. Institute, 2004).

SUMMARY

✓ Craniofacial anomalies such as cleft lip and palate are due mostly to genetic factors, although environmental and mechanical factors may also play a role.

✓ People with clefts of the palate have communication disorders associated with the clefts; the disorders include hearing loss and disorders of language, articulation, resonance, and voice.

✓ When assessing children with clefts, it is important to assess velopharyngeal incompetence as well as articulation, language, phonatory, and resonance disorders.

✓ Treatment of children with clefts usually consists of surgical management combined with treatment of disorders of language, articulation, resonance, and voice.

✓ Many genetic syndromes are associated with communication disorders. Those syndromes often cause disorders of articulation, language, voice, and resonance.

CHAPTER HIGHLIGHTS

◆ **CLIENTS AND THEIR FAMILIES** sometimes experience emotional reactions related to communicative disorders and their effects. Clinicians can make referrals to mental health professionals when warranted. In many cases, however, clinicians can provide the support and release families need.

◆ **VARIOUS APPROACHES TO COUNSELING** (client-centered, behavioral, and cognitive-behavioral) may be combined to provide the most appropriate support for the stage that clients and families are currently in. Special issues can make counseling challenging. Such issues include culture, gender, and age of clients and clinicians. Clients may also demonstrate emotional reactions and defense mechanisms during counseling situations. Clinicians who are aware of and prepared for these special issues are generally successful in dealing with them.

◆ **SPEECH–LANGUAGE PATHOLOGISTS SOMETIMES WORK** in medical settings, where they have a wide scope of professional responsibilities. They work on interdisciplinary teams that may consist of dieticians, infectious disease specialists, neurosurgeons, nurses, occupational therapists, otolaryngologists or head and neck surgeons, pediatricians, pharmacists, physical therapists, plastic surgeons, prosthodontists, psychiatrists, pulmonary specialists, radiologists, and social workers.

◆ **SPEECH–LANGUAGE PATHOLOGISTS SOMETIMES WORK** with patients who may transmit infectious diseases through the bodily fluids of blood, cerumen, mucous, and saliva. It is important to take precautions when serving such patients, some of whom are HIV positive or have AIDS. Patients with AIDS manifest a wide range of communicative disorders. Children with AIDS have special problems that must be addressed.

◆ **MANY MEDICAL SETTINGS USE** special imaging techniques to diagnose a variety of problems and diseases. Techniques include computerized axial tomography, electroencephalography, fluoroscopy, magnetic resonance imaging, and positron emission tomography.

◆ **SPEECH–LANGUAGE PATHOLOGISTS SOMETIMES DEAL** with clients who have craniofacial anomalies associated with clinical conditions and syndromes. Some clients have a cleft lip or palate. Others have a specific syndrome associated with disorders of language, articulation, voice, or resonance. Assessment and treatment may involve traditional methods as well as surgical intervention.

CHAPTER HIGHLIGHTS

✎ **ADD YOUR OWN CHAPTER HIGHLIGHTS HERE:**

Study & Review Questions

Essay

1. Discuss various approaches to counseling clients and families with communicative disorders.

2. Clinicians are increasingly working in medical settings where they need to be aware of infectious disease control procedures, especially when they work with patients who are HIV-positive or have AIDS. Describe these procedures that clinicians need to be aware of.

3. Outline the embryonic growth of the facial structures. What anatomical structures need to develop normally when a baby is in utero for the hard and soft palate and lip to be normal?

4. Describe surgical management of children with clefts of the palate, lip, or both. What procedures are often used with these children?

5. Describe Moebius syndrome and Williams syndrome. What are the characteristics of these syndromes?

Multiple Choice

6. An SLP is conferencing with the family of a 16-year-old girl with severe language-learning disabilities. The girl reads at a third-grade level and has been in special education placements since first grade. At an IEP meeting, the girl's parents say that they want her to attend college and eventually medical school, adding, "We are a family of doctors." The SLP tells the family, in a kind way, that their goal of their daughter attending medical school is unattainable. The family lashes out in anger against the SLP, saying that he is wrong, pessimistic, and negative about their daughter and her abilities. In this situation, the family is utilizing the defense mechanism of:

   A. repression.
   B. reaction formation.
   C. displacement.
   D. suppression.
   E. projection.

Questions 7–9 *refer to the following scenario:*

7. A clinician in a private practice is approached by the parents of Tommy D., a 5-year-old boy. They want to place Tommy in kindergarten in the fall, but share that "we know there's something wrong with him—we're just not sure what." According to Tommy's parents, he is a "sweet, lovable boy who will go to anybody. He likes to sing a lot, too." Because the parents live in a rural area, health-care access has been limited. After seeing Tommy for the first time, the clinician refers his parents to a neurologist because she suspects that Tommy has a syndrome. Tommy is small for his age and has an elfin-like appearance characterized

by a small chin, turned-up nose, puffiness around the eyes, a long upper lip, and a wide mouth. Tommy's teeth are small and widely spaced. The clinician suspects that Tommy has:

A. Williams syndrome.
B. Apert syndrome.
C. Moebius syndrome.
D. Turner syndrome.
E. Hurler syndrome.

8. This syndrome is caused by a rare genetic disorder that impacts an estimated one out of every 20,000 babies. It is caused by:

A. a missing part of chromosome 22, known as 22q11.
B. an expanded number of Cytosine-Guanine-Guanine (CGG) nucelic acid repeats on a specific gene on one of the distal ends of the X chromosome.
C. a spontaneous autosomal dominant mutation, whose gene and locus is FGR2 at 10q25–26.
D. autosomal dominant inheritance and deletion in the region of the long arm of chromosome 15 (15q11–15q13).
E. An abnormality on chromosome 7, including a gene that makes the protein elastin.

9. The clinician knows that she will probably end up seeing Tommy for intervention if his parents are able to bring him on a weekly basis. The clinician will probably be working on which of the following goals?

A. pragmatics, to increase Tommy's ability to interact with others
B. oral motor coordination, because children with this syndrome usually have oral-motor coordination problems which contribute to decrease intelligibility
C. overall expressive and receptive language, because children with this syndrome generally have IQs between 50–70 (although some of these children have good language skills)
D. morphological skills, because although children with this syndrome usually have above-average IQs, they frequently delete bound morphemes from the beginnings and ends of words
E. feeding, because children with this syndrome tend to have feeding problems

10. A condition in which the surface tissues of the soft or hard palate fuse but the underlying muscle or bone tissues do not is called:

A. fusion disorder.
B. submucous or occult cleft palate.
C. class III palatal cleft.
D. submucosal cleft class IV.
E. occult palate class I.

11. A clinician who is using a client-centered approach to counseling a client with a communicative disorder will:

A. be very directive, making specific recommendations for behavioral changes.
B. help the client understand repressed conflicts between the id, ego, and superego.
C. help the client to overcome faulty thinking that is causing distress.
D. respond with acceptance and empathic listening to both the content and the feeling of what the client is saying.
E. give specific advice and look for measurable behavioral changes that occur as a result of the client implementing that advice.

12. Speech–language pathologists working in medical settings frequently see patients who have been assessed with medical imaging techniques. A technique that uses emission-computed tomography that allows imaging of metabolic activity through measurements of radioactivity in the section of the body being viewed is called:

A. fluoroscopy.
B. MRI.
C. PET scan.
D. EEG.
E. CT scan.

13. The surgical method of cleft palate repair that involves raising two bipedicled flaps of mucoperiosteum, bringing them together, and attaching them to close the cleft is called the:

A. von Langenbeck surgical method.
B. V-Y retroposition.
C. Veau-Wardill-Kilner method.
D. pharyngeal flap procedure.
E. pharyngoplasty.

14. A child comes to a clinic with her mother for articulation therapy. The mother tells the clinician that her daughter has Hurler's syndrome. Hurler's syndrome is caused by:

A. autosomal recessive deficiency of X-L iduronidase.
B. a spontaneous autosomal dominant mutation of FGR2 at 10q25–26.
C. autosomal dominant inheritance and deletion in the region of the long arm of chromosome 15 (15q11–15q13).
D. an expanded number of Cytosine-Guanine-Guanine (CGG) nucelic acid repeats on a specific gene on one of the distal ends of the Y chromosome.
E. an extra whole number chromosome 21, resulting in 47, rather than the normal 46 chromosomes.

15. A school-based clinician is assessing the velopharyngeal adequacy of Janie K., a 17-year-old immigrant high school student from the Philippines. Janie was born with a cleft of the palate and lip; there was no repair until Janie's family came to the United States when Janie was 16 years old. In the Philippines, Janie and her family lived on Tablas, a small and rural island, where surgery was unavailable. Though the repair surgery in the United States a year ago was successful and Janie now has a more aesthetically pleasing appearance and better speech, there is still audible nasal emission and hypernasality when she speaks. The clinician plans to refer Janie to a local craniofacial team, but he still wants to conduct as thorough an examination as he can despite the lack of instrumentation available at his school site. The clinician does have access to an oral manometer. He uses this to provide a beginning point from which to refer Janie to the craniofacial team. After obtaining a ratio by comparing pressures achieved in the nostrils-occluded and the nostrils-open conditions, the clincian concludes that Janie especially needs to be referred to the craniofacial team for possible further surgery or a pharyngeal flap. When he did oral manometry, the clinician probably found that Janie:

A. had a ratio of 1.0.
B. had a ratio of 1.2.
C. had a ratio of .96.
D. had a ratio of .92.
E. had a ratio of .87.

16. In infants and children with cleft palates, eustachian tube dysfunction is probably mostly related to the lack of contraction of the:

A. levator veli palatini muscle.
B. veli palatini muscle.
C. tensor veli palatini muscle.
D. palatopharyngeus muscle.
E. superior constrictor.

17. A new clinician gets a job in a large hospital that serves many patients with HIV/AIDS. She will need to keep many factors in mind to provide sensitive and appropriate services to these patients. Which one of the following factors is FALSE in terms of what the clinician needs to remember?

   A. She needs to use universal precautions, which include wearing gowns if clothes are likely to become soiled; washing her hands before and after contact with patients, using antibacterial soap, hot water, and paper towels; and wearing gloves if there is to be contact with bodily fluids, broken skin, or mucous membranes.

   B. HIV and AIDS only rarely attack the nervous system, so most manifestations will be below the head and neck.

   C. Many adults with AIDS experience auditory dysfunction, which can stem from opportunistic infections as well as drug treatments that are potentially ototoxic.

   D. Patients may have articulation, swallowing, respiration, and voice problems due to candidiasis that can occur in the esophagus, mouth, lungs, trachea, and bronchial tubes.

   E. Children with AIDS may manifest language delays, elective mutism, and hysterical aphonia.

18. A child from Apple City transfers to Middleton City, and his file indicates that he has been receiving speech–language services in Apple City. To the chagrin of the Middleton City clinician, some pages of the report from the SLP in Apple City are missing. However, on the first page, it is indicated that this child has Moebius syndrome. He also has a history of frequent hospitalizations. The Middleton City clinician can probably expect to find that this child:

   A. has low muscle tone, a history of early feeding difficulties, initial failure to thrive, obesity after the first year, and underdeveloped genitals.

   B. has underdeveloped facial bones, including mandibular hypoplasia, malar hypoplasia, dental malocclusion, and downwardly slanted palpebral fissures.

   C. has a small maxillary structure, sphenoethmoidal synchondroses, ocular hypertelorism, facial asymmetry including a tall forehead, and brachycephaly.

   D. may have syndactyly, cranial synostosis resulting in smaller anterior-posterior skull diameter, high forehead, an arched and grooved hard palate, class III malocclusion, and possible cleft of the hard palate.

   E. may have delayed language and an articulation disorder as well as bilabial paresis and weak tongue control for lateralization, elevation, depression, and protrusion, a mask-like face, a history of feeding problems in infancy, and unilateral or bilateral paralysis of the abductors of the eye.

19. A clinician is a member of a cleft palate team that asks her to conduct an objective assessment of an 8-year-old child's velopharyngeal mechanism. The clinician decides to do nasopharyngoscopy, where the nasopharyngoscope is passed through the middle meatus and back to the area of velopharyngeal closure. This will enable the clinician to observe the child's:

   A. adenoid pads and anterior pharyngeal walls as the child prolongs /s/.

   B. posterior and lateral pharyngeal walls as well as the adenoid pad as the child sustains /ɑ/.

   C. nasal aspect of the velum and the adenoid pad as the child produces CVC words.

   D. posterior and lateral pharyngeal walls, as well as the nasal aspect of the velum and the adenoid pad as the child produces sentences .

   E. posterior and lateral pharyngeal walls, as well as the nasal aspect of the velum and the adenoid pad as the child produces nasals /n/ and /m/.

20. An 82-year-old man, John R., has had a stroke and now has aphasia. The doctor consults with the SLP because John cannot tolerate the MRI machine. However, the doctor wishes to diagnose the neuropathology associated with John's stroke. The SLP and doctor decide upon a radiographic imaging procedure

where x-ray beams will circle through segments of John's brain and pass through tissue. A camera will take pictures of sections of the structure being scanned. The scanner will detect density differences, and a computer will analyze the images generated by the scanning machine and produce pictures of the scanned structures. The procedure that will be used to diagnose the neuropathology associated with John's stroke is:

A. computerized axial tomography.
B. positron emission tomography.
C. single-photon emission computed tomography.
D. electroencephalography.
E. axial emission electrotomography.

REFERENCES AND RECOMMENDED READINGS

American Speech-Language-Hearing Association (2001). *Scope of practice in speech–language pathology.* Rockville, MD: Author.

American Speech-Language-Hearing Association (2004). *Communication disorders and HIV: A guide for audiologists and speech–language pathologists.* Rockville, MD: Author.

Benninger, M. S., & Gardner, G. M. (1998). Medical and surgical management in otolaryngology. In A. F. Johnson & B. H. Jacobson (Eds.), *Medical speech–language pathology: A practitioner's guide* (pp. 497–528). New York: Thieme Medical Publishers.

Berman, P. S. (2005). *Interviewing and diagnostic exercises for clinical and counseling skills building.* Mahwah, NJ: Lawrence Erlbaum Associates.

Buckholz, P., & Roseberry-McKibbin, C. (1997). *A case study of a child with Russell-Silver syndrome.* Paper presented at the annual meeting of the American Speech-Language-Hearing Association, Boston, MA.

Bzoch, K. (Ed.). (2004). *Communicative disorders related to cleft lip and palate* (5th ed.). Austin, TX: PRO-ED.

Case, L. (2002). *Clinical management of voice disorders* (4th ed.). Austin, TX: PRO-ED.

Clark, J. G. (2004). *Counseling in audiologic practice: Helping patients and families adjust to hearing loss.* Boston: Allyn & Bacon.

Cleft Lip and Palate Association of Ireland (2005). *Velocardiofacial syndrome.* Retrieved January 3, 2005, from http://www.cleft.ie/related/vcfs.htm

Dworkin, J. P., Marunick, M. T., & Krouse, J. H. (2004). Velopharyngeal dysfunction: Speech characteristics, variable etiologies, evaluation techniques, and differential treatments. *Language, Speech, and Hearing Services in Schools, 35,* 333–352.

Enerson, O. D. (2001). *Hurler's syndrome.* Retrieved December 27, 2004, from http://www.whonamedit.com/synd.cfm/1111.html

English, K. M. (2002). *Counseling children with hearing impairment and their families.* Boston: Allyn & Bacon.

Flasher, L. V., & Fogle, P. T. (2004). *Counseling skills for speech–language pathologists and audiologists.* Clifton Park, NY: Thomson/Delmar Learning.

George, K. P., Vikingstad, E. M., & Cao, Y. (1998). Brain imaging in neurocommunicative disorders. In A. F. Johnson & B. H. Jacobson (Eds.), *Medical speech–language pathology: A practitioner's guide* (pp. 285–336). New York: Thieme Medical Publishers.

Golper, L.A.C. (1998). *SourceBook for medical speech pathology* (2nd ed.). Clifton Park, NY: Delmar Learning.

Golding-Kushner, K. J. (2001). *Therapy techniques for cleft palate speech and related disorders.* San Diego, CA: Singular/Thomson Learning.

Haynes, W. O., & Pindzola, R. H. (2004). *Diagnosis and evaluation in speech pathology* (6th ed.). Boston: Allyn & Bacon.

Hegde, M. N. (2001a). *Pocketguide to assessment in speech–language pathology* (2nd ed.). San Diego, CA: Singular/Thomson Learning.

Hegde, M. N. (2001b). *Pocketguide to treatment in speech–language pathology* (2nd ed.) San Diego, CA: Singular/Thomson Learning.

Johnson, A. F., & Jacobson, B. H. (Eds.). (1998). *Medical speech–language pathology: A practitioner's guide.* New York: Thieme Medical Publishers.

Jung, J. H. (1989). Genetic syndromes in communication disorders. Austin, TX: PRO-ED.

Kahn, C. E. (2004). *Hurler's syndrome.* Retrieved December 27, 2004, from http://chorus.rad.mcw.edu/doc/00165.html

Kemker, B. E., & Antonelli, P. J. (2004). Audiologic management of patients with cleft palate and related disorders. In K. R. Bzoch (Ed.), *Communicative disorders related to cleft palate* (pp. 353–376). Austin, TX: PRO-ED.

Kummer, A. W., & Marsh, J. H. (1998). Pediatric voice and resonance disorders. In A. F. Johnson and B. H. Johnson (Eds.), *Medical speech–language pathology: A practitioner's guide* (pp. 613–633). New York: Thieme Medical Publishers.

Lewis, B. A., Freebairn, L., Heeger, S., & Cassidy, S. B. (2002). Speech and language skills of individuals with Prader-Willi Syndrome. *American Journal of Speech–Language Pathology, 11,* 285–294.

Luterman, D. M. (2001). *Counseling the communicatively disordered and their families* (4th ed.). Austin, TX: PRO-ED.

McWilliams, B. J., Morris, H. L., & Shelton, R. l. (1990). *Cleft palate speech* (2nd ed.). Philadelphia: B. C. Decker.

Mervis, C. B. (2003). *Williams Syndrome: A special double issue of Developmental Neuropsychology.* Mahwah, NJ: Lawrence Erlbaum Associates, Inc.

Miller, R. M., & Groher, M. E. (1990). *Medical speech pathology.* Rockville, MD: Aspen Publishers.

M.I.N.D. Institute (2004). *Neurodevelopmental disorders.* Davis, CA: Author.

Mosheim, J. (2004). Personal adjustment counseling. *ADVANCE for Speech–Language Pathologists and Audiologists, 14*(37), 13–14.

Nicolosi, L., Harryman, E., & Kresheck, J. (2004). *Terminology of communication disorders: Speech-language-hearing* (5th ed.). Baltimore: Williams & Wilkins.

Okun, B. F. (2002). *Effective helping: Interviewing and counseling techniques* (6th ed.). Pacific Grove, CA: Brooks/Cole.

Pannbacker, M. (2004). *Velopharyngeal incompetence: The need for speech standards. American Journal of Speech–Language Pathology, 13,* 195–201.

Roberts, J. E., Mirrett, P., Anderson, K., Burchinal, M., & Neebe, E. (2002). Early communication, symbolic behavior, and social profiles of young males with Fragile X syndrome. *American Journal of Speech–Language Pathology, 11,* 295–304.

Rollin, W. J. (2000). Counseling individuals with communication disorders: *Pyschodynamic and family aspects* (2nd ed.). Woburn, MA: Butterworth-Heinemann.

Sapienza, C. M., & Casper, J. (Eds.) (2004). *Vocal rehabilitation for medical speech–language pathology.* Austin, TX: PRO-ED.

Scott, A., & Johnson, H. (2004). *A practical approach to the management of saliva* (2nd ed.). Austin, TX: PRO-ED.

Semel, E., & Rosner, S. R. (2003). *Understanding Williams Syndrome: Behavioral patterns and interventions.* Mahwah, NJ: Lawrence Erlbaum Associates.

Shames, G. H. (2000). *Counseling the communicatively disabled and their families: A manual for clinicians.* Boston: Allyn & Bacon.

Shipley, K. G., & Roseberry-McKibbin, C. (2006). *Interviewing and counseling in communicative disorders: Principles and procedures* (3rd ed.). Austin, TX: PRO-ED.

Shprintzen, R. J. (1997). *Genetics, syndromes, and communication disorders.* San Diego, CA: Singular Publishing Group.

Shprintzen, R. J., & Bardach, J. (1995). *Cleft palate speech management: A multidisciplinary approach.* St. Louis, MO: Mosby.

Stewart, C. J., & Cash, W. B. (2003). *Interviewing: Principles and procedures* (10th ed.). New York: McGraw-Hill

Sue, D. W., & Sue, D. (2003) *Counseling the culturally diverse: Theory and practice* (4th ed.). New York: John Wiley & Sons.

Vogel, D., Carter, J., & Carter, P. (2000). *The effects of drugs on communication disorders* (2nd ed.) San Diego: Singular Publishing Group.

Volden, J. (2004). Nonverbal learning disability: A tutorial for speech–language pathologists. *American Journal of Speech–Language Pathology, 13,* 128–141.

Wallace, G. J. (1998). Adult neurogenic disorders. In D. E. Battle (Ed.), *Communicative disorders in multicultural populations* (2nd ed., pp. 309–304). Stoneham, MA: Andover Medical Publishers.

Woodnorth, G. H. (2004). Assessing and managing medically fragile children: Tracheostomy and ventilatory support. *Language, Speech, and Hearing Services in Schools, 35,* 363–372.

Zemlin, W. (1998). *Speech and hearing science: Anatomy and physiology* (4th Ed.). Boston: Allyn & Bacon.

Study & Review
Answers

6. C. In displacement, the client or family transfers their feelings of anger about a situation onto a safe object or person (frequently the clinician).

7. A. Because Tommy is small for his age and has an elfin-like appearance characterized by a small chin, turned-up nose, puffiness around the eyes, a long upper lip, and a wide mouth with small and widely spaced teeth, he probably has Williams syndrome.

8. E. Williams syndrome is caused by an abnormality on chromosome 7, including a gene that makes the protein elastin.

9. C. The clinician will probably work on increasing overall expressive and receptive language, because children with Williams syndrome generally have IQs between 50–70 (although some of these children have good language skills).

10. B. A condition in which the surface tissues of the soft or hard palate fuse but the underlying muscle or bone tissues do not is called submucous or occult cleft palate.

11. D. In the client-centered approach, the clinician does not give advice or specific recommendations for behavioral changes. Rather, he or she responds with acceptance and empathic listening to both the content and the feeling of what the client is saying, trusting that this will eventually lead to behavioral changes.

12. C. A type of emission-computed tomography that allows imaging of metabolic activity through measurements of radioactivity in the section of the body being viewed is called a PET scan.

13. A. The surgical method of cleft palate repair that involves raising two bipedicled flaps of mucoperiosteum, bringing them together, and attaching them to close the cleft is called the von Langenbeck surgical method.

14. A. Hurler's syndrome is caused by autosomal recessive deficiency of X-L iduronidase.

15. E. When the clinician did oral manometric testing, he probably found that Janie had a ratio of .87. Anything below .89 is especially indicative of problems.

16. C. In infants and children with cleft palates, eustachian tube dysfunction is mostly related to the lack of contraction of the tensor veli palatini muscle.

17. B. It is not true that HIV and AIDS only rarely attack the nervous system, so most manifestations will be below the head and neck. Rather HIV and AIDS almost always attack the nervous system, so almost 100% of the manifestations are at the level of the head and neck.

18. E. A child with Moebius syndrome can be expected to have possible delayed language and an articulation disorder as well as bilabial paresis and weak tongue control for lateralization, elevation, depression, and protrusion, a mask-like face, a history of feeding problems in infancy, and unilateral or bilateral paralysis of the abductors of the eye.

19. D. Nasopharyngoscopy enables the clinician to observe the posterior and lateral pharyngeal walls, as well as the nasal aspect of the velum and the adenoid pad as the child produces sentences.

20. A. The procedure that will be used to diagnose the neuropathology associated with John's stroke is computerized axial tomography (CAT).

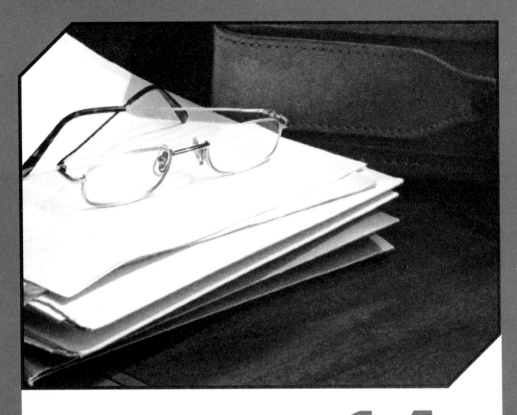

CHAPTER 14

PROFESSIONAL

ISSUES

At the beginning of the 20th century, there

were no professionally trained speech–language pathologists or audiologists in the United States. There were no educational or professional training programs in the country. In Europe, the treatment of speech disorders was a domain of medicine. In the United States, it was the public schools that took a leading role in providing special teaching programs for children with communicative disabilities. By 1910 Chicago public schools began to hire specialists who worked with children with disorders of speech. These specialists, called speech correction teachers, worked mostly with children who stuttered or had disorders of articulation. Other disorders of communication began to be treated only later. In the early 1920s, the University of Wisconsin and the University of Iowa began to offer doctoral programs with an emphasis on speech disorders. Soon other universities across the country, such as Northwestern University, instituted degree programs in speech disorders.

Today, in the twenty-first century, the profession of communicative sciences and disorders continues to undergo rapid changes and expansion. Such expansion is due in large part to a phenomenal growth in the amount of research information on communication and its disorders. In this chapter, we discuss the following professional issues: the American Speech-Language-Hearing Association (ASHA) and its professions of speech–language pathology and audiology, issues in certification and licensure, and legislative issues in regulation of the professions.

ASHA AND THE PROFESSIONS

INTRODUCTION

The American Speech-Language-Hearing Association (ASHA) is the national organization that fulfills many functions in research, legislation that affects the profession, regulation of the profession, academic training, and public information. Most speech–language pathologists and audiologists are members of ASHA. Speech–language pathologists and audiologists are professionals who deal with typical development and disorders of communication, including language, speech, and hearing. ASHA and the professions of speech–language pathology and audiology are continually expanding to serve greater numbers of clients who need services related to communicative disorders.

In this section, we discuss various ways in which ASHA helps ensure that the students who become speech–language pathologists or audiologists are well trained, that the professionals practice their specialty ethically, that the various government agencies support the services offered to people with communication disorders, and that the profession generates knowledge that advances its scientific base.

The American Speech-Language-Hearing Association

- The American Speech-Language-Hearing Association has undergone several name changes. In 1925, when it was established by a handful of people at the University of Iowa, it was called the American Academy of Speech Correction. In 1927 it was renamed the American Society for the Study of Speech Disorders. In 1934 the name was changed to the American Speech Correction Association.

- In 1947, the organization was renamed the American Speech and Hearing Association (ASHA). The addition of "hearing" to the name was significant, recognizing the intertwined nature of speech–language pathology and audiology.

- In 1978 the name was changed to the American Speech-Language-Hearing Association to reflect the field's deeper involvement in language and its disorders. This name stands today, although the acronym is still ASHA.

- Most members of ASHA are speech–language pathologists and audiologists living in the United States; however, ASHA is also open to international membership. ASHA represents the interests of 350 international affiliates in 38 countries. Therefore, ASHA is the leading international organization of speech–language pathologists and audiologists.

- ASHA has grown dramatically in recent decades. In 1935, the organization had fewer than 100 members; at the time of this publication, its membership exceeds 110,000 speech–language pathologists, audiologists, and speech–language and hearing scientists (American Speech-Language-Hearing Association, 2006). About 12,638 individuals who belong to ASHA are audiologists; their number has been decreasing annually. In addition, there are approximately 40,000–50,000 speech–language pathologists, many of whom work in public schools, who are not members of ASHA. Between 2003 and 2004, the membership increased by 1.7%. For the latest figures on membership, check asha.org.

- Only 4.5% of current ASHA members are males, compared to 8.3% in 1997 (American Speech-Language-Hearing Association, 2004a). Approximately 7.1% of ASHA members, international affiliates, and nonmember certificate holders are members of an ethnic or racial minority group. This percentage is far below the distribution of minorities in the general population.

■ Both the professional organization and the range of professional services offered to the public are growing. At the time of this writing, 72% of audiologists are employed in health care facilities such as medical clinics, 23% in hospitals, and the rest in residential health care facilities (American Speech-Language-Hearing Association, 2004a).

■ Currently, over 54% of speech–language pathologists work in educational settings, including special schools, preschools, grade schools, and colleges or universities. Thirty-nine percent work in health-care facilities.

■ ASHA is a national scientific and professional organization whose headquarters are located in the Washington, DC, metropolitan area (in Rockville Pike, Maryland). As a scientific and professional organization, ASHA plays a major role in promoting awareness of communicative disorders in the public and the government.

■ ASHA (2004b, p. 1) lists the following as its purposes:

- "encourage basic scientific study of the processes of individual human communication, with special reference to speech, language, and hearing;
- promote appropriate academic and clinical preparation of individuals entering the discipline of human communication sciences and disorders and to promote the maintenance of current knowledge and skills of those within the discipline;
- promote investigation and prevention of disorders of human communication;
- foster improvement of clinical services and procedures addressing such disorders;
- stimulate exchange of information among persons and organizations thus engaged and to disseminate such information;
- advocate for the rights and interests of persons with communication disorders; and
- promote the individual and collective professional interests of the members of the Association."

■ ASHA (2004b, p. 1) lists the following as its major activities:

- "sponsoring national conferences, institutes, and workshops each year as part of its continuing professional education program
- maintaining programs related to research, education, and delivery of clinical services
- conducting an Annual Convention at which scientific sessions, exhibits, short courses, and other educational and professional programs and a placement center are offered
- maintaining a national career information program, a governmental affairs program, and a public information program
- carrying out a continuing program of data collection related to professional training, human resource needs, and membership characteristics and activities
- sponsoring a voluntary continuing education program that approves providers of continuing education activities and offers an Award for Continuing Education to certified individuals and members
- publishing several professional journals and other professional materials
- providing technical support to practitioner members on issues affecting the delivery of services
- maintaining a computerized database that provides information about federal and private funding sources in the United States and Canada (includes abstract; amount; funding

source; and contact person's address, telephone number, and email address)
- protecting the public interest by maintaining high standards for members, certificate holders, accredited clinics, and accredited graduate educational programs."

■ ASHA has several membership categories:

- *Membership with certification* is open to those who have a master's degree from an ASHA-accredited university program with a major emphasis in speech–language pathology or audiology and have completed all requirements for the Certificate of Clinical Competence. To continue in this category, a member must meet the mandatory continuing education requirements.
- *Membership without certification* is open to U.S. residents who have a master's degree in speech–language pathology, audiology, or speech, language, and hearing sciences but are not involved in providing clinical services or clinical supervision.
- *Membership without certification (research or allied professional)* is open to individuals who hold a graduate degree and are involved in human communication research. These individuals do not provide clinical services.
- *International affiliates* is open to those who hold a graduate degree and reside abroad. These members are not eligible for clinical certification.
- *Certificate holders* are those who maintain their clinical certification but do not become members of the association. They do not enjoy the memberhip benefits.
- *Life membership* is open to those who are 65 years or older and have been members of the association for 25 consecutive years.

■ Students who have declared their major as speech–language pathology or audiology may become members of the National Student Speech-Language-Hearing Association (NSSLHA), which is recognized by ASHA.

■ Benefits of membership in NSSLHA include reduced fees for conventions and scientific journals. Many colleges and universities have active local chapters of NSSLHA that sponsor professional and social events.

■ Within the last several years, ASHA has created a number of *special interest divisions* (SIDs) for members who wish to interact with other members who have similar interests. Each division sponsors special presentations at ASHA and many hold their own national conferences. Any ASHA member may join one or more SID for an additional annual fee. As of 2004, there are sixteen special interest divisions:

- Division 1. Language Learning and Education
- Division 2. Neurophysiology and Neurogenic Speech and Language Disorders
- Division 3. Voice and Voice Disorders
- Division 4. Fluency and Fluency Disorders
- Division 5. Speech Science and Orofacial Disorders
- Division 6. Hearing and Hearing Disorders: Research and Diagnosis
- Division 7. Aural Rehabilitation and Its Instrumentation
- Division 8. Hearing Conservation and Occupational Audiology
- Division 9. Hearing and Hearing Disorders in Adults
- Division 10. Issues in Higher Education
- Division 11. Administration and Supervision
- Division 12. Augmentative and Alternative Communication
- Division 13. Swallowing and Swallowing Disorders (Dysphagia)

- Division 14. Communication Disorders and Sciences in Culturally and Linguistically Diverse Populations
- Division 15. Gerentology
- Division 16. School-Based Issues

■ Some (not all) SIDs offer a Clinical Specialty Recognition (e.g., Child Language, Fluency, Neurogenic Communiation Disorders, and Dysphagia) that confers the status of a specialist. This recognition, however, is not necessary to assess and treat clients with a given disorder. Each recognition requires ASHA members to fulfill additional requirements. See asha.org for details.

The Professions of Speech–Language Pathology and Audiology

■ Speech–language pathology is the scientific profession concerned with normal development and disorders of human communication (speech and language) and the assessment and treatment of those disorders.

■ The term speech–language pathologist is preferred among members of the profession. However, some people use the terms speech therapist and speech–language clinician.

■ Audiologists are specialists who are concerned with hearing, its disorders, and the assessment and rehabilitation of persons with hearing loss. Educational audiologists may be found in such educational settings as public schools, and industrial audiologists are those who work in the industrial sector.

■ Speech–language pathologists and audiologists work in a variety of professional settings such as hospitals, schools, private practices, rehabilitation clinics, skilled nursing facilities, and others.

■ Speech–language and hearing scientists generally work in research laboratories and university departments. Their primary task is to generate new knowledge through research.

The Scope of Practice: Speech–Language Pathology

ASHA is the main regulatory body that develops policies on the scope of practice of the profession (American Speech-Language-Hearing Association, 2001). The scope of practice document specifies what the clinicians can and cannot do; it is a guideline for ethical practice of the profession. When scientific evidence and expertise of the profession warrants it, the scope of practice may be expanded, as in the case of swallowing disorders and literacy skills. Students and clinicians should be fully aware of this document as it restricts practice to certain domains while opening possibilities for new services. A few highlights of the document include:

■ It is presumed that one can practice the profession only with required qualifications, certification, licensure, and credential when necessary.

■ The domain of practice includes human communication behaviors and disorders, as well as swallowing disorders and upper aerodigestive disorders.

■ Speech–langauge pathology practice involves offering prevention, screening, consultation, assessment and diagnosis, treatment, management, counseling, and follow-up services for disorders of:

- speech, including articulation, fluency, resonance, and voice
- language, including, phonological, morphologial, syntactic, and pragmatic aspects of language; comprehension and production of language; and literacy skills
- swallowing and upper aerodigestive disorders (e.g., infant feeding)
- cognitive aspects of communication, including memory and attention
- sensory awareness related to communication or swallowing
- developing and implementing augmentative and alternative forms of communication (AAC) and prescribing AAC devices and systems
- screening hearing and offering auditory training and speech–language services to the deaf and the hard of hearing
- using such instruments as videofluoroscopy, EMG, nasendoscopy, stroboscopy, and computerized instruments to observe, collect, and analyze data relative to communication and swallowing functions
- selecting, fitting, and training in the use of prosthetic devices for communication and swallowing; this excludes the prescription of hearing aids
- collaborating in the assessment and treatment of central auditory disorders associated with communication disorders
- educating and counseling individuals, families, co-workers, educators, and other professionals about communication disorders and swallowing
- promoting community awareness about communication disorders and their assessment and treatment and about removing barriers to individuals with such disorders
- working with other professionals and making referrals when they are in the best interests of individuals being served
- serving ethnoculturally diverse populations with communication and swallowing disorders with procedures that are suited or modified for their cultural background (American Speech-Language-Hearing Association, 2001).

■ The settings in which speech–language pathology may be practiced consist of a variety of educational and health-care facilites, including public and private schools, hospitals, rehabilitation facilities, long-term care facilities, home-health agencies, and behavioral and mental health facilities, private practices, university clinics, correctional institutions, military establishments, research facilities, and corporate and industrial settings.

ASHA Accreditation

■ ASHA has established standards of scientific and professional education in speech–language pathology and audiology. The standards include the kinds and variety of academic courses that must be offered and the amount and quality of supervised clinical practice student clinicians must complete.

■ Through its *Council on Academic Accreditation in Audiology and Speech–Language Pathology* (CAA), ASHA accredits master's degree programs in speech–language pathology and audiology that meet its minimum standards. A national team visits graduate degree programs in audiology or speech–langauge pathology and evaluates their quality.

■ Through its *Council for Clinical Certification,* ASHA evaluates and approves clinical certification standards (described in a later section).

CONCEPTS TO CONSIDER

Summarize the ASHA membership categories and requirements.

_____

_____

_____

_____

_____

SUMMARY

✓ ASHA, the national professional and scientific organization of communicative disorders professionals, has an interesting history, which includes phenomenal growth and change.

✓ With over 110,000 members, ASHA continually works to promote high ethical standards, pertinent legislation, and regulation of the professions of speech–language pathology and audiology. ASHA accredits graduate academic programs that meet its academic and scientific standards and certifies individuals who meet its clinical standards.

✓ ASHA offers various kinds memberships with and without clinical certification.

✓ Students may join the ASHA-affiliated NSSLHA, the national student organization, which provides many benefits. Members of ASHA include speech–language pathologists and audiologists who work in a variety of professional settings to provide comprehensive services to individuals with disorders of language, speech, and hearing.

ISSUES IN CERTIFICATION AND LICENSURE

INTRODUCTION

ASHA-administered certification helps ensure the quality of services provided to individuals with communication disorders. Individual states also have licensing and certification requirements for their clinicians. The necessity of holding a state license, state certificate, ASHA certificate, or all three, depends upon (a) the individual state, and (b) the professional setting in which the clinician works. In this section we discuss ASHA certification, state regulation of the professions, and issues regarding support personnel.

Clinical Certification

- To ensure the quality of speech–language and hearing services offered to the public, ASHA has developed two clinical certificates that are issued to members who meet the academic and clinical standards of the association.

- ASHA certifies speech–language pathologists and audiologists separately, although the requirements are parallel. The *Certificate of Clinical Competence in Speech–Language Pathology* (CCC-SLP) is issued to those individuals who have:

  - earned their master's degree or its equivalent in speech–language pathology at an accredited institution and have fulfilled clinical practicum and fellowship requirements. A minimum 75 semester hours of coursework must be completed in speech–language pathology and related disciplines; a minimum of 36 of the 75 hours must be at the graduate level.
  - demonstrated the acquisition of knowledge and clinical skill adequate for entry into professional practice. Required knowledge pertains to basic scientific understanding of communication and its disorders, research methods and evaluation of research evidence, the code of ethics, and professional issues and credentials. The students should acquire clinical skills as well as oral and written presentation skills. Students enrolled in graduate programs are expected to document when and how they acquired the necessary knowledge and skill. ASHA provides a Knowledge and Skills Acquisition (HASA) form to facilitate this task.
  - completed their clinical practicum with a minimum of 400 hours of supervised clinical work out of which 25 hours are set aside for preclinical observation of clinical work.
  - obtained a passing score on the National Examination in Speech–Language Pathology and Audiology (NESPA; also referred to as PRAXIS). See the Appendix for information on NESPA/PRAXIS.
  - completed a supervised clinical fellowship within 4 years of the date when the academic coursework and clinical practicum were completed. The fellowship may be completed in a full-time job of 30 hours a week for 36 weeks or up to 72 weeks of part-time work (15–19 hours per week).

- The *Certificate of Clinical Competence in Audiology* (CCC-A) has similar requirements, with the academic coursework, clinical practicum, and clinical fellowship completed in audiology.

- For students to be able to count their clinical practicum hours, all supervisors should hold a clinical certification in their speciality (speech–language pathology or audiology).

- The clinical certificates are renewable every 3 years. To maintain clinical certifications, all certificate holders must accumulate 30 contact hours of professional development (continuing education units) over the 3-year period.

- ASHA's certificates are not legal documents comparable to a state license. However, they are recognized by most employers, including hospitals, clinics, public school districts, and universities throughout the country. Many employers consider the certificates favorably in promotion and salary increases. Many state licensure laws are modeled after the ASHA requirements.

- Individuals who hold ASHA membership and clinical certification are committed to uphold the highest standards of clinical services. Treating people with communicative disorders is an ethical and socially responsible activity. Therefore, speech–language pathologists and audiologists who hold a certificate from ASHA are committed to its Code of Ethics. Violation of the code has serious consequences, including revocation of the clinical certificate and cancellation of membership in ASHA.

Speech–Language Pathology Assistants

■ ASHA supports the use of speech–language pathology assistants (SLPAs) who have received training according to its guidelines. ASHA's current position is not to require SLPAs to register with ASHA and not to review their academic and clinical program to give approval. ASHA recommends that the assistants complete an approved training program that includes coursework and fieldwork (American Speech-Language-Hearing Association, 2004c); on-the-job training may be acceptable. SLPAs should be supervised by ASHA-certified clinicians. ASHA specifies what SLPAs may or may not do; for instance, they may:

- implement treatment plans the supervising speech–language pathologist develops
- assist with speech–language and hearing screenings, formal and informal assessments, clerical duties, research projects, inservice training, public relations programs, and such departmental operations as scheduling and record keeping
- document client performance (prepare charts, records, and graphs)
- check and maintain equipment
- collect and document data for quality improvement

■ SLPA's *may not*:

- administer standardized or nonstandardized tests or interpret the results; screen or diagnose patients for feeding or swallowing disorders
- participate in parent or case conferences, nor can they counsel parents or clients unless supervised by a speech–language pathologist
- write or modify treatment plans; offer treatment that is not developed by a speech–language pathologist, and offer any treatment without supervision; sign treatment plans or assessment reports
- select, refer, or discharge clients
- disclose confidential information
- demonstrate swallowing strategies or precautions

State Regulation of the Profession

■ The state governments have laws and regulations that affect the work of speech–language pathologists and audiologists. Most states regulate the practice of speech–language pathology or audiology in the following ways:

- The state departments of education give credentials to their speech–language pathologists and audiologists working in the public schools. Generally, the requirements are similar to those of ASHA except some state regulations require coursework in education.
- A few states also combine a teaching credential with a credential in speech–language pathology, resulting in more coursework in education, because the professional in this case is both a teacher and a speech–language pathologist. State credentials may or may not

transfer to another state's public schools. State public school credentials are specific to the public school setting only. They do not allow private practice, work in a hospital or clinic, or supervision of clinical practice in university speech and hearing centers.

- Most state governments issue licenses to practice speech–language pathology or audiology. Most state licensure requirements are similar to those of ASHA. Professional settings other than public schools (e.g., hospitals and private clinics) usually require either the ASHA Certificate of Clinical Competence, state licensure if it exists, or both. However, in many states, public school districts are also beginning to require, or at least strongly encourage, speech–language pathologists to possess state licensure and ASHA certification.

■ By meeting the ASHA requirements, graduates in most states also meet the requirements for a credential to work in schools and license to practice speech–language pathology or audiology in non-school settings.

■ An important difference between a license and an ASHA certificate is that only the license carries the force of law. The state licensure is administered by a board or committee created by the state legislature.

SUMMARY

✓ ASHA regulates the quality of services offered to the public through its clinical certifications.

✓ States regulate the quality of services offered in different professional settings through their education credential and state licensure.

✓ ASHA has specific dos and don'ts for speech–language pathology assistants who should work under the supervision of a certified clinician.

LEGISLATIVE REGULATION OF THE PROFESSION

INTRODUCTION

Both state and federal laws affect the services offered in various professional settings. In this section, we summarize some of the key national laws that have affected service delivery in the public schools, employment, and health-care settings.

Federal Legislation Affecting School Settings

Public Law 94-142

Enacted in 1975, the Education of the Handicapped Act (later retitled the Individuals with Disabilities Education Act) mandated free and appropriate education for disabled students from ages 3 to 21. Basic tenets of this law included the following:

- Disabled children and youth from ages 3 to 21 years were guaranteed free and appropriate public education in the "least restrictive environment," including special education and related services. (In some states, due to conflicts with state laws and court orders, children under age 5 and over age 18 were excluded.)

- All students receiving special education services were to have individualized education programs (IEPs), determined by parents and professionals, that served as written records of commitments to meet students' goals.
- Students and parents were guaranteed protection of their rights through due legal process, including the right to an impartial due process hearing and the right to examine all relevant records.
- The federal government was to provide funds for local and state agencies to carry out prescribed programs and to monitor and evaluate those programs.

Public Law 99-457

- These amendments to P.L. 94-142, enacted in 1986, were intended to provide early intervention that would reduce the number of children requiring special education services in later years.
- P.L. 99-457 increased federal monetary support for states to provide services for disabled children between the ages of 3 and 6 years. It also created a new program that provided funds for services to infants and toddlers (up to 2 years) with disabilities.
- An important tenet of P.L. 99-457 is that all school service providers must meet their state's highest requirements for their discipline (in many states, that meant a master's degree, which fulfilled the academic criteria for state licensing).
- P.L. 99-457 established mandated development of individualized family service plans (IFSPs), requiring, among other things, information about:

  - the child's present level of development
  - the family's needs and strengths relating to the child's development
  - the major goals for the child and family, and services to be provided
  - a review of the plan at 6-month intervals or more frequently if needed

- A major provision of P.L. 99-457 is multidisciplinary programming for infants and toddlers with disabilities and their families. This includes involvement of agencies outside the education setting (e.g., community programs).
- Under P.L. 99-457, states were no longer required to report preschool children by disability category (e.g., hearing loss, mental retardation, learning disability). At-risk preschool children also became eligible for special education services, including children who had experienced traumatic life events, depression, child abuse, and substance abuse.

Individuals with Disabilities Education Act (IDEA)

- The IDEA (P.L. 101-476), enacted in 1990, reauthorized P.L. 94-142 and altered the language used in referring to its beneficiaries. Specifically, the term "disability" replaced the word "handicap."

- The IDEA also expanded the number of categories of disabilities. Originally, P.L. 94-142 consisted of 11 disability categories; the IDEA created 13 categories, newly including autism and traumatic brain injury.

- The definition of special education was expanded to include instruction in all settings (not just the school), including training centers and workplaces.

■ The Amendments of 1997, Public Law 105-17, constitute the reauthorization of the IDEA. This reauthorization was signed into law by President Clinton on October 22, 1997. This reauthorization included (California Speech-Language-Hearing Association, 1997; Miller & Hoffman, 2002):

- increased, meaningful parental involvement in evaluations, including parental access to reports, test instruments, and other interpretative materials that contain personally identifiable information
- improved educational results for children with disabilities
- increased participation of special educators in the general classroom setting, including involvement with curriculum
- increased participation of children with learning problems in the regular classroom activities
- prevention of inappropriate identification and mislabeling of children who are ethnically, linguistically, and racially diverse
- improved use of alternative assessments for children who cannot participate in standard assessments

■ On December 3, 2004, President Bush signed into law the new IDEA reforms, making it officially known as Public Law No. 108-446. The signing marked the end of a three-year reauthorization process and represented the first update to the country's special education law in seven years. The effective date for most changes in the law was July 1, 2005.

■ Foundational to this new law are the findings of the 2002 President's Commission on Excellence in Special Education, which recommended special education reforms based on paperwork reduction, parental choice, early intervention, and academic results for students.

■ The new IDEA puts a greater emphasis on using prereferral services to prevent unnecessary referrals to special education. Under the new IDEA, states are required to provide coordinated, comprehensive, early-intervention programs for children in groups that are overrepresented in special education.

Federal Legislation Affecting Employment Settings

■ The Americans with Disabilities Act (ADA, Public Law 101-336), enacted in 1990, provides civil rights protection relative to employment, state and local government services, telecommunications, and public accommodations to all individuals with disabilities.

■ The ADA bars employment discrimination against qualified people with mental or physical disabilities, or disabilities that substantially limit one or more of the basic activities of life such as talking or walking.

■ The ADA requires that employers make "reasonable accommodations" for workers with disabilities. This includes making existing facilities such as public buildings and mass transportation accessible and arranging modified or part-time work schedules.

■ Employers must also provide special equipment for workers with disabilities. Examples include the availability of relay stations for users of telecommunication devices for the deaf (TDDs), ramps for people in wheelchairs, and addition of auditory signals to visual signs so that blind people may know when an elevator door is open.

■ According to the ADA, employers do not have to provide accommodations that impose an "undue hardship" on business operations. The meaning of the term "undue hardship" has been the subject of much discussion and some law suits.

CONCEPTS TO CONSIDER

Describe one important point of each law: P.L. 99-457, IDEA, and ADA.

_____

_____

_____

_____

_____

Federal Legislation Affecting Health-Care Settings

Health-care legislation is under constant revision in the United States. One reason is that millions of Americans do not receive adequate health care. Statistics show that groups that are especially affected are children, low-income people, and people from culturally and linguistically diverse backgrounds.

Several key pieces of health-care legislation have been passed in preceding decades, but the entire health-care system is still in flux. This has service provision ramifications for the communicative disorders professions. Two key pieces of federal legislation affecting speech–language pathologists and audiologists in health-care settings are discussed below.

Social Security Act (SSA)

■ Passed in 1935, during the Depression, the SSA expanded the federal government's grant-in-aid assistance to the states. It was the federal government's first major step toward involvement in a widespread program of living and medical assistance to people at large.
■ The SSA provided the foundation for Medicaid and Medicare. It also provided for the general welfare of the public by establishing federal benefits for older people. Further, the SSA helped states provide more services for public health, maternal and child welfare, blind people, and dependent children and children with disabilities.
■ The SSA undergoes periodic ammendments. The amendments of 1983 had a significant effect on speech–language pathology and audiology services. They offered incentive reimbursements for hospitals to provide more "efficient" and "cost-effective" treatment for patients.
■ Unfortunately, although inpatient rehabilitation units and rehabilitation hospitals were exempt from some of the flat-payment regulations imposed on other services, cost limits were

placed on services provided. These limits have resulted in fewer speech–language pathology and audiology services being offered to patients.

Health Insurance Portability and Accountability Act (HIPAA)

- In 1996, Congress called on the U.S. Department of Health and Human Services to issue patient privacy protections as part of the Health Insurance Portability and Accountability Act (HIPAA). Health-care providers were mandated to comply with these protections starting April 14, 2003.
- HIPAA involves a set of rules followed by doctors, health plans, hospitals, and health-care providers. HIPAA is the first-ever set of federal privacy standards to protect patients' medical records and other health information provided to health plans, hospitals, doctors, and other health-care providers (covered entities).
- These new standards represent a uniform set of federal privacy protections for American consumers by limiting the ways that pharmacies, health plans, hospitals, and other covered entities can use and share patients' personal medical information. HIPAA's regulations protect medical records and other individually identifiable health information in any form—information communicated on paper, electronically, or orally. Key provisions of HIPAA's privacy standards are described below (U.S. Department of Health and Human Services, 2004).
- Patients generally should have access to their medical records. If there are mistakes, patients should be able to request corrections. Doctors, hospitals, clinics, nursing homes, health plans, and other covered entities generally must provide access to these records within 30 days, and they may charge patients for the cost of copying and sending the records.
- Health care providers and all covered entities must provide a notice to their patients about how they may use personal medical information as well as patients' rights under the new privacy regulation. This generally should happen on the first visit. Patients are asked to initial, sign, or otherwise acknowledge that they have received this notice.
- HIPAA's privacy rule sets limits on how covered entities may use personally identifiable health information. Covered entities may share information with each other related to patients' treatment. For example, a doctor may talk with a clinician about swallowing treatment for a patient with dysphagia. However, these entities may not share personal health information for purposes unrelated to health care unless the patient specifically signs an authorization. For example, without signed authorization from the patient, a hospital could not release the patient's medical information to a marketing firm, bank, or life insurance agency for purposes not related to the patient's health care.
- Under the privacy rule, patients may request that covered entities take reasonable steps to make sure that their communications with patients are confidential. For example, a patient with mild aphasia who has been discharged from treatment can ask the doctor or speech–language pathologist to call him at home, not at work. The patient's request should be reasonably accommodated.
- Consumers may file a formal complaint regarding the privacy practices of a covered provider such as a doctor, speech–language pathologist, hospital, or clinic. Such complaints may be made directly to the covered provider or to the Department of Health and Human Services' Office for Civil Rights (OCR). The OCR is charged with investigating complaints and enforcing the privacy regulation.
- If covered entities misuse personal health information, civil and criminal penalties may be imposed. For civil violations of the standards, OCR can fine a covered entity up to $25,000 a year. If a covered entity knowingly obtains protected health information in violation of the law, criminal penalties can range between $50,000 and $250,000 accompanied by 1–10 years in prison depending upon the nature and extent of the violation.

- Speech–language pathologists and audiologists must be sure to follow HIPAA regulations in all their dealings with clients and their families.

Future Trends

■ Health-care policy and special education policies that affect speech–language pathology and audiology services are constantly evolving. There is an increased emphasis on showing that services offered to children and adults with communication disorders make a difference in the lives of the individuals who receive them.

■ This means that there will be an increased emphasis on documentation of treatment outcomes and evidence-based practice. ASHA's *National Outcome Measurement System* (NOMS) will play an increasingly important role in selecting and evaluating treatment procedures.

■ Limited financial resources will call for collaborative efforts, resulting in cost savings and improved outcomes for the clients. In the public schools, emphasis on literacy skills of children will make additional demands on speech–language pathologists. Children with varied ethnocultural backgrounds provide both challenges and exciting opportunities to serve them.

■ An aging population in the United States will escalate demands for services that specialize in geriatric communication disorders. Doing all this in a cost-effective manner will be a pervasive theme.

SUMMARY

✓ **State and federal legislation has a major effect on speech–language pathology and audiology services provided in public school, employment, and health-care settings. Such legislation can expand or limit the services provided to clients with communicative disorders.**

✓ **The Health Insurance Portability and Accountability Act (HIPAA) is a new set of federal privacy regulations that protect patients' personal medical information and help ensure confidentiality.**

✓ **Future trends affecting health-care settings include increased accountability for documenting functional gains and providing measurable outcomes of services provided.**

CHAPTER HIGHLIGHTS

◆ **THE AMERICAN-SPEECH-LANGUAGE-HEARING ASSOCIATION (ASHA)** is a national professional and scientific organization that regulates the quality of service offered, promotes relevant legislation, encourages research, and facilitates exchange of information. Most speech–language pathologists and audiologists are members of ASHA.

◆ **ASHA AWARDS NATIONAL CERTIFICATION** when its members meet certain requirements. Many states also have credentialing and licensing requirements that clinicians must meet, depending upon the professional setting.

◆ **ASHA SUPPORTS THE USE** of speech–language pathology assistants (SLPAs) who have received training according to its guidelines. ASHA recommends that these assistants complete an approved training program that includes coursework and fieldwork; on-the-job training may be acceptable.

◆ **STATE AND FEDERAL LAWS** regulate service provision in public schools, employment settings, and health-care settings. All communicative disorders professionals and clients are affected by those laws, which are primarily influenced by the availability of funding. A new law affecting speech–language pathologists and audiologists is HIPAA, the Health Insurance Portability and Accountability Act of 1996, which took effect April 14, 2003.

◆ **BECAUSE OF LEGISLATION AND** resulting budget cuts, speech–language pathology and audiology services are often curtailed in many settings. Clinicians increasingly need to make the public aware of the communicative professions and the services offered. This can be done through marketing research and advertising. ASHA provides educational opportunities to teach its members about those areas.

✐ **ADD YOUR OWN CHAPTER HIGHLIGHTS HERE:**

_____

_____

_____

_____

Study & Review Questions

Essay

1. Describe the nature and purposes of ASHA.

2. Discuss the activities that may be undertaken by speech–language pathology assistants (SLPAs). What is ASHA's position on SLPAs?

3. Describe key pieces of federal legislation that have impacted school settings.

4. Discuss the scope of practice for speech–language pathologists (SLPs). What types of activities may SLPs engage in? What types of activities may SLPs not engage in?

5. What is HIPAA? What are the ramifications of HIPAA for speech–language pathologists and audiologists?

Multiple Choice

6. It would be considered ethical for a speech–language pathologist to:
   A. guarantee the results of a treatment program to a worried patient.
   B. make a reasonable statement of prognosis when the spouse of a woman with aphasia asks about his wife's potential for improvement.
   C. make a diagnosis through the mail when he or she receives a letter from a friend in a distant state who is concerned about her son's articulation.
   D. allow an unsupervised assistant who is in the certification process to provide clinical services.
   E. carry out a physician-recommended program of therapy with a head-injured patient even though the speech–language pathologist disagrees with the physician's recommendation.

7. Public Law 99-457:
   A. increased federal support for services to disabled children 3–6 years of age and provided funding for infants and toddlers.
   B. requires the development of individualized family service plans.
   C. allows at-risk preschool children (not just those with documented disabilities) to be eligible for special education services.
   D. A, B
   E. A, B, C

8. In most states, to work in the public schools, speech–language pathologists and audiologists **need:**

    A. a state license.
    B. ASHA certification.
    C. a state-issued credential from an agency such as the department of education.
    D. A, B
    E. A, B, C

9. Which one of the following is NOT TRUE?

    A. Many state licensure laws are modeled after ASHA's requirements.
    B. Violation of ASHA's Code of Ethics can have major consequences, including revocation of ASHA's clinical certificate and cancelation of ASHA membership.
    C. A Certificate of Clinical Competence and state license are not necessarily required in order to practice in public school settings.
    D. Some states require coursework in education or even a teaching credential for speech–language pathologists and audiologists who work in public school settings.
    E. In order to receive a Certificate of Clinical Competence in speech–language pathology or audiology, a speech–language pathologist or audiologist needs only to have a state-granted credential to work in public schools.

10. P.L. 94-142, the Education of the Handicapped Act, was later reauthorized and retitled as:

    A. the Americans with Disabilities Act.
    B. the Education of Disabled Individuals Act.
    C. the Handicapped Individuals Education Act.
    D. the Individuals with Disabilities Education Act.
    E. none of the above.

11. Activities that may be carried out by a trained SLPA (according to ASHA) include:

    A. implementing treatment plans developed by the supervising SLP, checking and maintaining equipment, and collecting and documenting data for quality improvement.
    B. demonstrating swallowing strategies or precautions, collecting and documenting data for quality improvement, and assisting with speech-language and hearing screenings.
    C. writing and modifying treatment plans, assisting with clerical duties and inservice training, and checking and maintaining equipment.
    D. signing treatment plans or assessment reports when the SLP is not available, assisting with speech–language and hearing screenings, and assisting with clerical duties.
    E. referring clients in need of speech–language services, assisting with clerical duties and in-service training, and checking and maintaining equipment.

12. Parents in a local school district have asked a clinician to give an inservice on the IDEA (1997). The parents are interested in the content of the IDEA, their parental rights, etc. Which one of the following would NOT be accurate for the clinician to tell the parents in the inservice?

    A. The IDEA discourages serving children with disabilities in general education classroom settings; rather, the IDEA encourages school districts to create more specialized pull-out programs for such children to best serve their needs.
    B. The IDEA promotes increased, meaningful parental involvement in evaluations, including access to reports and test instruments.
    C. The IDEA mandates the development of alternative assessments for children who cannot participate in standard assessments.

D. One goal of the IDEA is to promote increased participation of special educators in general classroom settings, including involvement with curriculum.

E. Another goal of the IDEA is to prevent inappropriate identification and mislabeling of children who are ethnically, linguistically, and racially diverse.

13. Speech–language pathologists and audiologists have been impacted by the Health Insurance Portability and Accountability Act (HIPAA). The main set of HIPAA standards that impacts these communicative disorders professionals deals with:

A. protecting patients from being assessed and treated by professionals who are not qualified.

B. protecting patients' privacy by putting limits on use of personal medical information and notifying patients of privacy practices, etc.

C. ensuring that covered entities such as clinics, hospitals, and other care providers inform patients if they are being used as subjects in a treatment efficacy research project.

D. making sure that patients are able to obtain two to three different opinions from qualified professionals about their medical condition.

E. making sure that covered entities make a prognostic statement about patients' potential to improve their communication skills after participating in treatment programs.

14. According to ASHA standards, which one of the following activities would NOT be within the scope of practice of a speech–language pathologist?

A. assessing and treating swallowing and upper aerodigestive disorders (e.g., infant feeding)

B. developing and implementing augmentative and alternative forms of communication (AAC) and prescribing AAC devices and systems

C. prescribing hearing aids for children and adults with hearing losses

D. screening hearing and offering auditory training and speech–language services to the deaf and the hard of hearing

E. using such instruments as videofluoroscopy, EMG, nasendoscopy, stroboscopy, and computerized instruments to observe, collect, and analyze data relative to communication and swallowing functions

15. P.L. 99-457 established mandated development of individualized family service plans (IFSPs), requiring, among other things, information about:

A. the child's present level of development.

B. the family's needs and strengths relating to the child's development.

C. the major goals for the child and family, and services to be provided.

D. a review of the plan at 6-month intervals or more frequently if needed.

E. all of the above.

REFERENCES AND RECOMMENDED READINGS

American Speech-Language-Hearing Association (2001). *Scope of practice in speech–language pathology.* Rockville, MD: Author.

American Speech-Language-Hearing Association (2004a). Highlights and trends: *ASHA counts for 2004.* Retrieved October 2, 2004, from http://www.asha.org.

American Speech-Language-Hearing Association (2004b). *Membership and certification handbook of the American Speech-Language-Hearing Association.* Retrieved October 2, 2004, from http://www.asha.org.

American Speech-Language-Hearing Association (2004c). *Guidelines for the training, use, and supervision of speech–language pathology assistants* [*Guidelines*]. Available at: http://www.asha.org/members/deskref-journals/deskref/default

California Speech-Language-Hearing Association (1997). Substantive and subtle changes for federal IDEA. *CSHA Magazine, 26*(4), 14.

Frattali, C., Curl, B., & Bevan, M. (1994). Health care legislation: Implications for financing and service delivery. In R. Lubinski & C. Frattali (Eds.), *Professional issues in speech–language pathology and audiology: A textbook* (pp. 173–177). San Diego, CA: Singular Publishing Group.

Meyer, S.M. (2004). *Survival guide for the beginning speech–language clinician* (2nd ed.). Austin, TX: PRO-ED.

Montgomery, J. B. (1994). Federal legislation affecting school settings. In R. Lubinski & C. Frattali (Eds.), *Professional issues in speech–language pathology and audiology: A textbook* (pp. 201–217). San Diego, CA: Singular Publishing Group.

Miller, L., & Hoffman, L. (2002). *Linking IEPs to state learning standards: A step-by-step guide.* Austin, TX: PRO-ED.

Nicolosi, L., Harryman, E., & Kresheck, J. (2004). *Terminology of communication disorders: Speech-language-hearing* (5th ed.). Baltimore: Williams & Wilkins.

United States Department of Health and Human Services (2004). *Fact sheet: Protecting the privacy of patients' health information.* Retrieved December 26, 2004, from http://www.hhs.gov/new/facts/privacy/html.

Study & Review
Answers

6. B. Principle of Ethics 1, Rule F, states that individuals may make a reasonable statement of prognosis. All other choices are forbidden by the rules in Principles of Ethics I, II, and IV.

7. E. P.L. 99-457 does all of the above, including mandating services for at-risk children.

8. C. In most states, public school systems require only a state-issued credential. Licensure and certification are required by many other settings such as hospitals and clinics.

9. E. In order to receive a Certificate of Clinical Competence in speech–language pathology or audiology, clinicians need a master's degree or its equivalent in speech–language pathology and must have fulfilled clinical practicum and fellowship requirements.

10. D. In 1990, the Individuals with Disabilities Education Act (IDEA) reauthorized and retitled P.L. 94-142 and made some changes in it.

11. A. According to ASHA, SLPAs may be involved in implementing treatment plans developed by the supervising SLP, checking and maintaining equipment, and collecting and documenting data for quality improvement.

12. A. It is not true that the IDEA discourages serving children with disabilities in general education settings and encourages school districts to create more specialized pull-out programs for such children to best serve their needs. It is the reverse; the IDEA encourages districts to serve children with disabilities in general classroom settings

13. B. The main set of HIPAA standards that impacts speech–language pathologists and audiologists deals with protecting patients' privacy by putting limits on use of personal medical information, notifying patients of privacy practices, etc.

14. C. According to ASHA standards, prescribing hearing aids for children and adults with hearing losses would NOT be within the scope of practice of a speech–language pathologist.

15. E. All of the above. P.L. 99-457 mandated the use of IFSPs, which require information about the child's present level of development, the family's needs and strengths relating to the child's development, major goals for the child and family, and services to be provided, and a review of the plan at 6-month intervals or more frequently if need.

APPENDIX

STUDY AND TEST-

TAKING TIPS

FOR THE PRAXIS

Most readers of this book are preparing for the National Examination in Speech Pathology and Audiology (NESPA). Today, people know the NESPA as the PRAXIS, so the term *PRAXIS* is used in this appendix. The purpose of this appendix is to provide you with a brief orientation to the PRAXIS and to give study and test-taking tips to help you pass the PRAXIS. (*Note:* Some of these suggestions may also be applied to studying for and passing comprehensive examinations in graduate programs; readers may apply the information to their individual programs as needed.) At the time of this writing, a very helpful website is http://www .asha.org/students/PRAXIS/overview.htm. Another informative website is http://www.ets.org/PRAXIS/ index.html. If these websites change, the reader is encouraged to use google.com as a search engine and type in "speech–language pathology PRAXIS examination."

NATURE AND PURPOSE OF THE PRAXIS

- Essentially, the purpose of the PRAXIS is to ask questions in all areas of speech–language pathology to assess whether or not examinees are prepared to competently serve as speech–language pathologists in a variety of clinical settings.

- The PRAXIS is administered at least 5 times a year at over 400 test centers throughout the United States. The exam "Registration Bulletin" and "Tests at a Glance" (TAAG), which contains the content outline and sample questions for the examination, may be obtained directly from Educational Testing Services (ETS):

  The PRAXIS Series Educational Testing Service
  P.O. Box 6051
  Princeton, NJ 08541-6051
  800-772-9476
  (TTY: 800-272-1391)

- The PRAXIS is "a set of rigorous and carefully validated assessments that provides accurate, reliable information for use by state education agencies in making licensing decisions" (Educational Testing Services, 2005). Speech–language pathologists (SLPs) take the PRAXIS-II "Subject Assessments" in the area of speech–language pathology (which at the time of this writing is 0330).

- According to ASHA (2005), the PRAXIS Examinations in Speech–Language Pathology and Audiology make up a major component of ASHA certification as well as most state licensing requirements. The PRAXIS Series Specialty Area Tests in Speech–Language Pathology and Audiology are owned by Educational Testing Services (ETS).

- There are several versions for each PRAXIS examination in speech–language pathology and audiology. The passing score for ASHA certification is 600 out of a possible 800. It is typical for 80% of students in both audiology and speech–language pathology to pass the PRAXIS examination on their first attempt (ASHA, 2005).

- Test takers in both speech–language pathology and audiology who have not earned a passing score can retake the PRAXIS an unlimited number of times over the next 2 years. If a person does not pass the PRAXIS within a 2-year period, his or her certification file will be closed. If the person passes the PRAXIS at a later date (after the 2-year period), the person has to reapply for certification under the standards in effect at the time of reapplication.

- ASHA (2005) recommends that students take the PRAXIS *no earlier* than at the completion of their graduate clinical practicum and graduate coursework or during their clinical fellowship year. (*First author's note:* It is the first author's experience that students who take the PRAXIS before these timelines almost invariably fail the exam. Though the exam can be retaken, it is expensive and time consuming. The first author heartily agrees with ASHA's recommendation based upon experience working with students at several universities.)

- The PRAXIS consists of 120 multiple-choice questions, which are to be answered within 2 hours. Table A.1 shows the content categories, approximate number of questions in each category, and approximate percentage of the examination devoted to each area (ETS, 2005).

- Questions on the PRAXIS are gathered from courses in undergraduate and graduate programs in speech–language pathology. The questions cover all age levels from newborns to geriatric patients.

- Passing the PRAXIS is one of the requirements for obtaining a Certificate of Clinical Competence issued by the American Speech-Language-Hearing Association. Individual states may use the PRAXIS as part of their licensing requirements. Some graduate programs may use the PRAXIS as part of the requirements to obtain a master's degree.

- In terms of reporting scores, exam results must be sent directly from ETS in order to be applicable toward certification. When you register to take the exam, be sure to request that your score be reported directly to ASHA. ETS charges an additional fee to report scores after you have taken the examination.

- To have ETS report your score to ASHA, use the code *R-5031 for Certification* on the exam registration form as indicated in the ETS "Registration Bulletin." Your score will be sent to the ASHA national office within 8 weeks of the exam date. The national office is able to automatically match scores with individuals *only if* your application for certification is on file

Table A.1   PERCENTAGE OF QUESTIONS IN VARIOUS TOPIC AREAS

Content Categories	Approximate # of Questions	Approximate Percentage of Examination
Basic Human Communication Processes	20	17%
Phonological and Language Disorders	23	19%
Speech Disorders	15	13%
Neurogenic Disorders	23	19%
Audiology/Hearing	6	5%
Clinical Management	23	19%
Professional Issues/Psychometrics/Research	10	8%

with the certification office at the time the score is received and if a computer record has been established for you.

■ To assist the national office in processing your exam information, it is helpful if you submit a copy of the report sent to you by ETS when you submit your application for certification. However, please note that this copy will not be used as official verification of completion of the examination requirement.

■ If you are applying for ASHA certification and you have a disability that impairs your ability to take the examination under standard conditions, contact ETS directly to arrange for appropriate accommodations. Write to: The PRAXIS Series, Nonstandard Testing Accommodations, Educational Testing Service, P.O. Box 6054, Princeton, NJ 08541-6054.

■ If you speak English as a second or foreign language, you may be able to obtain extended time to take the PRAXIS. For information regarding accommodations (in addition to the above address), a helpful website is: http://www.ets.org/praxis/prxplne.html

■ If you request nonstandard testing arrangements (e.g., extended time), you must complete and submit to ETS the following items: (a) exam registration form, (b) eligibility questionnaire, and (c) Certification of Documentation Form. Appropriate forms and additional information regarding the requirements for nonstandard testing accommodations can be found in the examination Registration Bulletin as well as on the ETS website.

■ It is important to save your exam score. ETS only retains an exam score for 5 years. If in the future you apply for certification or state licensure and cannot provide a copy of your exam score, you may be required to take the exam again and obtain a passing score on that exam. ASHA's national office is not responsible for maintaining exam scores after certification has been awarded (ASHA, 2005).

STUDY TIPS FOR PREPARING FOR THE PRAXIS

■ Many test takers, being human, attempt to memorize a great deal of information right before the examination. Research indicates that ideal learning does not occur under those conditions.

■ It is best to start studying at least several months before you take the PRAXIS. Ideally, you should try to study a little bit each day. Many examinees attempt to study for several hours only on weekends. It is optimal to study a little bit daily rather than try to "cram in" studying on weekends only.

■ If you studied 15 minutes a day 6 days a week, that would equal 1.5 hours of study a week. If that was done for 3 months, you would have studied for 18 hours total.

■ When it comes to studying, more is usually better. However, reality dictates that 15 minutes of studying a day for several months is the most many people can manage. When you do a little studying each day, you learn more than if studying was crammed into large blocks of time right before the examination.

■ Many adults learn best in a multimodal fashion. That is, they retain information best if they read it, write it, say it aloud, and discuss it with others, as opposed to just passively reading it. Thus, it is ideal to study both alone and with other people if possible. You should try to form study groups that meet once or twice a week. Many adults learn best in a study group format.

■ It is very helpful, in trying to retain information, to write the information down. You might make flash cards with pertinent information. These flash cards can be carried in a purse or pocket and pulled out during "dead time," when you are waiting in line at the supermarket or at a red light, for example. It is surprising how much dead time most of us have that we are not aware of.

■ It is extremely helpful to take a practice PRAXIS examination. The websites mentioned before will guide you to practice examinations. In addition, a CD is available from PRO-ED with three practice examinations with 120 questions each. At the time of this writing, this CD is the only product on the market in the United States based on the new speech–language pathology PRAXIS, which was changed and updated in fall 2004.

■ It is best to set aside 2 hours and take a practice examination with no interruptions. While it is challenging for many busy people to find a 2-hour uninterrupted time block, we have found that this is the very best situation for preparing to actually take the PRAXIS.

■ Many students have told us over the years, after taking the examination, that they ran out of time at the end because they worked too slowly. They had never before been required to answer 120 multiple-choice questions in 2 hours. Thus, taking a practice examination in an uninterrupted 2-hour time block is the very best way for you to be prepared for the actual situation ahead.

■ Many examinees stay up late the night before an examination. They spend those late hours "cramming" for the examination the next day. For many people, this does not work well when taking the PRAXIS. The PRAXIS questions (unlike some essay and fill-in-the-blank questions) do not necessarily require rote, pre-memorized answers. Rather, many questions require a great deal of reading, careful thought, and subjective clinical judgment decisions.

■ Such higher-level thought questions are usually best and most accurately answered if you have had a good night's sleep before the examination. In our opinion, the night before the PRAXIS is best spent sleeping and attempting to wake up refreshed to answer challenging questions the next day.

TIPS FOR TAKING THE PRAXIS

■ Right before taking the examination, it is best to go to the bathroom. While you may find this tip humorous, laughter quickly fades when you discover that if you take 10 minutes during the PRAXIS to go to the bathroom, that is 10 minutes lost during the examination.

■ In other words, if the PRAXIS is administered from 8:00 to 10:00 in the morning, you do not get to take 10 minutes in the bathroom during the examination and then continue taking the test until 10:10. Time spent in the bathroom is time lost in test-taking!

■ It is best to wear loose, comfortable clothing during the examination. Wear light clothing, but bring a sweater or wrap, even if the weather outside is warm. We have found that room temperatures may be too hot or cold for everyone's comfort and may distract from thinking and doing your best. You don't want to be so cold from a super-airconditioned room in July that you cannot concentrate on the exam!

■ Many examinees feel very nervous. Deep breathing is an excellent way to deal with feelings of nervousness. Deep breathing also enhances concentration by providing increased oxygen to the brain.

■ Bring a watch to have out on your desk during the examination. We have found that some testing rooms do not have clocks (which can be very distressing for those not wearing watches).

■ Be constantly mindful of time. You have approximately one minute to answer each question. As stated earlier, we have found that many examinees' greatest problem was that they ran out of time at the end. It is quite upsetting to have 10 minutes left with 35 questions still to answer. *Keep moving along,* even if you are unsure of each answer. At the end of the first hour of the test, you should be on #60.

■ Occasionally, you will encounter a question that seems deceptively simple and quick (as in the following example). There are a few of these on the PRAXIS. Answer them as best you can, and use the time you saved on those questions to answer the questions requiring more reading.

Which is the primary cranial nerve involved in innervation of the muscles of the larynx?

A. cranial nerve VIII
B. cranial nerve IX
C. cranial nerve II
D. cranial nerve X
E. cranial nerve XII

The answer is D, cranial nerve X.

■ Many PRAXIS questions require a great deal of reading. Those questions involve cases in which a clinical decision is necessary. Examinees have shared with us that they were unhappily surprised by the sheer number of these complicated questions. Knowing that such questions exist is very helpful. Remember that you can write in the test booklet if you need to! An example of a complicated clinical scenario follows:

> A 6-year-old child with a repaired posterior cleft palate has been referred to you by her teacher. The child's speech is hypernasal with numerous articulatory errors, including glottal stops, distortions of sibilants, and substitutions of w/r and j/l. The cleft palate team, consisting of an orthodontist, plastic surgeon, pediodontist, and oromaxillofacial surgeon, is involved in consulting with you in this case. During phonation of /u/, a palatopharyngeal gap exceeding 15 millimeters is observed. The parents are eager for their child to get as much assistance as possible and have indicated their willingness to provide as much support as is necessary. Given this information, which of the following will be your first priority in clinical management of this case?

> A. therapy beginning with the easy initiation /u/ blended with stop consonants to lower tongue position, reduce nasality, and eliminate glottal stops
> B. blowing exercises to strengthen velopharyngeal valving
> C. therapy to remediate the w/r and j/l substitutions
> D. ear training to identify distortion of sibilants
> E. referral to the appropriate specialists to determine physical management of the palatopharyngeal gap

> The answer is E.

■ Read all choices before you decide on the best answer. Reading all choices increases the chances of answering the question accurately.

■ Never leave any questions blank. Always answer each question. You are never penalized for guessing incorrectly, but you are always penalized for leaving items blank and unanswered in that you have no chance to get an unanswered question right.

■ If you do not know the answer to a question, guess. Your first guess is usually the right one. We have heard dozens of times over the years that examinees changed their answers, only to find later that the first guess was actually the right one.

■ If you are unsure of your answer on an item, answer it as best you can, circle that item in the test booklet (not on the answer sheet) and, if time permits, come back to that item after you have completed the examination. In this way, you keep moving forward. Always remember that you are allowed to write in the test booklet.

■ Constantly check your answer sheet to make sure you are filling in the right bubble for the item you think you are on. It is horrifying to come to question #115 and find that you are one item "off" because you accidentally skipped a question on the Scantron answer sheet. Keep checking!

■ If you erase an answer, erase very thoroughly. The Scantron machines that score the examinations are quite sensitive, and may pick up and score your erasure rather than your actual answer. Some examinees find it helpful to fill in the bubbles adequately but not so firmly that erasure is almost impossible.

■ Bring three or four sharpened pencils with good erasers to the examination. Do not assume that the PRAXIS proctor has extra pencils or a pencil sharpener.

■ Try to relax as much as possible. This is easier said than done, but the more relaxed you are, the higher your likelihood of passing the examination. Remember that if you should fail the PRAXIS, you can take it again. (*Note:* Policies about the number of retakes change occasionally, so check into the latest available information about this.)

REFERENCES

American Speech-Language-Hearing Association. (2005). *About the PRAXIS exam.* Retrieved January 2, 2005, from http://www.asha.org/students/praxis/overview.htm

Educational Testing Services. (2005). *The PRAXIS series: Professional assessments for beginning teachers.* Retrieved January 2, 2005, from http://www.ets.org/praxis/index.html

A

B

G

M

N

Q

R

S

T

U

X

Z

ABOUT THE AUTHORS

CELESTE ROSEBERRY-McKIBBIN received her Ph.D. from Northwestern University. She is a professor in the Department of Speech Pathology and Audiology at California State University, Sacramento. She also serves as a part-time itinerant speech–language pathologist in the Elk Grove Unified School District, where she provides direct services to elementary school students. She has worked in educational and medical settings with a wide variety of clients ranging from preschool-aged children through geriatric patients. She has copresented a number of workshops on taking and passing the PRAXIS.

Dr. Roseberry-McKibbin's research interests are in the areas of second-language acquisition and bilingualism, multiculturalism, and assessment and treatment of culturally and linguistically diverse students with communicative disorders. She has written over 30 publications and has made over 200 presentations at the local, state, national, and international levels. She lived in the Philippines from the age of 6 to the age of 17, when she came to live in the United States permanently.

M. N. (GIRI) HEGDE is a professor of Communicative Sciences and Disorders at California State University, Fresno. He holds a master's degree in experimental psychology from the University of Mysore, India, and a post-master's diploma in medical psychology from Bangalore University, India. His doctoral degree in speech–language pathology is from Southern Illinois University in Carbondale.

Dr. Hegde is a specialist in research methods, fluency disorders, language, and treatment procedures in communicative disorders. He has made many professional and scientific presentations to national and international audiences on a wide variety of topics in communicative disorders. He has published many research articles and over 18 books on a wide range of subjects in speech–language pathology. He has received numerous local, state, and national professional accolades and honors, including the ASHA Fellow Award.